Bioceramics and Biocomposites

Bioceramics and Biocomposites

From Research to Clinical Practice

Edited by
Iulian Antoniac, PhD
University Politehnica of Bucharest

The American Ceramic Society

WILEY

Published by John Wiley & Sons, Inc., Hoboken, New Jersey.
Published simultaneously in Canada.

Registered Office
John Wiley & Sons, Inc., 111 River Street, Hoboken, NJ 07030, USA

Editorial Office
111 River Street, Hoboken, NJ 07030, USA

For details of our global editorial offices, customer services, and more information about Wiley products visit us at www.wiley.com.

Wiley also publishes its books in a variety of electronic formats and by print-on-demand. Some content that appears in standard print versions of this book may not be available in other formats.

Library of Congress Cataloging-in-Publication Data

Names: Antoniac, Iulian, editor.
Title: Bioceramics and biocomposites : from research to clinical practice / edited by Iulian Antoniac.
Description: First edition. | Hoboken, New Jersey : John Wiley & Sons, Inc., [2019] | Includes bibliographical references and index. |
Identifiers: LCCN 2018056452 (print) | LCCN 2018058843 (ebook) | ISBN 9781119372134 (AdobePDF) | ISBN 9781119372141 (ePub) | ISBN 9781119049340 (hardcover : alk. paper)
Subjects: | MESH: Biocompatible Materials | Ceramics | Tissue Engineering | Bone and Bones
Classification: LCC R857.M3 (ebook) | LCC R857.M3 (print) | NLM QT 37 | DDC 610.28–dc23
LC record available at https://lccn.loc.gov/2018056452

Cover Design: Wiley
Cover Image: © danielzgombic/Getty Images

Set in 10/12pt WarnockPro by SPi Global, Chennai, India

Printed in the United States of America

V10009001_032219

Contents

List of Contributors

Simeon Agathopoulos
Materials Science and Engineering Department,
University of Ioannina,
Ioannina, Greece

Ika D. Ana
Department of Dental Biomedical Sciences,
Faculty of Dentistry,
Universitas Gadjah Mada,
Yogyakarta 55281, Indonesia

Maidaniuc Andreea
Department of Metallic Materials Science,
Physical Metallurgy,
Faculty of Material Science and Engineering,
Politehnica University of Bucharest,
Bucharest, Romania

Ilia Y. Bozo
Human Stem Cells Institute,
Moscow, Russia

A.I. Evdokimov Moscow State University of Medicine and Dentistry,
Moscow, Russia

A.I. Burnazyan Federal Medical and Biophysical Center,
Moscow, Russia

Vladimir Bystrov
Institute of Mathematical Problems of Biology,
Keldysh Institute of Applied Mathematics,
Russian Academy of Sciences,
142290, Pushchino, Russia

Anna Bystrova
Institute of Biomedical Engineering and Nanotechnologies,
Riga Technical University,
Riga, Latvia

Mocanu A. Cătălina
Department of Metallic Materials Science,
Physical Metallurgy,
Faculty of Material Science and Engineering,
Politehnica University of Bucharest,
Bucharest, Romania

Daniel Chappard
GEROM Groupe Etudes Remodelage Osseux et bioMatériaux – NextBone and SCIAM,
Service Commun d'Imagerie et Analyses Microscopiques,
Institut de Biologie en Santé,
CHU d'Angers,
Université d'Angers,
49933 Angers Cedex, France

Roman V. Deev
Human Stem Cells Institute,
Moscow, Russia

A.I. Burnazyan Federal Medical and Biophysical Center,
Moscow, Russia

Kazan (Volga region) Federal University,
Kazan, Russia

Yuri Dekhtyar
Institute of Biomedical Engineering and Nanotechnologies,
Riga Technical University,
Riga, Latvia

Petr S. Eremin
A.I. Burnazyan Federal Medical and Biophysical Center,
Moscow, Russia

Ilya I. Eremin
A.I. Burnazyan Federal Medical and Biophysical Center,
Moscow, Russia

Anna Eroshenko
Institute of Strength Physics and Materials Science SB RAS,
2/4 Akademicheskii prospekt, Tomsk, 634055 Russia

Miculescu Florin
Department of Metallic Materials Science,
Physical Metallurgy,
Faculty of Material Science and Engineering,
Politehnica University of Bucharest,
Bucharest, Romania

Stan E. George
Laboratory of Multifunctional Materials and Structures,
National Institute of Materials Physics,
Măgurele-Bucharest, Romania

Irina M. Gheorghiu
Department of Endodontology,
"Carol Davila" University of Medicine and Pharmacy,
Bucharest, Romania

Vasily I. Grachev
X-ray Diagnostics Laboratories "3D Lab",
Moscow, Russia

Sri Hinduja
The University of Manchester,
School of Mechanical, Aerospace and Civil Engineering,
Manchester, United Kingdom

Boyang Huang
The University of Manchester,
School of Mechanical,
Aerospace and Civil Engineering,
Manchester,
United Kingdom

Alexandru A. Iliescu
Department of Oral Rehabilitation,
University of Medicine and Pharmacy of Craiova,
Craiova, Romania

Mihaela G. Iliescu
Department of Endodontology,
"Carol Davila" University of Medicine and Pharmacy,
Bucharest, Romania

Voicu S. Ioan
Department of Analytical Chemistry and Environmental Engineering,
Faculty of Applied Chemistry and Material Science,
Politehnica University of Bucharest,
Bucharest, Romania

Iulian Antoniac
Department of Metallic Materials Science,
Physical Metallurgy,
Faculty of Material Science and Engineering,
Politehnica University of Bucharest,
313 Splaiul Independentei, District 6, JA 104-106 Building, 060042 Bucharest, Romania

Igor A. Khlusov
Department of Morphology and General Pathology,
Siberian State Medical University,
634050, Tomsk, Russia

National Research Tomsk Polytechnic University,
Research School of Chemistry & Applied Biomedical Sciences,
634050, Tomsk, Russia

Marina Yu. Khlusova
Department of Morphology and General Pathology,
Siberian State Medical University,
634050, Tomsk, Russia

National Research Tomsk Polytechnic University,
Research School of Chemistry & Applied Biomedical Sciences,
634050, Tomsk, Russia

Ekaterina Komarova
Institute of Strength Physics and Materials Science SB RAS,
2/4 Akademicheskii prospekt, Tomsk, 634055 Russia

Vladimir S. Komlev
A.A. Baikov Institute of Metallurgy and Materials Science,
Russian Academy of Sciences,
Moscow, Russia

Institute of Laser and Information Technologies,
Russian Academy of Sciences,
Moscow, Russia

Larisa Litvinova
Laboratory of Immunology and Cellular Biotechnology,
Immanuel Kant Baltic Federal University,
14 A. Nevskogo Street, 236041 Kaliningrad, Russia

Fengyuan Liu
The University of Manchester,
School of Mechanical, Aerospace and Civil Engineering,
Manchester, United Kingdom

Horia O. Manolea
Department of Oral Rehabilitation,
University of Medicine and Pharmacy of Craiova,
Craiova, Romania

Miculescu Marian
Department of Metallic Materials Science,
Physical Metallurgy,
Faculty of Material Science and Engineering,
Politehnica University of Bucharest,
Bucharest, Romania

Gujie Mi
Department of Chemical Engineering,
Northeastern University,
Boston, MA 02115, USA

Lupescu Olivera
Department of Orthopaedics,
Faculty of Medicine,
"Carol Davila" University of Medicine and Pharmacy of Bucharest,
37 Dionisie Lupu Street, District 2, 020021 Bucharest, Romania

Paola Palmero
Department of Applied Science and Technology,
INSTM R.U. PoliTO,
LINCE Laboratory,
Politecnico di Torino,
Corso Duca degli Abruzzi, 24, 10129 Torino, Italy

Paula Perlea
Department of Endodontology,
"Carol Davila" University of Medicine and Pharmacy,
Bucharest, Romania

Vladimir Pichugin
National Research Tomsk Polytechnic University,
Research School of Chemistry & Applied Biomedical Sciences,
634050, Tomsk, Russia

Konstantin Prosolov
National Research Tomsk Polytechnic University,
Research School of High-Energy Physics,
634050, Tomsk, Russia

Institute of Strength Physics and Materials Science of SB RAS,
Russia

Andrey A. Pulin
A.I. Burnazyan Federal Medical and Biophysical Center,
Moscow, Russia

Sergey I. Rozhkov
A.I. Evdokimov Moscow State University of Medicine and Dentistry,
Moscow, Russia

Maria Sedelnikova
Institute of Strength Physics and Materials Science
SB RAS,
2/4 Akademicheskii prospekt, Tomsk, 634055 Russia

Yurii Sharkeev
National Research Tomsk Polytechnic University,
Research School of High-Energy Physics,
634050, Tomsk, Russia

Institute of Strength Physics and Materials Science of SB RAS,
Russia

Di Shi
Department of Chemical Engineering,
Northeastern University,
Boston, MA 02115, USA

Valeria Shupletsova
Laboratory of Immunology and Cellular Biotechnology,
Immanuel Kant Baltic Federal University,
14 A. Nevskogo Street, 236041 Kaliningrad, Russia

Paulo J. da Silva Bartolo
The University of Manchester,
School of Mechanical, Aerospace and Civil Engineering,
Manchester, United Kingdom

Izabela-Cristina Stancu
APMG Advanced Polymer Materials Group,
Faculty of Applied Chemistry and Materials Science,
Faculty of Medical Engineering,
University Politehnica of Bucharest,
1–7 Gh Polizu Street, Sector 1, 011061 Bucharest, Romania

Evgeniy N. Toropov
A.I. Burnazyan Federal Medical and Biophysical Center,
Moscow, Russia

Gabriel Tulus
European Society of Endodontology,
Viersen, Germany

Dilhan U. Tulyaganov
Turin Polytechnic University in Tashkent,
Niyazova, Uzbekistan

Grigory A. Volozhin
A.I. Evdokimov Moscow State University of Medicine and Dentistry,
Moscow, Russia

Thomas J. Webster
Department of Chemical Engineering,
Northeastern University,
Boston, MA 02115, USA

Center of Excellence for Advanced Materials Research,
King Abdulaziz University,
Jeddah, Saudi Arabia

Vadim L. Zorin
Human Stem Cells Institute,
Moscow, Russia

A.I. Burnazyan Federal Medical and Biophysical Center,
Moscow, Russia

1

Multifunctionalized Ferri-liposomes for Hyperthermia Induced Glioma Targeting and Brain Drug Delivery

Di Shi[1], Gujie Mi[1], and Thomas J. Webster[1,2]

[1] Department of Chemical Engineering, Northeastern University, Boston, MA 02115, USA
[2] Center of Excellence for Advanced Materials Research, King Abdulaziz University, Jeddah, Saudi Arabia

1.1 Introduction

1.1.1 Blood–brain Barrier

1.1.1.1 What is the Blood–brain Barrier (BBB)?

The discovery of the blood–brain barrier (BBB) traces back to more than 100 years ago [1, 2]. However, it was not until the 1960s when electron microscopes became available in medical research that the endothelial cells and the actual BBB were observed and confirmed [3]. Compared to "ordinary" endothelial cells that line blood vessels in the rest of the body, endothelial cells in the brain microvessels exhibit highly extensive tight junctions and thus lower endocytosis or transcytosis activities more than peripheral endothelial cells [3, 4]. Besides the existence of the tight junctions, the endothelial cells in the BBB are distinct from the peripheral endothelial cells by processing much fewer pinocytic vesicles, producing high electrical resistance for over 0.1 Ω m and the absence of fenestration [5]. In addition, what also makes them distinguishable from peripheral endothelial cells is that several cytoplasmic adaptors are enriched at the BBB [6].

Generally, there are three different transport systems for compounds to pass through the BBB. Nutrients (such as glucose and amino acids) are transported by transport proteins, while larger molecules including insulin and iron transferrin are carried by receptor-mediated endocytosis or transcytosis [7]. The other transcytosis is called adsorptive-mediated transcytosis, which helps albumin and other native plasma protein transportation by cationization [5, 8]. While it is worth mentioning that since more than 98% of hydrophilic agents, including polar drugs, are blocked by tight junctions, most of the central nervous system (CNS) drugs penetrate the BBB using either transcellular lipophilic pathways or one of the transportation routes (Table 1.1 and Figure 1.1).

Together with these highly selective tight junctions and transcellular transportation pathways, the brain endothelial cells scrupulously regulate brain homeostasis and the microenvironment, and limit the penetration of a majority of the microorganisms and compounds including potentially toxic compounds that circulate in the blood [4, 9].

1.1.1.2 The BBB Formation and Composition

The basic building blocks of the BBB are formed by endothelial cells surrounded by the basal lamina (not shown in Figure) and are attached by pericytes, astrocyte endfeet, and neurons (Figure 1.2) [10]. As seen from Figure 1.5, the basement membrane of capillaries in the BBB are ensheathed with astrocyte end-feet and are attached by pericytes, which for larger blood vessels (such as arteries and veins), will be replaced by a continuous layer of smooth muscle [12]. It is a consensus that all of the components in the BBB are important for stability and daily functions and among them endothelial cells and astrocytes are the most important building blocks.

1.1.1.3 Endothelial Cell and Tight Junctions

Endothelial cells of the capillaries continuously envelop the inner surface of the blood vessel and act as the first wall facing the circulating blood in the brain. As mentioned previously, this active interface shows several unique features not only as an endothelium, such as highly controlled paracellular and transcellular pathways, but also shows a high value of transepithelial electrical resistance (TEER) of 1500–2000 $\Omega\,cm^2$ compared to less than 30 $\Omega\,cm^2$ in other tissues [13, 14].

TEER is a typical and straightforward method being used to assess the tightness of the BBB both *in vivo* and *in vitro*, since the tightness of the BBB is correlated to the flux of all the ions that go through the membrane [15]. The experiment is carried out by applying

Bioceramics and Biocomposites: From Research to Clinical Practice, First Edition. Edited by Iulian Antoniac.

Table 1.1 Nutrient transportation pathways in the BBB.

Pathways	Paracellular or transcellular	Molecules being transported	Available for drug delivery
Hydrophilic pathway	Paracellular	Water-soluble small molecules (water, ethanol)	No
Lipophilic pathway	Transcellular	Lipid-soluble small molecules (caffeine)	Yes
Transport proteins	Transcellular	Glucose, amino acids, vitamins, fatty acids	Yes
Receptor-mediated transcytosis	Transcellular	Insulin, tranferin	Yes
Adsorptive-mediated transcytosis	Transcellular	Plasma proteins (albumin)	Yes

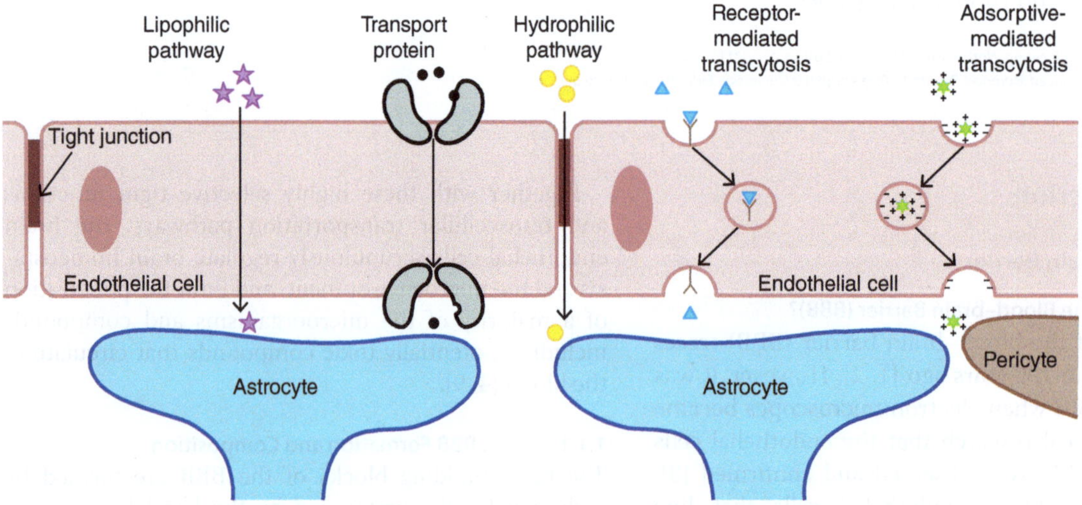

Figure 1.1 Transportation pathways across the BBB. Source: Abbott et al. 2006 [9]. Adapted with permission of Springer Nature.

a transepithelial current to the membrane and then test the membrane potential that is being generated, and finally translate the value into resistance (current, Ohm [Ω]) multiplied by the area (cm^2) of the endothelial monolayer (expressed as $\Omega\,cm^2$). For instance, as for the *in vitro* model that will be discussed later, the surface area of the transmembrane is 0.32 cm^2 for 24-well plates and 1.1 cm^2 for 12-well plates. Therefore, if the resistance of the measurement is 100 Ω, it will be 32 $\Omega\,cm^2$ for the 24-well plate and 110 $\Omega\,cm^2$ for the 12-well plate [16]. Such a discussion is important for *in vitro* models on the blood barrier. Tight junctions and adherent junctions are the interconnectors of cerebral endothelial cells [17] (Figure 1.3). There are basically four important integral membrane proteins being expressed in the tight junctions and basically they can be all divided into two categories [18]: transmembrane proteins (including occludin, claudin, and junctional adhesion molecules [JAMs]) and cytoplasmic proteins (including zonula occludens). These tight junctional proteins together

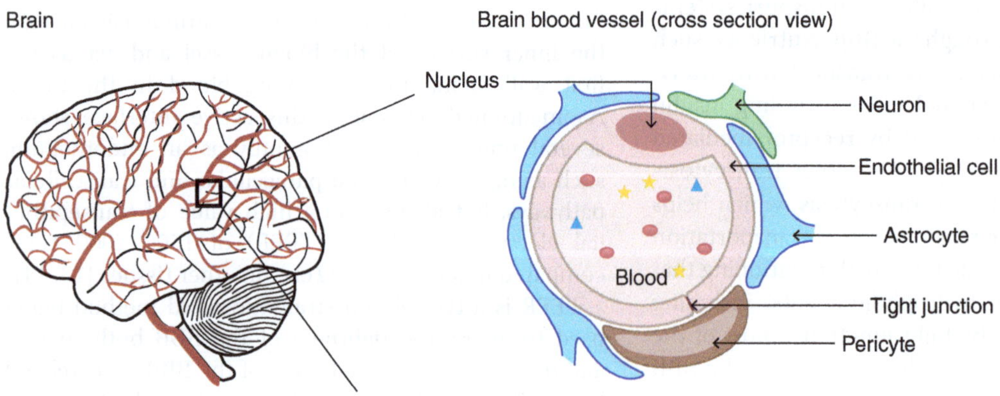

Figure 1.2 Cellular components of the blood–brain barrier (cross-section view).

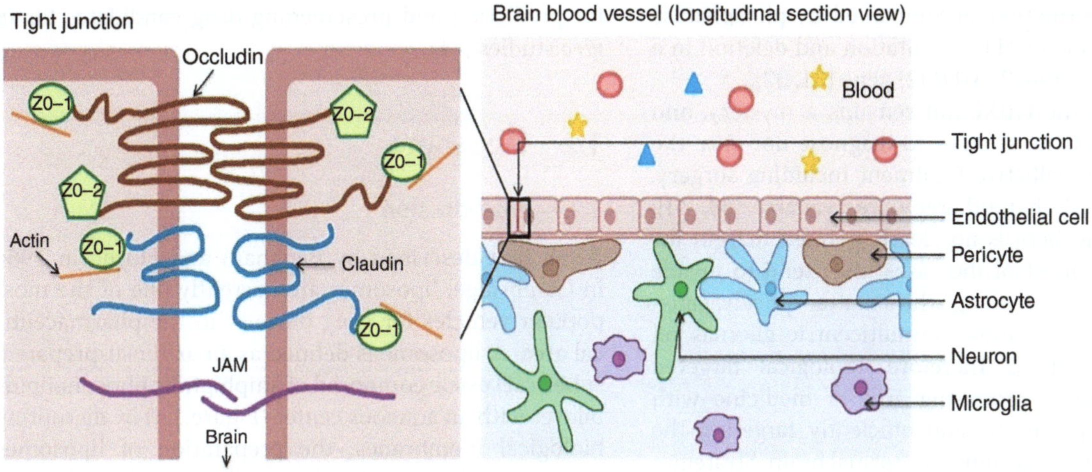

Figure 1.3 Molecular components of endothelial tight junctions.

form the super restrictive paracellular pathways, which represents one of the hallmarks of the BBB phenotype, and are discussed in greater detail subsequently [19, 20].

Both tight junctions and adherens junctions are composed of transmembrane proteins and cytoplasmic proteins. The difference is that transmembrane proteins such as JAM will physically associate with their counterparts on the plasma membrane and form dimers, whereas cytoplasmic proteins will not only connect tight junctional/adherens junctional proteins and the actin cytoskeleton but are also involved in intracellular signaling [17].

1.1.1.4 Astrocytes

Astrocytes, also known as astroglia, ensheath more than 99% of the endothelium. They are one of the major subtypes of glial cells and play an important role for providing cellular links to neurons in the CNS (Figures 1.5 and 1.6). These star-shaped glial cells have been shown to perform many functions, including structurally supporting the endothelial cells to form the BBB. Since they are able to carry out glycogenesis, astrocytes can provide neurons with glucose when glucose consumption rate is high or during glucose shortage periods [21]. They are also involved in the transmission of neuronal synapses and regulate ion concentrations of extracellular space [22]. Since they provide a connection between neurons and the vascular endothelium, they are able to deliver signals and thus regulate blood flow by controlling the contraction and dilation of the smooth muscles and/or pericytes that surround the blood vessels [23]. In addition, if the brain or spinal cord undergoes traumatic injury, astrocytes will then execute a scar repairing process and form glial scars to heal the wound by transforming into neurons [24, 25]. Astrocytes are also suggested to be an important mediator and regulate endothelial functions during BBB formation and development. For example, they are believed to be involved in vascular growth by secreting vascular endothelial growth factors (VEGF). However, a recent study showed that these cells might not be involved in the initial generation of the BBB but only maintain and regulate the BBB after it is formed. Research carried out at the University of California, San Francisco, showed that astrocytes are not required to induce BBB formation initially [26], but to act as a regulator that maintains BBB function and response to neural diseases or after injury when necessary as mentioned [27].

1.1.1.5 Glioma

Usually appearing inside the brain, glioblastoma multiformes (GBMs) are one of the most common brain tumors that arise mainly from astrocytes, which are the star-shaped glial cells that support the tissues of the brain. GBM, also known as Grade IV glioma, accounts for more than 50% of all astrocytomas and has been considered as the most aggressive tumors of the brain due to their highly malignant (cancerous) base on the rapid cell reproduce rate supported by the large network of blood vessels inside the brain [28]. Patients receiving this diagnosis are most likely having an average of 15 months or less to live, and even those who survived from first-line therapy will usually face long-term neurologically impairment or be debilitated [29, 30]. In recent years, increasing evidence indicates that primary and secondary GBMs exhibit distinct disease entities and therefore probably involve different genetic pathways and mutations, despite the fact that they both behave in a clinically indistinguishable manner and share the similar survival rates. For primary GBM, epidermal growth factor receptor (EGFR) and loss of heterozygosity (LOH) are shown to be the major genes that are amplified during tumor formation, accompanied by phosphatase and tensin homolog (PTEN) mutation and deletion in a mouse double-minute 2 (MDM2) gene [31, 32].

The cause of the GBM still remains a mystery, and currently, there is no strategy to diagnose nor cure the tumor, but only palliative treatment including surgery, radiotherapy, and chemotherapy are available [33, 34]. Moreover, since there is no clearly defined margin for those GBMs in most of the cases, they tend to invade locally and spread out along white matter quickly, causing multi-GBM formation or multicentric gliomas on imaging studies [35]. Therefore, biological targeted therapy becomes a promising area of medicine with a purpose of specifically and efficiently targeting the tumor area without harming the normal brain. Strategies include altering the natural behavior of tumor cells, such as angiogenic pathways. Several genetic pathways in the brain, such as the relevant growth factor pathways in malignant glioma include platelet-derived growth factor (PDGF), VEGF, and epidermal growth factor (EGF), are under investigation recently based on the fact that they will undergo mutation and increase survival of abnormal cells and blood supply to the tumor [36, 37]. Take EGF as an example, EGFR has been found to overexpress in more than 60% of GBM, and it mainly acts through the tyrosine kinase (RTK) pathways [38].

1.1.2 New Strategies for Measuring Drug Transport Across the BBB

Since it is that fact that over 98% of small molecule drugs cannot penetrate through the BBB due to the presence of the tight junctions, not only the hydrophilic but also hydrophobic ones, the BBB becomes the fundamental barrier that prevents progress in the development of new therapeutics for brain diseases and/or radiopharmaceuticals for imaging the brain, and the prospect for neuropharmaceuticals has become a promising global pharmaceutical market. Traditional pharmacokinetic techniques for measuring pharmaceutical agent transport across the BBB *in vivo*, such as intravenous administration and tissue sampling, are more sensitive and represent the full physiological conditions [39]. However, these kinds of methods are yet to be more time-consuming and based on trial and error. Compared to traditional methods, there are emerging types of *in vitro* BBB models that can rapidly assess the potential permeability of drugs and screening procedures such as active efflux and carrier-mediated uptake. This method is more accessible and repeatable to discover the molecular transport mechanism of pharmaceutical agents across the BBB and have an advantage of evaluating systemic drugs more efficiently with much less time and labor [40]. Therefore, this *in vitro* BBB model is now often used for predicting and prescreening drug candidates for *in vivo* studies [41].

1.2 Liposome

1.2.1 Introduction

Being first described by Bangham and Horne in 1964 in Cambridge, liposomes are currently one of the most popular vehicles for drug delivery in the pharmaceutical area. A liposome is defined as an artificial-prepared, spherical vesicle composed of amphiphilic phospholipids bilayer with an aqueous center (Figure 1.4) by disrupting biological membranes, the preparation of liposomes from natural nontoxic phospholipids and cholesterol can be simply conducted by sonication [42, 43]. With hydrophilic groups facing outside, this self-closed bilayer structure is formed due to the accumulation of lipids that interact with one another in a specific manner. The assembled liposome is then able to protect therapeutic molecules inside the core from aqueous environments and go through the cell membrane.

The size of liposomes can vary from ~50 nm to several micrometers, and there are also some different types of liposomal vesicles according to their diameters. The major types include multilamellar vesicle (MLV) which is composed of several concentric bilayers and ranging from 500 to 5000 nm; small unilamellar vesicle (SUV) 100 nm in size and consisting of a single bilayer; and a large unilamellar vesicle (LUV) with sizes ranging from 200 to 800 nm [44].

According to a report in 2005 [44], the current marketed liposomal products used for cancer therapy include Doxil® (PEGylated liposomal formulation of doxorubicin [DOX] for cancer treatment), DaunoXome® (liposomal formulation of daunorubicin to treat

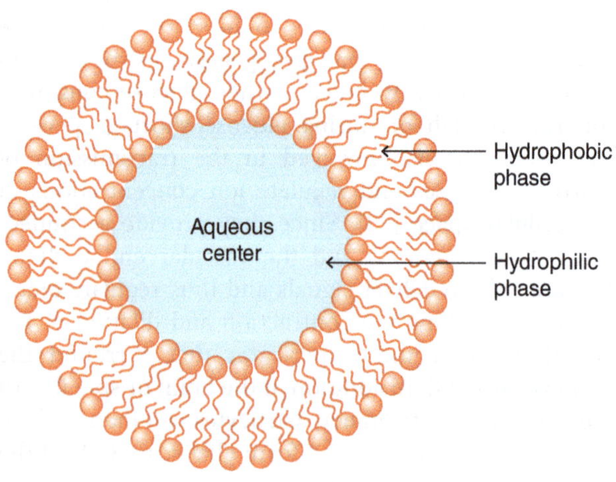

Figure 1.4 Schematic drawing of a liposome.

AIDS-related Kaposi's sarcoma and leukemia), and DepoCyt® (cytarabine to treat cancers of white blood cells such as acute myeloid leukemia) [45]. Drugs (such as DOX) that have severe side effects on normal tissues usually intend to choose liposomes and other nanocarriers to shield itself from undesirable release and increase the applicable dosage.

Other than commercialized products, researchers in the University of Shizuoka indicated that liposomes as drug carriers could be used for cancer anti-neovascular therapy. Regarding this liposome-drug combinational delivery, liposome-encapsulated DOX significantly inhibited the VEGF-induced mitogen-activated protein kinase (MAPK) pathway and suppressed VEGF-induced human umbilical vein endothelial cell (HUVEC) proliferation *in vivo*. Consequently, tumor growth and surviving time were significantly suppressed [46].

1.2.2 Functionalization of Liposomes

Liposomes have been studied for a long time according to their attractive biological properties such as biocompatibility, biodegradability, controllable release, and ability to carry both hydrophilic pharmaceutical agents inside the aqueous internal area and hydrophobic ones into the membrane as well as protect the pharmaceutical agents from the external environment without having undesirable side effects [47]. However, there are limitations on the other side. Compared to other delivery systems, the drawbacks of using liposomes as drug carriers include fast elimination from the blood, relatively low encapsulation efficacy, poor storage stability, and the capture of the liposomes by the cells in the liver before it reaches the target [44]. Therefore, a number of developments have been developed in order to solve these problems.

1.2.2.1 PEGylation

To increase liposome circulation time and stability, attention has been given to the surface modification approaches that form stealth liposomes and therefore protect liposomes from the external bioenvironment after administration and prolong their residence time [48, 49]. One of the most popular approaches is, according to Yuta Yoshizawa's research in 2011, by conjugating polyethylene glycol (PEG) units to liposomalization drugs such as paclitaxel (PTX). The author compared PEGylated-liposome (also known as "stealth" or sterically stabilized liposome) to a naked liposome and O/W emulsion and indicated that after intravenous injection, area under the concentration-time curve (AUC) of the PEG-liposome was almost four times higher than the uncoated liposome. Also, pharmacokinetics and the release rate of PEG-liposome were much better than the emulsion and naked liposome. For the most important, it was confirmed that the PEG-liposome formation would deliver larger amounts of drugs to the target area, in this case tumor tissue, *in vivo*, and hence it was suggested that PEG-coated liposomes could be treated as a potential drug carrier in cancer chemotherapy [45].

In addition, besides efficacy, a previous study showed that there was a significant reduction of adverse effects on PEG-liposome–encapsulated drug compared to other entrapped drugs. For instance, in a study in 2001, Gerald Batist et al. indicated that PEG-liposome–encapsulated DOX increased the therapeutic index of DOX by decreasing irreversible cardiotoxicity [50]. Also, similar to Doxil, a study showed that PEGylated liposomes efficiently blocked its interaction with plasma proteins as well as mononuclear phagocytes and exhibited significantly prolonged system-circulation time as a result.

1.2.2.2 Ligand-mediated Liposome Targeting

On the other hand, since optimization of immunoliposomes properties remains a big concern, conjugating specific ligands such as monoclonal antibodies have been shown to be a promising way to selectively deliver liposomes to many targets. Mostly in cancer research, the optimization of immunoliposomes properties is an ongoing concern. For instance, as reported by Zhang et al. [51], PEGylated OX26 (monoclonal antibody to the rat transferrin receptor)-immunoliposomes loaded with expression plasmids of gene encoding tyrosine hydroxylase (TH) showed promising results in a rat model for Parkinson's disease. Puja Sapra, and Theresa M. Allen also demonstrated that antibody-involved liposomes (such as anti-CD19-targeted liposomes) were able to be internalized into human B-lymphoma (Namalwa) cells rapidly and achieved a much more enhanced therapeutic efficacy [52]. Moreover, due to the fact that folate receptors (FR) are usually overexpressed in a range of tumor cells, delivering folate-modified liposomes has been assessed by different groups as a promising approach. For example, oligonucleotide (ON)-encapsulated in folate-targeted liposomes to FR-positive tumor cells have been recently evaluated both *in vitro* and *in vivo* by Leamon et al., and revealed that the functionalized liposome delivered about twofold more oligonucleotides to the livers of nude mice than nontargeted formulations [53]. FR-targeted liposomes have also been demonstrated to have great capability in delivering DOX both *in vitro* and *in vivo*, and havealso indicated being able to inhibit multidrug-resistant tumor cells [54].

Similar to folate-targeted liposome, transferrin (Tf)-mediated liposome targeting is another approach that has been investigated for tumor targeting, since the transferring receptor (TfR) is frequently overexpressed on the surface of many tumor cells. As a result, TfR antibodies become one of the most popular ligands for liposomes to target tumor cells [55]. Studies show that Tf-modified DOX-liposomes exhibit increased binding efficiency and selectively cytotoxicity toward C6 glioma cells [56] and Tf/anti TfR antibodies also display an enhanced gene delivery ability to endothelial cells with cationic liposomes as carriers [57, 58].

1.2.2.3 Cell-penetrating Peptide (CPP) Modification

Different from most of the peptides, cell-penetrating peptides (CPPs) are a class of short peptides, typically around 5–30 amino acids that can cross the cellular membrane. There are basically two main types of CPP: one is the polypeptide motifs that are derived from natural proteins that exhibit penetrating functions (such as TAT) [59], VP_{22} [60], Antp [61], gH_{625} [62, 63], etc.; and the other type is artificially synthesized polypeptides that are being designed based on the structure of naturally derived CPPs, such as mTAT(C-5H-TAT-5H-C) [64]. Based on its ability to facilitate cellular uptake and accessibility by incorporating functional motifs [65, 66], CPP has been used as a vector for delivering various cargos such as chemical molecules, siRNA [67], contrast (imaging) agents, and proteins both *in vitro* and *in vivo* [68, 69]. The discovery of CPP can be traced back to 1988, when Frankel and Pabo [70], together with Green and Loewenstein [71], reported that the viral trans-activator of transcription protein (TAT) encoded by HIV-1 was able to cross biological membranes and dramatically enhance viral transcription efficiency [72]. Currently, the amino acid sequence of the protein transduction domain of TAT has been narrowed down to YGRKKRRQRRR (amino acids 47–57), in which the arginine and lysine-rich motif GRKKR was found to be the nuclear localization sequences (NLSs) responsible for nuclear localization and thus mediates further translocation of TAT into the nucleus [73–75].

Within the last several decades, more than hundreds of CPPs have been discovered, but the application of those CPPs in biomedical and clinical research has been retained due to their nonspecific targeting and weak stability [76]. Other than adding, replacing, or other methods to modify amino acid sequences of CPP itself to enhance its integrity, it draws people's attention that CPP is also able to combine with other drug carriers and hence integrate with various characteristics associated with different drug-deliver techniques for developing innovative multifunctional drug delivery systems (MDDS). Major MDDSs based on CPPs combined with other drug carriers include CPP-liposome, CPP-polymers, and CPP-nanoparticles (such as magnetic nanoparticles and nanogold Table 1.2).

Among all the MDDS, the CPP-liposome is one of the most utilized systems due to its ability to be manipulated in many different ways and its good biocompatibility. CPP coupled liposomes, especially sterically stabilized liposomes, are under investigation by many researchers. For example Yun-Long Tseng et al. indicated that, compared to the control peptide group, both penetratin (PEN) and TAT displayed improved translocation ability of liposomes and the more peptides attached onto the liposomal surface, the better the translocation effect would show, and the peptide number could be as few as five to enhance intracellular delivery of liposomes [88]. Moreover, an arginine-rich-peptide conjugated liposome was evaluated by Soon Sik Kwon et al. for its ability to deliver an antioxidant, *Polygonum aviculare* L. extract transdermally. Results indicated that CPP-liposomes presented improved cellular uptake activity and skin permeability compared to antioxidant agents only [89]. In addition to intracellular drug delivery, CPP-conjugated liposome also plays an important role in siRNA translocation. In this case, CPP-liposomes entrapped with nona-arginine (R_9) and NF-κB decoy

Table 1.2 Major MDDSs based on CPPs combined with other drug carriers.

Drug carriers		CPPs	Purpose	References
Liposome		R_8	Deliver siRNA into cells and gene silencing	[77]
		Gh_{625}	Anti-cancer drug delivery	[78]
Polymers	PEI	TAT	Gene delivery	[79]
	CBA-DAH	TAT	Increase the delivery of siRNA to cardiomyocytes	[80]
	PNVA-*co*-AA	D-R_8	Mucosal vaccine deliver	[81]
Nanoparticles	PEI-MNP	G_3R_6-TAT	Gene transfer	[82]
	Gold	TAT	For intracellular localization studies	[83, 84]
	Nanomicelle	TAT	Anti-cancer drug delivery	[85]
Others	Cholesterol	G_3R_6-TAT	Antimicrobial application	[86]
	Dendrimer	TAT	Deliver oligonucleotide into cells	[87]

PEI, polyethylenimine; CBA-DAH, cystamine bisacrylamide-diaminohexane; PNVA-*co*-AA, poly(*N*-vinylacetamide)-*co*-acrylic acid; PEI-MNP, polyethylenimine coated magnetic nanoparticles.

oligodeoxynucleotides have been evaluated for their intracellular uptake efficiency as well as anti-glioma ability *in vitro* [90]. Results showed that the CPP-liposomes were successfully and effectively taken up by U87MG glioblastoma cells and facilitated tumor cell death.

1.2.3 Physiologically Modified Liposomes

1.2.3.1 PH-sensitive Liposome

Since the 1970s, pH-sensitive drug delivery system (DDS) in biomedical treatments have been extensively investigated [91]. A majority of the early work was to propose a kind of PSL formed with pH-responsive phospholipids, such as dioleylphosphoethanolamine (DOPE), which contains unsaturated acyl chains that destabilize the liposomes at low pH spots and release the encapsuled drug/DNA as a result [92, 93]. To achieve the localized release of the liposome content, PSL consisting of DOPE was demonstrated to be endocytosed and fused with the endovascular membrane due to the low pH inside the endosome and released its contents into the cytoplasm as a result [94]. Selvam et al. indicated that anionic polyelectrolyte (PE) containing immuno-PSL showed successful release of antisense oligonucleotides (ONs) and suppressed by 85% HIV-1 replication *in vitro*, which was much higher than the control group [95]. Furthermore, in the *in vivo* evaluation, liposomes consisting of DOPE and oleic acid was indicated as an efficient and stable immune-PSL with the addition of cholesterol [96]. In other cases, the PH value around the tumor tissue was not much lower than normal tissue and usually around a pH of 6.5 [97]. In this scenario, fusogenic lipids are therefore introduced and DOPE together with cholesteryl hemisuccinate (CHEMS) have become a popular combination for synthesizing fusogenic PSL for endosomal/lysosomal escape [98]. CHEMS is a kind of acidic cholesterol ester which undergoes self-assembly and forms bilayers under high or neutral pH [99]. In slightly acidic pH values, CHEMS with the inverted conical shape and a large headgroup will lose its original shape and lead to membrane destabilization due to the disruption of ionized headgroup [100]. Consequently, the cargos (such as anticancer drugs and genes) will then be released under mild acidic pH.

1.2.3.2 Thermosensitive Liposomes

Thermosensitive liposomes (TSLs) are another stimuli-triggered localized drug delivery strategy that has been frequently explored for cancer and antimicrobial therapies. First introduced in 1978, when Yatvin et al. formulated a kind of liposome that released a hydrophilic antibiotic neomycin *in vitro* at specific temperatures and inhibited bacteria protein synthesis [101]. This kind of liposome with its ability to release hydrophilic drugs when the temperature increased to a few degrees higher than physiological temperature was then known as a traditional thermosensitive liposome (TTSL). TTSLs were later developed over decades and have become one of the most commonly used techniques in cancer therapies when combined with mild hyperthermia [102]. Lipids with appropriate phase transition temperatures (T_m) have been used to synthesize TSLs. Briefly, T_m is the temperature at which the lipid membrane undergoes phase transitions from a gel to a liquid in response to heating. The orientation of the C—C single bonds in each lipid molecule will then switch from *trans* to *gauche* due to the increased temperature. As a result, leaky interface domains begin to form at the "melting" boundaries and the lipid membrane will show much higher permeability at these locations, which can lead to the release of encapsulated drugs [103]. Basically different lipids have different T_m, and among all kinds of thermosensitive lipids, dipalmitoylphosphatidylcholine (DPPC), are currently highly investigated since they have an ideal gel-to-liquid T_m of around 41 °C [104, 105]. DPPC lipids are usually combined with either 1,2-distearoyl-*sn*-glycero-3-phosphocholine (DSPC) or hydrogenated soy phosphocholine (HSPC) in order to increase its T_m to ~43 °C for better drug release at the tumor site.

However, although supplementing DPPC (16-carbon chains) with DSPC (18-carbon chains) or HSPC (18-carbon chains) that has a positive effect on the drug-releasing rate, the addition of lipids with longer carbon chains than DPPC showed an undesireable side-effect on its phase transition activity [11]. For instance as measured by differential scanning calorimetry, the T_m of a DPPC/DSPC liposome was shown to increase proportionally to the molar fraction of the DSPC being added [106]. Moreover, the range of the T_m became wider with the inclusion of DSPC or HSPC [106, 107]. By examining different molar ratios between the lipids, Gaber et al. found that the T_m of DPPC/HSPC liposomes had a peak value at 46 °C but exhibited temperature ranges between 43 and 48 °C, which was significantly different from the sharp peaks of DPPC at 41 °C [108]. In recent years, the original formulation based on DPPC and DSPC was modified with various compositions to overcome several limitations such as relatively short-circulation times and high DSPC molar ratios that induced necrosis of healthy tissues surrounding the tumor [11, 108]. Specifically, in 1999, Needham and coworkers together with Anyarambhatla came out with the idea of substituting DSPC with lysolipids – monopalmitoyl phosphocholine (MPPC) that contained only one acyl chain. Due to the fact that MPPC lipids have a relatively larger head group than the two hydrocarbon tail lipids, they were more favorable to become micelles with the curvature-forming intuition and consequently, those MPPC inside the bilayers

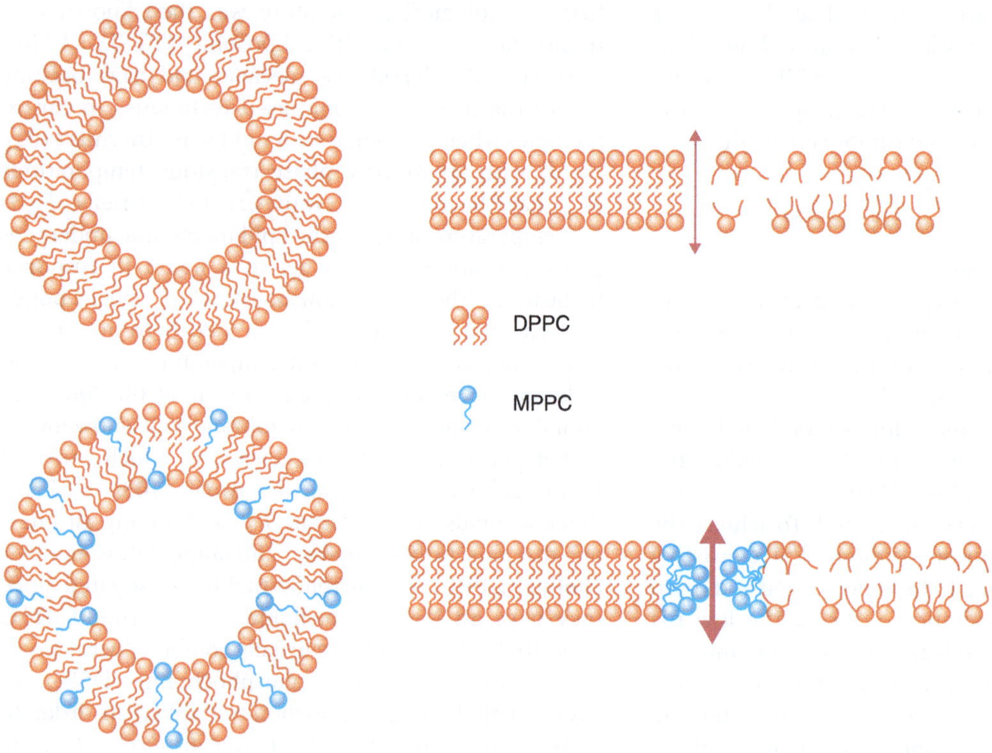

Figure 1.5 Mechanisms of drug release from TTSL and the LTSL. Source: Ta and Porter 2013 [11]. Adapted with permission of Elsevier.

tended to from highly curved micelles and lead to the pore-forming phenomenon that increases cargo release from the liposome lumen [109]. Needham and coworkers hence incorporated MPPC with a molar ratio of 10% into PEGylated TTSL and narrowed down the T_m range while promoting the drug release rate from lower than 40% to 50–60% (Figure 1.5) [11].

In addition, as demonstrated in several human tumor xenograft models, lysolipid containing low temperature-sensitive liposomes (LTSLs) presented a significantly higher efficiency than either TTSL, nonthermosensitive (NTSL), or free drugs (DOX) in tumor cell uptake experiments and tumor cell growth inhibition experiments when combined with mild hyperthermia (42 °C for one hour immediately after tail vein injection, T43 °C = 15 minutes) [110]. Furthermore, Garheng Kong et al. indicated that combining LTSL with hyperthermia resulted in significant amounts of DNA-bound DOX in tumor tissues from animal models [91].

1.2.4 Liposome in Combinational Therapies

1.2.4.1 CPP and Antibody Co-delivery System

To further solve the problem that CPPs do not exhibit specific targeting capabilities, ligands or antibodies have been applied together with CPPs to form dually modified nanostructures on the drug carrier's surface, and therefore allow synergistic effects for tumor targeting delivery. For instance two different types of CPPs have been dual-functionalized with transferrin (Tf), a serum glycoprotein that facilitates iron transcytosis across the BBB, on the liposome surface and form Tf-CPP-liposomes. Studies showed that, although both of the CPPs exhibited good BBB penetrating effect, poly-L-arginine with a long peptide chain has greater cationic charge and thus showed higher cytotoxicity than TAT-based short peptide chains. Moreover, compared to single ligand or unmodified liposomes, Tf-TAT-liposomes exhibited great translocation of DOX across the brain endothelial barrier with no hemolytic activity up to a 200 nM phospholipid concentration [111, 112]. In addition, Taili Zong et al. demonstrated enhanced glioma targeting and cell membrane penetration when combining the nonspecific TAT penetrating peptide with T7, a specific ligand that targets BBB and brain glioma tumor cells together [113].

1.2.4.2 Superparamagnetic Iron Oxide Nanoparticles-Induced Hyperthermia Treatment

Among several intriguing nanoparticles, superparamagnetic iron oxide nanoparticles (SPIONs) have been extensively studied because of their ability to be controlled by magnetic fields [114]. Superparamagnetism is a phenomenon that usually appears among nanoparticles with a diameter smaller than 20 nm. Briefly, when applying an external magnetic field, superparamagnetism nanoparticles will be magnetized up to their saturation of magnetization just as other magnetic particles. However, the nanoparticles with superparamagnetism will no longer display any residual or delayed magnetic interaction after the external magnetic field is removed, which also can be reflected by the hysteresis figures [115]. SPION is therefore a kind of magnetic nanoparticle that can exhibit superparamagnetism. One of the outstanding properties of SPIONs is that when combined with external alternating magnetic fields (AMF), these magnetic materials will exhibit magnetic hysteresis. Consequently, the area close to the hysteresis cycle will generate irreversible work that is being released as thermal energy [116]. The released thermal energy was first discovered as undesirable heat in many industrial applications, yet shows a great profile in magnetic-induced hyperthermia treatment in biomedical fields. The application of SPIONs as hyperthermia agents was once stranded due to their extremely small sizes. Since SPIONs usually share a size range from 5 to 20 nm, which is smaller than the pores of fenestrated capillaries in normal tissues, they were found to leak from circulating blood to normal tissues than target tumors and sometimes resulted in undesired accumulation [117]. To solve this problem, researchers began to use carriers to directly send theses nanoparticles to the target site while protecting them from leaking into normal tissues. One of the most popular delivery systems is to use a liposome. In addition to the plain liposomes, studies indicated that, with SPIONs loaded inside and AMF-introduced hyperthermia on the target site, multifunctional magnetic liposomes conjugated with specific ligands exhibited more specific cell targeting and drug delivery results compared to the control groups [118, 119].

In conclusion, targeting of malignant brain tumors such as GBM and the delivery of therapeutic agents into the brain remains a big concern because of the existence of the BBB and the difficulties in finding suitable candidates for specific tumor locating. Based on the fact that CPP has the capability to penetrate through the BBB and locate the tumor site when combining with tumor-specific ligands, SPIONs loaded thermosensitive liposomes are under investigation for better BBB penetration and selective targeting of brain glioma under mild hyperthermia conditions in the current study. This innovative multifunctionalized liposome is promising because it has the ability to not only target the tumor site inside BBB but also shows controllable release effect when releasing the drugs on site when combined with magnetic field.

1.3 Experimental

1.3.1 *In Vitro* BBB Model Set Up

To assess the effect of astrocytes cocultured in the BBB model, together with trans-endothelial electrical resistance (TEER) assessment, paracellular permeability of 3 kDa fluorescein isothiocyanate-conjugated (FITC) dextran was measured for both the endothelial cell-only model and the astrocyte cocultured model on transwell membranes. Results showed that the BBB model with astrocyte cocultures had a permeability 15% lower than those of the b.End3 monoculture in FITC-Dextran permeabiltiy, but this difference was not significant ($p > 0.1$) (Figure 1.6a). Also the cocultures tended to have significantly higher TEER values (~120 Ω cm^2) than monolayers (~105 Ω cm^2) (Figure 1.6b). Therefore, results suggested that both of the BBB models were confirmed, yet the cocultured BBB model indicated lower paracellular permeability.

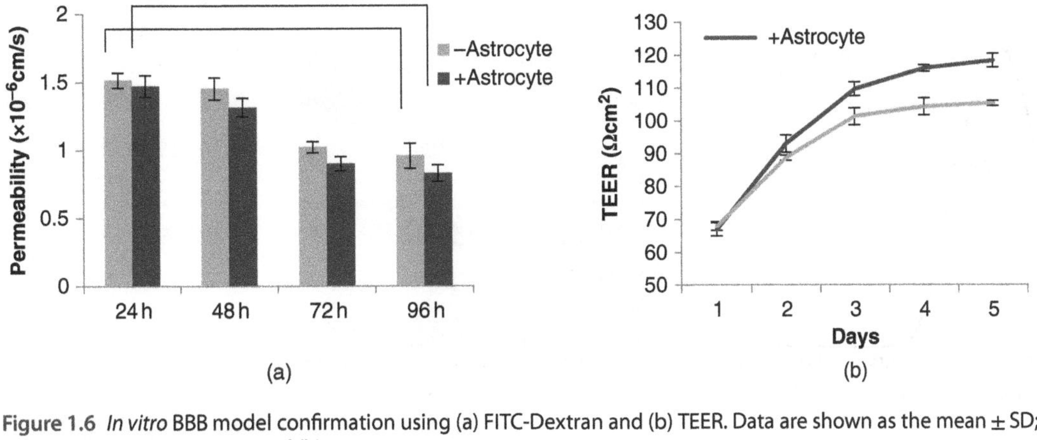

Figure 1.6 *In vitro* BBB model confirmation using (a) FITC-Dextran and (b) TEER. Data are shown as the mean ± SD; $N = 3$, *$p < 0.05$ compared with (a) 24 hours and (b) −Astrocyte.

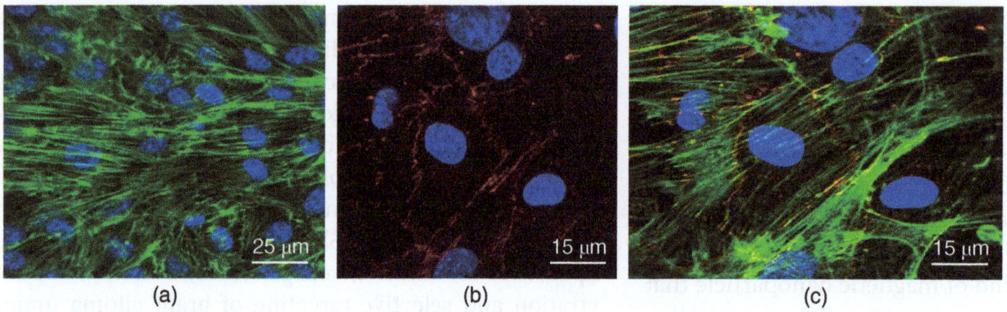

Figure 1.7 Comparison of essential junction proteins expressed by bEnd.3 cells when cocultured with astrocytes: (a) 4′,6-diamidino-2-phenylindole (DAPI) (blue), rhodamine (green); (b) anti-ZO 1 conjugated FITC; (c) DAPI (blue), rhodamine (green), and anti-ZO 1-FITC (red).

1.3.2 Immunostaining and Confocal Imaging

Confocal imaging protocols were administered with immunostaining. The expression of tight junction proteins in the *in vitro* BBB models was examined. Figure 1.7 shows images of the tight junction cytoplasmic protein ZO-1 expressed in the cell layer. From the images we can see that the bEnd.3 cells formed confluent monolayers on the luminal side of the inserts when cocultured with astrocytes and successfully expressed tight junction proteins.

1.4 Liposome Synthesis

1.4.1 Material Characterization

Earlier transmission electronic microscopy (TEM) images characterized the iron oxide core with a result of 5–10 nm [120]. Plain liposome, ferri-liposome, and PEGylated ferri-liposome appeared with slightly different diameters at ∼120, ∼105, and ∼115 nm separately under dynamic light scattering (DLS) (Figure 1.8a) and TEM (Figure 1.8b). Zeta values revealed that most of the liposomes are neutrally charged. X-ray diffraction (XRD) peaks of the SPIONs matched with iron oxide standard peaks.

1.4.2 DOX Release and Loading Efficiency

A representative set of data from the DOX release is shown in Figure 1.9a as a percentage of DOX released compared to positive controls (100% release) versus time in seconds at 42 °C, and as a percentage of LTSL liposome DOX released at 42 °C vs. 37 °C (Figure 1.9b). Results revealed that DOX-LTSL, compared to TTSL, released DOX that is more efficient when the liposomes were heated to their T_m. NTSL served as a negative control with no significant difference in release rate throughout the time. In addition, from Figure 1.9b it is obvious that LTSL played an important role in keeping the pharmaceutical cargos inside the liposome lumen at normal body temperature and thus protect the drugs from premature release.

1.4.3 Liposome Permeability Study

To test the final iron oxide concentration, iron in the receiving wells was collected, and the concentration was

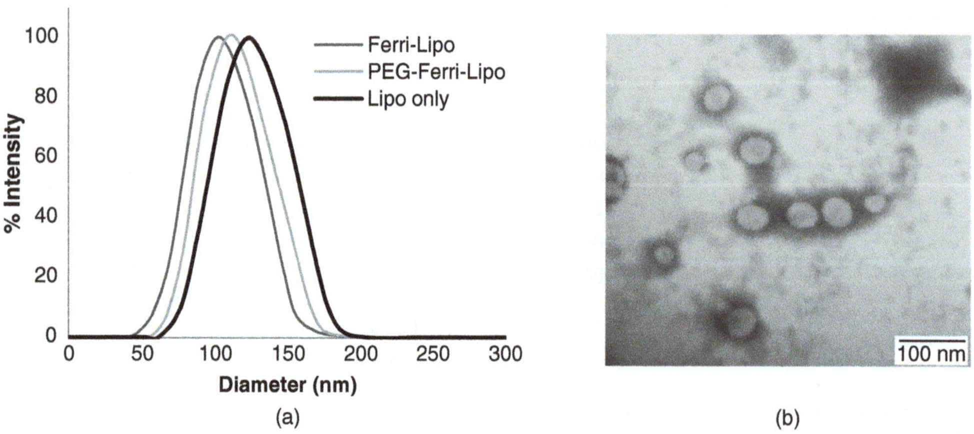

Figure 1.8 Material characterization. (a) Dynamic light scattering (DLS) data of three samples; (b) TEM image of PEGylated ferri-liposomes.

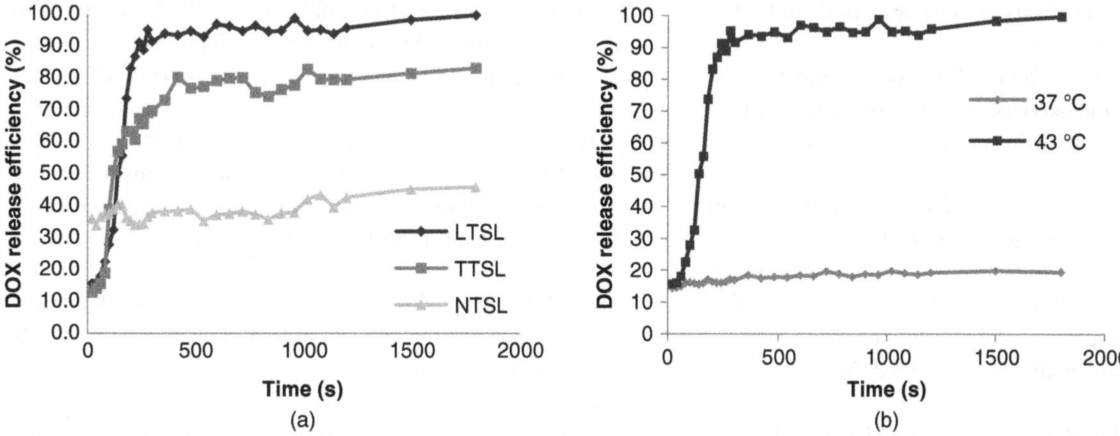

Figure 1.9 DOX release over time: (a) DOX release data from different liposome compositions; (b) DOX-LTSL release at different temperature.

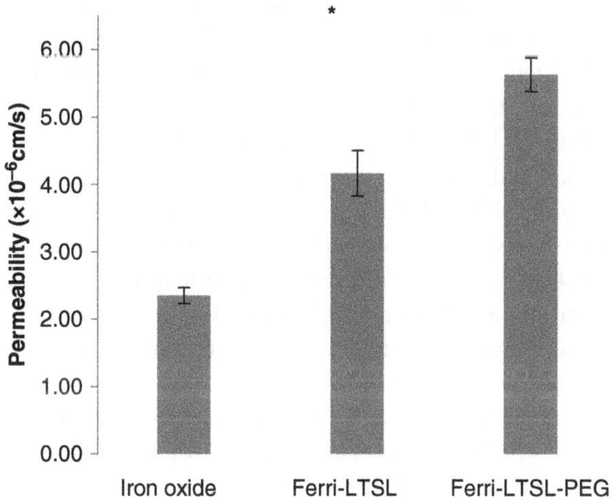

Figure 1.10 Permeability of the ferri-liposomes across the BBB model. Data are shown as the mean ± SD; $N = 3$, *$p < 0.05$ compared with the bare iron oxide.

measured by an iron assay kit. Basically, iron in the sample was released by the addition of an acidic buffer, then the released iron reacted with a chromagen would result in a colorimetric (593 nm) product, proportional to the iron presented in the samples. As the final results shown in Figure 1.10, PEGylated LTSL has double the permeability as bare iron oxide or non-PEGylated liposomes from the permeability chart.

Thus far, this project on the characterization of functionalized liposomes as antitumor drug carriers for BBB delivery has shown that SPION-loaded thermosensitive liposomes, especially LTSL, not only exhibited greater drug release rates and efficiency but also reduced the cytotoxicity of DOX to normal tissues. In addition, the successfully established *in vitro* BBB model shows a promising way to assess the permeability for the functionalized liposomes and hence provide an opportunity to locate the most appropriate candidates for future *in vivo* studies. However, functionalization experiments on the synthesized liposomes have not yet been conclusive to this point. Therefore, in order to optimize the modification of liposome as well as the *in vitro* brain tumor targeting experiments, further work on this project will be aimed at conjugating functional groups (such as CPP and anti-glioma antibody) onto ferri-liposome, and investigating the antitumor ability of the multi-functionalized ferri-liposome under hyperthermia treatment.

References

1 Davson, H. (1989). History of the blood–brain barrier concept. In: *Implications of the Blood–Brain Barrier and Its Manipulation: Basic Science Aspects*, vol. **1** (ed. E.A. Neuwelt), 27–52. Boston, MA: Springer.

2 Banks, W.A. (1995). Physiology and pathology of the blood–brain barrier: implications for microbial pathogenesis, drug delivery and neurodegenerative disorders. *J. Neurovirol.* **5**: 538–555.

3 Ballabh, P., Braun, A., and Nedergaard, M. (2004). The blood–brain barrier: an overview: structure, regulation, and clinical implications. *Neurobiol. Dis.* **16** (1): 1–13.

4 Daneman, R. and Prat, A. (2015). The blood–brain barrier. *Cold Spring Harbor Perspect. Biol.* **7** (1): a020412.

5 Butt, A.M., Jones, H.C., and Abbott, N.J. (1990). Electrical resistance across the blood–brain barrier

in anaesthetized rats: a developmental study. *J. Physiol.* **429**: 47–62.

6 Groothuis, D.R. (2000). The blood–brain and blood–tumor barriers: a review of strategies for increasing drug delivery. *Neuro-Oncology* **2** (1): 45–59.

7 Pardridge, W.M. (2007). Blood–brain barrier delivery. *Drug Discov. Today* **12** (1–2): 54–61.

8 Triguero, D., Buciak, J.B., Yang, J., and Pardridge, W.M. (1989). Blood–brain barrier transport of cationized immunoglobulin G: enhanced delivery compared to native protein. *Proc. Natl. Acad. Sci. U.S.A.* **86** (12): 4761–4765.

9 Abbott, N.J., Ronnback, L., and Hansson, E. (2006). Astrocyte-endothelial interactions at the blood–brain barrier. *Nat. Rev. Neurosci.* **7** (1): 41–53.

10 Hawkins, B.T. and Davis, T.P. (2005). The blood–brain barrier/neurovascular unit in health and disease. *Pharmacol. Rev.* **57** (2): 173–185.

11 Ta, T. and Porter, T.M. (2013). Thermosensitive liposomes for localized delivery and triggered release of chemotherapy. *J. Controlled Release* **169** (1–2): 112–125.

12 Iadecola, C. (2004). Neurovascular regulation in the normal brain and in Alzheimer's disease. *Nat. Rev. Neurosci.* **5** (5): 347–360.

13 Butt, H.J., Downing, K.H., and Hansma, P.K. (1990). Imaging the membrane protein bacteriorhodopsin with the atomic force microscope. *Biophys. J.* **58** (6): 1473–1480.

14 Crone, C. and Christensen, O. (1981). Electrical resistance of a capillary endothelium. *J. Gen. Physiol.* **77** (4): 349–371.

15 Huber, J.D., Egleton, R.D., and Davis, T.P. (2001). Molecular physiology and pathophysiology of tight junctions in the blood–brain barrier. *Trends Neurosci.* **24** (12): 719–725.

16 Deli, M.A., Ábrahám, C.S., Kataoka, Y., and Niwa, M. Permeability studies on in vitro blood–brain barrier models: physiology, pathology, and pharmacology. *Cell. Mol. Neurobiol.* **25** (1): 59–127.

17 Stamatovic, S.M., Keep, R.F., and Andjelkovic, A.V. (2008). Brain endothelial cell–cell junctions: how to "open" the blood brain barrier. *Curr. Neuropharmacol.* **6** (3): 179–192.

18 Fink, C., Weigel, R., Hembes, T. et al. (2006). Altered expression of ZO-1 and ZO-2 in sertoli cells and loss of blood-testis barrier integrity in testicular carcinoma *in situ*. *Neoplasia (New York, NY)* **8** (12): 1019–1027.

19 Anderson, J.M. and Van Itallie, C.M. (2009). Physiology and function of the tight junction. *Cold Spring Harbor Perspect. Biol.* **1** (2): a002584.

20 Wolburg, H. and Lippoldt, A. (2002). Tight junctions of the blood–brain barrier: development, composition and regulation. *Vasc. Pharmacol.* **38** (6): 323–337.

21 Turner, D.A. and Adamson, D.C. (2011). Neuronal-astrocyte metabolic interactions: understanding the transition into abnormal astrocytoma metabolism. *J. Neuropathol. Exp. Neurol.* **70** (3): 167–176.

22 Walz, W. (2000). Role of astrocytes in the clearance of excess extracellular potassium. *Neurochem. Int.* **36** (4–5): 291–300.

23 Su, Z., Niu, W., Liu, M.-L. et al. (2014). In vivo conversion of astrocytes to neurons in the injured adult spinal cord. *Nat. Commun.* **5** (1). https://doi.org/10.1038/ncomms4338.

24 Gordon, A.M., Hung, Y.-C., Brandao, M. et al. (2011). Bimanual training and constraint-induced movement therapy in children with hemiplegic cerebral palsy: a randomized trial. *Neurorehabil. Neural Repair* **25** (8): 692–702.

25 Attwell, D., Buchan, A.M., Charpak, S. et al. (2010). Glial and neuronal control of brain blood flow. *Nature* **468** (7321): 232–243.

26 Bush, T.G., Puvanachandra, N., Horner, C.H. et al. (1999). Leukocyte infiltration, neuronal degeneration, and neurite outgrowth after ablation of scar-forming, reactive astrocytes in adult transgenic mice. *Neuron* **23** (2): 297–308.

27 Daneman, R., Zhou, L., Kebede, A.A., and Barres, B.A. (2010). Pericytes are required for blood–brain barrier integrity during embryogenesis. *Nature* **468** (7323): 562–566.

28 Buckner, J.C., Brown, P.D., O'Neill, B.P. et al. (2007). Central nervous system tumors. *Mayo Clin. Proc.* **82** (10): 1271–1286.

29 Hanson, J.A., Hsu, F.P.K., Jacob, A.T. et al. (2013). Antivascular endothelial growth factor antibody for treatment of glioblastoma multiforme. *Perm. J.* **17** (4): 68–74.

30 Clarke, J., Butowski, N., and Chang, S. (2010). Recent advances in therapy for glioblastoma. *Arch. Neurol.* **67** (3): 279–283.

31 Keating, R.F., Goodrich, J.T., and Packer, R.J. (2001). *Tumors of the Pediatric Central Nervous System.* Thieme.

32 Ohgaki, H. and Kleihues, P. (2007). Genetic pathways to primary and secondary glioblastoma. *Am. J. Pathol.* **170** (5): 1445–1453.

33 Glantz, M., Chamberlain, M., Liu, Q. et al. (2003). Temozolomide as an alternative to irradiation for elderly patients with newly diagnosed malignant gliomas. *Cancer* **97** (9): 2262–2266.

34 Scott, J., Tsai, Y.-Y., Chinnaiyan, P., and Yu, H.-H.M. (2011). Effectiveness of radiotherapy for elderly patients with glioblastoma. *Int. J. Radiat. Oncol. Biol. Phys.* **81** (1): 206–210.

35 Malmström, A., Grønberg, B.H., Marosi, C. et al. (2012). Temozolomide versus standard 6-week radiotherapy versus hypofractionated radiotherapy in patients older than 60 years with glioblastoma: the Nordic randomised, phase 3 trial. *Lancet Oncol.* **13** (9): 916–926.

36 Raizer, J.J., Abrey, L.E., Lassman, A.B. et al. (2010). A phase II trial of erlotinib in patients with recurrent malignant gliomas and nonprogressive glioblastoma multiforme postradiation therapy. *Neuro Oncol.* **12** (1): 95–103.

37 Stommel, J.M., Kimmelman, A.C., Ying, H. et al. (2007). Coactivation of receptor tyrosine kinases affects the response of tumor cells to targeted therapies. *Science* **318** (5848): 287–290.

38 Carrasco-García, E., Saceda, M., and Martínez-Lacaci, I. (2014). Role of receptor tyrosine kinases and their ligands in glioblastoma. *Cells* **3** (2): 199–235.

39 Bickel, U. (2005). How to measure drug transport across the blood–brain barrier. *NeuroRx* **2** (1): 15–26.

40 Upadhyay, R.K. (2014). Drug delivery systems, CNS protection, and the blood brain barrier. *BioMed Res. Int.* **2014**: 37.

41 Cecchelli, R., Dehouck, B., Descamps, L. et al. (1999). In vitro model for evaluating drug transport across the blood–brain barrier. *Adv. Drug Delivery Rev.* **36** (2–3): 165–178.

42 Bangham, A.D. and Horne, R.W. (1964). Negative staining of phospholipids and their structural modification by surface-active agents as observed in the electron microscope. *J. Mol. Biol.* **8** (5): 660–IN10.

43 Sahoo, S.K. and Labhasetwar, V. (2003). Nanotech approaches to drug delivery and imaging. *Drug Discov. Today* **8** (24): 1112–1120.

44 Torchilin, V.P. (2005). Recent advances with liposomes as pharmaceutical carriers. *Nat. Rev. Drug Discov.* **4** (2): 145–160.

45 Yoshizawa, Y., Kono, Y., Ogawara, K.-I. et al. (2011). PEG liposomalization of paclitaxel improved its in vivo disposition and anti-tumor efficacy. *Int. J. Pharm.* **412** (1–2): 132–141.

46 Katanasaka, Y., Ishii, T., Asai, T. et al. (2010). Cancer antineovascular therapy with liposome drug delivery systems targeted to BiP/GRP78. *Int. J. Cancer* **127** (11): 2685–2698.

47 Lasic, D.D. and Papahadjopoulos, D. (1998). General introduction. In: *Medical Applications of Liposomes*, Chapter 1.1, 1–7. Amsterdam: Elsevier Science B.V.

48 Klibanov, A.L., Maruyama, K., Torchilin, V.P., and Huang, L. (1990). Amphipathic polyethyleneglycols effectively prolong the circulation time of liposomes. *FEBS Lett.* **268** (1): 235–237.

49 Blume, G. and Cevc, G. (1993). Molecular mechanism of the lipid vesicle longevity in vivo. *Biochim. Biophys. Acta, Biomembr.* **1146** (2): 157–168.

50 Batist, G., Ramakrishnan, G., Rao, C.S. et al. (2001). Reduced cardiotoxicity and preserved antitumor efficacy of liposome-encapsulated doxorubicin and cyclophosphamide compared with conventional doxorubicin and cyclophosphamide in a randomized, multicenter trial of metastatic breast cancer. *J. Clin. Oncol.* **19** (5): 1444–1454.

51 Zhang, Y., Calon, F., Zhu, C. et al. (2003). Intravenous nonviral gene therapy causes normalization of striatal tyrosine hydroxylase and reversal of motor impairment in experimental parkinsonism. *Hum. Gene Ther.* **14** (1): 1–12.

52 Sapra, P. and Allen, T.M. (2002). Internalizing antibodies are necessary for improved therapeutic efficacy of antibody-targeted liposomal drugs. *Cancer Res.* **62** (24): 7190–7194.

53 Leamon, C.P., Cooper, S.R., and Hardee, G.E. (2003). Folate-liposome-mediated antisense oligodeoxynucleotide targeting to cancer cells: evaluation in vitro and in vivo. *Bioconjugate Chem.* **14** (4): 738–747.

54 Immordino, M.L., Dosio, F., and Cattel, L. (2006). Stealth liposomes: review of the basic science, rationale, and clinical applications, existing and potential. *Int. J. Nanomed.* **1** (3): 297–315.

55 Hatakeyama, H., Akita, H., Maruyama, K. et al. (2004). Factors governing the in vivo tissue uptake of transferrin-coupled polyethylene glycol liposomes in vivo. *Int. J. Pharm.* **281** (1–2): 25–33.

56 Lv, Q., Li, L.-M., Han, M. et al. (2013). Characteristics of sequential targeting of brain glioma for transferrin-modified cisplatin liposome. *Int. J. Pharm.* **444** (1–2): 1–9.

57 Xu, L., Huang, C.-C., Huang, W. et al. (2002). Systemic tumor-targeted gene delivery by anti-transferrin receptor scFv-immunoliposomes 1 This work was supported in part by National Cancer Institute Grant R01 CA45158 (to E. C.), National Cancer Institute Small Business Technology Transfer Phase I Grant R41 CA80449 (to E. C.), and a grant from SynerGene Therapeutics, Inc.1. *Mol. Cancer Ther.* **1** (5): 337–346.

58 Tan, P.H., Manunta, M., Ardjomand, N. et al. (2003). Antibody targeted gene transfer to endothelium. *J. Gene Med.* **5** (4): 311–323.

59 Fittipaldi, A. and Giacca, M. (2005). Transcellular protein transduction using the Tat protein of HIV-1. *Adv. Drug Delivery Rev.* **57** (4): 597–608.

60 Okada, A., Kodaira, A., Hanyu, S. et al. (2014). Intracellular localization of Equine herpesvirus type 1 tegument protein VP22. *Virus Res.* **192**: 103–113.
61 Derossi, D., Chassaing, G., and Prochiantz, A. (1998). Trojan peptides: the penetratin system for intracellular delivery. *Trends Cell Biol.* **8** (2): 84–87.
62 Galdiero, S., Falanga, A., Morelli, G., and Galdiero, M. (2015). gH625: a milestone in understanding the many roles of membranotropic peptides. *Biochim. Biophys. Acta, Biomembr.* **1848** (1, Part A): 16–25.
63 Tarallo, R., Carberry, T.P., Falanga, A. et al. (2013). Dendrimers functionalized with membrane-interacting peptides for viral inhibition. *Int. J. Nanomed.* **8**: 521–534.
64 Yamano, S., Dai, J., Hanatani, S. et al. (2014). Long-term efficient gene delivery using polyethylenimine with modified Tat peptide. *Biomaterials* **35** (5): 1705–1715.
65 Taylor, B.N., Mehta, R.R., Yamada, T. et al. (2009). Noncationic peptides obtained from azurin preferentially enter cancer cells. *Cancer Res.* **69** (2): 537–546.
66 Johansson, H.J., El-Andaloussi, S., Holm, T. et al. (2007). Characterization of a novel cytotoxic cell-penetrating peptide derived from p14ARF protein. *Mol. Ther.* **16** (1): 115–123.
67 Eguchi, A. and Dowdy, S.F. (2009). siRNA delivery using peptide transduction domains. *Trends Pharmacol. Sci.* **30** (7): 341–345.
68 Mäe, M. and Langel, Ü. (2006). Cell-penetrating peptides as vectors for peptide, protein and oligonucleotide delivery. *Curr. Opin. Pharmacol.* **6** (5): 509–514.
69 Järver, P., Mäger, I., and Langel, Ü. (2010). In vivo biodistribution and efficacy of peptide mediated delivery. *Trends Pharmacol. Sci.* **31** (11): 528–535.
70 Frankel, A.D. and Pabo, C.O. (1988). Cellular uptake of the tat protein from human immunodeficiency virus. *Cell* **55** (6): 1189–1193.
71 Green, M. and Loewenstein, P.M. (1988). Autonomous functional domains of chemically synthesized human immunodeficiency virus tat trans-activator protein. *Cell* **55** (6): 1179–1188.
72 Debaisieux, S., Rayne, F., Yezid, H., and Beaumelle, B. (2012). The ins and outs of HIV-1 Tat. *Traffic* **13** (3): 355–363.
73 Schwarze, S.R., Hruska, K.A., and Dowdy, S.F. (2000). Protein transduction: unrestricted delivery into all cells? *Trends Cell Biol.* **10** (7): 290–295.
74 Ruben, S., Perkins, A., Purcell, R. et al. (1989). Structural and functional characterization of human immunodeficiency virus tat protein. *J. Virol.* **63** (1): 1–8.
75 Hauber, J., Malim, M.H., and Cullen, B.R. (1989). Mutational analysis of the conserved basic domain of human immunodeficiency virus tat protein. *J. Virol.* **63** (3): 1181–1187.
76 Zhang, D., Wang, J., and Xu, D. (2016). Cell-penetrating peptides as noninvasive transmembrane vectors for the development of novel multifunctional drug-delivery systems. *J. Controlled Release* **229**: 130–139.
77 Zhang, C., Tang, N., Liu, X. et al. (2006). siRNA-containing liposomes modified with polyarginine effectively silence the targeted gene. *J. Controlled Release* **112** (2): 229–239.
78 Perillo, E., Allard-Vannier, E., Falanga, A. et al. (2015). Quantitative and qualitative effect of gH625 on the nanoliposome-mediated delivery of mitoxantrone anticancer drug to HeLa cells. *Int. J. Pharm.* **488** (1–2): 59–66.
79 Hu, Y., Xu, B., Ji, Q. et al. (2014). A mannosylated cell-penetrating peptide-graft-polyethylenimine as a gene delivery vector. *Biomaterials* **35** (13): 4236–4246.
80 Nam, H.Y., Kim, J., Kim, S. et al. (2011). Cell penetrating peptide conjugated bioreducible polymer for siRNA delivery. *Biomaterials* **32** (22): 5213–5222.
81 Sakuma, S., Suita, M., Inoue, S. et al. (2012). Cell-penetrating peptide-linked polymers as carriers for mucosal vaccine delivery. *Mol. Pharm.* **9** (10): 2933–2941.
82 Song, H.P., Yang, J.Y., Lo, S.L. et al. (2010). Gene transfer using self-assembled ternary complexes of cationic magnetic nanoparticles, plasmid DNA and cell-penetrating Tat peptide. *Biomaterials* **31** (4): 769–778.
83 Tkachenko, A.G., Xie, H., Liu, Y. et al. (2004). Cellular trajectories of peptide-modified gold particle complexes: comparison of nuclear localization signals and peptide transduction domains. *Bioconjugate Chem.* **15** (3): 482–490.
84 de la Fuente, J.M. and Berry, C.C. (2005). Tat peptide as an efficient molecule to translocate gold nanoparticles into the cell nucleus. *Bioconjugate Chem.* **16** (5): 1176–1180.
85 Kanazawa, T., Morisaki, K., Suzuki, S., and Takashima, Y. (2014). Prolongation of life in rats with malignant glioma by intranasal siRNA/drug codelivery to the brain with cell-penetrating peptide-modified micelles. *Mol. Pharm.* **11** (5): 1471–1478.
86 Liu, L., Xu, K., Wang, H. et al. (2009). Self-assembled cationic peptide nanoparticles as an efficient antimicrobial agent. *Nat. Nano* **4** (7): 457–463.

87 Juliano, R.L. (2006). Intracellular delivery of oligonucleotide conjugates and dendrimer complexes. *Ann. N.Y. Acad. Sci.* **1082** (1): 18–26.

88 Tseng, Y.-L., Liu, J.-J., and Hong, R.-L. (2002). Translocation of liposomes into cancer cells by cell-penetrating peptides penetratin and Tat: a kinetic and efficacy study. *Mol. Pharmacol.* **62** (4): 864–872.

89 Kwon, S.S., Kim, S.Y., Kong, B.J. et al. (2015). Cell penetrating peptide conjugated liposomes as transdermal delivery system of *Polygonumaviculare* L. extract. *Int. J. Pharm.* **483** (1–2): 26–37.

90 Saw, P.E., Ko, Y.T., and Jon, S. (2010). Efficient liposomal nanocarrier-mediated oligodeoxynucleotide delivery involving dual use of a cell-penetrating peptide as a packaging and intracellular delivery agent. *Macromol. Rapid Commun.* **31** (13): 1155–1162.

91 Kong, G., Anyarambhatla, G., Petros, W.P. et al. (2000). Efficacy of liposomes and hyperthermia in a human tumor xenograft model: importance of triggered drug release. *Cancer Res.* **60** (24): 6950–6957.

92 Torchilin, V. (2009). Multifunctional and stimuli-sensitive pharmaceutical nanocarriers. *Eur. J. Pharm. Biopharm.* **71** (3): 431–444.

93 Connor, J. and Huang, L. (1986). pH-sensitive immunoliposomes as an efficient and target-specific carrier for antitumor drugs. *Cancer Res.* **46** (7): 3431–3435.

94 Simões, S., Moreira, J.N., Fonseca, C. et al. (2004). On the formulation of pH-sensitive liposomes with long circulation times. *Adv. Drug Delivery Rev.* **56** (7): 947–965.

95 Selvam, M.P., Buck, S.M., Blay, R.A. et al. (1996). Inhibition of HIV replication by immunoliposomal antisense oligonucleotide. *Antiviral Res.* **33** (1): 11–20.

96 Liu, D. and Huang, L. (1989). Role of cholesterol in the stability of pH-sensitive, large unilamellar liposomes prepared by the detergent-dialysis method. *Biochim. Biophys. Acta, Biomembr.* **981** (2): 254–260.

97 Andresen, T.L., Jensen, S.S., and Jørgensen, K. (2005). Advanced strategies in liposomal cancer therapy: problems and prospects of active and tumor specific drug release. *Prog. Lipid Res.* **44** (1): 68–97.

98 Deshpande, P.P., Biswas, S., and Torchilin, V.P. (2013). Current trends in the use of liposomes for tumor targeting. *Nanomedicine (London, England)* **8** (9). https://doi.org/10.2217/nnm.13.118.

99 Hafez, I.M. and Cullis, P.R. (2000). Cholesteryl hemisuccinate exhibits pH sensitive polymorphic phase behavior. *Biochim. Biophys. Acta, Biomembr.* **1463** (1): 107–114.

100 Farhood, H., Serbina, N., and Huang, L. (1995). The role of dioleoyl phosphatidylethanolamine in cationic liposome mediated gene transfer. *Biochim. Biophys. Acta, Biomembr.* **1235** (2): 289–295.

101 Yatvin, M., Weinstein, J., Dennis, W., and Blumenthal, R. (1978). Design of liposomes for enhanced local release of drugs by hyperthermia. *Science* **202** (4374): 1290–1293.

102 Kneidl, B., Peller, M., Winter, G. et al. (2014). Thermosensitive liposomal drug delivery systems: state of the art review. *Int. J. Nanomed.* **9**: 4387–4398.

103 Kim, K.Y. (2007). Nanotechnology platforms and physiological challenges for cancer therapeutics. *Nanomed. Nanotechnol. Biol. Med.* **3** (2): 103–110.

104 Zhu, L. and Torchilin, V.P. (2013). Stimulus-responsive nanopreparations for tumor targeting. *Integr. Biol.* **5** (1). https://doi.org/10.1039/c2ib20135f.

105 Kono, K. (2001). Thermosensitive polymer-modified liposomes. *Adv. Drug Delivery Rev.* **53** (3): 307–319.

106 Nibu, Y., Inoue, T., and Motoda, I. (1995). Effect of headgroup type on the miscibility of homologous phospholipids with different acyl chain lengths in hydrated bilayer. *Biophys. Chem.* **56** (3): 273–280.

107 Ganesan, M.G., Schwinke, D.L., and Weiner, N. (1982). Effect of Ca^{2+} on thermotropic properties of saturated phosphatidylcholine liposomes. *Biochim. Biophys. Acta, Biomembr.* **686** (2): 245–248.

108 Gaber, M.H., Hong, K., Huang, S.K., and Papahadjopoulos, D. Thermosensitive sterically stabilized liposomes: formulation and in vitro studies on mechanism of doxorubicin release by bovine serum and human plasma. *Pharm. Res.* **12** (10): 1407–1416.

109 Landon, C.D., Park, J.-Y., Needham, D., and Dewhirst, M.W. (2011). Nanoscale drug delivery and hyperthermia: the materials design and preclinical and clinical testing of low temperature-sensitive liposomes used in combination with mild hyperthermia in the treatment of local cancer. *Open Nanomed. J.* **3**: 38–64.

110 Needham, D., Anyarambhatla, G., Kong, G., and Dewhirst, M.W. (2000). A new temperature-sensitive liposome for use with mild hyperthermia: characterization and testing in a human tumor xenograft model. *Cancer Res.* **60** (5): 1197–1201.

111 Sharma, G., Modgil, A., Zhong, T. et al. (2013). Influence of short-chain cell-penetrating peptides on transport of doxorubicin encapsulating receptor-targeted liposomes across brain endothelial barrier. *Pharm. Res.* **31** (5): 1194–1209.

112 Sharma, G., Modgil, A., Sun, C., and Singh, J. (2012). Grafting of cell-penetrating peptide to receptor-targeted liposomes improves their transfection efficiency and transport across blood–brain barrier model. *J. Pharm. Sci.* **101** (7): 2468–2478.

113 Zong, T., Mei, L., Gao, H. et al. (2014). Enhanced glioma targeting and penetration by dual-targeting liposome co-modified with T7 and TAT. *J. Pharm. Sci.* **103** (12): 3891–3901.

114 Plank, C., Zelphati, O., and Mykhaylyk, O. (2011). Magnetically enhanced nucleic acid delivery. Ten years of magnetofection—progress and prospects. *Adv. Drug Delivery Rev.* **63** (14–15): 1300–1331.

115 Wahajuddin, A.S. (2012). Superparamagnetic iron oxide nanoparticles: magnetic nanoplatforms as drug carriers. *Int. J. Nanomed.* **7**: 3445–3471.

116 Kumar, C.S.S.R. and Mohammad, F. (2011). Magnetic nanomaterials for hyperthermia-based therapy and controlled drug delivery. *Adv. Drug Delivery Rev.* **63** (9): 789–808.

117 Hayashi, K., Nakamura, M., Sakamoto, W. et al. (2013). Superparamagnetic nanoparticle clusters for cancer theranostics combining magnetic resonance imaging and hyperthermia treatment. *Theranostics* **3** (6): 366–376.

118 Darwish, M.S.A., Nguyen, N.H.A., Ševců, A. et al. (2016). Dual-modality self-heating and antibacterial polymer-coated nanoparticles for magnetic hyperthermia. *Mater. Sci. Eng., C* **63**: 88–95.

119 Kang, L., Gao, Z., Huang, W. et al. (2015). Nanocarrier-mediated co-delivery of chemotherapeutic drugs and gene agents for cancer treatment. *Acta Pharm. Sin., B* **5** (3): 169–175.

120 Di, S., Linlin, S., Gujie, M. et al. (2014). Controlling ferrofluid permeability across the blood–brain barrier model. *Nanotechnology* **25** (7): 075101.

2

Biofabrication Techniques for Ceramics and Composite Bone Scaffolds

Fengyuan Liu, Boyang Huang, Sri Hinduja, and Paulo J. da Silva Bartolo

The University of Manchester, School of Mechanical, Aerospace and Civil Engineering, Manchester, United Kingdom

2.1 Introduction

Bone is a vascular and highly specialized form of connective tissue playing a very demanding biomechanical and metabolic role [1]. It maintains the shape of the skeleton, protects soft tissues in the cranial, thoracic and pelvic cavities, transmits the forces of muscular contraction during movement, serves as a reservoir for ions and contributes to the regulation of the extracellular matrix (ECM) composition, blood production, and blood pH regulation [2]. Most of bone properties depend on its composition, which consist of 60–70% mineral, 10–20% collagen, and 9–20% water by weight [3]. As shown by Currey [4], the Young's modulus value increases significantly with increased Ca content (Figure 2.1). Additionally, the strain at yield decreases with increasing mineral content. However, this correlation is not conclusive, as it has not taken account of the variations in the porosity, the direction of loading, and the relative proportions of woven and lamellar bone. Other organic materials such as growth factors, cytokines, osteonectin, osteopontin, osteocalcin, bone sialoprotein, hyaluronan thrombospondin, proteoglycans, phospholipids, and phosphoproteins are also present, playing an important role in bone remodeling and osteogenesis [5].

Macroscopically, bone is made up of very dense cortical or compact bone (porosity of 5–10%), representing 80% of the total bone mass, and cancellous or spongeous bone (porosity of 50–95%), representing 20% of the bone mass [6]. Bone's structure is highly anisotropic and it remodels itself along local stress lines [7].

Bone is able to heal and remodel without leaving any scar in cases of very limited damage or fracture. However, in pathological fractures, traumatic bone loss or primary tumor resection, where the bone defect exceeds a critical size, bone is no longer able to heal itself [8, 9]. Moreover, this regenerative ability reduces with age [10]. In these cases, the clinical approach is the use of bone grafts, defined as an implanted material that promotes bone healing alone or in combination with other materials, through osteogenesis, osteoinduction, and osteoconduction [11]. Bone grafts can be divided into autografts, allografts, and xenografts [8, 9, 11–16]. Autografts, the gold standard in reconstructing small bone defects, are harvested from one site and implanted into another site within the same individual. They can be cancellous or cortical (nonvascularized or vascularized) bone, and in some cases, a combination of both. Autografts are osteogenic, osteoinductive, osteoconductive, and have no risks of immunogenicity and disease transmission [9, 12]. Main complications are related to pain and morbidity in the donor site, limited quantity and availability, prolonged hospitalization time, the need for general sedation or anaesthesia, and risk of deep infection and haematoma [9, 11, 12, 14]. They can be obtained from the iliac wring or crest, distal radius or tibia, and proximal tibia or humerus or ribs [11].

Allografts are harvested from one individual and implanted into another individual of the same species. They can be obtained from cadavers or living donors and can be either cortical or cancellous bone and are prepared in fresh, frozen, and freeze-dried forms. Allograft's major limitations are associated with the risk of rejection, transmission of diseases and infections from donor to recipient, limited supply, and loss of biological and mechanical properties due to its processing and cost [9–12]. Additionally, the rate of healing is generally lower than autografts.

Xenografts are harvested from one individual and transplanted into another individual of a different species. They are osteoinductive and osteoconductive, low cost, and highly available grafts. Major limitations are related to their lack of osteogenic properties, risk of immunogenicity and transmission of infections and zoonotic diseases, and poor clinical outcome [10–12].

Bioceramics and Biocomposites: From Research to Clinical Practice, First Edition. Edited by Iulian Antoniac.

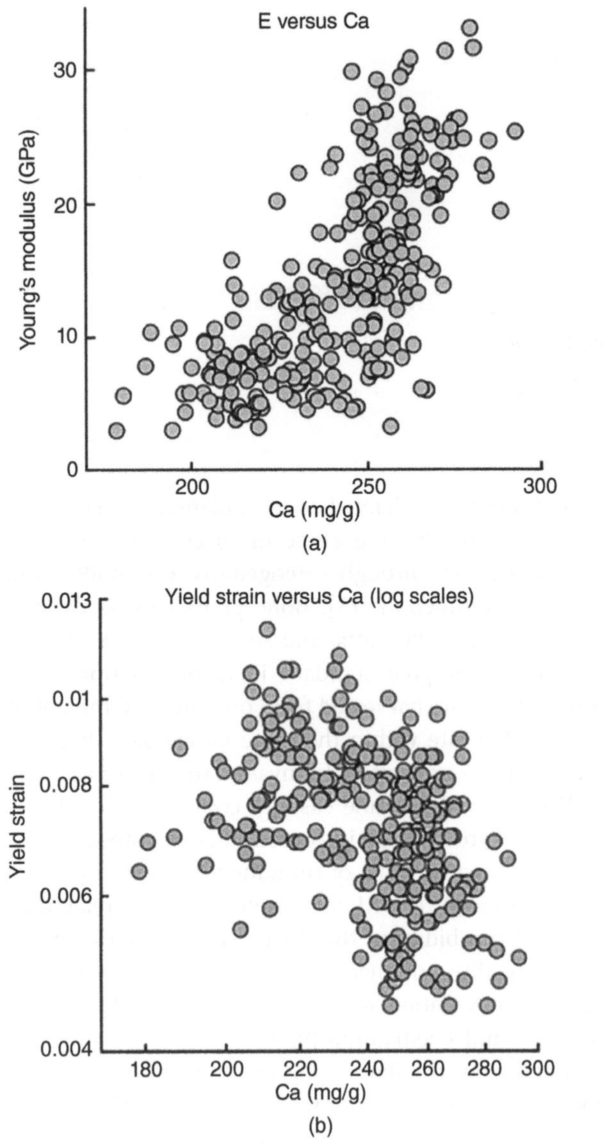

Figure 2.1 Variation of bone elastic modulus and yield strain as a function of mineral content. Source: Currey 2003 [4]. Reproduced with permission of Elsevier.

For larger bone damage or diseases, besides the abovementioned limitations, bone grafts face difficulties. Therefore, biofabrication, the combined use of additive manufacturing techniques, biocompatible and biodegradable materials, cells, growth factors, etc., for the fabrication of bioactive scaffolds (synthetic grafts), is becoming a promising alternative for grafting [17]. These scaffolds can be designed to match the defect site and are able to incorporate growth factors and cells. However, they are usually associated with poor neovascularization, limited mechanical properties, and variable biodegradability [10].

This chapter reviews major additive manufacturing technologies used to produce ceramic and composite scaffolds, highlighting main advantages and limitations.

2.2 Scaffolds

Scaffolds provide an initial biochemical substrate for the novel tissue until cells can produce their own extracellular matrix. Scaffolds not only define the 3D space for the formation of new tissues but also serve to provide tissues with appropriate functions. Scaffolds are often critical, both *ex vivo* as well as *in vivo*, as they serve some of the following purposes [17–20]:

- Allow cell attachment, proliferation, and differentiation;
- Deliver and retain cells and growth factors;
- Enable diffusion of cell nutrients and oxygen;
- Enable an appropriate mechanical and biological environment for tissue regeneration in an organized way.

To achieve these goals, an ideal scaffold for bone regeneration must satisfy some biological and mechanical requirements [17, 19, 21–29]:

***Biological requirements*:**

- Biocompatibility – the scaffold material must be nontoxic and allow cell attachment, proliferation, and differentiation.
- Biodegradability – the scaffold material must degrade into nontoxic products.
- Controlled degradation rate – the degradation rate of the scaffold must be adjustable in order to match the rate of tissue regeneration. Controlling the degradation process and the effects of its degradation products

Table 2.1 Hierarchical pore size distribution for an ideal scaffold.

Pore size	Biomechanical effect or function
<1 μm	Interaction with proteins
	Responsible for bioactivity
1–20 μm	Type of cells attracted
	Cellular development
	Orientation and directionality of cellular ingrowth
100–1000 μm	Cellular growth
	Bone ingrowth
	Predominant function in the mechanical strength
>1000 μm	Implant functionality
	Implant shape

Source: From Sanchez-Salcedo et al. 2008 [30].

is crucial to avoid tissue necrosis or inflammation. Scaffolds should also promote osteointegration, which corresponds to the formation of a chemical bond between bone and the surface of the implanted scaffold without the formation of fibrous tissue.

- Appropriate porosity, pore size (Table 2.1), pore shape, and pore distribution to allow tissue in-growth and vascularization. As reported by Bose et al. (2012), pores smaller than 75 μm favor the formation of fibrous tissue, pores in the range of 75–100 μm support the formation of tissue with un-mineralized osteoid and pores greater than 200 μm facilitate enhanced bone ingrowth and vascularization.
- Osteoconduction and osteogenesis – the scaffold must induce chemical stimulation of human mesenchymal stem cells into bone-forming osteoblasts. An ideal scaffold should have macroporous of 150–500 μm in diameter and 60–80% interconnected porosity to induce osteoconduction.
- Ability to delivery growth factors, cytokines, and antibacterial materials – growth factors represent a family of proteins controlling the activity of tissue-specific cells through a complex regulating system. In bone tissue engineering, a wide range of growth factors are used to regulate cell differentiation, proliferation, and expression of ECM proteins of the cells, including transforming growth factor (TGF-β), insulin-like growth factor (IGF), platelet-derived growth factor (PDGF), basic fibroblast growth factor (bFGF), and bone morphogenetic proteins (BMPs). Angiogenic growth factors like vascular endothelial growth factor (VEGF) are also used. Techniques used to incorporate growth factors into the scaffold include soaking the scaffold in a growth factor-containing solution or through a covalent linkage of the growth factors to the scaffold. Cells modified to express and secrete osteoinduction growth factors may also be seeded in the scaffold.

***Mechanical and physical requirements*:**

- Sufficient strength and stiffness to withstand stresses in the host tissue environment. For load-bearing applications such as bone, the scaffold must be strong enough to withstand physiological stresses. However, transfer of load to the scaffold (stress shielding) may result in lack of sufficient mechanical stimulation to the ingrowing tissue.
- Adequate surface properties like wettability and surface roughness (Figure 2.2) guaranteeing that a good biomechanical coupling is achieved between the scaffold and the tissue.

Easily sterilized either by exposure to high temperatures or by immersion in a sterilization agent, remaining unaffected by either of these processes.

2.2.1 Materials

From a material point, scaffolds for bone tissue engineering can be classified as ceramic scaffolds, polymeric scaffolds, and composite scaffolds [17, 32, 33].

Bioceramics used for tissue engineering are classified as nonresorbable (relatively inert), bioactive or surface active (semi-inert), and biodegradable or resorbable (noninert). The various bioresorbable ceramic materials used in bone applications include calcium phosphates (CaP) (hydroxyapatite [HA], and tricalcium phosphate [TCP]) and bioglasses (amorphous ceramics) [11, 17, 34]. Calcium phosphates (CaP) enhance bone formation depending on crystallinity, crystalline phase, and Ca/P ratio [12, 35]. Hydroxyapatite is the most commonly used bioceramic. It presents a similar mineral structure to natural bone. It is an osteoconductive

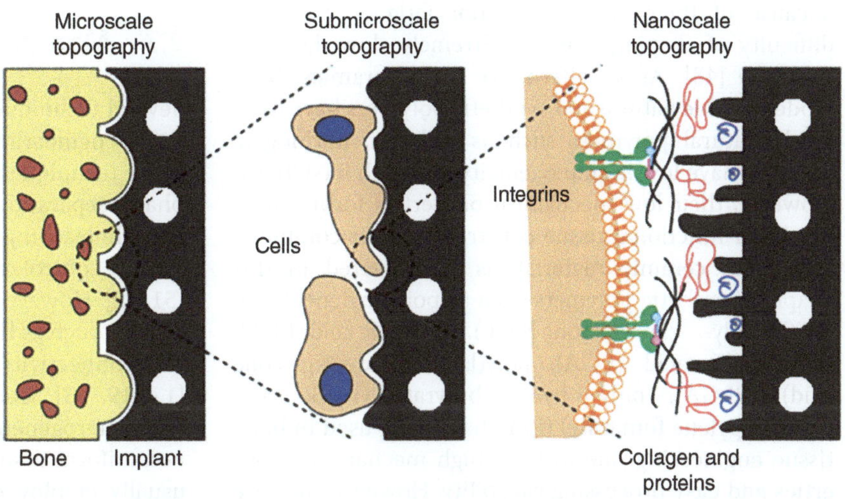

Figure 2.2 Interactions between bone and the scaffold surface at different topographical scales. Source: Gittens et al. 2011 [31]. Reproduced with permission of Elsevier.

material that allow the formation of a high connection with the surrounding bone tissues. The major drawbacks are their brittleness and low mechanical stability, which prevent their use in large bone tissue regeneration [36]. Nano-scale HA powders, produced through sol–gel synthesis, co-precipitation, hydrothermal reaction, and microemulsion synthesis, are gaining importance to improve the mechanical properties of HA ceramics [37]. Nano-hydroxyapatite in the size range of 20–80 nm shows high cell adhesion, proliferation, and differentiation [38]. The nanoscale features of HA allow the crystals to act as direct building blocks for biomineralization.

TCP has four forms including α-TCP, β-TCP, α′-TCP, and super α-TCP. The α′-TCP is a high-pressure phase, and the super α-TCP is only observed at approximately 1500 °C. Therefore, α-TCP and β-TCP are the most frequently observed polymorphs. The rate of biodegradation of different CaP compounds, which is directly related to their Ca/P is α-TCP > β-TCP > HA.

Biphasic calcium phosphate (BCP) compounds are made of variable amounts of β-TCP and HA. The dissolution rate can be controlled by adjusting the ratio between HA and β-TCP.

Bioactive glasses, based on acidic oxides (e.g. phosphorus pentoxide, silicon dioxide, and aluminum oxide) and basic oxides (e.g. calcium oxide, magnesium oxide, and zinc oxide), have also been successfully used for bone tissue engineering applications [3, 9, 17, 39, 40]. They have controlled biodegradability, low fracture toughness, stimulate both gene expression of osteoblasts and angiogenesis *in vitro* and *in vivo*, and they favor the formation of bone-mineral like phases and have antibacterial and inflammatory effects [3, 5, 17, 39–41]. Drug loading of bioglasses is also possible. The degradation of bioglass, through a dissolution-based procedure, is very slow and influenced by the particle size, glass type, and type of medium [42].

Clinical applications of bioceramics have been limited because of their brittleness, poor fatigue resistance, difficulty of shaping, and an extremely slow degradation rate [43]. As an alternative to bioceramics, both biodegradable natural and synthetic polymers have been used. Natural polymers such as collagen, fibrinogen, chitosan have low immunogenicity and high bioactivity. However, their low mechanical properties forbid them to obtain functional tissue constructs. Their combined used with ceramic materials is not covered in this chapter. Synthetic polymers such as polyethylene glycol (PEG), poly-ε-caprolactone (PCL), polylactic acid (PLA), polyglycolic acid (PGA), poly(lactic acid-*co*-glycolic acid) (PLGA), poly-β-hydroxybutyrate (PHB), and poly(propylene fumarate) (PPF) have been used in bone tissue engineering due to their high mechanical properties and easy processing capability. However, they are

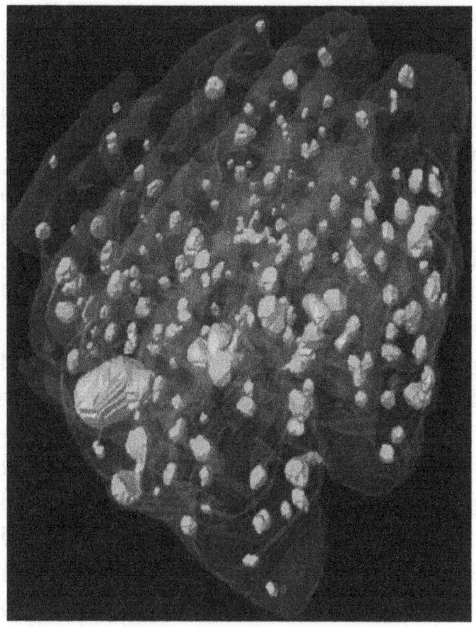

Figure 2.3 μCT image of a PCL-HA scaffold.

hydrophobic, have limited capabilities in achieving a strong bonding and integration with bone, exhibit weak mechanical properties, and are prone to creep [44, 45]. Polymers degrade primary by hydrolysis and also by enzymatic and cellular pathways [46, 47]. Development of composite materials consisting of a biodegradable matrix incorporating rigid bioactive particles (Figure 2.3) combines the reinforcement activity provided by bioactive ceramic particles with the tailored degradation kinetics of biodegradable polymers [48]. Figure 2.4 compares the mechanical properties of different ceramic, polymeric, and composite materials with the mechanical properties of cortical and trabecular bone. Table 2.2 summarizes the most commonly used materials to produce composite scaffolds for bone applications.

2.3 Manufacturing Processes

Several techniques can be used to produce scaffolds for tissue engineering applications. Conventional or nonadditive techniques such as solvent casting, freeze-drying, phase separation, gas foaming, melt moulding, and particle-leaching are used to produce 3D scaffolds with relative control over the micro- and macro-scale features [51, 52]. However, these techniques present several limitations, such as the lack of control over the pore size and interconnectivity, porosity, and pore spatial distribution [17, 19, 53], leading to an inadequate vascularization and heterogeneous distribution of cells, promoting a nonuniform tissue growth. In addition, these techniques usually employ toxic organic solvents, which prevent

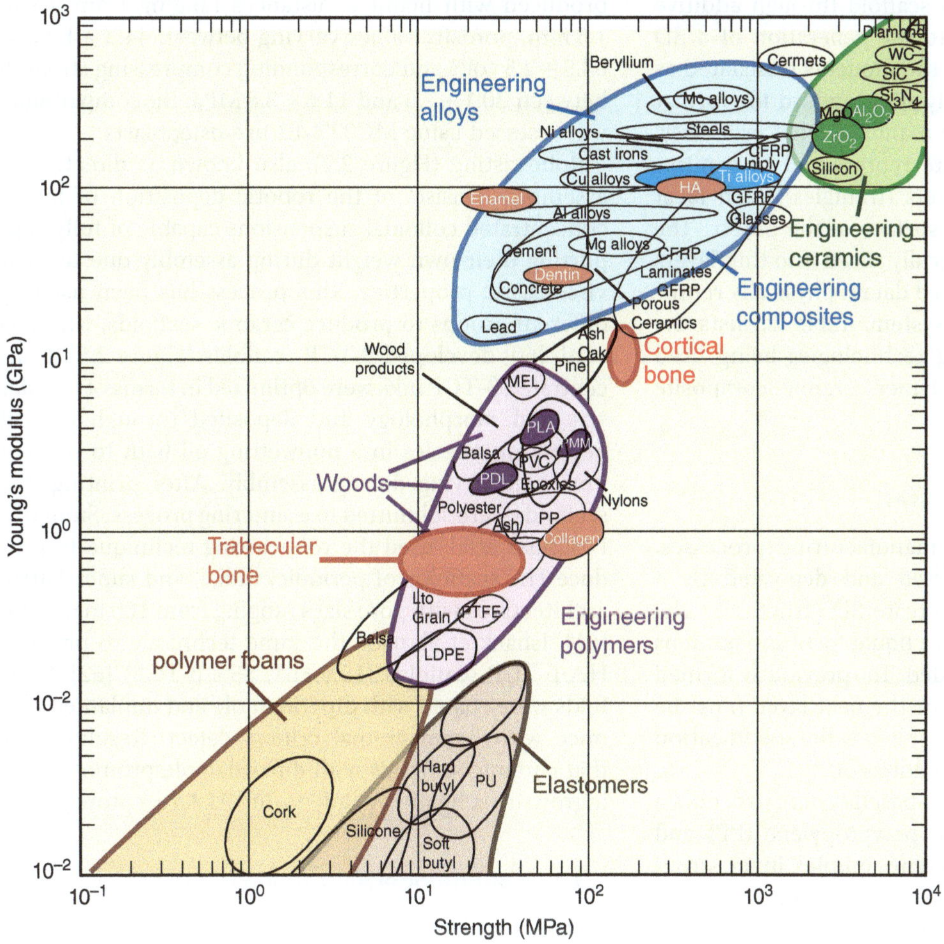

Figure 2.4 Young's modulus versus strength for different materials. Source: Wegst and Ashby 2004 [49]. Reproduced with permission of Taylor & Francis.

Table 2.2 Materials commonly used to produce bioceramic composite scaffolds for bone applications.

Material	Advantages	Disadvantages
Synthetic polymers • Poly-glycolic acid (PGA) • Poly-lactic acid (PLA) • Poly(lactide-*co*-glycolide) (PLGA) • Poly(ε-caprolactone) (PCL)	• Biocompatibility • Biodegradability • Versatility	• Low mechanical strength • High local concentration of acidic degradation products
Ceramics • Hydroxyapatite • Tricalcium phosphate *Bioglasses* • Silicate bioactive glasses (45S5, 13–93) • Borosilicate bioactive glasses (13–93B2, 13–93B3)	• Biocompatibility • Biodegradability • Bioactivity • Osteoconductivity (depending on structural and chemical properties)	• Brittleness • Low fracture strength • Degradation rates difficult to predict

Source: Garcia-Gareta et al. 2015 [50].

the incorporation of cells and other biological molecules during fabrication [19, 53]. Biomanufacturing represents a new group of nonconventional fabrication techniques for the production of 3D scaffolds through the use of additive technologies, biodegradable and biocompatible materials, cells, and growth factors [17, 54, 55], providing precise control over the pore size, porosity, and pore interconnectivity [17, 53].

The first step to produce a scaffold through additive manufacturing corresponds to the generation of a 3D computer solid model. Then, the model is tessellated as an STL file, which is currently the standard file format for data input for all additive manufacturing processes. In this format, 3D models are represented by a number of three-sided planar facets (triangles), each facet defining part of the external surface of the object. The STL model is then mathematically sliced into thin layers (sliced model). Finally, the sliced data is physically reproduced using an appropriate system. Table 2.3 lists the main additive manufacturing technologies being used to produce ceramic and polymer/ceramic composite scaffolds.

2.3.1 Extrusion-based Processes

In extrusion-based additive manufacturing processes, pellets or filaments are melted and deposited by a controlled robotic device to create 3D structures. The material leaves the extruder in a liquid form and hardens immediately after being extruded. The previously formed layer, which is the substrate for the next layer, must be maintained at a temperature just below the solidification point to assure good interlayer adhesion.

Kalita et al. used an extrusion-based system to produce composite scaffolds based on polypropylene (PP) and TCP [56]. Scaffolds with different complex inner structures were fabricated as shown in Figure 2.5. The average pore size was 160 μm, and samples with 36% of porosity showed the best compressive strength of 12.7 MPa. Scaffolds were biologically tested with a modified human osteoblast cell-line (HOB). The results showed that the samples were nontoxic with excellent cell growth during the first two weeks.

Bose et al. [57] produced alumina and β-TCP ceramic scaffolds with pore size in the range of 300–480 μm and porosity of 25–45%. The biological performance of these scaffolds was assessed using OPC1 human osteoblasts during 28 days. No cytotoxicity effects were observed. Similarly, Kim et al. produced poly(D,L-lactide:glycolide) (DL-PLGA) and β-TCP scaffolds with 0/90° and 0/45° lay-down patterns, coated with HA. The surface morphology of the scaffolds was assessed before and after HA coating using scanning electron microscopy [58]. The scaffolds were implanted into rabbit femoral bone defects.

Jo et al. developed the concept of rapid direct deposition of ceramic paste (RDD-C process) to produce porous BCP scaffolds (Figure 2.6) [59]. The process is based on the rapid solidification of BCP filaments through the precipitation of a methylcellulose (MC) polymer used as the binder in aqueous BCP paste, via solvent extraction mechanism. Different scaffolds were produced with filament distances ranging from 0.5 to 1.5 mm, porosity values varying between 44.3 ± 4.9 and 63.5 ± 2.5 vol% and corresponding compressing strength between 30.1 ± 7.6 and 11.6 ± 3.8 MPa. Biocompatibility was assessed using MC3T3-E1 pre-osteoblasts.

Robocasting (Figure 2.7), also known as direct-write assembly, consists of the robotic deposition of highly concentrated colloidal suspensions capable of fully supporting their own weight during assembly due to their viscoelastic properties. This process has been used by different groups to produce ceramic scaffolds. Miranda et al. [60] developed β-TCP scaffolds (Figure 2.8). Concentrated β-TCP inks were optimized in terms of powder size and morphology and deposited through conical deposition nozzles in a nonwetting oil bath to prevent unwanted drying during assembly. After printing, the scaffolds were submitted to a sintering process. Similarly, Dellinger et al. used the robocasting technique to produce HA scaffolds of periodic, radial, and super-lattice architectures with pore sizes ranging from 100 to 600 μm [61]. Ishack et al. used the same technique to produce HA/β-TCP scaffolds (15% HA, 85% β-TCP) [62]. Scaffolds were coated with dipyridamole and implanted into mice with 3 mm cranial critical defect. Results show that ceramic scaffolds with dipyridamole promote bone ingrowth via ligation of adenosine A2A receptors.

2.3.2 Vat-photopolymerization Processes

Vat-photopolymerization or stereolithographic processes produce three-dimensional solid objects in a multilayer procedure through the selective photoinitiated cure reaction of a photosensitive material [17, 19, 63–67]. These processes usually employ two distinct methods of irradiation [66]. The first method is the mask-based method in which an image is transferred to a liquid polymer by irradiating through a patterned mask. The irradiated part of the liquid polymer is then solidified. In the second method, a direct writing process using a focused UV beam produces polymer structures.

The direct or laser writing approach consists of a vat containing a photosensitive material, a moveable platform on which the model is built, a laser to irradiate and cure the material, and a dynamic mirror system to direct the laser beam over the polymer surface "writing" each layer. After drawing a layer, the platform dips into the material vat, leaving a thin film from which the next layer will be formed. Mask-based writing systems build models by shining a flood lamp through a mask, which lets light pass through it [68].

Vat-photopolymerization processes are commonly used to produce a negative replica of the scaffold that is filled with ceramic slurries and burnt away during sintering [17, 53, 69, 70]. Chu et al. developed a lost-mold

Table 2.3 Additive manufacturing processes classification according to the American Society for Testing and Materials (ASTM) International Committee F42.

Vat-photopolymerization

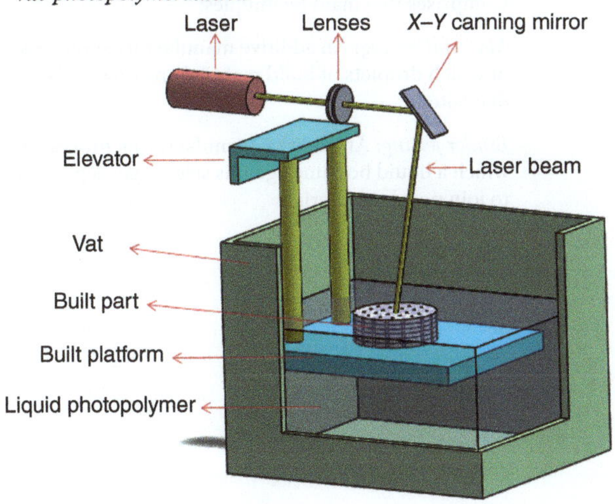

An additive manufacturing process in which a liquid photopolymer in a vat is selectively cured by light-activated polymerization.

Material extrusion

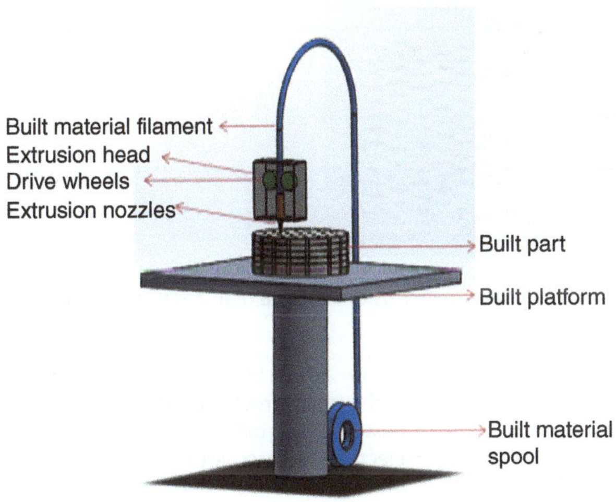

An additive manufacturing process in which material is selectively dispensed through a nozzle or orifice.

Powder bed fusion

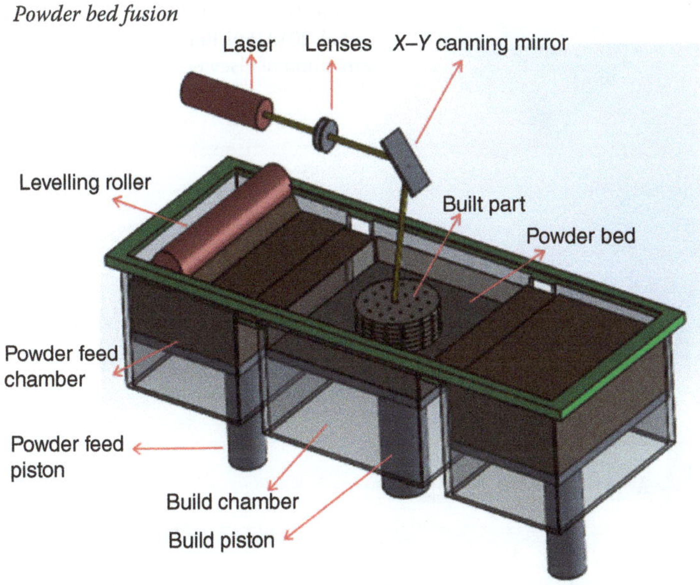

An additive manufacturing process in which thermal energy selectively fuses regions of a powder bed.

Table 2.3 (Continued)

Inkjet printing processes 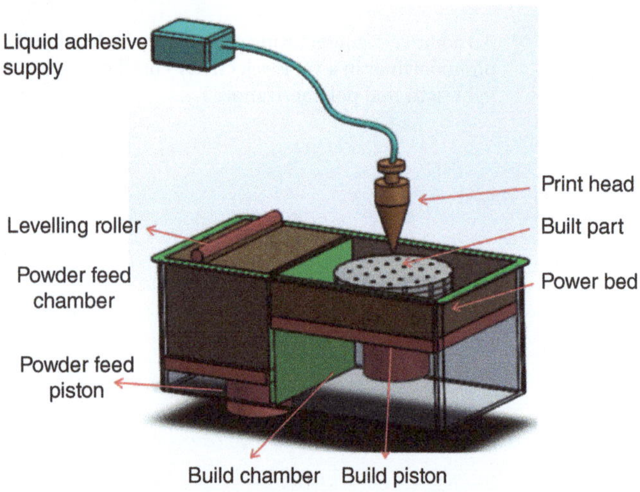	Comprises two main techniques: *Material jetting*: An additive manufacturing process in which droplets of build material are selectively deposited. *Binder jetting*: An additive manufacturing process in which a liquid bonding agent is selectively deposited to join powder materials.

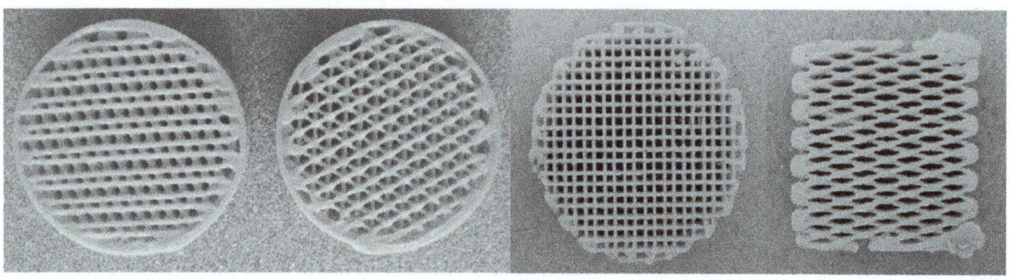

Figure 2.5 Porous composite scaffold of different inner structure designs produced through extrusion additive manufacturing. Source: Kalita et al. 2003 [56]. Reproduced with permission of Elsevier.

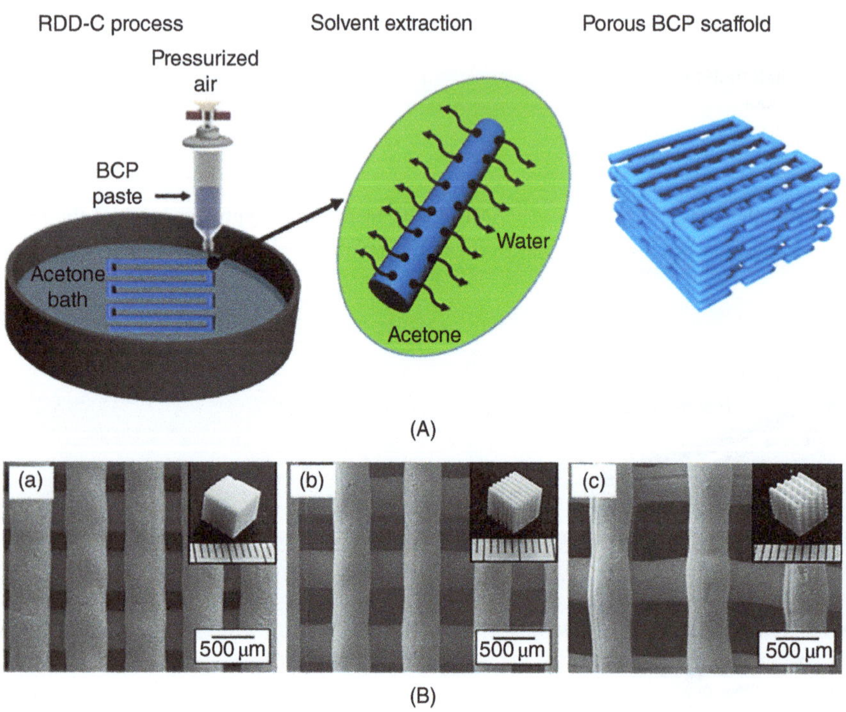

Figure 2.6 (A) Schematic representation of the rapid direct deposition of ceramic paste (RDD-C) process. (B) Scanning electron microscopy (SEM) images of porous BCP scaffolds produced using different distances between filaments ((a) 0.5 mm, (b) 1 mm, and (c) 1.5 mm). Source: Jo et al. 2014 [59]. Reproduced with permission of Elsevier.

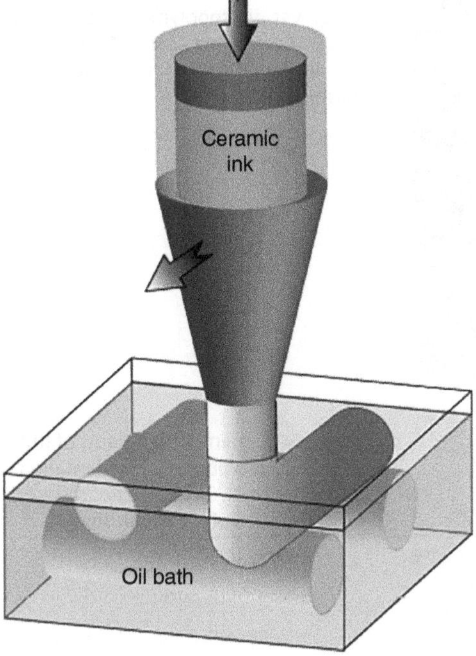

Figure 2.7 Schematic representation of the robocasting process. Source: Miranda et al. 2006 [60]. Reproduced with permission of Elsevier.

technique to produce implants with designed channels and connection pattern [71]. Vat-photopolymerization was used to create epoxy molds designed from the negative image of implants. A highly loaded HA-acrylate suspension was cast into the mold. The mold and the acrylic binder were removed by pyrolysis and the HA green scaffold submitted to a sintering process. The finest channel size achieved was about 366 μm and the range of implant porosity between 26% and 52%.

Bian et al. produced an osteochondral β-TCP/collagen scaffold containing a bone phase with a 3D channel network composed of β-TCP, a cartilage phase consisting of collagen and a transitional interface between the bone and cartilage (Figure 2.9) [69]. Vat-photopolymerization was used to produce both bone and transitional phase, through the polymerization of a ceramic suspension. After processing, the binder was removed by pyrolysis, and the porous structure sintered. To produce the cartilage phase, a solution of type-I collagen was casted into a cylindrical mold on the surface of the ceramic scaffold, and then freeze-dried. Finally, the scaffold was immersed into a glutaraldehyde solution (0.5 wt%) to allow the cross-linking of collagen. Bone marrow stromal cells, cultured on the porous scaffolds under perfusion attached well, cover about 60% of the structure after seven days.

Bian et al. also produced β-TCP scaffolds for the treatment of an early femoral head necrosis [69]. Scaffolds were produced through a sequence of processes including photocuring, dehydration, rinsing, drying, and sintering. The compression strength of the scaffolds was 23.54 MPa, close to that of natural cancellous bone. The scaffolds were designed with a preset channel structure for blood vessel implantation. According to this design, a small artery and vein can be implanted into the preset channel structure and sutured to form the arteriovenous loop pathway (Figure 2.10). The revascularized implant

Figure 2.8 SEM micrographs of a TCP scaffold: (a) general view. (b) *XY* plane view. (c) TCP filaments. (d) Filament surface. Source: Miranda et al. 2006 [60]. Reproduced with permission of Elsevier.

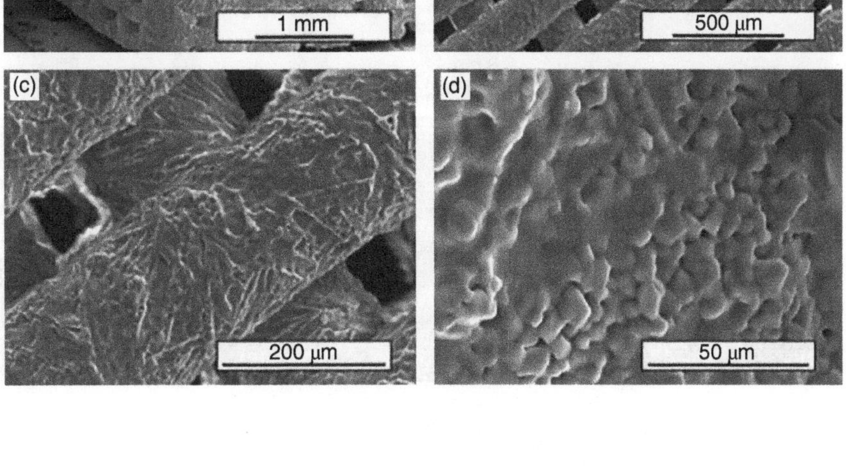

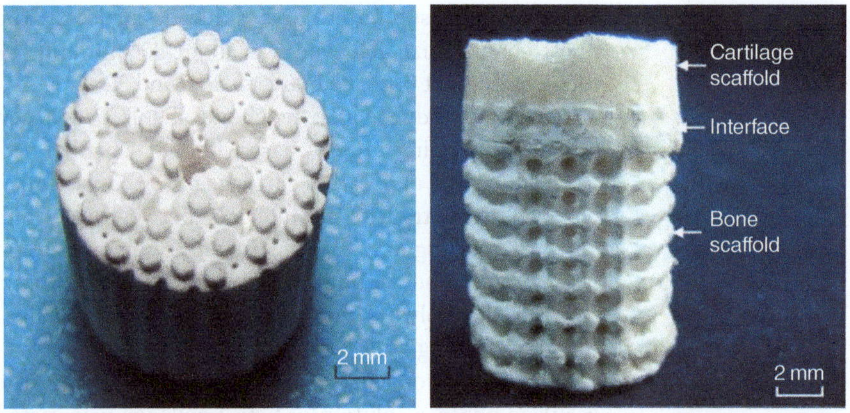

Figure 2.9 β-TCP/collagen scaffold built through vat-photopolymerization and gel casting. Source: Bian et al. 2011 [69]. Reproduced with permission of IOP Publishing.

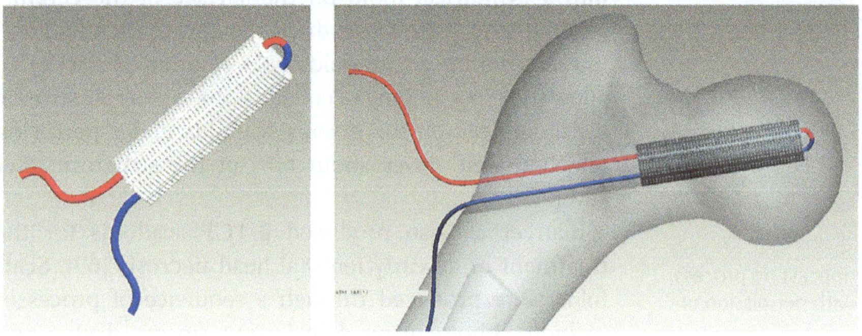

Figure 2.10 Schematic diagrams of the scaffold and the proposed implantation. Source: Bian et al. 2011 [69]. Reproduced with permission of IOP Publishing.

can be implanted into the core decompression hole of the necrotic femoral head (Figure 2.10).

Chopra et al. [72] produced glass–ceramic (apatite–mullite glass–ceramic, LG112) scaffolds with simple cubic structure, by gel-casting into moulds produced by vat-photopolymerization (Figure 2.11a). The molds were produced by the polymerization of an acrylate polymer, removed prior to sintering. Primary human osteoblasts, cultured on the scaffolds composed of only a few slices (Figure 2.11b) and square channels of 400 or 600 μm of width, showed good adhesion and proliferation. Despite the fact that cells readily proliferate on the scaffold surface, its penetration into the structure was limited, as observed by confocal microscopy (Figure 2.11c–e).

Bartolo proposed a multiphoton and multimaterial stereolithographic system called stereo-thermal-lithography (STLG) [67, 73]. This system (Figure 2.12) uses a mercury lamp of 350 W as a light source and optical filters to split the radiation into two different wavelengths: UV radiation and near-infrared (near-IR) radiation. Optical fibers, projection, and focal lenses

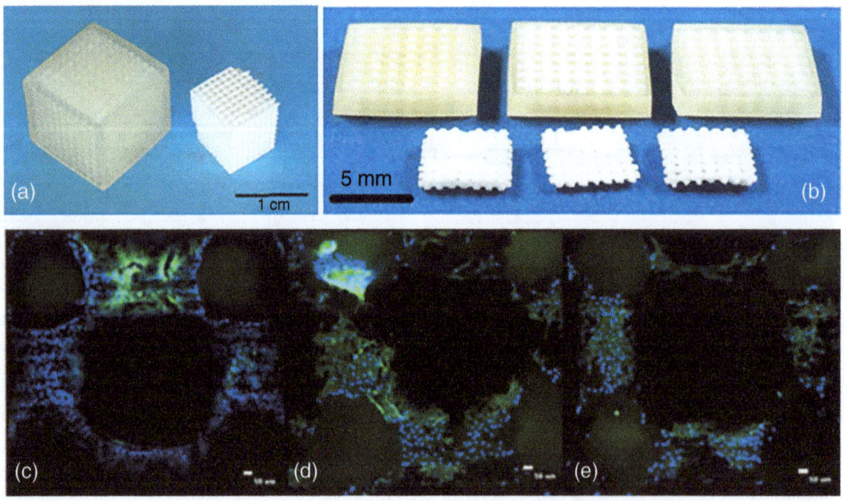

Figure 2.11 (a) Mould built by vat-photopolymerization and respective sintered glass–ceramic scaffold obtained by gel-casting; (b) scaffolds used in the cell culture studies; confocal fluorescence micrographs of osteoblasts, stained with fluorescein isothiocyanate-conjugated (FITC) phalloidin for f-actin and 4′,6-diamidino-2-phenylindole (DAPI) for nuclei on the top (c), middle (d), and bottom (e) of the scaffold. Source: Chopra et al. 2012 [72]. Reproduced with permission of IOP Publishing.

Figure 2.12 Stereo-thermal-lithography system.

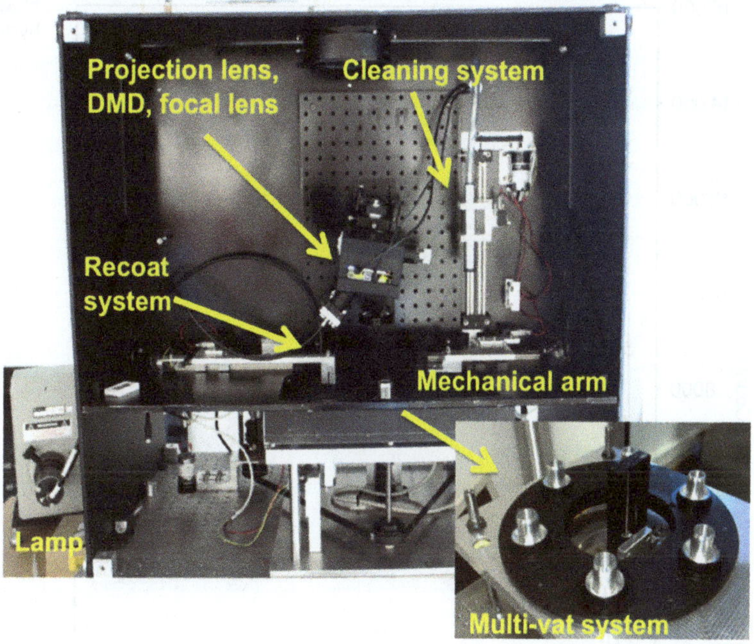

irradiate a ultra violet-digital micromirror devices (UV-DMDs) and a infra red-digital micromirror devices (IR-DMDs). A dichroic mirror captures the images projected on both DMDs (1024 × 768 pixels, 14 mm in size), combining them into a single image that is transferred to the liquid polymer. The equipment also includes a multivat system enabling the fabrication of multimaterial constructs. The vertical displacement of the platform is secured by a positioner uniaxial MYCOSIS® Translation Stage VT-80. This positioner allows vertical increments of 1 μm, at a speed ranging between 0.001 and 20 mm/s.

The STLG system was used to produce poly(ethylene glycol) dimethacrylate (PEGDMA)/HA scaffolds [74]. Energy dispersive spectroscopy (EDS) was used to quantify the elemental composition of polymer/ceramic scaffolds as shown in Figure 2.13, revealing that the PEGDMA/HA scaffolds present four characteristic peaks, corresponding to the C, O, P, and Ca elements, which confirm the presence of HA at the surface of the scaffolds. EDS results also show the absence of impurities like carbonaceous species within the HA nanoparticles.

Lee et al. [100] produced PPF/DEF (diethyl fumarate) scaffolds containing 7% of HA nanopowder and bis-acylphosphine oxide (BAPO) as a photoinitiator. MC3T3-E1 preosteoblasts, cultured on these scaffolds during two weeks, showed better adhesion and proliferation in the composite scaffolds than on scaffolds without HA. Sharifi et al. produced soft nanocomposite hydrogel structures by the polymerization of a solution, consisting of methacrylate-functionalized triblock copolymers of PEG with poly(trimethylene carbonate) (PTMC) with colloidal dispersions of clay nanoparticles (Laponite XLG) at different concentrations (2.5 and 5 wt%) [75]. Unconfined compression tests were performed regarding the swollen hydrogels, showing that an increasing on the concentration of the Laponite nanoclay improved the compressive modulus. In another work, bioactive glass S53P4 was combined with a methacrylated PCL polymer to produce porous scaffolds [76]. Bioactive glass was homogeneously distributed through the scaffold and its surface, improving the compression modulus of the construct and the cellular activity of seeded fibroblasts.

2.3.3 Powder Bed Fusion Processes

Powder bed fusion processes use a laser to selectively heat and melt powder material. The laser traces the shape of each cross-section of the model to be built, sintering powder in a thin layer. It also supplies energy that not only fuses neighboring powder particles but also bonds each new layer to those previously sintered. After each layer is solidified, the piston over the model retracts to a new position and a new layer of powder is supplied using a mechanical roller. The powder that remains unaffected by the laser acts as a natural support for the model and remains in place until the model is complete.

The properties of scaffolds obtained by powder bed fusion processes strongly depend on the powder properties (e.g. particle size and powder morphology) and operational parameters, such as spot diameter, laser power, scanning speed, and layer thickness [77–79]. Savalani et al. investigated the effect of processing parameters on the physical properties of HA/polyamide structures [78]. Results show that the layer thickness

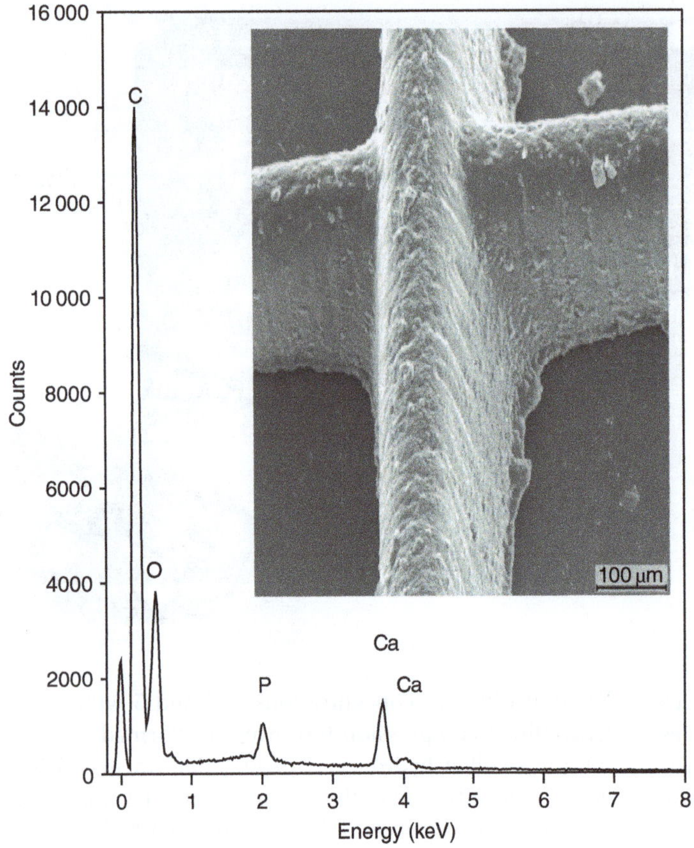

Figure 2.13 EDS and SEM micrograph of PEGDMA/HA hydrogel scaffolds.

is the most critical parameter, strongly influencing the physical properties and the pore morphology. The use of high values of layer thickness results in structures with higher open porosity, and increased average pore width and proportion of pores of a suitable size to enable bone regeneration. This is due to the specific heat capacity of the composite material, which leads to a lesser conduction of heat and lesser fusion between particles during the sintering process.

Wiria et al. produced composite scaffolds consisting of PCL and HA at different percentages (10, 20, and 30 wt%). Scaffolds soaked in a simulated body fluid during 16 days, induced the formation of a hydroxy carbonate apatite layer, indicating the bioactivity of the material [80]. Osteoblast-like SaOS-2 cells attach to the construct and spread well along 12 days of culture. Lindner et al. produced TCP/PDLLA (poly-DL lactic acid) composite scaffolds (Figure 2.14) with 90 μm of pore size and compressive strength of 23 MPa [81]. Liu et al. investigated TCP scaffolds with different amounts (0.5–3 wt%) of poly-L-lactic acid (PLLA) aiming to improve the mechanical properties [44]. Results show that the scaffold present high compressive performance (17.67 MPa) and fracture toughness (1.43 MPa) when 1 wt% of PLLA was used. Above these values, an increase of PLLA decreases the mechanical properties.

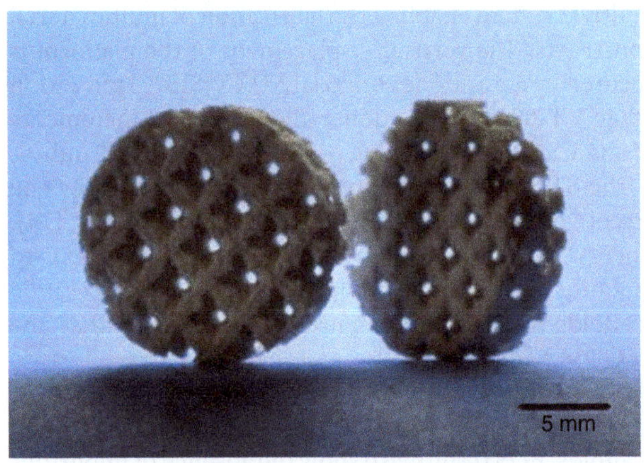

Figure 2.14 Composite scaffolds containing 50% of β-TCP and 50% PDLLA. Source: Lindner et al. 2011 [81]. Reproduced with permission of John Wiley & Sons.

Lohfeld et al. evaluated the *in vivo* performance of a commercial β-TCP implant and a composite PCL/TCP scaffold produced by laser sintering (Figure 2.15a,b) [82]. Constructs were implanted into a critical size bone defect created in a sheep tibia during 14 weeks. Results showed the formation of both higher mineralized callus

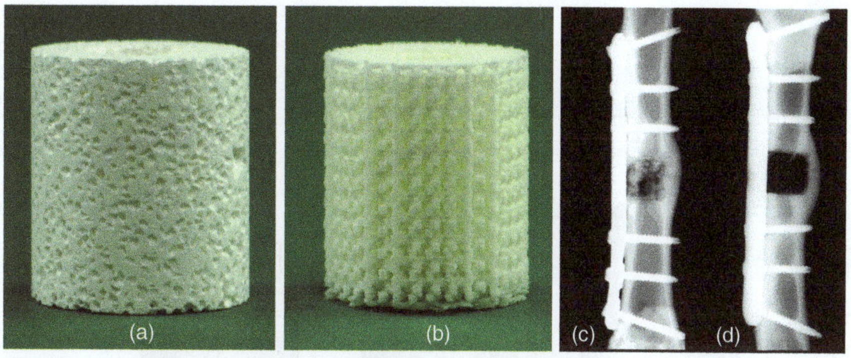

Figure 2.15 Commercial β-TCP implant (a) and PCL/TCP scaffolds built by SLS (b). X-rays images of the tibia defects treated with β-TCP (c) and PCL/TCP (d) scaffolds, after 14 weeks of implantation. Source: Lohfeld et al. 2011 [82]. Reproduced with permission of Elsevier.

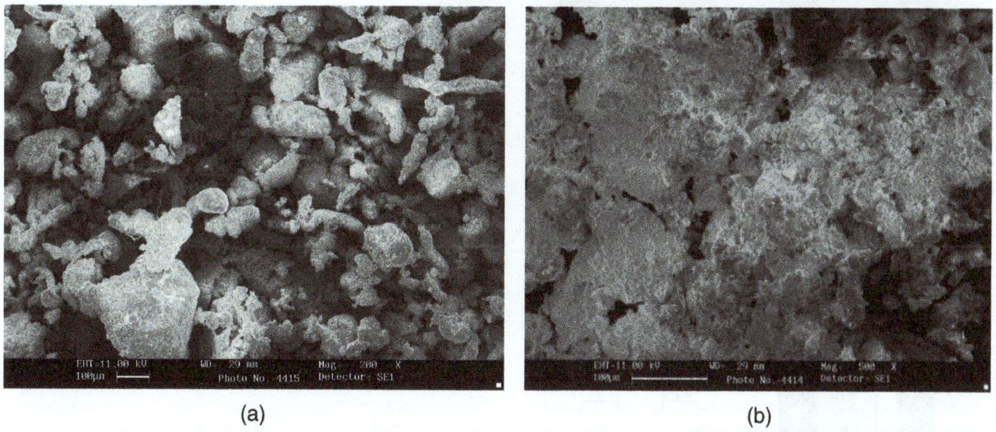

Figure 2.16 SEM micrograph of sintered layer's surface with irradiated at 1200 mm/s of scanning speed and different laser power: (a) 3.6 W. (b) 7.2 W. Source: Hao et al. 2006 [83]. Reproduced with permission of SAGE Publications.

and bending stiffness in the β-TCP scaffolds, comparatively to the PCL/TCP scaffolds produced by laser sintering (Figure 2.15c,d). β-TCP scaffolds induced the formation of large amounts of new bone in the defect area after eight weeks of implantation.

Hao et al. investigated the effect of process parameters on the fabrication of HA/high-density polyethylene (HDPE) scaffolds [83]. Different scanning speeds and laser power values were considered. HA and HDPE powders with 40% HA by volume ratio were mixed using a high-speed blender. Different process parameters resulted in different sintered morphologies (Figure 2.16). The results revealed that for low power or high-scanning speed, the layers were in general not sintered or very fragile. Powder blends of polyetheretherketone (PEEK)/HA have also been processed experimentally by Tan et al. and Naing et al. [84, 85]. Powders were obtained through mechanical blending using a roller-mixer. The studies were carried out to determine the potential of sintering a high melting point biopolymer in lower temperature environment.

Eosoly et al. investigated the performance of PCL/HA scaffolds with different compositions (PCL/HA powder blends containing 15 and 30 wt% of HA) seeded with MC 3T3 osteoblast-like cells [86]. Cells steadily grew on the scaffolds for 21 days with preferential distribution around the macropores and initially PCL/HA (15%) composites had higher cell numbers. Removal of loosely sintered parts was observed during the culturing period. Cell culture conditions did not change the compressive moduli significantly but had a distinct effect on compressive strength (Figure 2.17). For PCL/HA (15%) composites, an initial loss in strength caused by cell culture was reversed by longer cell exposure, with compressive strength of the structures restored to the initial properties. In general, in the initial period, composites with lower HA content (15 wt%) showed better metabolic activity compared to the higher HA content, however, by day 14, the performance of the two compositions was equal (Figure 2.18). The results suggest that changes in sintering due to the differences in powder composition can have profound effects on the short- and long-term mechanical properties of the scaffold particularly under cell culture conditions.

Goodridge et al. produce porous apatite–mullite glass–ceramic constructs [87]. Ceramic particles were mixed with a commercially available acrylic binder, which was subsequently removed by heating.

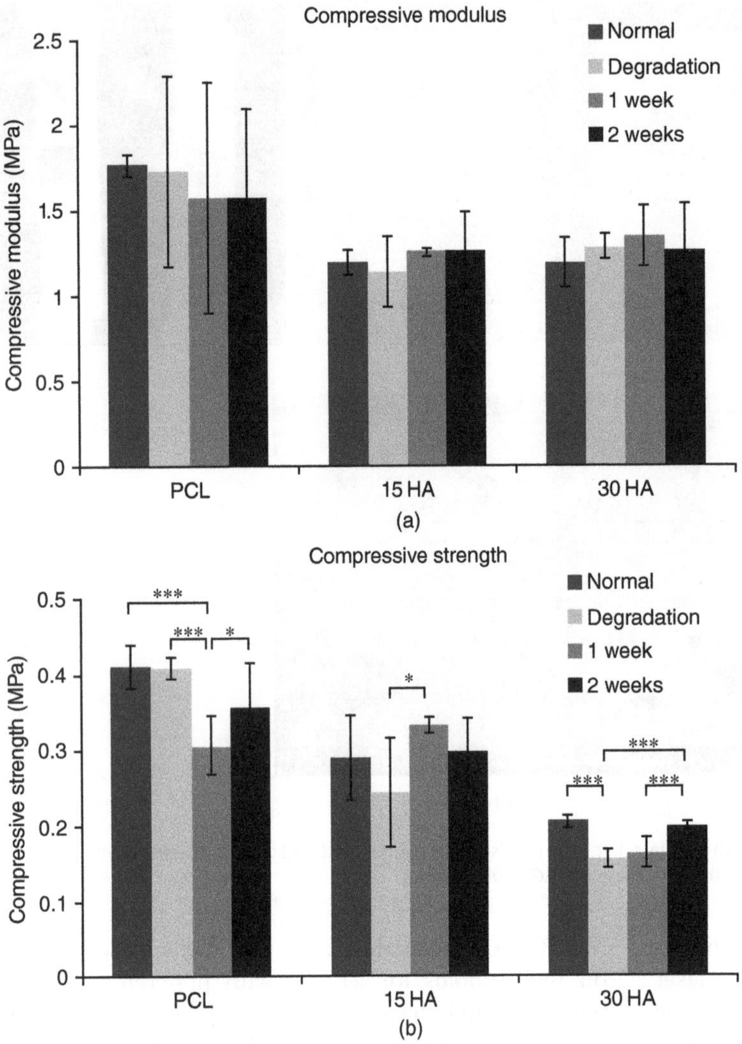

Figure 2.17 (a) Effect of degradation tests and cell culturing on the compressive modulus of scaffolds, and (b) compressive strength of the scaffolds (*, **, and *** indicate significance at $p < 0.1$, $p < 0.05$, and $p < 0.01$, respectively). Sintered samples without degradation tests and cell culturing are included as controls. Source: Eosoly et al. 2012 [86]. Reproduced with permission of Elsevier.

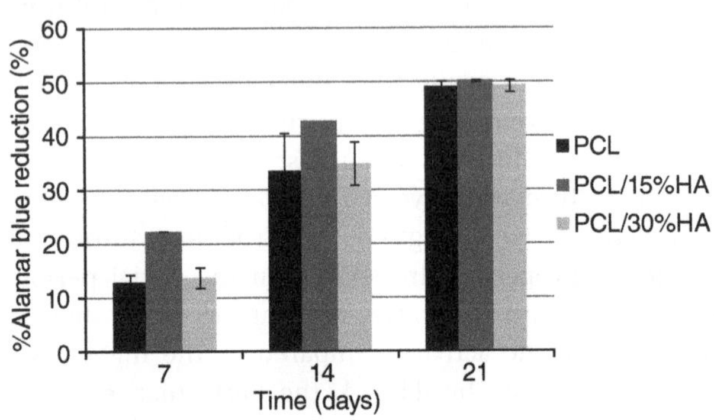

Figure 2.18 Alamar blue assay for different scaffold compositions after 7, 14, and 21 days of culturing. Source: Eosoly et al. 2012 [86]. Reproduced with permission of Elsevier.

Cytotoxicity studies, using human dermal fibroblasts and MG-63 osteoblasts, revealed the ability of the material to support cell growth without cytotoxic effects. Constructs were implanted into a defect created on a rabbit tibiae during four weeks, inducing the formation of new bone into the construct pores. Kolan et al. fabricated 13–93 bioactive glass scaffolds by using stearic acid as a polymer binder [88]. The binder was burnout, and the construct sintered at temperatures in the range of 675–695 °C. Scaffolds were obtained with an apparent porosity of 50%, pore sizes in the range of 300–800 μm and an average compressive strength of 20.4 MPa. Scaffolds containing bioactive molecules were also fabricated, using nanocomposite microspheres as protective carriers to maintain the bioactivity of these molecules [89]. Three-dimensional–porous scaffolds were produced by sintering Ca–P/poly(hydroxybutyrate-*co*-hydroxyvalerate) (PHBV) nanocomposite microspheres loaded with bovine serum albumin (BSA). After sintering, 50% of the encapsulated BSA maintained the bioactivity without denaturation.

Duan et al. produced 3D interconnected porous scaffolds based on calcium phosphate (CaP)/PHBV and carbonated hydroxyapatite (CHA)/PLLA nanocomposite using selective laser sintering [90]. The morphology and mechanical properties of CaP/PHBV and CHA/PLLA scaffolds as well as PHBV and PLLA polymer scaffolds were investigated. Compression tests under wet conditions showed that the mechanical properties of both the polymer and composite scaffolds decreased gradually after their immersion in phosphate-buffered saline (PBS) at 37 °C. *In vitro* biological evaluation showed that SaOS-2 cells had high cell viability and normal morphology and phenotype after three and seven days of culture on all scaffolds (Figure 2.19). The incorporation of Ca–P nanoparticles significantly improved cell proliferation and alkaline phosphatase activity for CaP/PHBV scaffolds, whereas CHA/PLLA nanocomposite scaffolds exhibited a similar level of cell response compared with

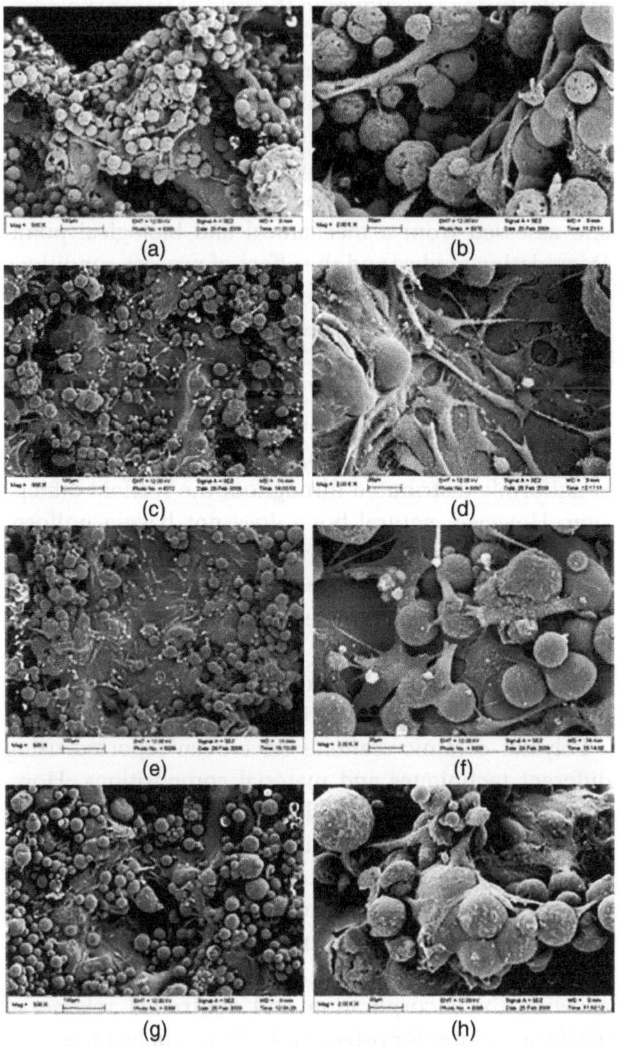

Figure 2.19 Morphology of SaOS-2 cells cultured on different scaffolds for 7 days. (a,b) PHBV; (c,d) Ca-P/PHBV; (e,f) PLLA; (g,h) CHA/PLLA. Source: Duan et al. 2010 [90]. Reproduced with permission of Elsevier.

PLLA polymer scaffolds. Zhou et al. studied the use of bio-nano-composite microspheres, consisting of CHA nanospheres within a PLLA matrix to produce scaffolds (Figure 2.20) [91]. PLLA microspheres and PLLA/CHA nanocomposites microspheres were prepared by emulsion techniques. The resultant microspheres had a size of 5–30 μm, suitable for the laser sintering process. The use of PLLA/CHA nanocomposite microspheres seems to offer a solution to the problem of removing the excessive powder from the pores after fabrication.

2.3.4 Inkjet Printing Processes

Seitz et al. produced HA scaffolds using an inkjet printing system. The HA powder was bounded using a polymer-based binder printed layer-by-layer [92]. After the printing process, the unbounded powder was removed and the scaffolds sintered to remove the binder. The pore size ranged between 450 and 470 μm, and this is closed to the optimum channel size (565 μm). Leukers et al. also used HA powder and a water-soluble polymer binder to produce bone scaffolds [93]. Scaffolds with a pore size of 500 μm were sintered at 1300 °C, during two hours, to improve the strength and remove the binder agent. The overall shrinkage after sintering was about 18–20%. Scaffolds, seeded with MC3T3-E1 murine fibroblasts, were cultured in static and dynamic conditions (perfusion system), showing ability to support the cell attachment and proliferation in both methods.

Vorndran et al. used a multijet-3D printing system to produce TCP scaffolds containing biologically active drugs and proteins with a spatial resolution of 300 μm [94]. During the fabrication process, vancomycin, heparin, and rhBMP-2 were deposited with high spatial accuracy at different locations of the construct. The effect of the polymer modification on the release kinetics of the biologically active compounds was tested by mixing TCP with hydroxypropylmethylcellulose (HPMC) or by printing polymer solutions of chitosan on TCP powder.

Zhou et al. investigated the use of calcium sulfate powders to produce scaffolds through an inkjet printing system [95]. Calcium phosphate powders were blended with calcium sulfate-based powders and glued by printing a water-based binder. Higher compressive strength was obtained for powders with the higher calcium phosphate/calcium sulfate ratio. HA/calcium sulfate powders showed better results than β-TCP/calcium sulfate.

Inzana et al. evaluated *in vivo* the regenerative potential of calcium phosphate scaffolds in a 2 mm critically sized murine femoral defect [96]. Results, confirmed that the resorbable scaffolds were osteoconductive. X-ray analysis and 3D micro-CT scans nine weeks postoperatively show

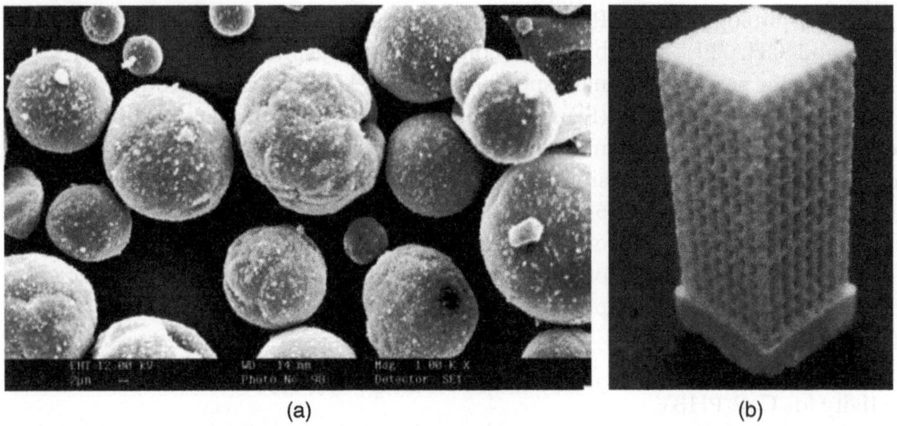

Figure 2.20 (a) SEM image of PLLA/CHA nanocomposite microspheres. (b) PLLA/CHA nanocomposite scaffolds. Source: Duan et al. 2010 [90]. Reproduced with permission of Elsevier.

similar levels of new bone formation in the allografts and calcium phosphate scaffolds. Ceramic scaffolds were also produced with 1 wt% collagen dissolved into the binder solution. However, these scaffolds appeared to be associated with less new bone formation.

Inkjet printing has also been used to produce lost moulds for the fabrication of scaffolds [97–99]. Wilson et al. used this method to produce HA scaffolds for bone tissue engineering [99]. The ModelMaker II system was employed to produce lost molds, in which an aqueous HA slurry was casted to obtain porous scaffolds with defined porous architecture. After fabrication, the molds were removed by pyrolysis, and the ceramic constructs sintered at 1250 °C. Bone-marrow stromal cells were seeded into the constructs, cultured *in vitro* during seven days and implanted subcutaneously in nude mice. Scaffolds supported the formation of mineralized bone without significant difference in the percentage of new bone after four and six weeks of implantation. A similar approach was used by Li et al. to produce composite scaffolds with a woodpile structure. In this research work, a slurry composed of PLLA, chitosan, and HA microspheres was casted into lost molds [97]. Afterward, the scaffolds were obtained through a freeze-drying method to induce microporosity. MC3T3-E1 preosteoblastic cells were seeded into the constructs and cultured *in vitro* conditions, during five weeks. The produced scaffolds showed excellent biocompatibility, supporting cell proliferation on both macro and micropores. Alkaline phosphatase showed the differentiation of MC3T3-E1 preosteoblastic cells into mature osteoblasts.

2.4 Conclusion

Although great progress has been made in the field of bone regeneration, current clinical therapies based on bone autografts, allografts, and xenografts still have many limitations. The introduction of additive manufacturing techniques in the field of tissue engineering enabled the quick fabrication of personalized 3D synthetic bone grafts (scaffolds) to promote bone regeneration of tissues and organs. Different techniques have been used to directly or indirectly produce ceramic and composite scaffolds. Several compositions and scaffold with different topologies and pore sizes were produced and assessed from a mechanical and biological point. Degradation studies and the effect of process conditions on the performance of these scaffolds were also investigated. Table 2.4 summarizes the main characteristics of the additive manufacturing processes discussed in this chapter.

Mechanical properties are the major drawback of porous composite scaffolds. Porosity in most scaffolds is uniformly distributed throughout the scaffold dimension. However, natural bone does not have a uniform distribution of porosity. A gradient distribution of porosity from the center to the periphery of the scaffold can be achieved through complex design and manufacturing that will ensure mechanical integrity and scaffold interconnectivity. Hierarchical scaffolds can be produced by combining multiple fabrication techniques.

Polymer-ceramic scaffolds have been reported using different techniques and material compositions. However, polymeric materials degrade faster than most of the ceramic materials, making the scaffold degradation uneven. To achieve a uniform resorption of the scaffolds, degradation of polymer and ceramic materials should match. Controlling the degradation rate is also critical to create scaffolds that also act as drug-delivery system, allowing the incorporation and controlled release of bisphosphonates for osteoporotic bone applications.

Bone is a vascularized tissue and angiogenesis occurs spontaneously upon implantation of a scaffold. However, the vascularization of thick and large scaffolds is a remaining problem.

Table 2.4 Main characteristics of the additive manufacturing processes for tissue engineering.

Additive manufacturing process	Accuracy (μm)	Advantages	Limitations
Vat photopolymerization	0.5–50	High accuracy and precision; fabrication of complex geometries with high resolution; easy to achieve small features	Limited number of available photo-crosslinkable materials; requires postprocessing and support structures; and cytotoxic phot-initiators
Powder bed fusion processes	50	Support structures are not required; fast processing; solvent free; induce microporosity, which can be advantageous for tissue ingrowth; wide range of materials; high mechanical strength	Requires the use of powder materials; high processing temperatures, which can lead to material degradation; difficult to remove the entrapped powder; accuracy limited by particle size
Extrusion-based processes	100	Good mechanical properties; wide range of processable materials; low cost fabrication approach	Some techniques require the use of organic solvents and high temperatures; postprocessing operations are required to produce ceramic scaffolds; low accuracy
Inkjet printing processes (binder jetting)	50	No requires support structures; fast processing; possibility of use nonorganic binders; low temperature process; fast fabrication process	Uses powder materials; low mechanical properties; high porosity; low-surface quality; difficult to remove the trapped nonbound powder; might require postprocessing; accuracy limited by particle size

References

1 Salgado, A.J., Coutinho, O.P., and Reis, R.L. (2004). Bone tissue engineering: state of the art and future trends. *Macromol. Biosci.* **4**: 743–765.

2 Dorati, R., Colonna, C., and Conti, B. (2011). Polymer scaffolds for bone tissue regeneration. In: *Studies in Mechanobiology, Tissue Engineering and Biomaterials*, vol. **8** (ed. A. Gefen). Springer.

3 Wu, S., Liu, X., Yeung, K.W.K. et al. (2014). Biomimetic porous scaffolds for bone tissue engineering. *Mater. Sci. Eng. R* **80**: 1–36.

4 Currey, J.D. (2003). The many adaptations of bone. *J. Biomech.* **36** (10): 1487–1495.

5 Bose, S. and Tarafder, S. (2012). Calcium phosphate ceramic systems in growth factor and drug delivery for bone tissue engineering: a review. *Acta Biomater.* **8**: 1401–1421.

6 Sikavitsas, V.I., Temenoff, J.S., and Mikos, A.G. (2001). Biomaterials and bone mechanotransduction. *Biomaterials* **22**: 2581–2593.

7 Andersen, M.R. and Petersen, M.M. (2016). Adaptive bone remodelling of the femoral bone after tumor resection arthroplasty with an uncemented proximally hydroxyapatite-coated stem. *J. Clin. Densitom.* **19**: 202–207.

8 Lee, J., Farag, M.M., Park, E.K. et al. (2014). A simultaneous process of 3D magnesium phosphate scaffold fabrication and bioactive substance loading for hard tissue regeneration. *Mater. Sci. Eng., C* **36**: 252–260.

9 Lichte, P., Pape, H.C., Pufe, T. et al. (2011). Scaffolds for bone healing: concepts, materials and evidence. *Injury* **42**: 569–573.

10 Tang, D., Tare, R.S., Yang, L.Y. et al. (2016). Biofabrication of bone tissue: approaches, challenges and translation for bone regeneration. *Biomaterials* **83**: 363–382.

11 Oryan, A., Alidati, S., Moshiri, A., and Maffulli, N. (2014). Bone regenerative medicine: classic options, novel strategies, and future directions. *J. Orthop. Surg. Res.* **9**: 18–45.

12 Denry, I. and Kuhn, L. (2016). Design and characterization of calcium phosphate ceramic scaffolds for bone tissue engineering. *Dent. Mater.* **32**: 43–53.

13 Sanz, M. and Vignoletti, F. (2015). Key aspects on the use of bone substitutes for bone regeneration of endentulous ridges. *Dent. Mater.* **31**: 640–647.

14 Arvidson, K., Abdallah, B.M., Applegate, L.A. et al. (2011). Bone regeneration and stem cells. *J. Cell. Mol. Med.* **15**: 718–746.

15 Dimitriou, R., Jones, E., McGonagle, D., and Giannoudis, P.V. (2011). Bone regeneration: current concepts and future directions. *BMC Med.* **9**: 66–76.

16 Gomes, K.U., Carlini, J.L., Biron, C. et al. (2008). Use of allogeneic bone graft in maxillary reconstruction for installation of dental implants. *J. Oral Maxillofac. Surg.* **66**: 2335–2338.

17 Bartolo, P., Kruth, J.P., Silva, J. et al. (2012). Biomedical production of implants by additive electro-chemical and physical processes. *CIRP Ann.–Manuf. Technol.* **61**: 635–655.

18 Pereira, R.F. and Bartolo, P.J. (2014). Recent advances in additive biomanufacturing. In: *Biomedical Applications – Comprehensive Materials Processing*, vol. **10** (ed. S. Masood).

19 Bartolo, P.J., Chua, C.K., Almeida, H.A. et al. (2009). Biomanufacturing for tissue engineering: present and future trends. *Virtual Phys. Prototyping* **4**: 203–216.

20 Leong, K.F., Cheah, C.M., and Chua, C.K. (2003). Solid freeform fabrication of the three-dimensional scaffolds for engineering replacement tissues and organs. *Biomaterials* **24**: 2363–2378.

21 Kumar, A., Mandal, S., Barui, S. et al. (2016). Low temperature additive manufacturing of three dimensional scaffolds for bone-tissue engineering applications: processing related challenges and property assessment. *Mater. Sci. Eng. R* **103**: 1–39.

22 Amini, A.R., Laurencin, C.T., and Nukavaparu, S.P. (2012). Bone tissue engineering: recent advances and challenges. *Crit. Rev. Biomed. Eng.* **40**: 363–408.

23 Jeong, I., Yu, H.S., Kim, M.K. et al. (2010). FGF2-adsorbed macroporous hydroxyapatite bone granules stimulate in vitro osteoblastic gene expression and differentiation. *J. Mater. Sci. Mater. Med.* **21**: 1335–1342.

24 Drosse, I., Volkmer, E., Capanna, R. et al. (2008). Tissue engineering for bone defect healing: an update on a multi-component approach. *Injury* **39**: S9–S20.

25 Albrektsson, T. and Johansson, C. (2001). Osteoinduction, osteoconduction and osteointegration. *Eur. Spine J.* **10**: S96–S109.

26 Diaz-Rodriguez, P., Gonzalez, P., Serra, J., and Landin, M. (2014). Key parameters in blood-surface interactions of 3D bioinspired ceramic materials. *Mater. Sci. Eng. C Mater. Bio. Appl.* **41**: 232–239.

27 Barrera, F., van Blitterswijk, C.A., and de Groot, K. (2006). Bone regeneration: molecular and cellular interactions with calcium phosphate ceramics. *Int. J. Nanomed.* **1**: 317–332.

28 Almeida, H.A. and Bartolo, P.J. (2014). Design of tissue engineering scaffolds based on hyperbolic surfaces: structural numerical evaluation. *Med. Eng. Phys.* **36**: 1033–1040.

29 Almeida, H.A. and Bartolo, P.J. (2010). Virtual topological optimisation of scaffolds for raid prototyping. *Med. Eng. Phys.* **32**: 775–782.

30 Sanchez-Salcedo, S., Arcos, D., and Vallet-Regi, M. (2008). Upgrading calcium phosphate scaffolds for tissue engineering applications. *Key Eng. Mater.* **377**: 19–42.

31 Gittens, R.A., McLachlan, T., Olivares-Navarrete, R. et al. (2011). The effects of combined micron-/submicron-scale surface roughness and nanoscale features on cell proliferation and differentiation. *Biomaterials* **32**: 3395–3403.

32 Salamon, D., Teixeira, S., Dutczak, S.M., and Stamatialis, D.F. (2014). Facile method of building hydroxyapatite 3D scaffolds assembled from porous hollow fibers enabling nutrient delivery. *Ceram. Int.* **40**: 14793–14799.

33 Roohani-Esfehani, S.I., Chen, Y., Shi, J., and Zreiqat, H. (2013). Fabrication and characterization of a new, strong and bioactive ceramic scaffold for bone regeneration. *Mater. Lett.* **107**: 378–381.

34 Gao, C., Deng, Y., Feng, P. et al. (2014). Current progress in bioactive ceramic scaffolds for bone repair and regeneration. *Int. J. Mol. Sci.* **15**: 4714–4732.

35 Dorozhkin, S.V. (2013). Calcium orthophosphate-based bioceramics. *Materials* **6**: 3840–3942.

36 Adams, C.S., Mansfield, K., Perlot, R.L., and Shapiro, I.M. (2001). Matrix regulation of skeletal cell apoptosis – role of calcium and phosphate ions. *J. Biol. Chem.* **276**: 20316–20322.

37 Yang, Y., Kang, Y., Sen, M., and Park, S. (2011). Bioceramics in tissue engineering. In: *Biomaterials for Tissue Engineering Applications* (ed. J.A. Burdick and R.L. Manck). Springer.

38 Billström, G.H., Blom, A.W., Larsson, S., and Beswick, A. (2013). Application of scaffolds for bone regeneration strategies: current trends and future directions. *Injury* **44**: S28–S33.

39 Chen, Q., Baino, F., Spriano, S. et al. (2014). Modelling of the strength-porosity relationship in glass-ceramic foam scaffolds for bone repair. *J. Eur. Ceram. Soc.* **34**: 2663–2673.

40 Li, W., Nooeaid, P., Roether, J.A. et al. (2014). Preparation and characterization of vacomycin releasing PHBV coated 45S5 Bioglass-based glass-ceramic scaffolds for bone tissue engineering. *J. Eur. Ceram. Soc.* **34**: 505–514.

41 Gorustovich, A.A., Roether, J.A., and Boccaccini, A.R. (2010). Effect of bioactive glasses on angiogenesis: a review of in vitro and in vivo evidences. *Tissue Eng. Part B* **16**: 199–207.

42 Habraken, W.J.E.M., Wolke, J.G.C., and Jansen, J.A. (2007). Ceramic composites as matrices and scaffolds for drug delivery in tissue engineering. *Adv. Drug Delivery Rev.* **59**: 234–248.

43 Wu, C. (2009). Methods of improving mechanical and biomedical properties of Ca-Si-based ceramics and scaffolds. *Expert. Rev. Med. Devices* **6**: 237–241.

44 Liu, Y., Lim, J., and Teoh, S.H. (2013). Review: development of clinically relevant scaffolds for vascularized bone tissue engineering. *Biotechnol. Adv.* **31**: 688–705.

45 William, D. and Callister, J. (2007). *Materials Science and Engineering: An Introduction*. Wiley.

46 Breche, Q., Chagnon, G., Machado, G. et al. (2016). Mechanical behaviour's evolution of a PLA-b-PEG-b-PLA triblock copolymer during hydrolytic degradation. *J. Mech. Behav. Biomed. Mater.* **60**: 288–300.

47 Malwela, T. and Ray, S.S. (2015). Enzymatic degradation behaviour of nanoclay reinforced biodegradable PLA/PBSA blend composites. *Int. J. Biol. Macromol.* **77**: 131–142.

48 Venkatesan, J., Bhatnagar, I., Manivasagan, P. et al. (2015). Alginate composites for bone tissue engineering: a review. *Int. J. Biol. Macromol.* **72**: 269–281.

49 Wegst, U.G.K. and Ashby, M.F. (2004). The mechanical efficiency of natural materials. *Philos. Mag. A* **84** (21): 2167–2186.

50 Garcia-Gareta, E., Coathup, M.J., and Blunn, G.W. (2015). Osteoinduction of bone grafting materials for bone repair and regeneration. *Bone* **81**: 112–121.

51 Macchieta, A., Turner, I.G., and Bowen, C.R. Fabrication of HA/TCP scaffolds with a graded and porous structure using a camphene-based freeze-casting method. *Acta Biomater.* **5**: 1319–1327.

52 Deville, S., Saiz, E., and Tomsia, A.P. Freeze casting of hydroxyapatite scaffolds for bone tissue engineering. *Biomaterials* **27**: 5480–5489.

53 Peltola, S.M., Melchels, F.P.W., Grijpma, D.W., and Kellomak, M. (2008). A review of rapid prototyping techniques for tissue engineering purposes. *Ann. Med.* **40**: 268–280.

54 Moroni, L., Nandakumar, A., de Groot, F.B. et al. (2015). Plug and play: combining materials and technologies to improve bone regeneration strategies. *J. Tissue Eng. Regener. Med.* **9**: 745–759.

55 Stevens, B., Yang, Y.Z., Mohandas, A. et al. (2008). A review of materials, fabrication methods and strategies used to enhance bone regeneration in engineered bone tissues. *J. Biomed. Mater. Res.B Appl. Biomater.* **85**: 573–582.

56 Kalita, S.J., Bose, S., Hosick, H.L., and Bandyopadhyay, A. (2003). Development of controlled porosity polymer-ceramic composite scaffolds via fused deposition modelling. *Mater. Sci. Eng., C* **23**: 611–620.

57 Bose, S., Darsell, J., Kintner, M. et al. (2003). Pore size and pore volume effects on alumina and TCP ceramic scaffolds. *Mater. Sci. Eng.* **23** (4): 479–486.

58 Kim, J., McBride, S., Tellis, B. et al. (2012). Rapid-prototyped PLGA/β-TCP/hydroxyapatite nanocomposite scaffolds in a rabbit femoral defect model. *Biofabrication* **4**: 025003.

59 Jo, I.H., Ahn, M.K., Moon, Y.W. et al. (2014). Novel rapid direct deposition of ceramic paste for porous biphasic calcium phosphate (BCP) scaffolds with tightly controlled 3-D microchannels. *Ceram. Int.* **40**: 11079–11084.

60 Miranda, P., Saiz, E., Gryn, K., and Tomisa, A.P. (2006). Sintering and robocasting of β-tricalcium phosphate scaffolds for orthopaedic applications. *Acta Biomater.* **2** (4): 457–466.

61 Dellinger, J.G., Cesarano, J., and Jamison, R.D. (2007). Robotic deposition of model hydroxyapatite scaffolds with multiple architectures and multiscale porosity for bone tissue engineering. *J. Biomed. Mater. Res. A* **82** (2): 383–394.

62 Ishack, S., Mediero, A., Wilder, T. et al. (2015). Bone regeneration in critical bone defects using three-dimensionally printed β-tricalcium phosphate/hydroxyapatite scaffolds is enhanced by coating scaffolds with either dipyridamole or BMP-2. *J. Biomed. Mater. Res. B Appl. Biomater.* **20**: 1–10.

63 Kim, H., Moon, S.K., and Seo, M. (2016). Hybrid layering scanning-projection micro-stereolithography for fabrication of conical microlens array and hollow microneedle array. *Microelectron. Eng.* **153**: 15–19.

64 Kanai, T. and Tsuchiya, M. (2016). Microfluidic devices fabricated using stereolithography for preparation of monodisperse double emulsions. *Chem. Eng. J.* **290**: 400–404.

65 Song, X., Chen, Y., Lee, T.W. et al. (2015). Ceramic fabrication using mask-image-projection-based stereolithography integrated with tape-casting. *J. Manuf. Processes* **20**: 456–464.

66 Bartolo, P.J. (2011). *Stereolithography: Materials, Processes and Applications*. Springer.

67 Bartolo, P.J. (2001). Optical approaches to macroscopic and microscopic engineering. PhD thesis. University of Reading, UK.

68 Ali, Z., Tureyen, E.B., Karpat, Y., and Cakmakci, M. (2016). Fabrication of polymer micro needles for transdermal drug delivery system using DLP based

projection stereo-lithograhy. *Procedia CIRP* **42**: 87–90.

69 Bian, W., Li, D.H., Lian, Q. et al. (2011). Design and fabrication of a novel porous implant with pre-set channels based on ceramic stereolithography for vascular implantation. *Biofabrication* **3**: 034103.

70 Levy, R.A., Chu, T.G., Holloran, J.W. et al. (1997). CT-generated porous hydroxyapatite orbital floor prosthesis as a prototype bioimplant. *Am. J. Neuroradiol.* **18**: 1522–1525.

71 Chu, T.G., Halloran, J.W., Hollister, S.J., and Feinberg, S.E. (2001). Hydroxyapatite implants with designed internal architecture. *J. Mater. Sci. - Mater. Med.* **12**: 471–478.

72 Chopra, K., Mummery, P.M., Derby, B., and Gough, Y.E. (2012). Gel-cast glass-ceramic tissue scaffolds of controlled architecture. *Biofabrication* **4** (4): 045002.

73 Bartolo, P.J. and Mitchell, G. (2003). Stereo-thermal-lithography: a new principle for rapid prototyping. *Rapid Prototyping J.* **9**: 150–156.

74 Patricio, T., Pereira, R., Oliveira, L., and Bartolo, P.J. (2013). Polyethylene glycol and polyethylene glycol/hydroxyapatite constructs produced through stereo-thermal-lithography. *Adv. Mater. Res.* **749**: 87–92.

75 Sharifi, S., Blanquer, S.B.G., van Kooten, T.G., and Grijpma, D.W. (2012). Biodegradable nanocomposite: hydrogel structures with enhanced mechanical properties prepared by photo-crosslinking solutions of poly(trimethylene carbonate)-poly(ethylene glycol)-poly(trimethylene carbonate) macromonomers and nanoclay particles. *Acta Biomater.* **8**: 4233–4243.

76 Elomaa, L., Kokkari, A., Narhi, T., and Seppala, J.V. (2013). Porous 3D modeled scaffolds of bioactive glass and photocrosslinkable poly(ε-caprolactone) by stereolithography. *Compos. Sci. Technol.* **74**: 99–106.

77 Kolan, K.C.R., Leu, M.C., Hilmas, G.E., and Velez, M. (2012). Effect of material, process parameters, and simulated body fluids on mechanical properties of 13-93 bioactive glass porous constructs made by selective laser sintering. *J. Mech. Behav. Biomed. Mater.* **13**: 14–24.

78 Savalani, M.M., Hao, L., Dickens, P.M. et al. (2012). The effects and interactions of fabrication parameters on the properties of selective laser sintered hydroxyapatite polyamide composite biomaterials. *Rapid Prototyping J.* **18**: 16–27.

79 Beal, V.E., Paggi, R.A., Salmoria, G.V., and Lago, A. (2009). Statistical evaluation of laser energy density effect on mechanical properties of polyamide parts manufactured by selective laser sintering. *J. Appl. Polym. Sci.* **113**: 2910–2919.

80 Wiria, F.E., Leong, K.F., Chua, C.K., and Liu, Y. (2007). Poly-ε-caprolactone/hydroxyapatite for tissue engineering scaffold fabrication via selective laser sintering. *Acta Biomater.* **3**: 1–12.

81 Lindner, M., Hoeges, S., Meiners, W. et al. (2011). Manufacturing of individual biodegradable bone substrate implants using selective laser melting technique. *J. Biomed. Mater. Res. A* **97**: 466–471.

82 Lohfeld, S., Cahill, S., Barron, V. et al. (2012). Fabrication, mechanical and in vivo performance of polycaprolactone/tricalcium phosphate composite scaffolds. *Acta Biomater.* **8**: 3446–3456.

83 Hao, L., Savalani, M.M., Zhang, Y. et al. (2006). Selective laser sintering of hydroxyapatite reinforced polyethylene composites for bioactive implants and tissue scaffold development. *Proc. Inst. Mech. Eng. H* **220**: 521–531.

84 Tan, K.H., Chua, C.K., Leong, K.F. et al. (2003). Scaffold development using selective laser sintering of polyetheretherketone-hydroxyapatite biocomposite blends. *Biomaterials* **24**: 3115–3123.

85 Naing, M.W., Chua, C.K., and Leong, K.F. (2008). Computer aided tissue engineering scaffold fabrication. In: *Virtual Prototyping & Biomanufacturing in Medical Applications* (ed. B. Bidanda and P.J. Bártolo). Springer.

86 Eosoly, S., Vrana, N.E., Lohfeld, S. et al. (2012). Interaction of cell culture with composition effects on the mechanical properties of polycaprolactone-hydroxyapatite scaffolds fabricated via selective laser sintering (SLS). *Mater. Sci. Eng., C* **32**: 2250–2257.

87 Goodridge, R.D., Wood, D.J., Ohtsuki, C., and Dalgarno, K.W. (2007). Biological evaluation of an apatite-mullite glass ceramic produced via selective laser sintering. *Acta Biomater.* **3**: 221–231.

88 Kolan, K.C.R., Leu, M.C., Hilmas, G.E. et al. (2011). Fabrication of 13-93 bioactive glass scaffolds for bone tissue engineering using indirect selective laser sintering. *Biofabrication* **3**: 025004.

89 Duan, B. and Wang, M. (2010). Encapsulation and release of biomolecules from Ca–P/PHBV nanocomposite microspheres and three-dimensional scaffolds fabricated by selective laser sintering. *Polym. Degrad. Stab.* **95**: 1655–1664.

90 Duan, B., Wang, M., Zhou, W.Y. et al. (2010). Three-dimensional nanocomposite scaffolds fabricated via selective laser sintering for bone tissue engineering. *Acta Biomater.* **6**: 4495–4505.

91 Zhou, W.Y., Lee, S.H., Wang, M. et al. (2008). Selective laser sintering of porous tissue engineering scaffolds from poly(L-lactide)/carbonated hydroxyapatite nanocomposite microspheres. *J. Mater. Sci. Mater. Med.* **19**: 2535–2540.

92 Seitz, H., Rieder, H., Irsen, S. et al. (2005). Three-dimensional printing of porous ceramic scaffolds for bone tissue engineering. *J. Biomed. Mater. Res. B Appl. Biomater.* **74**: 782–788.

93 Leukers, B., Guikan, H., Irsan, S.H. et al. (2005). Hydroxyapatite scaffolds for bone tissue engineering made by 3D printing. *J. Mater. Sci. - Mater. Med.* **15**: 1121–1124.

94 Vorndran, E., Klammert, U., Ewald, A. et al. (2010). Simultaneous immobilization of bioactives during 3D powder printing of bioceramic drug-release matrices. *Adv. Funct. Mater.* **20**: 1585–1591.

95 Zhou, Z., Buchanan, F., Mitchell, C., and Dunne, N. (2014). Printability of calcium phosphate: calcium sulfate powders for the application of tissue engineered bone scaffolds using the 3D printing technique. *Mater. Sci. Eng., C* **38**: 1–10.

96 Inzana, J., Olvera, D., Fuller, S.M. et al. (2014). 3D printing of composite calcium phosphate and collagen scaffolds for bone regeneration. *Biomaterials* **35**: 4026–4034.

97 Li, L.H., Kommareddy, K.P., Pilz, C. et al. (2010). In vitro bioactivity of bioresorbable porous polymeric scaffolds incorporating hydroxyapatite microspheres. *Acta Biomater.* **6**: 2525–2531.

98 Park, C.H., Rios, H.F., Jin, Q. et al. (2010). Biomimetic hybrid scaffolds for engineering human tooth-ligament interfaces. *Biomaterials* **31**: 5945–5952.

99 Wilson, C.E., de Bruijn, J.D., van Blitterswijk, C.A. et al. (2004). Design and fabrication of standardized hydroxyapatite scaffolds with a defined macro-architecture by rapid prototyping for bone-tissue-engineering research. *J. Biomed. Mater. Res. A* **68**: 123–132.

100 Lee, J.W., Ahn, G.S., Kim, D.S., and Cho, D.-W. (2009). Development of nano- and microscale composite 3D scaffolds using PPF/DEF-HA and micro-stereolithography. *Microelectron. Eng.* **86** (4–6): 1465–1467.

3

Developments in Hydrogel-based Scaffolds and Bioceramics for Bone Regeneration

Izabela-Cristina Stancu[1] *and Daniel Chappard*[2]

[1] *APMG Advanced Polymer Materials Group, Faculty of Applied Chemistry and Materials Science, Faculty of Medical Engineering, University Politehnica of Bucharest, 1-7 Gh Polizu Street, Sector 1, 011061 Bucharest, Romania*
[2] *GEROM Groupe Etudes Remodelage Osseux et bioMatériaux – NextBone and SCIAM, Service Commun d'Imagerie et Analyses Microscopiques, Institut de Biologie en Santé, CHU d'Angers, Université d'Angers, 49933 Angers Cedex, France*

3.1 Introduction

Methodologies in biomimetic and bioinspired biomaterials and scaffolds have been continuously developed and their potential in replicating advantageous structural, architectural, and mechanical characteristics of the extracellular matrix (ECM), in order to promote desired biointeractions with cells and physiological media with the ultimate goal of tissue regeneration. Generally ECM is used as a model and various parameters are artificially designed to promote and assist an accelerated regeneration of the damaged tissue. As previously emphasized, a natural ECM or its derivatives do not always provide the best solution for tissue regeneration [1] and the development of extracellular matrix analogs (EMAs) remains a challenging task. Scaffold requirements are already overviewed in other works [2]. The correlation composition–structure–properties–functionality becomes mandatory since it allows the understanding and control of the performances of a biomaterial through material factors and fabrication parameters. Bone is a complex tissue that contains cells embedded in a hydrated biocomposite matrix mainly formed by macromolecular fibers of collagen type I (diameters of 50–500 nm) and nanocrystals of nonstoichiometric hydroxyapatite (HA) (100 nm length, 20–30 nm widths, 3–6 nm thick) [3]. The high amount of mineral phase (roughly 65%) and the intimate interaction of the latter with the fibrillary collagen result in assembled mineralized fibrils responsible for the specific mechanical properties of bones. Bone ECM also contains several protein types including proteoglycans and glycoproteins coexisting with mineralized collagen fibrils and such constituents are also considered in the design of bioinspired/biomimetic EMA for bone.

From a material perspective and considering the above, biomaterials based on collagen (or its derivatives) and/or calcium phosphates are especially appealing for bone regeneration and bone tissue engineering since they mimic structural components of the natural tissue. The use of bone-like apatite as key surface component promoting superior binding to living bone represents nowadays a common procedure for bioactivation of orthopedic scaffolds [4–6]. However, the number of materials proposed for bone regeneration is much more important and it includes natural and synthetic polymers, bioceramics, and combinations. Fibrous and nanostructured scaffolds become interesting since they recapitulate structural features of the natural tissue, while an interconnected porosity of a certain size is critical to promote cell infiltration and angiogenesis phenomena required for new tissue formation in three-dimensional (3D) matrices. Bioactive, stimuli responsive, smart, biodegradable are only few examples of key characteristics to be balanced by materials scientists in order to produce advanced materials with bone regenerative properties. Surface engineering has recently received increased attention due to the potential to stimulate improved tissue–biomaterial interactions. In addition, practical aspects related to fabrication techniques, handling properties, shape, application methods, and cost also represent challenging issues to be optimized [7]. For a more comprehensive overview of bioinspired and biomimetic approaches in the design of tissue regenerative biomaterials and scaffolds, several excellent works are available [1, 5, 7–19].

This chapter will discuss different approaches in the design and development of scaffolds for bone regeneration. Inspired by the presence of two main phases (organic and mineral) of bone ECM, we will initially present aspects in the engineering of hydrogels, followed

Bioceramics and Biocomposites: From Research to Clinical Practice, First Edition. Edited by Iulian Antoniac.

by the analysis of current challenges in the preparation of Ca/P bioceramic materials for bone regeneration.

3.2 Directions in the Design of Hydrogels for Bone Regeneration

3.2.1 On the Preparation of Bioinspired and Biomimetic Hydrogels

Naturally derived and synthetic polymers inspired from the natural ECM have been extensively investigated to develop 3D scaffolds with improved cell interactivity and bone regeneration potential. The study of macromolecules, their chemistry, the possibility to tailor their physical and mechanical properties as well as their stability in physiological media represent interesting tools for the design of biomaterials and the fabrication of 3D scaffolds inspired from bone ECM. In the last years 10 years, the conventional polymer chemistry (including polymerization, polymer analogous and cross-linking reactions) has been combined with bioconjugation techniques, biochemistry, chemical peptide synthesis and recombinant peptide synthesis, supramolecular chemistry, and nanotechnology to obtain a new generation of macromolecular matrices adapted for predefined physicochemical, mechanical, and functional characteristics.

To develop 3D matrices recapitulating bone ECM, simplified designs often include hydrated macromolecular matrices (usually hydrogel networks), eventually containing biomimetic biodegradable components, decorated with cell recognition motifs, adapted to a fabrication method leading to structural/architectural features critical for bone regeneration (i.e. interconnected porosity, pores of specific sizes, fibrillary structures, nanostructured materials).

Hydrogels are used to fabricate bioinspired and biomimetic fibrous and porous scaffolds due to their advantageous similarity with the organic component of bone ECM in terms of macromolecular nature, elasticity, permeability for hydrosoluble compounds, and water affinity. Relevant aspects on hydrogels are excellently overviewed in Refs. [1, 2, 9, 16, 20–30]. Natural or naturally derived and naturally inspired hydrogels such as those based on collagen, gelatin, alginate, chitosan, hyaluronic acid, polylysine, polyglutamic acid (PGA) have confirmed their potential for bone regenerative scaffolds. In addition, synthetic hydrogels such as poly(2-hydroxyethyl methacrylate) (PHEMA), polyethylene glycol (PEG), oligo(poly[ethylene glycol] fumarate) (OPF), poly(propylene fumarate) (PPF), poly(acrylic acid) (PAA), poly(*N*-isopropylacrylamide), poly(vinyl alcohol) (PVA) have also been successfully used for bone repair and regeneration. Such polymer networks may be generated by cross-linking hydrophilic macromolecules and their properties can be rationally controlled by material factors and synthesis parameters (Figure 3.1) to optimally respond predefined functionality for a specified application such as bone repair and regeneration.

Mabilleau et al. [31] demonstrated the influence of the cross-linker type and length on key properties such as water affinity, surface roughness, and biomechanical properties of PHEMA, using four cross-linking agents: divinyl benzene, ethylene glycol dimethacrylate (EGDMA), tetraethylene glycol diacrylate, and polyethylene glycol diacrylate. The last two compounds, with longer molecules, generated longer spacer arms between the PHEMA chains and have been associated with the most suitable cross-linking with respect to uses in bone sites and for controlled release of bioactive molecules in hard tissues [31].

Two main chemical routes are generally used to prepare hydrogels:

(a) starting from macromolecules (usually natural or naturally derived) by different cross-linking reactions (Figure 3.2a).
(b) starting from monomers (usually synthetic or, eventually, naturally derived), followed by network-forming

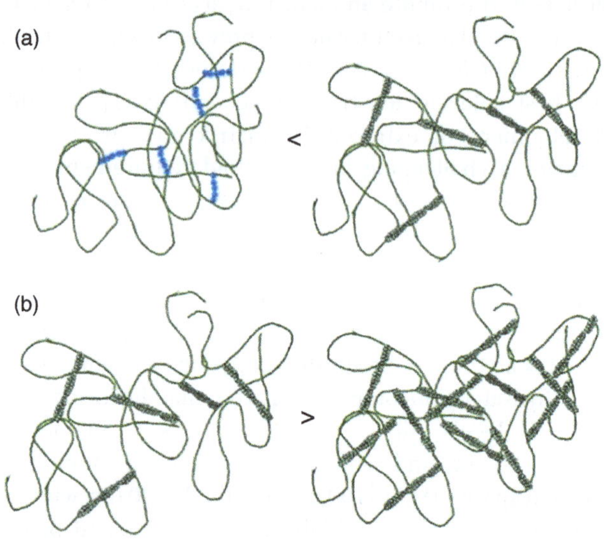

Figure 3.1 Hydrogels with properties controlled by the nature and length of the cross-linking agent and by the degree of cross-linking: the use of cross-linking agent with small molecules (blue) leads to denser networks, with lower affinity for water when compared to networks having the same cross-linking degree but longer intermacromolecular bridges (a) while higher amount of crosslinker leads to denser networks, with lower water affinity when compared to less cross-linked networks obtained using the same cross-linking agent (b).

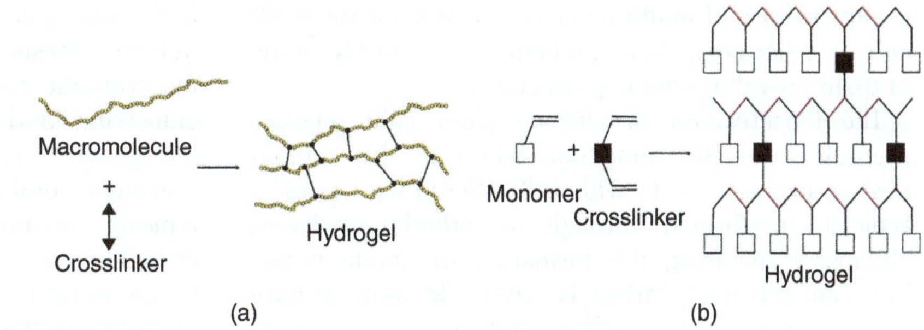

Figure 3.2 Hydrogel formation by (a) cross-linking of macromolecules; (b) polymerization with network formation, starting from monomers and cross-linkers.

polymerization (usually leading to synthetic materials) (Figure 3.2b).

The cross-linking method is critical for the properties of the resulting hydrogel and can be mainly performed (i) in bulk, when the cross-linker is added into the reaction system and leads to an *in situ* network formation and (ii) through diffusion, when the cross-linker diffuses into a macromolecular matrix progressively forming the hydrogel. The selection of the cross-linking method may be a challenging task since advantages and drawbacks are associated to each technique. Bulk network formation is suitable for network-forming polymerizations starting from monomers and cross-linking agents, such as the free-radical polymerization of (meth)acrylate monomers (2-hydroxyethyl methacrylate [HEMA]), in the presence of dimethacrylates such as EGDMA. In some situations, the polymerizations are performed in the presence of water to generate networks with predefined intrinsic porosity or containing water-soluble ingredients (bioactive molecules, mineral precursors, drugs). Special consideration should be given to avoid the synthesis of nonhomogeneous products when a cross-linking agent is added to a hydrophilic polymer solution (i.e. the cross-linking of collagen with glutaraldehyde added into the protein aqueous solution). To avoid such problems, the concentration of the cross-linker should be adjusted to allow homogeneous network formation.

While natural or naturally derived polymers present advantages such as biocompatibility, biodegradability, cell adhesion motifs, synthetic polymers are appealing due to their wide range of compositions, controlled properties, versatility, and availability. In addition to advantageous features, natural materials usually lack mechanical strength and often present difficult processing, while the synthetic counterparts lack cell recognition elements. To overcome eventual drawbacks and take advantage of other convenient properties, hydrogel engineering by combinatorial synthesis and fabrication are often performed, leading to complex biomaterials with personalized characteristics adapted to a specific functionality under *in vivo* conditions in bone.

3.2.2 Biofunctionalization of Non-adhesive Macromolecules with Cell-adhesive Peptides or Other Bioactive Molecules

Bioactive hydrogels may be generated by biofunctionalization with cell adhesion peptide sequences. The list of cell-interactive peptides includes Arg-Gly-Asp (RGD) tripeptide [32–39], Lys-Arg-Ser-Arg (KRSR) [40], Phe-His-Arg-Arg-Ile-Lys-Ala (FHRRIKA) [40], Pro-His-Ser-Arg-Asn (PHSRN) and colocalized RGD and PHSRN spaced by 13-mer of glycine ($RGDG_{13}PHSRN$) [39], and GFOGER (incorporated in a 20 Gly-Pro-Pro sequence) [41]. Alternative approaches involve the bioactivation of hydrogels with growth factors [42, 43] or other biomolecules, such as alkaline phosphatase [44–47]. Numerous studies report physical entrapment of bioactive cues in hydrogels through absorption or immobilization during hydrogel formation. Most of the physical methods, despite their facility, do not provide a stability of the functionalization and therefore the development of chemical methods has been justified. The access of cells to chemically bioactivated materials depends on the distribution of the bioactive moieties in the final products. Two types of topochemistry are possible:

- at the surface of the materials,
- on the polymer backbone, followed by further processing of the biomaterial.

The surface functionalization of scaffolds has recently gained increased interest since it allows direct cell adhesion onto an implanted product at the interface with the host tissue. It can be realized by reactions at the liquid–scaffold interface or on the macromolecular backbone prior to scaffold fabrication, followed by the surface decoration with such activated polymers. Most of the bioconjugation strategies used to bioactivate hydrogels target the carbodiimide-mediated coupling of amino groups of the peptide/protein (usually $—NH_2$ from the side chain of lysine residues) with carboxyls from the scaffold. Such approach is facilitated by the fact that Lys residues are exposed to the surface of peptides/proteins often leading to randomly cross-linked groups in case of multifunctional reaction partners. Of course, other cross-linking schemes are available, some of them providing coupling selectivity.

The bioactivation of alginate (Alg) is a relevant example here. The functionalization of this nonadhesive macromolecule with cell adhesion peptides is typically performed through a carbodiimide-based chemistry involving the formation of amide bonds between activated carboxyls from Alg and primary amines from peptides. Other strategies are presented in detail in other works [48, 49]. The polysaccharide has been successfully decorated with adhesive peptides also by a more selective bioconjugation strategy involving the coupling of —COOH from Alg with —SH groups from thiol-ended peptides [40]. In the first step, —COOH groups in alginate have been activated with 1-ethyl-3-(3-dimethylaminopropyl)carbodiimide hydrochloride (EDC)/N-hydroxysulfosuccinimide (S-NHS) and then a bioconjugation intermediate has been obtained through the reaction between activated carboxyls in alginate and amines in 2-(2-pyridyldithio) ethyleneamine (PDEA). In the next step, the reaction with thiol terminal group of the peptides has been performed leading to alginate–peptide conjugates with adhesive properties with respect to MC3T3 osteoblast cells [40]. Another interesting example of bioinspired chemistry devoted to the synthesis of bioactive hydrogels is represented by the use of an elastin-mimetic polypeptide with the amino acid sequence GRDPSS [VPGVG VPGKG VPGVG VPGVG VPGEG VPGIG](7) for the chemical conjugation of various integrin ligands (RGD peptides). It was demonstrated that cell adhesion with mouse osteoblasts was influenced by the ligand type, ligand density, and the use of a spacer [39]. Pectin hydrogels have also been recently bioactivated with RGD, by carbodiimide chemistry, and the resulting microspheres promoted enhanced adhesion and spreading of MC3T3-E1 cElls as well as mineralization, when compared to unmodified control [48]. While providing appealing routes for the stimulation of cell interaction, bioconjugation strategies are still under optimization/development to remove cost limitations and sometimes lack of specificity or stability.

3.2.3 Engineering of Synthetic Hydrogels with Bioactive or Biodegradable Sites

In addition to the incorporation of bioadhesive components, bioinspired and biomimetic materials may also mimic specific ECM responsiveness to proteolytic or hydrolytic activity.

The combination of synthetic hydrogels with naturally derived hydrogels such as those obtained from collagen and gelatin is a widely used approach. *Interpenetrated hydrophilic macromolecular networks* play a leading role in the synthesis of natural–synthetic hydrogels combining synthetic and natural components with the aim of enhancing predefined biointeractions. They consist in interpenetrated polymer networks of distinct hydrophilic polymers combined at molecular level and can be typically obtained (i) by simultaneous/step-by-step cross-linking of the macromolecules of interest or (ii) by the network-forming polymerization of a synthetic monomer in the presence of macromolecules, followed by the cross-linking of the latter. Numerous works describe the potential of such materials to improve the tissue regeneration potential of some hydrogels [50]. From the wide range of explored hydrogels and strategies, *polymer analogous reactions decorating natural polymers with synthetic polymerizable (meth)acrylamide groups* have emerged as appealing chemical strategy to generate naturally derived hydrogels through *controlled network-forming polymerization*, similar to synthetic vinyl-based monomers. Gelatin, alginate, hyaluronic acid, dextran, gellan gum, chitosan, and tropoelastin have been modified to present (meth)acrylamide side chains and polymer networks have been obtained mainly by photopolymerization [51–53]. The main advantage of the method consists in the possibility to tune the properties of such hydrogels through the control of the (meth)acrylation degree and the composition of the polymerization mixture. Numerous studies investigated the behavior of such hydrogels for biomedical applications including tissue regeneration. It was demonstrated that polymerizable macromolecular derivatives can be used to fabricate cell-adhesive patterned surfaces, cell-laden scaffolds, 3D scaffolds, and coatings. Methacrylamide gelatin or gelatin methacryloyl (GelMA) has become the main actor of this family of macromolecules of semisynthetic origin since it generates by *network-forming polymerization* (sometimes combined with methacrylated hyaluronate or other compounds) a physiological microenvironment for cells adapted for the fabrication of cell-loaded 3D constructs or cell-interactive scaffolds [54–57]. Recently, bicomponent hydrogels have been prepared starting from a water-soluble synthetic monomer and GelMA, who acts both as a macromonomer and as a cross-linking agent. Following a one-pot network-forming radical polymerization, GelMA-synthetic hydrogels such as PHEMA and poly(acrylamide) (PAAm) have been obtained [58–60]. Such materials have interesting potential for tissue regeneration due to the possibility of controlling key features such as water affinity, capacity to generate porous structures, interaction with cells, degradability, and mechanical behavior, by adjusting the composition of the polymerization mixtures [59, 60]. The synthetic component modulates the density of the network and accordingly the water affinity impacting on both elasticity and degradability. Supplementary cross-linking of the synthetic component provided additional control over hydrophilicity and biodegradation rate and extent. The presence of GelMA macromolecules, covalently combined in a synthetic hydrogel generated not only cell-interactive sequences but also degradation sites by collagenase. Nondegradable synthetic components are "dispersed" by the biodegradable sequences. Hydrogels engineered with such bioactive and biodegradation sites are recognized for their potential to enhance cell invasion with progressive degradation of the matrix. The interaction with osteoblasts will be influenced by material factors such as cross-linking density, type of hydrogel, ratio between the bioadhesive and biodegradable inert components. A wide range of new synthetic–natural hydrogels may be developed by this strategy in order to combine the advantages of different polymers and overcome current drawbacks of individual components. Furthermore, the possibility to photopolymerize the reaction mixtures under mild conditions, eventually after the fabrication of 3D acellular or cell-loaded scaffolds, represents an appealing advantage of the described method.

Among other natural materials attracting increasing interest, biodegradable soybean-based biomaterials present bone regeneration potential as proved by *in vitro* and *in vivo* studies [61–63]. When used as a bone filler in rabbit distal femurs, the soybean-based biomaterial stimulated significantly higher outer bone formation and microhardness at 24 weeks, when compared to Fisiograft([R]) gel [63].

3.2.4 Nanoparticle-loaded Fibrous Hydrogels for Bone Regeneration

Recently, porous and fibrous hydrogel matrices have been fabricated and engineered using combinations of polymers and techniques. In some situations, hydrogel precursors are needed to fabricate the 3D scaffold, followed by subsequent cross-linking or network-forming polymerization of the components. The design and development of fibrous scaffolds has the potential to generate tissue mimetics when exposed to *in vivo* or in *ex vivo* tissue engineering. Unlike bulk materials, porous scaffolds have recognized architectural advantages such as interconnected porosity allowing colonization with cells and blood vessels. Fibrous meshes have a different kind of porosity when compared to other porous scaffolds. They do contain pores formed during the fabrication, through entanglement of micro- or nanofibers (eventually oriented along an axis), and often allow cell infiltration despite low dimensions of pores (Figure 3.3). Electrospinning is widely used to fabricate nano- and microfibers in an attempt to reproduce microenvironments that can be favorably recognized by osteoblasts. The principle of the method and the importance of the fabrication parameters do not need to be recalled. Details on electrospun nanofiber with high

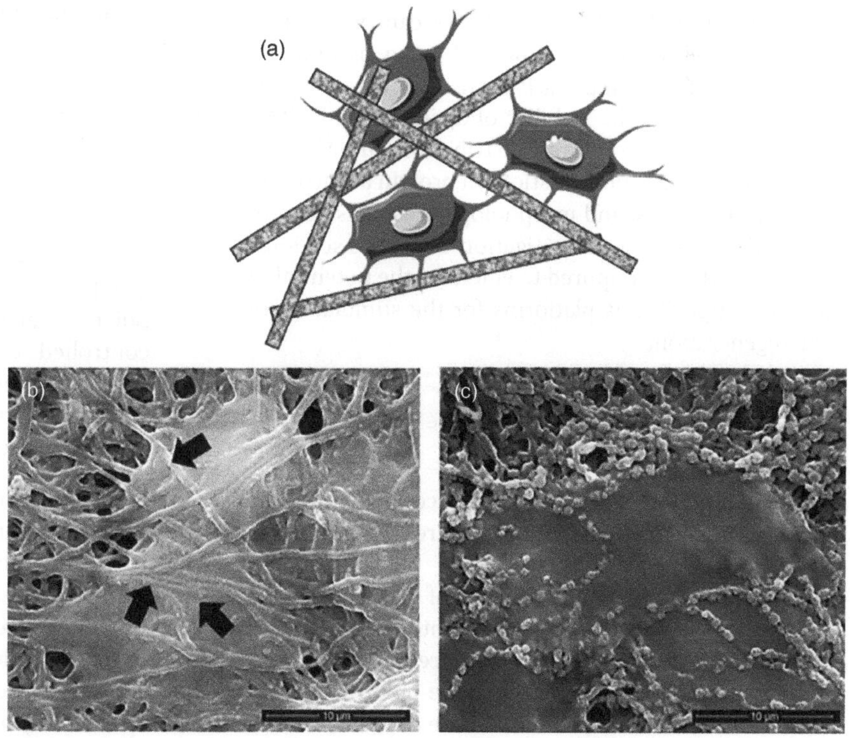

Figure 3.3 (a) Schematic representation of osteoblasts anchored on nanostructured fibers; (b) MG63 cells attached on electrospun fibers obtained from gelatin loaded with 1% COOH-modified NDPs, at 24 hours postseeding. Multiple adhesion points are formed with fibers, cells infiltrated between the fibers – analyzed by scanning electron microscopy; (c) multiple mineralized structures are formed in the fibers, in cell culture conditions (MG63 cells, 24 hours postseeding) – analyzed by scanning electron microscopy.

potential for tissue regeneration are excellently reviewed [15, 64–67]. Since osteoblasts are anchorage-dependent cells, nanostructure-loaded hydrogels have attracted increased interest in the fabrication of biomimetic fibrous scaffolds for bone regeneration.

Various nanospecies such as nanoapatite, carbon nanotubes, graphene, and graphene oxide have been investigated with respect to their ability to support bone formation when incorporated in hydrogel formulations. Nanodiamond particles (NDPs) have recently attracted attention as nanomaterials with high innovation potential for the development of matrices for tissue regeneration due to their including chemical stability, mechanical improvement, hydrophilicity, platform for controlled adsorption of proteins. Electrospun gelatin fibers loaded with NDPs have recently been fabricated by Serafim et al. [68]. NDPs surface functionalized with —COOH groups have been used as nanostructuring component in the fabricated fibers, in an attempt to locally improve the affinity of the substrate for ECM proteins and the mechanical properties.

This study suggested that 1% loading with nanoparticles enhanced the biointeractions of gelatin fibers both with MG63 osteoblast-like cells and with physiologically simulated media [68].

Control gelatin fibers stimulated adhesion but cells remained rounded and intercellular interactions were noticed. The cells firmly adhered and spread on the fibrous scaffolds loaded with NDPs (Figure 3.3a,b), and mineralized structures have been produced in cell culture conditions, as presented in Figure 3.3c. It has been also demonstrated that such matrixes can be successfully coated with bone-like mineral using biomimetic coating with alternating Ca/P baths and the presence of NDPs enhanced the stability of apatite coating [68]. The effect of nanostructures' distribution and agglomeration, surface functionalization on protein adsorption, mechanical features, and morphological aspects need to be established. Further investigation of fibrous scaffolds containing NDPs is required to elucidate the potential of such biocomposites as platforms for the stimulation of bone regeneration.

3.2.5 Biomineralization and Hydrogels Bearing Negatively Charged Groups

It is widely accepted that the presence of biomimetic mineral phase at the surface of bone regeneration biomaterials stimulates improved bone integration and osteoconduction. Functionalization of biomaterials to stimulate biomineralization at the interface with the surrounding bone emerged to enhance the stability of the binding between implants and the host tissue. The methods to stimulate such behavior are as follows:

- loading of the scaffold with ceramic particles,
- biomimetic coating with apatite layers,
- functionalization of polymers with groups promoting apatite nucleation through capturing Ca^{2+} and PO_4^{3-} ions from physiological fluids.

Some aspects related to the last method will be further presented. Inspiration came from phosphorylated and acidic biomolecules presenting affinity for calcium cations and thus being involved in the regulation of natural mineralization phenomena. Phosphatidylserine (PS) together with annexins have affinity for calcium cations. The role of phospholipids including PS in the stimulation of calcification has been extensively investigated [69, 70]. Noncollagenous proteins involved in physiological mineralization (bone sialoprotein) are rich in glutamate residues and therefore have the ability to capture calcium cations and lead Ca/P mineral nucleation. Macromolecules with pendant anionic groups such as phosphate, carboxylate, and sulfate have been investigated with respect to their affinity for calcium ions as chemical features inspired by the natural proteins involved in mineralization [71]. For an overview on strategies approached to promote mineralization by functionalization of hydrogels with negatively charged groups, the readers are directed to a review by Gkioni et al. [25] while aspects on phosphorus-containing polymers for biomedical applications are reviewed by Monge et al. [71] and Watson et al. [72]. Generally, hydrogels are excellent candidates to host mineral nucleation and growth in their intrinsic hydrated microenvironment. When the macromolecular backbone is decorated with pendant anionic groups, negatively charged at physiological pH, an enhanced capturing of calcium from physiological fluids is expected and mineral nucleation would lead to formation of Ca/P mineral phase. Negatively charged groups may be added to a polymer by:

(i) copolymerization with monomers bearing anionic groups,
(ii) polymer analogous reactions modifying, to a controlled extent, existing groups with anionic functionalities,
(iii) entrapment of a molecule containing the desired functional groups into a polymer network.

Despite experimental evidence on calcium capturing by anionic pendant groups, the design of hydrogel matrices with calcification potential is not fully understood yet. The chemical functionality of the scaffold, the density of negatively charged groups, their distribution, the length and nature of the spacer arm between the anionic group and the macromolecular backbone, the hydrophobic–hydrophilic balance, physical interactions in the hydrated matrix, the stability and the permeability of the scaffold for water-soluble species are few examples of factors involved in the biomineralization process.

3.2.5.1 Polymers Containing Acidic Functional Groups

It has been demonstrated that PHEMA surface functionalized with —COOH groups using a carboxymethylation reaction at —OH functions induces Ca/P nucleation and growth of apatite mineral after immersion in a synthetic body fluid [73]. PGA is a potential stimulator of biomimetic mineralization. Koh et al. reported that a 3-aminopropyltriethoxysilane PGA derivative pretreated with calcium chloride solution successfully accelerated the formation of bone-like apatite in a simulated body fluid [74]. In an attempt to develop hydrogels in which apatite grows in contact with self-assembling natural polymers, gelatin–calcium alginate freeze-dried scaffolds were investigated. The study demonstrated that the apatite-forming ability was favored by alginate-reinforced gelatin elastic chains. The biomineralization capacity of the bicomponent hydrogel was influenced by structural, compositional, and morphological features derived from the interaction between the two components [75]. More recently, polyamidoamine (PAMAM) dendrimers with —COOH groups on the reactive shell have been investigated with respect to their potential to stimulate biomimetic mineralization. Induction of bioinspired mineralization by PAMAM-COOH on human dentine was reported [76, 77]. Especially the fourth generation (G4-COOH) has the potential to prepare restorative materials for biomineralized hard tissues [77], while triclosan-loaded PAMAM-COOH has the ability to induce *in situ* remineralization on etched dentine, leading to regenerated apatite with a similar crystal structure with natural dentine [76]. It was also reported that gold nanoparticle–PAMAM dendrimer nanocomposites with succinamic acid terminal groups and dodecanediamine core induced calcification when immersed in simulated body fluids [78]. It is expected that dendrimers with anionic shells to be further investigated for such applications.

3.2.5.2 Phosphorus-containing Polymers Enhance Mineralization

Phoshorylated polymers have promising potential for bone regeneration. Penczek et al. reported the synthesis of poly(alkylene phosphates) mimicking biomacromolecules and their effect in controlling the crystallization of $CaCO_3$, in a process related to biomineralization [79]. Some studies were devoted to the calcification capacity of ethylene glycol methacrylate phosphate (MOEP) and ethylene glycol acrylate phosphate (MAEP). Stancu et al. [80] investigated the ability of MOEP to induce calcification in *in vitro* acellular conditions. The study based on two families of MOEP copolymers, with (diethylamino)ethyl methacrylate and 1-vinyl-2-pyrrolidinone suggested that the formation of Ca/P mineral is influenced not just by the presence of phosphate groups but also by its density and distribution [80]. Wang et al. reported that increased mineralization in both cellular and acellular constructs based on phosphoester–poly(ethylene glycol) polymer (PhosPEG) when compared with PEG gels [81]. Casein, a phosphorylated protein has induced mineral nucleation when immobilized in a hydrogel and immersed in simulated body fluids [82–84]. Cardoso et al. emphasized that surface treatment of implants with polyphosphoric acid (PPA) and phosphorylated pullulan (PPL) may positively influence osseointegration [85]. A poly(*N*-isopropylacrylamide)-based hydrogel promoting *in vitro* mineralization was obtained by Watson et al. starting from a macromer with pendant phosphate groups [86]. Among recently developed phosphorylated polymers, poly(sebacoyl diglyceride) phosphate (PSeD-P) was reported by Huang et al. [87] as the first polymer to integrate the osteoinductive moiety β-glycerol phosphate (β-GP). Remarkably, PSeD-P substantially induces mineralization of the ECM in MSCs without using β-GP, while PSeD does not promote mineralization under identical culture conditions. The authors concluded that PSeD-P provides a new strategy to integrate bioactive phosphates via β-GP into biomaterial and has promise for bone regeneration applications [87]. These examples illustrate the potential of phosphorylated macromolecules to control biomimetic mineralizations and continuation of the research in this direction is fully justified.

To conclude, hydrogel-based scaffolds for bone tissue engineering and bone regeneration are under continuous development, representing a main challenge in the field of biomaterials. The correlation design–properties–fabrication–functionality is of main importance and bioinspired and biomimetic approaches have attracted increased interest lately. However, despite obvious progress, unresolved problems justify the demand for even more complex scaffolds combining chemistry, fabrication, surface engineering for a predesigned functionality *in vivo*.

3.3 Ca/P Biomaterials for Bone Regeneration

3.3.1 Introduction: Remaining Challenges

The microarchitecture of bone makes it suitable to resist and adapt to muscle contractions and gravity [88]. It is a biphasic natural connective tissue composed of an elastic phase made of type I collagen microfibrils and noncollagenous proteins which confer to bone its elasticity. Moreover, this organic phase is rigidified by deposition of HA crystals between the collagen microfibrils. During aging, the osteoblasts (bone-forming cells) become less active leading to a progressive reduced bone volume but the microarchitecture of trabecular bone is optimized to maintain bone quality [89, 90].

In human pathology, localized bone defects can occur in bony cysts or are frequently observed after tooth extraction or during the revision of hip prosthesis. Valgization or vanization osteotomy is also routinely performed to correct the weight-bearing axis in case of unicompartmental osteoarthritis of the knee. In these cases, the use of a biomaterial is frequently used to help bone reconstruction [91]. Allogenic or xenogenic bone has been proposed as suitable biomaterials for filling these bone defects as an alternative to bone autografts. These bone grafts can be prepared by bone banks or companies and several processes have been developed, leading to different quality of materials [92]. One of the interests, of bone grafts, is that they are made of the same material than the receiver's bone and possess a 3D microarchitecture that makes the grafts suitable for osteoconduction while retaining biomechanical properties. However, the use of synthetic ceramics prepared with the same composition than the mineral phase of bone (i.e. calcium and phosphate) was reported about one century ago [93]. At the present time, the use of synthetic calcium phosphate ceramics tends to increase in the surgical practice: they can be prepared in large amounts by companies, they are relatively cheap, the exhibit good cytocompatibility, osteoconductive properties, and resorbability *in vivo*. In addition, such synthetic substitutes are safe and avoid the risk of nonconventional agents and virus which are extremely low but not equal to zero [94]. Among the calcium phosphate ceramics, HA, β-tricalcium phosphate (β-TCP), mixed formulations including HA + β-TCP have been developed extensively [95]. If the first clinical trials used dense or compact biomaterials, it became rapidly evident that preparing scaffolds, granules, or blocks with an open and interconnected porosity and with pores having 100–350 μm range in diameter could greatly enhance vascular sprout invasion carrying osteoprogenitor cells at the center of the grafted area. These ceramics based on calcium orthophosphates are well recognized by osteoblasts as they mimic bone surfaces. They are resorbed by macrophages and osteoclasts and have good osteoconductive properties. However, they can be brittle and some formulations are not adapted for repairing weight-bearing bones [96]. Some groups have claimed that they can be osteoinductive (i.e. they have the possibility to induce bone in ectopic sites such as muscles) [97]. However, this remains a subject of controversy [98] and most studies have been conducted in the sheep or the goat which have a propensity to develop ectopic calcifications [99].

3.3.2 Micro- and Nanocomputed Tomography for the Study of Porous Ca/P Biomaterials

Because the synthetic biomaterials can be prepared in the form of bone they are destined to replace, a considerable amount of literature is available on the different preparing process but also on the techniques to evaluate their microarchitecture. A significant advance in the bone field arose with the development of microcomputed tomography (micro-CT) around the 2000s. This method is superior to scanning electron microscopy (SCM) at low magnifications and allows direct 3D measurements of the bone mass, porosity, and microarchitecture [100–103]. The method is faster than morphometric analysis of histological sections and new micro-CTs have a resolution in the 2–3 μm/pixel range. In addition, micro-CT is nondestructive and the samples can be processed for additional histological studies. Because most Ca/P ceramics have a higher content than bone, they absorb X-ray more intensely, making a clear distinction between them and the bone matrix. This allows a separate measurement of bone and the grafted biomaterial, allowing the study of both osteoconduction and resorbability of the material (Figure 3.4) [104, 105]. The more recent development of nano-CT allows a precision close to the synchrotron and also offers to study soft tissues or thin polymer scaffolds (Figure 3.5b).

3.3.3 Preparation of 3D Porous Blocks and Granules of Ca/P Ceramics

Ca/P ceramics can be prepared in a variety of techniques. Pressing the Ca/P material with a porogen is a relatively old method that often leads to a noninterconnected porosity of the final block of biomaterial. For example HA can be mixed with naphthalene particles, pressed, and fired at high temperature to remove naphthalene [104, 106]. Polyester or glucose/sucrose fibers have also been used to prepare scaffolds having an interconnected porosity but it remains largely under the "normal" porosity of human bone (usually ~70–85% when such scaffold produce ~40–50% porosity [107]. It should also be noted that increasing the porosity considerably reduces the biomechanical properties of the scaffolds.

Other methods have also been proposed such as gas-foaming or freeze-drying but the pores' size and interconnectivity cannot be properly controlled. The

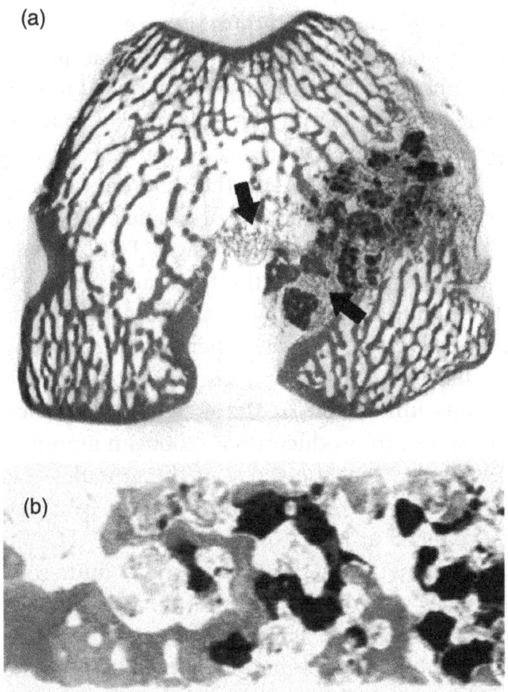

Figure 3.4 (a) μ-CT analysis of a rabbit femoral condyle grafted with β-TCP granules 28 days before sacrifice. The biomaterial granules having a higher Ca content than bone are clearly identified (in black on this inversed image). Note the thin less-mineralized trabeculae of woven bone developed by osteoconduction (arrows), which are less mineralized than the mature surrounding bone. The β-TCP granules are fragmented, indicating a resorption by osteoclasts and macrophages. (b) Bone biopsy in a patient having had a sinus lift with β-TCP granules six months before. Note the increased contrast of the granules (in black) with the bone matrix (in gray) and the direct apposition of bone at the surface of the granules (inverted image).

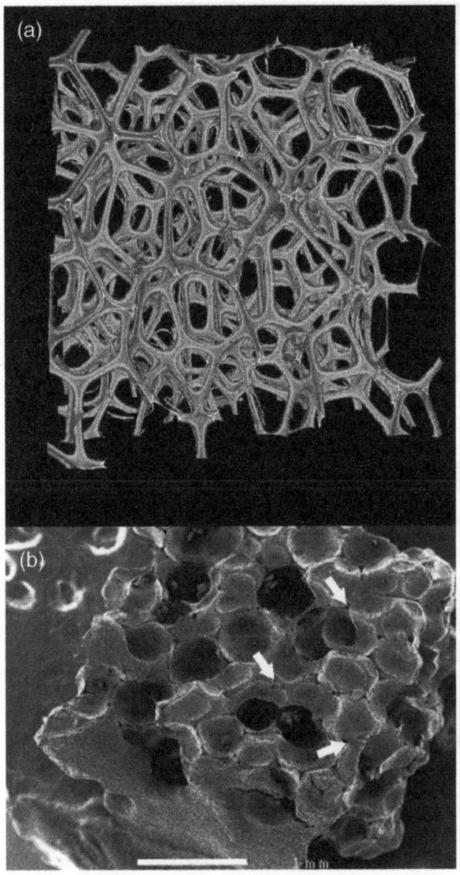

Figure 3.5 A wedge for tibial osteotomy prepared with HA and β-TCP by laser sintering. The block is 20 mm in height and as a 3D interconnected porosity. (a) The cubic wedge is imaged by micro-CT (Kasios, Duowedge). Porosity represents 50.38% of the volume of the block. (b) Same block analyzed by scanning electron microscopy.

recent development of 3D printing in the 1980s has led to new approaches of scaffolds fabrication which are computer-aided. Different methods for 3D printing are described in the literature, such as stereolithography, rapid prototyping, and laser sintering [108, 109]. Figure 3.6 illustrates a wedge for tibial osteotomy prepared with 60% HA and 40% β-TCP and having a 3D interconnected porosity.

This type of blocks is sufficiently hard to be placed in weight-bearing areas. However, the high amount of HA implies a long term of resorbability for this type of scaffold. Scaffolds of pure β-TCP can be prepared by the polyurethane foam technique. This type of block is friable but can be used in dental and maxillofacial surgery. The method was first developed by Schartzwalder and Somers and has been used to prepare a considerable number of porous materials including Ca/P and metallic foams [110]. Briefly, pieces of a polyurethane foam are used as a template which is impregnated with an aqueous slurry of β-TCP. The Ca/P material adheres onto the surface of the foam network made of thin trabeculae interconnected by triangular nodes. Once the foam is impregnated with the slurry, it is dried in an oven and then heated at >1200 °C. The polyurethane microarchitecture is known to have a tetrakaidecahedron 3D geometry (Figure 3.5a) and the image of a cube of β-TCP prepared by this manner exhibits a macroporosity (due to the cavities of the foam) and an inner porosity (due to the sublimation of the foam (Figure 3.5b).

Granules, one of the most suitable form usable in dental surgery, are obtained by crushing these blocks in a mortar. An additional sieving step allows the separation of granules with a calibrated size (Figure 3.7a,b,d). This type of granules is used to fill alveolar sockets or restoring a suitable bone volume at the maxilla before dental implant placement [111]. It should be kept in mind that

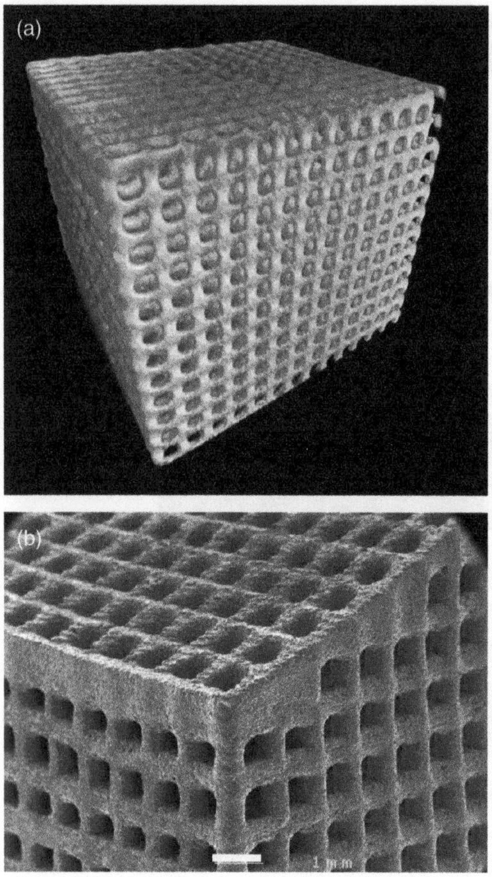

Figure 3.6 Preparation of blocks of β-TCP by the polyurethane foam method. (a) Nanotomographic aspect of the polyurethane foam with the typical tetrakaidecahedron structure. (b) Block of sintered β-TCP prepared with the polyurethane foam. Note the interconnected macroporosity due to the cellularization of the foam and the small internal porosity due to the sublimation of the polyurethane during sintering (arrows).

once placed in a bone defect, the granules occupy the 3D space according to their shape (Figure 3.7c). However, this aspect of the problem has received little consideration although their size, branching, and porosity that determine the 3D arrangement will strongly influence the circulation and penetration of biological fluids and cell invasion throughout the material [112, 113]. In fact, a set of granules placed in the grafted site behaves as if it have recreated its own macroporosity (intergranule porosity). So it was interesting to evaluate (i) if changing the amount of β-TCP in the slurry would lead to modification of the shape and biomechanical properties of the granules, (ii) what would be the effects of such changes on the 3D intergranule porosity, (iii) will these changes in the 3D intergranule porosity will affect the diffusion of body fluids in the grafted area. The effect of such factors is further described.

3.3.3.1 Changing the Shape of Ca/P Granular Biomaterial Affects its Biomechanical Resistance

It is possible to change the shape of Ca/P granules by reducing the amount of elementary powder used to prepare the slurry. This was verified by reducing the amount of β-TCP used to prepare granules as above from 25 g to 10 g/100 ml of distilled water. The different steps of the process using standardized polyurethane cubes were described by SEM and micro-CT. Low β-TCP dosages in the slurry readily infiltrated the foam and produced blocks with a thin and regular deposition along the polyurethane trabeculae. On the other hand, increasing the amount led to more viscous slurries producing an inhomogeneous infiltration of the cubes [100]. When crushed and sieved to produce 1000–2000 μm granules, nano-CT evidenced that the shape of the granules was considerably modified [114] (Figure 3.7a,b). Macroporosity was reduced at high concentration of β-TCP in the slurry and conversely, there were more numerous concave surfaces associated with thin branchings at the lowest concentrations. It should be noted that the internal porosity (due to sublimation of the polyurethane foam) was present in all types of granules. Careful 3D analysis of pores' diameter clearly identified a small peak corresponding to internal porosity on the frequency histograms determined by micro-CT [115]. One of the most interesting findings derived from nano-CT analysis was that granules presented a heterogeneous aspect due to variations in the mineralization degree of the sintered grains used to prepare the granules [114]. Similarly, in granules prepared with a mixture of HA and β-TCP, nano-CT evidenced the different Ca content of each of the components of Ca/P ratio ~1.67 for HA and 1.5 for β-TCP. It is likely that changing the shape of biomaterial granules affects the biomechanical resistance [116]. When compression analysis of stacks of granules was done, analysis of the curves revealed two domains: the first one being related to the rearrangement by sliding and rotation producing a denser stack collapse of granules; the second one being due to the destruction of the scaffold by compression. There is a direct relationship between the work to failure and the density of the granules and also an exponential relationship between stiffness and the amount of β-TCP used to prepare the granules (Figure 3.8a). Macroporosity, intergranule porosity and also internal porosity (microporosity) are parameters that affect the biomechanical properties of a material [117–119].

3.3.3.2 Changing the Shape of a Granular Biomaterial Affects its 3D Porosity

When a surgeon places granules of a material in a receptor site, they are gently packed together without crushing

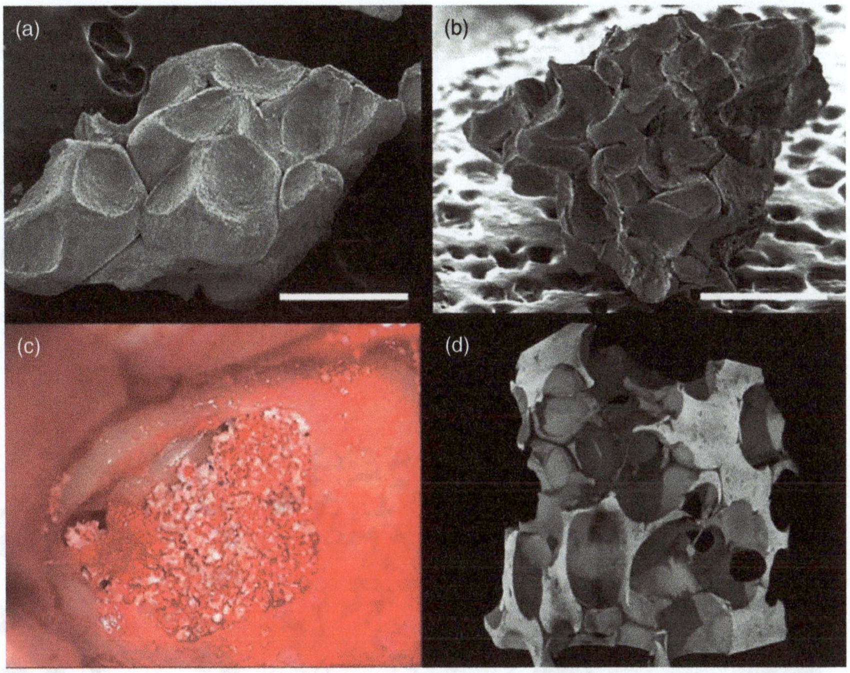

Figure 3.7 (a) SEM of a β-TCP granule prepared with 25 g Ca/P powder in the slurry. (b) SEM of a granule prepared with 12.5 g in the slurry. Note the modified architecture (the white bar stands for 500 μm); (c) A defect prepared in an edentulated maxilla for a sinus elevation. The subantral cavity created was filled with the β-TCP granules described in 4B after detachment of the Schneiderian membrane. Note the complex arrangement of the granules and the 3D intergranule porosity filled with blood. (d) Nano-CT analysis of a 1000–2000 μm granule of β-TCP prepared with 11 g of Ca/P powder in the slurry. Note the thin and fragile branchings determined by the polyurethane foam.

(Figure 3.7c). As mentioned above, this creates an intergranule 3D porosity well suitable for body fluids and cell invasion. However, the 3D arrangement of objects is only well known for particles with a well-defined and simple shape [120, 121]. We have developed several strategies to evaluate the complexity of porosity of porous biomaterials (synthetic or bone) with new algorithms used to characterize the mean size of the pores and their interconnectivity. Most of these methods are based on a stereological or mathematical morphological analysis of 2D sections either obtained by histology or by using 2D sections obtained from μCT stacks of images (Figure 3.8c–e) [122–125]. A new algorithm based on vector analysis of images was recently described to study the porosity of large blocks of porous biomaterials [126]. The method has been successfully applied to evaluate the porosity of complex porous objects such as the alveolar bone of the jaw [127], the porosity of the epiphyses of the long bones [128], and the intergranules porosity in stacks of biomaterials [129]. The principle of the Vectopor™ algorithm is to study the porosity of binarized images obtained by μCT. On each image, considered as an *x*–*y* map, pixels of the pores which belong to the same *x* column receive the same color according to a look-up table. This color is also used to build a frontal plane constructed line by line; each line resuming a single 2D image of the image stack. A measure of the complexity of the porosity can be obtained either by computing the fractal dimension of the gray image of the frontal plane [126] or by measuring the ratio of the red + green pixels over the total number of pixels of the colored image [128]. The method is rapid and is well adapted to the study of stacks of biomaterial granules (Figure 3.9). Linear correlations exist between the fractal dimension and the exact porosity measured in 3D.

3.3.3.3 Changing the 3D Porosity of a Porous Biomaterial Modifies Liquid Diffusion

The diffusion of a liquid in relation with porosity is a topic that is highly developed in geology and soil science [130, 131]. We have tried to see if image analysis techniques could be used to evaluate this parameter when applied to biomaterials. This would help to better characterize the scaffolds of granules and get indication of their invasion *in vivo* by biological fluids. The recent development of fractal geometry and its application to bone and biomaterials have been of considerable interest [132]. Fractal dimensions can evaluate the complexity of the material to fill the reference space [133, 134]. Recently, new fractal parameters (lacunarity and succolarity) have been proposed to better characterize the porosity of a biomaterial [135, 136]. Lacunarity describes the nature of the pores within an image and is influenced by their variation in size. It represents a measure of the complexity of these pores. Succolarity is another parameter which informs about connectivity intercommunication. The algorithms used to determine succolarity on a 2D image resemble a flooding procedure (i.e. similar to the penetration of a liquid according to the direction the liquid is poured in the image [136]. So, this parameter represents the degree of percolation of an image [137]. When these methods were applied to stacks of granules prepared with increasing concentration of β-TCP in the slurry, it was found that porosity decreased as the

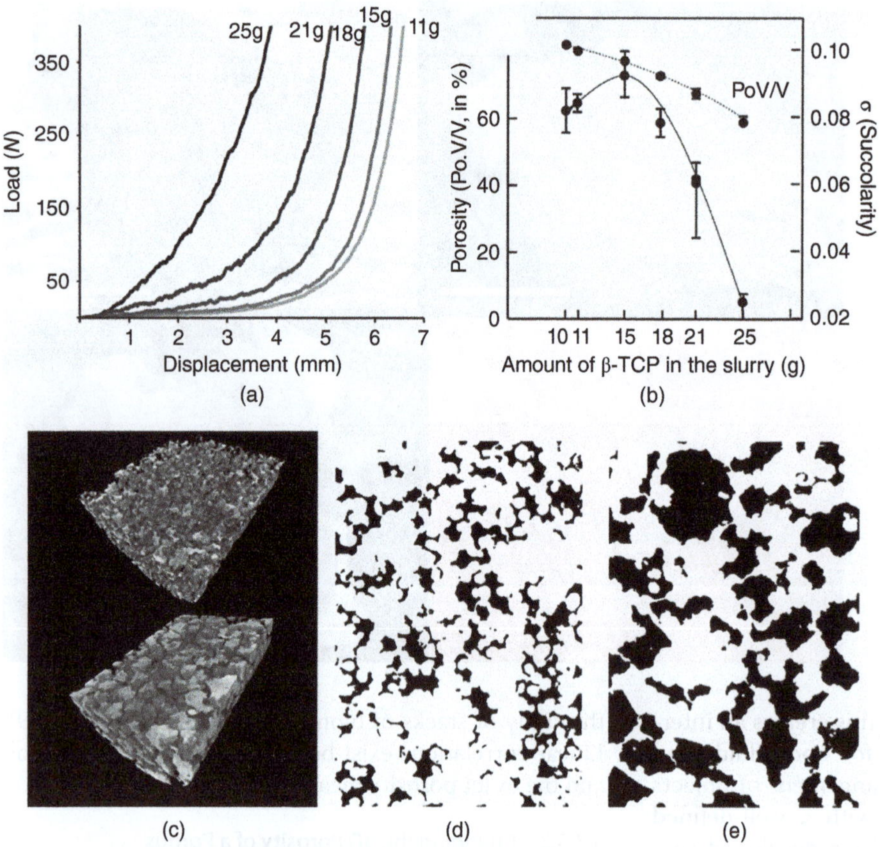

Figure 3.8 (a) Influence of increasing the concentration of β-TCP in the slurry on biomechanical properties studied in compression. (b) Relationship between the amount of β-TCP in the slurry with the intergranule 3D macroporosity of stacks of granules (plain line) and evolution of succolarity with an inverse U curve centered on the 15–18 g groups (dotted line). (c) μCT analysis of two stacks of granules prepared with 12 g/100 ml (upper image) and 25 g/100 ml in the slurry (lower image). (d) 2D section of a stack of granules figured in (c) (upper image) prepared with 12 g/100 ml; (e) 2D sections of the stack of granules figured in (c) (lower image) prepared with 25 g. In (c) and (d), note the interconnectivity of the pores and the differences in the branchings of the granules.

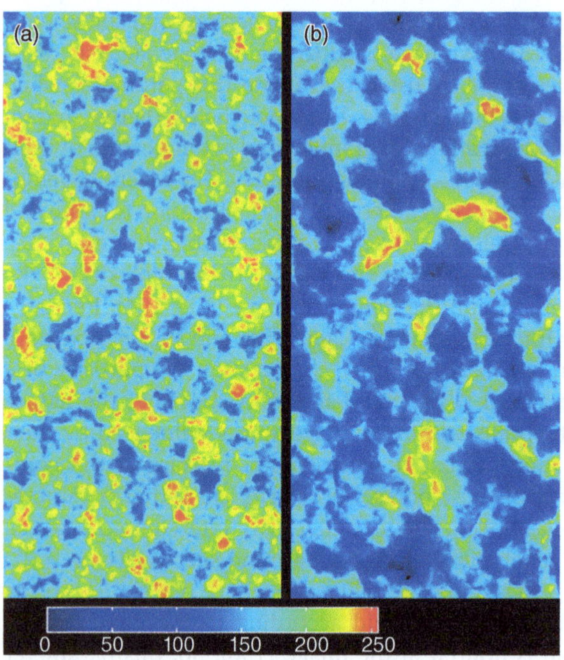

Figure 3.9 Vector analysis of the stacks of β-TCP granules illustrated in Figure 3.5c. (a) Granules prepared with 12 g/100 ml; (b) granules prepared with 25 g/100 ml in the slurry. The look up table is figured at the bottom of the image.

amount of material increased. In addition, nonlinear relationships were obtained between descriptors of the pores and porosity (Figure 3.8b). Lacunarity increased exponentially with the amount of material while succolarity had an inverse U curve with a maximum centered in the 15–18 g/100 ml of β-TCP [138].

3.4 Perspectives

Both hydrogels and bioceramics have become main actors in the design and fabrication of scaffolds for bone regeneration. Natural and naturally derived hydrogels are appealing mainly for their ability to provide cell interactivity and/or biodegradability, whereas synthetic hydrogels are typically responsible for structural stability and advanced control of properties. A wide range of hybrid hydrogels with tailored *in vitro* and *in vivo* functionality have been developed in the last years, with a shift to 3D constructs with predefined biointeractivity. Important progress has been recorded also in the field of bioceramics, while advanced manufacturing techniques and accurate complex characterization methods have been developed. Future research will have to include specific features leading to a concerted *in- vivo* functionality to obtain performant cell-interactive alternatives to bone regeneration.

Acknowledgments

The financial support from the project PNII PCCA 183/2012, Bioactive injectable macroporous biomaterials for bone regeneration is acknowledged. Dr. Eugeniu Vasile is kindly acknowledged for SEM analyses. Also thanks to Andrada Serafim, Sergiu Cecoltan, Diana-Maria Dragusin, and Adriana Lungu for their help with the synthesis and characterization of hydrogels.

This work was also made possible by grants from ANR (Agence Nationale de la Recherche), program LabCom "NextBone." Thanks to Hervé Nyangoga, Lisa Terranova, Romain Mallet, Guillaume Mabilleau, Bernard Guillaume, Eric Aguado for help with microphotographs, also Nadine Gaborit, Stéphanie Lemière for technical help with the μCT, and Laurence Lechat for secretarial assistance. Kasios SAS, 18 Chemin de la Violette, 31240 L'Union-France provided different types of β-TCP biomaterials.

References

1 Ma, P.X. (2008). Biomimetic materials for tissue engineering. *Adv. Drug Delivery Rev.* **60**: 184–198.
2 Short, A.R., Koralla, D., Deshmukh, A. et al. (2015). Hydrogels that allow and facilitate bone repair, remodeling, and regeneration. *J. Mater. Chem. B* **3**: 7818–7830.
3 Wang, P., Zhao, L., Liu, J. et al. (2014). Bone tissue engineering via nanostructured calcium phosphate biomaterials and stem cells. *Bone Res.* **2**: 14017.
4 Venugopal, J., Prabhakaran, M.P., Zhang, Y. et al. (2010). Biomimetic hydroxyapatite-containing composite nanofibrous substrates for bone tissue engineering. *Philos. Trans. R. Soc. A: Math. Phys. Eng. Sci.* **368**: 2065 2081.
5 Liu, Y., Wu, G., and de Groot, K. (2010). Biomimetic coatings for bone tissue engineering of critical-sized defects. *J. R. Soc. Interface* **7** (Suppl. 5): S631–S647.
6 Ohtsuki, C., Kamitakahara, M., and Miyazaki, T. (2009). Bioactive ceramic-based materials with designed reactivity for bone tissue regeneration. *J. R. Soc. Interface* **6** (Suppl. 3): S349–S360.
7 Bohner, M. (2010). Resorbable biomaterials as bone graft substitutes. *Mater. Today* **13**: 24–30.
8 Cordonnier, T., Sohier, J., Rosset, P., and Layrolle, P. (2011). Biomimetic materials for bone tissue engineering – state of the art and future trends. *Adv. Eng. Mater.* **13** (5): B135–B150.
9 Engel, E., Castano, O., Salvagni, E. et al. (2009). *Strategies in Regenerative Medicine. Integrating Biology with Materials Design* (ed. M. Santin), 56–96. Springer. 10.1007/978-0-387-74660-9_3.
10 Grayson, W.L., Martens, T.P., Eng, G.M. et al. (2009). Biomimetic approach to tissue engineering. *Semin. Cell Dev. Biol.* **20**: 665–673.
11 Green, D.W. (2008). Tissue bionics: examples in biomimetic tissue engineering. *Biomed. Mater.* **3**: 034010.
12 Green, D.W., Goto, T.K., Kim, K.-S., and Jung, H.-S. (2014). Calcifying tissue regeneration via biomimetic materials chemistry. *J. R. Soc. Interface* **11**: 20140537.
13 Holzwarth, J.M. and Ma, P.X. (2011). Biomimetic nanofibrous scaffolds for bone tissue engineering. *Biomaterials* **32**: 9622–9629.
14 Kim, T.G., Shin, H., and Lim, D.W. (2012). Biomimetic scaffolds for tissue engineering. *Adv. Funct. Mater.* https://doi.org/10.1002/adfm.201103083.
15 Liao, S., Li, B., Ma, Z. et al. (2006). Biomimetic electrospun nanofibers for tissue regeneration. *Biomed. Mater.* **1**: R45–R53.
16 Patterson, J., Martino, M.M., and Hubbell, J.A. (2010). Biomimetic materials in tissue engineering. *Mater. Today* https://doi.org/10.1016/S1369-7021(10)70013-4.
17 Sant, S., Hancock, M.J., Donnelly, J.P. et al. (2010). Biomimetic gradient hydrogels for tissue engineering. *Can. J. Chem. Eng.* **88**: 899–911.
18 Ruiz-Hitzky, E., Darder, M., Aranda, P., and Ariga, K. (2010). Advances in biomimetic and nanostructured biohybrid materials. *Adv. Mater.* **22**: 323–336.
19 Stancu, I.C., Lungu, A., and Iovu, H. (2014). *Biomaterials for Bone Regeneration: Novel Techniques and Applications*. Elsevier. https://doi.org/10.1533/9780857098104.1.62.
20 Lutolf, M.P. and Hubbell, J.A. (2005). Synthetic biomaterials as instructive extracellular microenvironments for morphogenesis in tissue engineering. *Nat. Biotechnol.* **23**: 47–55.
21 Niu, X., Wang, Y., Luo, Y., and Xin, J. (2005). Arg-Gly-Asp (RGD) modified biomimetic polymeric materials. *J. Mater. Sci.* **21**: 571–576.
22 Sadat-Shojai, M., Khorasani, M.T., and Jamshidi, A. (2015). 3-Dimensional cell-laden nano-hydroxyapatite/protein hydrogels for bone

regeneration applications. *Mater. Sci. Eng., C* **49**: 835–843.

23 Betz, M.W., Yeatts, A.B., Richbourg, W.J. et al. (2010). Macroporous hydrogels upregulate osteogenic signal expression and promote bone regeneration. *Biomacromolecules* **11**: 1160–1168.

24 Park, J.B. (2011). The use of hydrogels in bone-tissue engineering. *Med. Oral Patol. Oral Cir. Bucal* **16**: e115–e118.

25 Gkioni, K., Leeuwenburgh, S.C.G.G., Douglas, T.E.L.L. et al. (2010). Mineralization of hydrogels for bone regeneration. *Tissue Eng. Part B: Rev.* **16**: 577–585.

26 Lienemann, P.S., Lutolf, M.P., and Ehrbar, M. (2012). Biomimetic hydrogels for controlled biomolecule delivery to augment bone regeneration. *Adv. Drug Delivery Rev.* **64**: 1078–1089.

27 Killion, J.A., Geever, L.M., Devine, D.M. et al. (2011). Mechanical properties and thermal behaviour of PEGDMA hydrogels for potential bone regeneration application. *J. Mech. Behav. Biomed. Mater.* **4**: 1219–1227.

28 Patterson, J., Siew, R., Herring, S.W. et al. (2010). Hyaluronic acid hydrogels with controlled degradation properties for oriented bone regeneration. *Biomaterials* **31**: 6772–6781.

29 Moreira Teixeira, L.S., Patterson, J., and Luyten, F.P. (2014). Skeletal tissue regeneration: where can hydrogels play a role? *Int. Orthop.* **38**: 1861–1876.

30 Gibbs, D.M.R., Black, C.R.M., Dawson, J.I., and Oreffo, R.O.C. (2015). A review of hydrogel use in fracture healing and bone regeneration. *J. Tissue Eng. Regener. Med.* https://doi.org/10.1002/term.1968.

31 Mabilleau, G., Stancu, I.C., Honoré, T. et al. (2006). Effects of the length of crosslink chain on poly(2-hydroxyethyl methacrylate) (pHEMA) swelling and biomechanical properties. *J. Biomed. Mater. Res. A* **77**: 35–42.

32 Moshaverinia, A., Chen, C., Xu, X. et al. (2014). Bone regeneration potential of stem cells derived from periodontal ligament or gingival tissue sources encapsulated in RGD-modified alginate scaffold. *Tissue Eng. Part A* **20**: 611–621.

33 Tsai, W.B., Chen, Y.R., Liu, H.L., and Lai, J.Y. (2011). Fabrication of UV-crosslinked chitosan scaffolds with conjugation of RGD peptides for bone tissue engineering. *Carbohydr. Polym.* **85**: 129–137.

34 Kantlehner, M., Finsinger, D., Meyer, J. et al. (1999). Selective RGD-mediated adhesion of osteoblasts at surfaces of implants. *Angew. Chem. Int. Ed.* **38**: 560–562.

35 Tsai, W.B., Chen, Y.R., Li, W.T. et al. (2012). RGD-conjugated UV-crosslinked chitosan scaffolds inoculated with mesenchymal stem cells for bone tissue engineering. *Carbohydr. Polym.* **89**: 379–387.

36 Mas-Moruno, C., Dorfner, P.M., Manzenrieder, F. et al. (2013). Behavior of primary human osteoblasts on trimmed and sandblasted Ti6Al4V surfaces functionalized with integrin avb3-selective cyclic RGD peptides. *J. Biomed. Mater. Res. Part A* **101**: 87–97.

37 Comisar, W.A., Kazmers, N.H., Mooney, D.J., and Linderman, J.J. (2007). Engineering RGD nanopatterned hydrogels to control preosteoblast behavior: a combined computational and experimental approach. *Biomaterials* **28**: 4409–4417.

38 Benoit, D.S.W. and Anseth, K.S. (2005). The effect on osteoblast function of colocalized RGD and PHSRN epitopes on PEG surfaces. *Biomaterials* **26**: 5209–5220.

39 Kaufmann, D., Fiedler, A., Junger, A. et al. (2008). Chemical conjugation of linear and cyclic RGD moieties to a recombinant elastin-mimetic polypeptide – a versatile approach towards bioactive protein hydrogels. *Macromol. Biosci.* **8**: 577–588.

40 Bubenikova, S., Stancu, I.-C., Kalinovska, L. et al. (2012). Chemoselective cross-linking of alginate with thiol-terminated peptides for tissue engineering applications. *Carbohydr. Polym.* **88**: 1239–1250.

41 Reyes, C.D. and García, A.J. (2003). Engineering integrin-specific surfaces with a triple-helical collagen-mimetic peptide. *J. Biomed. Mater. Res. Part A* **65**: 511–523.

42 Mabilleau, G., Aguado, E., Stancu, I.-C. et al. (2008). Effects of FGF-2 release from a hydrogel polymer on bone mass and microarchitecture. *Biomaterials* **29**: 1593–1600.

43 Mantripragada, V.P. and Jayasuriya, A.C. (2016). Bone regeneration using injectable BMP-7 loaded chitosan microparticles in rat femoral defect. *Mater. Sci. Eng., C* **63**: 596–608.

44 Filmon, R., Baslé, M.F., Barbier, A., and Chappard, D. (2000). Poly(2-hydroxy ethyl methacrylate)-alkaline phosphatase: a composite biomaterial allowing in vitro studies of bisphosphonates on the mineralization process. *J. Biomater. Sci., Polym. Ed.* **11**: 849–868.

45 Filmon, R., Baslé, M.F., Atmani, H., and Chappard, D. (2002). Adherence of osteoblast-like cells on calcospherites developed on a biomaterial combining poly(2-hydroxyethyl) methacrylate and alkaline phosphatase. *Bone* **30**: 152–158.

46 Douglas, T.E.L., Messersmith, P.B., Chasan, S. et al. (2012). Enzymatic mineralization of hydrogels for bone tissue engineering by incorporation of alkaline phosphatase. *Macromol. Biosci.* **12**: 1077–1089.

47 Douglas, T.E.L., Wlodarczyk, M., Pamula, E. et al. (2014). Enzymatic mineralization of gellan gum

hydrogel for bone tissue-engineering applications and its enhancement by polydopamine. *J. Tissue Eng. Regener. Med.* **8**: 906–918.
48 Kim, H. and Lee, J. (2016). Strategies to maximize the potential of marine biomaterials as a platform for cell therapy. *Mar. Drugs* **14**: 29.
49 Bidarra, S.J., Barrias, C.C., Fonseca, K.B. et al. (2011). Injectable in situ crosslinkable RGD-modified alginate matrix for endothelial cells delivery. *Biomaterials* **32**: 7897–7904.
50 Dinescu, S., Galateanu, B., Radu, E. et al. (2015). A 3D porous gelatin-alginate-based-IPN acts as an efficient promoter of chondrogenesis from human adipose-derived stem cells. *Stem Cells Int.* **2015**: 252909.
51 Wang, H., Zhou, L., Liao, J. et al. (2014). Cell-laden photocrosslinked GelMA-DexMA copolymer hydrogels with tunable mechanical properties for tissue engineering. *J. Mater. Sci. - Mater. Med.* **25**: 2173–2183.
52 Van Vlierberghe, S., Dubruel, P., and Schacht, E. (2011). Biopolymer-based hydrogels as scaffolds for tissue engineering applications: a review. *Biomacromolecules* **12**: 1387–1408.
53 Aubin, H., Nichol, J.W., Hutson, C.B. et al. (2010). Directed 3D cell alignment and elongation in microengineered hydrogels. *Biomaterials* **31**: 6941–6951.
54 Loessner, D., Meinert, C., Kaemmerer, E. et al. (2016). Functionalization, preparation and use of cell-laden gelatin methacryloyl based hydrogels as modular tissue culture platforms. *Nat. Protoc.* **11**: 727–746.
55 Klotz, B.J., Gawlitta, D., Rosenberg, A.J.W.P. et al. (2016). Gelatin-methacryloyl hydrogels: towards biofabrication-based tissue repair. *Trends Biotechnol.* **34**: 394–407.
56 Yue, K., Trujillo-de Santiago, G., Alvarez, M.M. et al. (2015). Synthesis, properties, and biomedical applications of gelatin methacryloyl (GelMA) hydrogels. *Biomaterials* **73**: 254–271.
57 Visser, J., Peters, B., Burger, T.J. et al. (2013). Biofabrication of multi-material anatomically shaped tissue constructs. *Biofabrication* **5**: 035007.
58 Serafim, A., Tucureanu, C., Petre, D.-G. et al. (2014). One-pot synthesis of superabsorbent hybrid hydrogels based on methacrylamide gelatin and polyacrylamide. Effortless control of hydrogel properties through composition design. *New J. Chem.* **38**: 3112.
59 Serafim, A., Dragusin, D.-M., Butac, L.M. et al. (2013). New hydrogels based on gelatin and acrylamide. *UPB Sci. Bull., Ser. B Chem. Mater. Sci.* **75**: 3–14.
60 Dragusin, D.-M., Van Vlierberghe, S., Dubruel, P. et al. (2012). Novel gelatin–PHEMA porous scaffolds for tissue engineering applications. *Soft Matter* **8**: 9589.
61 Santin, M., Morris, C., Standen, G. et al. (2007). A new class of bioactive and biodegradable soybean-based bone fillers. *Biomacromolecules* **8**: 2706–2711.
62 Merolli, A., Nicolais, L., Ambrosio, L., and Santin, M. (2010). A degradable soybean-based biomaterial used effectively as a bone filler in vivo in a rabbit. *Biomed. Mater.* **5**: 15008.
63 Giavaresi, G., Fini, M., Salvage, J. et al. (2010). Bone regeneration potential of a soybean-based filler: experimental study in a rabbit cancellous bone defects. *J. Mater. Sci. - Mater. Med.* **21**: 615–626.
64 Sell, S.A., McClure, M.J., Garg, K. et al. (2009). Electrospinning of collagen/biopolymers for regenerative medicine and cardiovascular tissue engineering. *Adv. Drug Delivery Rev.* **61**: 1007–1019.
65 Lee, K.Y., Jeong, L., Kang, Y.O. et al. (2009). Electrospinning of polysaccharides for regenerative medicine. *Adv. Drug Delivery Rev.* **61**: 1020–1032.
66 Agarwal, S., Wendorff, J.H., and Greiner, A. (2008). Use of electrospinning technique for biomedical applications. *Polymer (Guildf)* **49**: 5603–5621.
67 Xie, J., MacEwan, M.R., Schwartz, A.G., and Xia, Y. (2010). Electrospun nanofibers for neural tissue engineering. *Nanoscale* **2**: 35–44.
68 Serafim, A., Cecoltan, S., Lungu, A. et al. (2015). Electrospun fish gelatin fibrous scaffolds with improved bio-interactions due to carboxylated nanodiamond loading. *RSC Adv.* **5**: 95467–95477.
69 Santin, M., Rhys-Williams, W., O'Reilly, J. et al. (2006). Calcium-binding phospholipids as a coating material for implant osteointegration. *J. R. Soc. Interface* **3**: 277–281.
70 Merolli, A. and Santin, M. (2009). Role of phosphatidyl-serine in bone repair and its technological exploitation. *Molecules* **14**: 5367–5381.
71 Monge, S., Canniccioni, B., Graillot, A., and Robin, J.-J. (2011). Phosphorus-containing polymers: a great opportunity for the biomedical field. *Biomacromolecules* **12**: 1973–1982.
72 Watson, B.M., Kasper, F.K., and Mikos, A.G. (2014). Phosphorous-containing polymers for regenerative medicine. *Biomed. Mater.* **9** (25014).
73 Filmon, R., Grizon, F., Baslé, M.F., and Chappard, D. (2002). Effects of negatively charged groups (carboxymethyl) on the calcification of poly(2-hydroxyethyl methacrylate). *Biomaterials* **23**: 3053–3059.
74 Koh, M.-Y., Ohtsuki, C., and Miyazaki, T. (2011). Modification of polyglutamic acid with silanol

groups and calcium salts to induce calcification in a simulated body fluid. *J. Biomater. Appl.* **25**: 581–594.
75 Stancu, I.-C., Dragusin, D.M., Vasile, E. et al. (2011). Porous calcium alginate-gelatin interpenetrated matrix and its biomineralization potential. *J. Mater. Sci. - Mater. Med.* **22**: 451–460.
76 Zhou, Y., Yang, J., Lin, Z. et al. (2014). Triclosan-loaded poly(amido amine) dendrimer for simultaneous treatment and remineralization of human dentine. *Colloids Surf., B* **115**: 237–243.
77 Li, J., Yang, J., Li, J. et al. (2013). Bioinspired intrafibrillar mineralization of human dentine by PAMAM dendrimer. *Biomaterials* **34**: 6738–6747.
78 Vasile, E., Serafim, A., Petre, D. et al. (2014). Direct synthesis and morphological characterization of gold-dendrimer nanocomposites prepared using PAMAM succinamic acid dendrimers: preliminary study of the calcification potential. *Sci. World J.* **2014**: 103462.
79 Penczek, S., Pretula, J., and Kaluzynski, K. (2005). Poly(alkylene phosphates): From synthetic models of biomacromolecules and biomembranes toward polymer - Inorganic hybrids (mimicking biomineralization). *Biomacromolecules* **6**: 547–551.
80 Stancu, I., Filmon, R., Cincu, C. et al. (2004). Synthesis of methacryloyloxyethyl phosphate copolymers and in vitro calcification capacity. *Biomaterials* **25**: 205–213.
81 Wang, D.-A., Williams, C.G., Yang, F. et al. (2005). Bioresponsive phosphoester hydrogels for bone tissue engineering. *Tissue Eng.* **11**: 201–213.
82 Dragusin, D.M., Serafim, A., Zecheru, T. et al. (2011). Casein - nanosized nucleator for in vitro mineralization. *Optoelectron. Adv. Mater. Rapid Commun.* **5**: 1320–1324.
83 Dragusin, D.M., Giol, D.E., Serafim, A. et al. (2011). Casein-PHEMA: in vitro formation of nanometric Ca-P nuclei. *Dig. J. Nanomater. Biostruct.* **6**: 1909–1918.
84 Serafim, A., Vasile, E., Cristescu, I. et al. (2014). Biomimetic apatite deposition within casein-loaded hydrogel scaffolds. *Key Eng. Mater.* **614**: 22–25.
85 Cardoso, M.V., Chaudhari, A., Yoshida, Y. et al. (2014). Bone tissue response to implant surfaces functionalized with phosphate-containing polymers. *Clin. Oral Implants Res.* **25**: 91–100.
86 Watson, B.M., Kasper, F.K., Engel, P.S., and Mikos, A.G. (2014). Synthesis and characterization of injectable, biodegradable, phosphate-containing, chemically cross-linkable, thermoresponsive macromers for bone tissue engineering. *Biomacromolecules* **15**: 1788–1796.
87 Huang, P., Bi, X., Gao, J. et al. (2016). Phosphorylated poly(sebacoyl diglyceride) – a phosphate functionalized biodegradable polymer for bone tissue engineering. *J. Mater. Chem. B* **4**: 2090–2101. https://doi.org/10.1039/c5tb02542g.
88 Chappard, D., Baslé, M.-F., Legrand, E., and Audran, M. (2008). Trabecular bone microarchitecture: a review. *Morphologie* **92**: 162–170.
89 Brandi, M.L. (2009). Microarchitecture, the key to bone quality. *Rheumatology* **48**: iv3–iv8.
90 Chappard, D., Baslé, M.F., Legrand, E. et al. (2011). New laboratory tools in the assessment of bone quality. *Osteoporos. Int.* **22**: 2225–2240.
91 Legeros, R.Z., Garrido, C.A., Lobo, S.E., and Turíbio, F.M. (2011). Biphasic calcium phosphate bioceramics for orthopaedic reconstructions: clinical outcomes. *Int. J. Biomater.* https://doi.org/10.1155/2011/129727.
92 Dumas, A., Gaudin-Audrain, C., Mabilleau, G. et al. (2006). The influence of processes for the purification of human bone allografts on the matrix surface and cytocompatibility. *Biomaterials* **27**: 4204–4211.
93 Albee, F.H. (1920). Studies in bone growth: triple calcium phosphate as a stimulus to osteogenesis. *Ann. Surg.* **71**: 32–39.
94 Laurencin, C., Khan, Y., and El-Amin, S.F. (2014). Bone graft substitutes. *Expert Rev. Med. Devices* **3**: 49–57.
95 Dorozhkin, S.V. (2012). Biphasic, triphasic and multiphasic calcium orthophosphates. *Acta Biomater.* **8**: 963–977.
96 Shavandi, A., Bekhit, A.E.-D.A., Sun, Z.F., and Ali, A. (2015). A review of synthesis methods, properties and use of hydroxyapatite as a substitute of bone. *J. Biomimetics Biomater. Biomed. Eng.* **25**: 98–117.
97 Fellah, B.H., Gauthier, O., Weiss, P. et al. (2008). Osteogenicity of biphasic calcium phosphate ceramics and bone autograft in a goat model. *Biomaterials* **29**: 1177–1188.
98 Ghanaati, S., Udeabor, S.E., Barbeck, M. et al. (2013). Implantation of silicon dioxide-based nanocrystalline hydroxyapatite and pure phase beta-tricalciumphosphate bone substitute granules in caprine muscle tissue does not induce new bone formation. *Head Face Med.* **9** (1).
99 Walton, M. and Rothwell, A.G. (1983). Reactions of thigh tissues of sheep to blunt trauma. *Clin. Orthop. Relat. Res.* 273–281.
100 Filmon, R., Retailleau-Gaborit, N., Grizon, F. et al. (2002). Non-connected versus interconnected macroporosity in poly(2-hydroxyethyl methacrylate) polymers. An X-ray microtomographic and histomorphometric study. *J. Biomater. Sci., Polym. Ed.* **13**: 1105–1117.
101 Ruhe, P.Q., Hedberg, E.L., Padron, N.T. et al. (2003). rhBMP-2 release from injectable poly(DL-lactic-co-glycolic acid)/calcium-phosphate

cement composites. *J. Bone Joint Surg. Am.* **85**: 75–81.

102 Guldberg, R.E., Duvall, C.L., Peister, A. et al. (2008). 3D imaging of tissue integration with porous biomaterials. *Biomaterials* **29**: 3757–3761.

103 Ho, S.T. and Hutmacher, D.W. (2006). A comparison of micro CT with other techniques used in the characterization of scaffolds. *Biomaterials* **27**: 1362–1376.

104 Jones, A.C., Arns, C.H., Sheppard, A.P. et al. (2007). Assessment of bone ingrowth into porous biomaterials using MICRO-CT. *Biomaterials* **28**: 2491–2504.

105 Nyangoga, H., Aguado, E., Goyenvalle, E. et al. (2010). A non-steroidal anti-inflammatory drug (ketoprofen) does not delay beta-TCP bone graft healing. *Acta Biomater.* **6**: 3310–3317.

106 De Oliveira, J.F., De Aguiar, P.F., Rossi, A.M., and Soares, G.A. (2003). Effect of process parameters on the characteristics of porous calcium phosphate ceramics for bone tissue scaffolds. *Artif. Organs* **27**: 406–411.

107 Chang, B.S., Lee, C.-K., Hong, K.-S. et al. (2000). Osteoconduction at porous hydroxyapatite with various pore configurations. *Biomaterials* **21**: 1291–1298.

108 Kim, K., Yeatts, A., Dean, D., and Fisher, J.P. (2010). Stereolithographic bone scaffold design parameters: osteogenic differentiation and signal expression. *Tissue Eng. Part B: Rev.* **16**: 523–539.

109 Bose, S., Vahabzadeh, S., and Bandyopadhyay, A. (2013). Bone tissue engineering using 3D printing. *Mater. Today* **16**: 496–504.

110 Schwartzwalder, K., Somers, H., and Somers, A.V. (1963). Method of making porous ceramic articles. US Patent 3,090,094.

111 Guillaume, B. (2016). Dental implants: a review. *Morphologie* https://doi.org/10.1016/j.morpho.2016.02.002.

112 Ripamonti, U. (1996). Osteoinduction in porous hydroxyapatite implanted in heterotopic sites of different animal models. *Biomaterials* **17**: 31–35.

113 Holmes, R.E., Bucholz, R.W., and Mooney, V. (1987). Porous hydroxyapatite as a bone graft substitute in diaphyseal defects: a histometric study. *J. Orthop. Res.* **5**: 114–121.

114 Terranova, L., Libouban, H., Mallet, R., and Chappard, D. (2015). Analysis of β-tricalcium phosphate granules prepared with different formulations by nano-computed tomography and scanning electron microscopy. *J. Artif. Organs* https://doi.org/10.1007/s10047-015-0838-9.

115 Filmon, R., Retailleau-Gaborit, N., Brosard, G. et al. (2009). Preparation of b-TCP granular material by polyurethane foam technology. *Image Anal. Stereol.* **28**: 1–10.

116 Wang, L., Barbieri, D., Zhou, H. et al. (2015). Effect of particle size on osteoinductive potential of microstructured biphasic calcium phosphate ceramic. *J. Biomed. Mater. Res. Part A* **103**: 1919–1929.

117 Groot, K. (1988). Effect of porosity and physicochemical properties on the stability, resorption, and strength of calcium phosphate ceramics. *Ann. N.Y. Acad. Sci.* **523**: 227–233.

118 Niu, W., Gill, S., Dong, H., and Bai, C. (2010). A two-scale model for predicting elastic properties of porous titanium formed with space-holders. *Comput. Mater. Sci.* **50**: 172–178.

119 Karageorgiou, V. and Kaplan, D. (2005). Porosity of 3D biomaterial scaffolds and osteogenesis. *Biomaterials* **26**: 5474–5491.

120 Aste, T., Saadatfar, M., and Senden, T.J. (2005). Geometrical structure of disordered sphere packings. *Phys. Rev. E: Stat. Nonlinear Soft Matter Phys.* **71**: 061302.

121 Jerram, D.a., Cheadle, M.J., Hunter, R.H., and Elliott, M.T. (1996). The spatial distribution of grains and crystals in rocks. *Contrib. Mineral. Petrol.* **125**: 60–74.

122 Chappard, D., Legrand, E., Pascaretti, C. et al. (1999). Comparison of eight histomorphometric methods for measuring trabecular bone architecture by image analysis on histological sections. *Microsc. Res. Tech.* **45**: 303–312.

123 Takemoto, M., Fujibayashi, S., Neo, M. et al. (2005). Mechanical properties and osteoconductivity of porous bioactive titanium. *Biomaterials* **26**: 6014–6023.

124 Libicher, M., Hillmeier, J., Liegibel, U. et al. (2006). Osseous integration of calcium phosphate in osteoporotic vertebral fractures after kyphoplasty: initial results from a clinical and experimental pilot study. *Osteoporos. Int.* **17**: 1208–1215.

125 N'Diaye, M., Degeratu, C., Bouler, J.M., and Chappard, D. (2013). Biomaterial porosity determined by fractal dimensions, succolarity and lacunarity on microcomputed tomographic images. *Mater. Sci. Eng., C* **33**: 2025–2030.

126 Chappard, D. and Stancu, I.-C. (2015). Porosity imaged by a vector projection algorithm correlates with fractal dimension measured on 3D models obtained by microCT. *J. Microsc.* **258**: 24–30.

127 Kün-Darbois, J.-D., Libouban, H., and Chappard, D. (2015). Botulinum toxin in masticatory muscles of the adult rat induces bone loss at the condyle and alveolar regions of the mandible associated with a

bone proliferation at a muscle enthesis. *Bone* **77**: 75–82.

128 Chappard, D. and Libouban, H. (2016). Bone loss also concerns the epiphysis in the BTX rat model of disuse osteoporosis. *J. Anat. Soc. Ind.* **65**.

129 Chappard, D., Terranova, L., Mallet, R., and Mercier, P. (2015). 3D porous architecture of stacks of β-TCP granules compared with that of trabecular bone: a microCT, vector analysis, and compression study. *Front. Endocrinol. (Lausanne)* **6**.

130 Beven, K. and Germann, P.F. (1982). Macropores and water flows in soils. *Water Resour. Res.* **18**: 1311–1325.

131 Bear, J. (2013). *Dynamics of Fluids in Porous Media.* Courier Corporation.

132 Chappard, D., Legrand, E., Haettich, B. et al. (2001). Fractal dimension of trabecular bone: comparison of three histomorphometric computed techniques for measuring the architectural two-dimensional complexity. *J. Pathol.* **195**: 515–521.

133 Haire, T.J., Hodgskinson, R., Ganney, P.S., and Langton, C.M. (1998). A comparison of porosity, fabric and fractal dimension as predictors of the Young's modulus of equine cancellous bone. *Med. Eng. Phys.* **20**: 588–593.

134 Hu, B.X., Meerschaert, M.M., Barrash, W. et al. (2009). Examining the influence of heterogeneous porosity fields on conservative solute transport. *J. Contam. Hydrol.* **108**: 77–88.

135 de Melo, R.H.C. and Conci, A. (2011). How succolarity could be used as another fractal measure in image analysis. *Telecommun. Syst.* **52**: 1643–1655.

136 De Melo, R.H.C. (2007). Using fractal characteristics such as fractal dimension, lacunarity and succolarity to characterize texture patterns on images. PhD thesis. Federal University of Fluminense.

137 Mandelbrot, B. (1977). The Fractal Geometry of Nature.

138 Ndiaye, M., Terranova, L., Mallet, R. et al. (2015). Three-dimensional arrangement of beta-tricalcium phosphate granules evaluated by microcomputed tomography and fractal analysis. *Acta Biomater.* **11**: 404–411.

4

Zirconia-Based Composites for Biomedical Applications

Paola Palmero

Department of Applied Science and Technology, INSTM R.U. PoliTO, LINCE Laboratory, Politecnico di Torino, Corso Duca degli Abruzzi, 24, 10129 Torino, Italy

4.1 Introduction

The most accepted definition of *biomaterial* is currently the one adopted by the National Institutes of Health Consensus Development Conference. According to this definition, a biomaterial is "any substance (other than a drug) or combination of substances, synthetic or natural in origin, which can be used for any period of time, as a whole or as a part of a system which treats, augments, or replaces any tissue, organ or function of the body" [1].

Medical practice today utilizes a large number of biomaterials for devices and implants to replace and/or restore the function of traumatized or degenerated tissues or organs and consequently to improve the quality of life of the patients. The key requirement is the biocompatibility, which means not only that the synthetic material has not to be harmful toward the body but also that the surrounding tissues must not alter the material. A material is "not biocompatible" if it is toxic or causes death of the surrounding tissues [2].

In this frame, the use of ceramic biomaterials has been growing in the past 40 years, especially for the repair and replacement of diseased and damaged parts of the musculoskeletal system. Besides their applications for hip, knee, and as bone gap filler, they are currently used as dental devices. An overview of the current biomedical applications of ceramics is given in Table 4.1.

Bioceramics are presently classified into three basic types, depending on their *in vivo* behavior: bioinert, bioactive, and/or bioresorbable [2], as shown in Table 4.2.

Bioinert refers to a material that retains its structure in the body after implantation, showing high chemical stability *in vivo*, as well as a high mechanical strength. At the same time, this kind of material shows a minimum interaction with the surrounding tissue and does not induce any immunologic host reactions. Bioinert is a term that should be used with care, since all materials introduced into the physiological environment elicit a response from living tissues [2]. However, for the purposes of biomedical implants, the term can be used to identify a minimal level of response from the host tissue. In this condition, the implant becomes covered

Table 4.1 Biomedical application of ceramics [1–4].

Application	Biomaterial
Artificial total hip, knee shoulder, elbow, wrist	High-density alumina, alumina–zirconia composites
Root repair material paste and sealer	Tricalcium silicate, dicalcium silicate, zirconia, calcium phosphate
Dental materials	Alumina; zirconia; bioactive glass; dense hydroxyapatite; alumina-, zirconia-, magnesia-based porcelain; leucite; lithium silicate
Maxillofacial reconstruction	Alumina, hydroxyapatite, hydroxyapatite-polylactic acid (HA-PLA) composites, bioactive glasses
Alveolar bone/ridge replacement	Porous alumina, dense apatite, bioactive glass, HA-PLA composites
Coating in orthopedic, dental, and maxillofacial prosthetic	Hydroxyapatite, bioactive glass, bioactive glass ceramics
Vertebrae spacers and extensors	Alumina
Temporary bone space fillers	Tricalcium phosphate Calcium and phosphate salts
Otolaryngology	Alumina, hydroxyapatite, bioactive glasses, and glass-ceramics

Bioceramics and Biocomposites: From Research to Clinical Practice, First Edition. Edited by Iulian Antoniac.

Table 4.2 Classification and examples of ceramics according to their *in vivo* behavior.

Type of ceramic	Examples	References
Inert	Alumina (Al_2O_3);	[2, 3, 5, 6]
	Zirconia (ZrO_2);	
	Carbon ceramics	
Bioactive	Bioglass®, glasses in the $Na_2O–CaO–SiO_2–P_2O_5$ system;	[2, 6, 7]
	Hydroxyapatite, $Ca_{10}(PO_4)_6(OH)_2$;	
	A-W glass-ceramics, which contains apatite and wollastonite in an $MgO–CaO–SiO_2–Al_2O_3$ glassy matrix;	
	Glass-ceramic Ceravital, in the system $SiO_2–CaO–Na_2O–P_2O_5–MgO–K_2O$	
Bioresorbable	α-/β-Tricalcium phosphate, α-/β-$Ca_3(PO_4)_2$	[2, 6, 8]
	Calcium sulfate, $CaSO_4 \cdot 0.5H_2O$	
	Calcium phosphate salts	

by a thin, nonadherent fibrous layer [9]. The thickness of such interfacial zone can be related to reactivity degree between tissue and device, as well as to motion and fit at the interface [2]. This interface is known to be a critical zone, with a remarkable effect on the durability of the implant. For nearly inert ceramics, the interface is free from chemical or biological bonds with the implants, allowing a relative movement and promoting the development of the fibrous capsule and eventually leading to deterioration of the implant. In the case of dense alumina (Al_2O_3) used as nearly interimplant, the fibrous tissue at the interface can be very thin. Consequently, if Al_2O_3 devices are implanted with a very tight mechanical fit and are loaded primarily in compression, they will be clinically successful. In contrast, if loading on an inert implant is such that interfacial movement can occur, the fibrous capsule can thicker till several hundred micrometers, and the implant loosens and fails [2]. According to Hench's classification [2], the attachment due to bone ingrowth into surface irregularities is named *morphological* fixation.

In the case of porous inert ceramics, there is an increased interfacial area between the implant and the natural tissue, resulting in an increased inertial resistance to movement of the device in the tissue. The ingrowth of bone into pores on the surface or throughout the implant and subsequent mechanical attachment to the device is named *biological* fixation [2].

Bioactive refers to materials that present the capability of inducing a favorable response from the host tissues, forming direct chemical bonds with bone or even with soft tissue, thus favoring bone ingrowth. They are generally regarded as ceramics that are designed to induce specific biological activity for repairing damaged organs, [10] but their mechanical properties are generally lower than those of bioinert ceramics. Attachment of such ceramics by chemical bonding with the bone is known as *bioactive* fixation [2].

Bioresorbable ceramics have the unique ability to degrade gradually, being replaced by regenerating natural tissue. This leads to a very thin or not existing interfacial layer. The chemical by-products of the degrading materials are absorbed and released via metabolic processes of the body. Major complications in the development of bioresorbable ceramics are (i) the maintenance of sufficient strength and stability of the interface during the degradation period and replacement by the natural host tissue and (ii) matching resorption rate of the implants with ingrowth rate of the natural tissue. In addition, because large quantities of material may be replaced, it is also essential that a resorbable material consists only of metabolically accepted substances, with considerable limitations on their compositional design.

This wide spectrum of biological interactions leads to a broad range of engineering design and strategies. In fact, bioactive materials (such as hydroxyapatite and tricalcium phosphate [TCP]) have poor mechanical properties, so their applicability is confined to implants that do not have to bear significant loadings, and the main requirement is to provide favorable surfaces for biological bonding and bone ingrowth. Otherwise, the critical conditions in joint replacement restrict the choice of materials to the harder and stronger ones, such as alumina (Al_2O_3) and zirconia (ZrO_2), even though they are not able to create (at least at the moment) a bone–implant interface and cannot be used as bone filler [2].

This chapter focuses on nearly inert ceramics and their clinical applications, and particularly on ZrO_2-based composites. The dissertation starts from monolithic Al_2O_3, which has been the first biomedical grade ceramic used for clinical applications. Al_2O_3 was introduced as a material for orthopedic bearings in the 1970s due to some outstanding properties, such as high strength and wear resistance, high corrosion resistance, and biocompatibility *in vivo*. Despite such good properties, Al_2O_3 is characterized by low fracture toughness, which limits its reliability and use in load-bearing applications.

ZrO_2 was introduced in the 1980s, in response to the brittleness of Al_2O_3 and the consequent potential failure of implants. ZrO_2 exhibits the best mechanical properties among oxide ceramics, well superior of those of Al_2O_3. However, some kinds of biomedical grade ZrO_2 and specifically those mostly used in orthopedic applications (3Y-TZP) showed degradation under *in vivo* conditions, which has caused the failure of some implants and consequently the disappearance of 3Y-TZP from the orthopedic field.

In order to overcome the low toughness of Al_2O_3 and the sensitivity to aging of ZrO_2, composites in the Al_2O_3–ZrO_2 system have been developed, moving from the Al_2O_3-rich side to the ZrO_2-rich one. The most common approach is to use ZrO_2 particles as reinforcement for the Al_2O_3 matrix, giving rise to zirconia-toughened alumina (ZTA) composites. The development of ZTA represents a key advancement in the ceramic implant field: due to the reduced risk of ceramics implant failure, ZTA is today one of the mostly used femoral head material.

A most innovative approach deals with the development of ZrO_2-based composites, which could be the way to fully exploit the outstanding properties of ZrO_2 without the major drawback associated with its degradation under *in vivo* conditions. Therefore, the last part of this chapter is dedicated to describe such more innovative composites, describing the role of selected second phases on the physical, mechanical, and biological behavior of the materials.

4.2 Inert Ceramics for Biomedical Applications: Monolithic Al_2O_3 and ZrO_2

4.2.1 Alumina (α-Al_2O_3)

High-density, high-purity (>99.5%) α-alumina (α-Al_2O_3) was the first bioceramic widely used for clinical applications. In orthopedic surgery, Al_2O_3 has been employed for nearly 45 years, because of combination of good biocompatibility, excellent corrosion resistance, high wear resistance, and high compressive strength.

The excellent wear and friction resistance of Al_2O_3 can be explained on the ground of the extremely smooth surface – which can be easily achieved by diamond polishing – the very high hardness and the surface wettability. Al_2O_3–Al_2O_3 bearing couples provide the lowest wear rate (linear wear <5 μm/yr [8]) among many tested couples, reaching values that could be 50 times lower than those of standard CoCr-UHMWPE (ultra high molecular weight polyethylene) couples [11].

The strong ionic bonds and oxygen-rich stoichiometry, which characterize the Al_2O_3 structure, make this ceramic chemically bioinert, unaffected by corrosive processes and exceptionally stable in the human body. Such stability is the key property in impeding Al-ion release from the bulk material and from wear debris, strengthening the biocompatibility of this ceramic and its safe use in the human body.

Concerning the mechanical properties, bulk Al_2O_3 ceramics are quite resistant under compressive loads but show a limited strength under tensile and bending stress. Therefore, through the years many efforts were made for improving the final density and decreasing the average grain size, thus to enhance the mechanical characteristics of biomedical grade Al_2O_3. In fact, the fabrication of dense Al_2O_3 bodies with fine grain size (about 1 μm) has become possible through many years of technological improvements, especially owing to two important findings both related to the sintering process:

(i) Use of sintering aids, such as small amount of MgO (<0.5 wt%). The addition of this dopant allowed Al_2O_3 ceramics to reach nearly full density at relatively low sintering temperature, with a beneficial effect on the final grain size. The optimization of the sintering aid amount was a further goal: it was found that excessive quantities of MgO should be avoided since their segregation at grain boundaries decreases the fatigue resistance, especially in corrosive physiological environment [2].

(ii) Use of posthot isostatic pressing (HIP) to push the final density close to the theoretical value at relatively low sintering temperatures, once again with a benefit on the final microstructure.

The improvement of the physical and mechanical properties of biomedical grade Al_2O_3 through the years is marked by the characteristics of first, second, and third generations of commercial Al_2O_3 bioceramics, as shown in Table 4.3 [12].

First-generation Al_2O_3 was introduced in the biomedical field in 1970, as an alternative to metal-UHMWPE bearing systems, and manufactured until 1992. Early clinical application of this ceramic showed a high failure rate (~13%) owing to incomplete densification during

Table 4.3 Characteristics of first-, second-, and third-generation Al_2O_3 and ISO requirements [2, 12, 13].

Property	First-generation Al_2O_3	Second-generation Al_2O_3	Third-generation Al_2O_3	ISO Al_2O_3 Standard 6474
Al_2O_3 content (wt%)	99.7	/	>99.8	≥99.5
Density (g/cm^3)	3.94	3.96	3.97–3.98	>3.90
Average grain size (μm)	<4.5	<3.2	<1.8	<7
Vickers hardness (HV)	1800	1900	2000	>2000
Bending strength (MPa)	400	500	580–630	>400 (in Ringer's solution
Fracture toughness (MPa $\sqrt{m}$)	2.8	2.8	2.8	/

air sintering, large grain size, and consequently low strength. Second-generation Al_2O_3 was introduced in 1992: as compared to previous products, there was an improvement in the selection of raw material: smaller grain size and higher purity. However, the ceramics were still processed by air sintering, therefore not reaching full densification. Third-generation Al_2O_3, introduced in 1995, was a further evolution regarding raw materials, manufacturing, and quality control. In particular, the introduction of a HIPping step after sintering allowed further reducing the grain size and enhancing the fired density, ultimately providing better wear properties, resistance to fracture, and durability [14]. This last generation of ceramics fulfilled the current International Standard Organization (ISO) requirements for medical grade Al_2O_3 implants and showed reduced fracture rate (of about 0.004–0.015%) as compared to previous devices.

The evolution of the grain size distribution from the first- to the third-generation Al_2O_3 is depicted in Figure 4.1 [15]. Besides the decrease of the average grain size, one can easily observe that the distribution becomes narrower moving from the first to the last generation. In particular, the size distribution of the early material was affected by a non-negligible amount of abnormally grown grains (AGG) of several microns in length.

Pezzotti and Yamamoto [15] investigated the correlation between grain size and strength in polycrystalline Al_2O_3, highlighting the role of the asymmetry (and associated anisotropy) of the crystalline corundum structure on such relationship. Al_2O_3 grains possess a pronounced thermal expansion mismatch between the *c*-axis and the axes lying on the basal plane. As a result, during cooling from the sintering temperature to room temperature, a larger shrinkage along the *c*-axis is produced as compared to the axes in the basal plane. This causes the creation of a certain fraction of "weak" grain boundaries, e.g. those comprised between grains sharing a common *c*-axis orientation and affected by high tensile residual stresses. Furthermore, it was demonstrated that

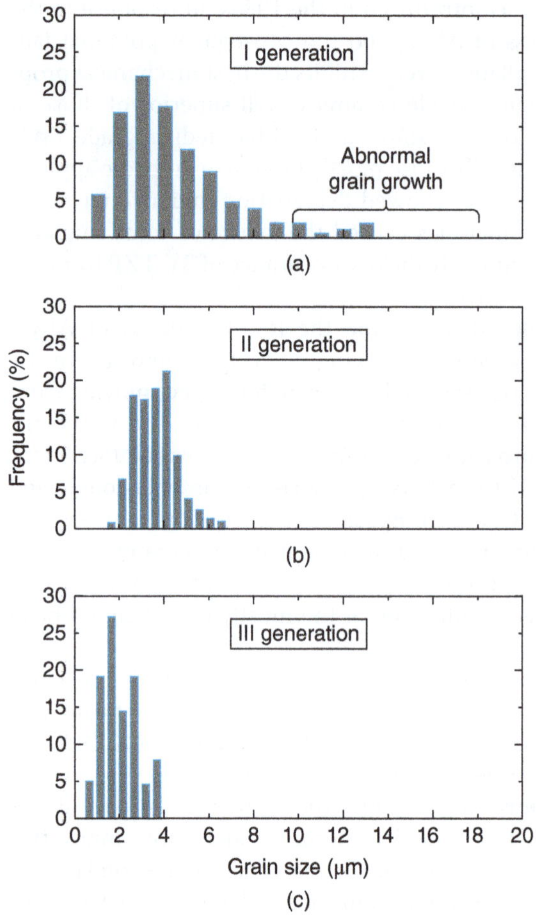

Figure 4.1 Grain size distribution as retrieved from Al_2O_3 femoral heads belonging to different manufacturing generations. Source: Pezzotti and Yamamoto 2014 [15]. Reprinted with the permission of Elsevier.

the residual stress magnitude increases with increasing grain size [16]. Weak grain boundaries act as preferential sites for the fracture origin when an external stress is applied, thus explaining the inverse relationship between grain size and material strength.

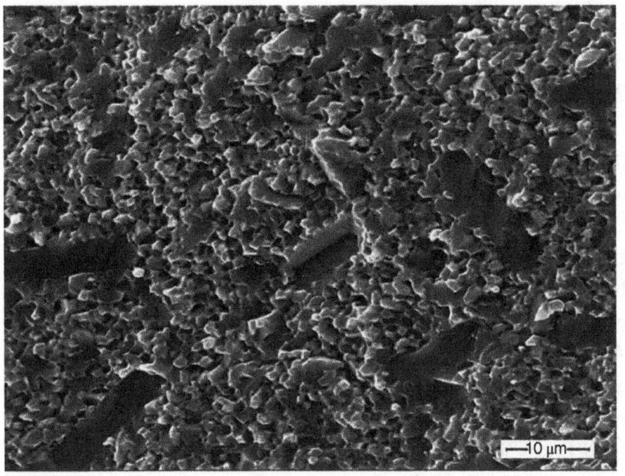

Figure 4.2 Field emission scanning electron microscopy (FESEM) micrograph of sintered Al_2O_3, showing several platelet-like grains (also known as abnormally grown grains, AGGs) embedded in a fine Al_2O_3 matrix.

In Al_2O_3, anisotropy also leads to AGG, recognized as large, platelet-like grains with a high aspect ratio embedded in a matrix of finer, equiaxed grains (Figure 4.2).

The occurrence of AGG is due to the faster growth of certain crystallographic planes as respect to others, with the higher growth rate being due to a relatively lower interfacial energy (i.e. higher driving force for growth). AGG are responsible, again, for "weak" grain boundaries, which could become the origin of fracture under an externally applied tensile load, therefore decreasing the overall mechanical properties of the specimen. With reference to Figure 4.1, we can observe a high cumulative fraction (≈5%) of AGG (from 10 to 18 μm) in first-generation Al_2O_3. In materials belonging to the second generation, we can find a quite high fraction of grains with size >4 μm: this fraction almost disappeared in third-generation materials, further explaining their increased mechanical performance.

Besides the important role of grain size, there are two major concerns for the reliability of Al_2O_3 bearings: the low fracture toughness (~3 MPa $\sqrt{m}$) and the susceptibility of Al_2O_3 to failure through slow crack growth at stresses well below to the ultimate fracture strength.

Under an applied stress σ, the stress at the tip of a crack can be described by the stress intensity K_I given by the following equation, as reviewed in [11]:

$$K_I = \sigma\sqrt{\pi a} \tag{4.1}$$

where $2a$ is the length of a crack. It is assumed that fast failure in brittle materials occurs when K_I becomes equal or greater that the critical intensity factor, K_{IC}, commonly named fracture toughness. Therefore, the fracture strength σ_f can be written as:

$$\sigma_f = \frac{K_{IC}}{\sqrt{\pi a}} \tag{4.2}$$

Equation (4.2) shows that the fracture strength of a brittle material depends on the fracture toughness and the flaw size, and represents the critical condition for the *fast crack growth*. However, brittle materials can also undergo a phenomenon known as *slow crack growth* (also referred to as *subcritical crack growth*, SCG) which can occur at values well below the σ_f value expressed by Eq. (2.2). In fact, besides the applied stress, ceramics can be also sensitive to environmental factors, such as water, water vapor, and temperature. The combined effect of high stress at the crack tip and reaction with water (or body fluids) allows the crack to grow, until reaching the critical length for failure. Thus, many efforts have been devoted to determine a threshold in stress intensity factor (K_{I0}), corresponding to the condition of zero crack velocity, at which subcritical crack propagation does not occur. K_{I0} values can be easily determined from crack velocity (V) versus K_I data, as schematically shown in Figure 4.3 [17]. In the scheme, we can observe three segments: the first (segment I) corresponds to chemically enhanced crack growth, which also allows the determination of K_{I0} below which cracks do not propagate. Segment II (plateau region) corresponds to region with a combination of stress and environment, where minor species in a liquid or gas control the crack tip reaction. Segment III is independent from the environment: microstructure, material thickness, and stress have a major influence on the crack growth rate within this segment. The toughness (K_{IC}) can be determined by

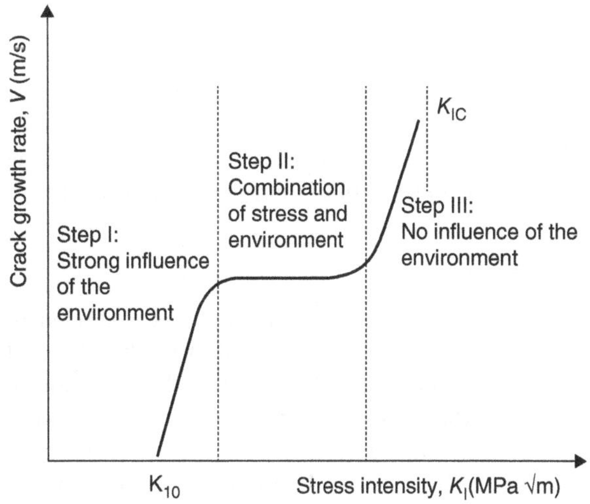

Figure 4.3 Scheme of crack growth rate–stress intensity behavior and determination of K_{I0} and K_{IC} values. Source: Adapted from Palmero 2015 [17].

extrapolation of the V–K_I curve to high crack velocities, as shown in the scheme.

For ceramics, K_{I0} is a key parameter since it determines the safe range for using the material in clinical applications: the higher K_{I0}, the higher the reliability and, hence, the higher the lifetime of the device. Seidel and Rödel [18] have experimentally measured K_{I0} for Al_2O_3 materials with different microstructures, giving rise to a mean value of 2.3 MPa $\sqrt{m}$, almost independent on the crack geometry.

SCG was a relevant problem in some Al_2O_3 devices used in joint replacements, especially for devices manufactured in the late 1970s, because of the impurity of alkali, calcium, and silicon oxides contained in precursors. Calcium segregation at grain boundaries and CaO interactions with the aqueous environment were the main reasons for strength degradation. In addition, silica impurities were found to limit densification and to promote grain growth during sintering, decreasing the material strength. Finally, segregation of alkalis at grain boundaries and their dissolution in physiologic liquids accelerated fatigue fracture [19]. It should be pointed out that the control of the strength degradation due to SGC and chemical impurities in Al_2O_3 was achieved only after the release of the standard ISO 6474 (Table 4.3) in 1980, which specified the minimum purity requirements of Al_2O_3 for clinical implants [20].

Besides the applications in orthopedics, Al_2O_3 has been also used for dental devices, starting from the work of Dr. Sami Sandhaus, a Swiss dentist, who developed a medical device entirely made of polycrystalline Al_2O_3, the CBS® dental implant [21]. This dental device enjoyed good clinical success, thus leading to the development of other highly pure Al_2O_3 implants. Besides the advantages of esthetic and biocompatibility, Al_2O_3 dental implants have shown some shortcomings in terms of design, stiffness, and modest fracture toughness, similarly to what already observed in orthopedics. The low flexural strength and the flaws introduced during the surface grinding have caused failures on these devices, leading to their demise in favor of titanium dental fixtures [21].

4.2.2 Zirconia (ZrO_2)

The research on ZrO_2 as a biomaterial was started in the late sixties. In 1969, Helmer and Driskell published the first paper concerning the biomedical application of ZrO_2 [22]. In the second half of the 1980s, ZrO_2 femoral heads were introduced in the market in response to the brittleness of Al_2O_3 and the consequent potential failure of implants [23, 24].

Biomedical grade ZrO_2 exhibits the best mechanical properties of oxide ceramics, well superior to those of Al_2O_3. In fact, the fracture toughness of ZrO_2 is almost the double than that of Al_2O_3 (6–8 MPa $\sqrt{m}$ versus 3–4 MPa $\sqrt{m}$) and the strength can reach values around 2 GPa for a fine-grained material [11, 25].

This exceptional mechanical strength is due to the phase transformation toughening mechanism, which is able to increase the crack propagation resistance in ZrO_2 [26]. To explain such phenomenon, we should introduce the three polymorphic ZrO_2 forms: monoclinic (m), tetragonal (t), and cubic (c). Pure ZrO_2 is monoclinic at room temperature, and this phase is stable up to 1170 °C. Above this temperature, it transforms into tetragonal and then into cubic phase at 2370 °C. During cooling, a martensitic tetragonal-to-monoclinic (t–m) transformation takes place in a temperature range of about 100 °C below 1070 °C. This phase transformation is associated with a volume expansion of approximately 3–4% and to large shear strain (~7%) [27]. The stress generated by such volume expansion originates cracks in pure ZrO_2 ceramics that on cooling from sintering temperatures breaks into pieces at room temperature.

However, by adding suitable stabilizers, the t-ZrO_2 phase can be retained at room temperature in a metastable phase, thus avoiding the negative – previously described – transformation. In fact, it was found that alloying with oxides whose cations have a lower valence as compared to Zr^{4+} (such as CaO, MgO, La_2O_3, and Y_2O_3), the strained m-ZrO_2 phase at room temperature is disfavored, whereas the more symmetric metastable c-ZrO_2 and t-ZrO_2 lattice structures are stabilized [28]. These c and t phases are analogous to those in pure ZrO_2 but have dopant ions substituted on Zr^{4+} sites and have a fraction of oxygen sites vacant to retain charge neutrality. The amount of dopant required for stabilization is substantial: for instance, the addition of 8 mol% of Y_2O_3 to ZrO_2 allows the stabilization of a cubic, fully stabilized zirconia (FSZ), in which one oxygen vacancy is created for every two yttrium ions [28]. Partial stabilization can be obtained at lower yttria content (4–7%) or by adding other stabilizing oxides (CaO, MgO, CeO_2) in proper amount to pure ZrO_2, generating multiphase materials known as partially stabilized zirconia (PSZ). The microstructure of PSZ at room temperature generally consists of c-ZrO_2 as the major phase, with m- and t-ZrO_2 precipitates as the minor phases. These precipitates, having a characteristic lenticular morphology (approximately 200 nm diameter and 75 nm thick) may exist at grain boundaries or within the cubic matrix grains.

The development of ZrO_2 as an engineering material was marked by Garvie et al. who in their paper "*Ceramic Steel?*" [29] clarified the role of the t–m transformation in improving the mechanical strength and toughness of PSZ ceramics. They observed that metastable t-ZrO_2 precipitates finely dispersed within the c matrix were

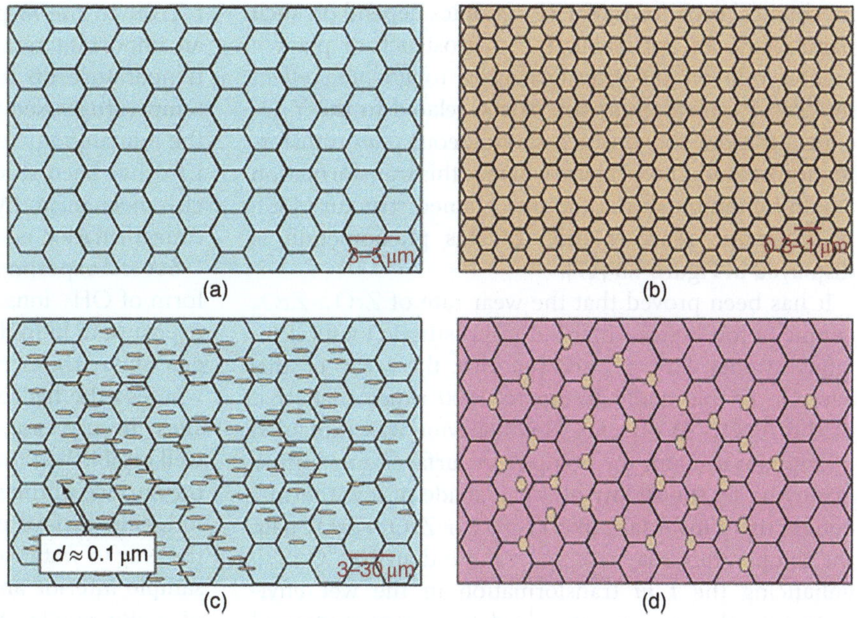

Figure 4.4 Schematic representation of the microstructures of the main types of ZrO_2 ceramics and composites: (a) cubic, fully stabilized zirconia (FSZ); (b) tetragonal zirconia polycrystal (TZP); (c) partially stabilized zirconia (PSZ), with tetragonal precipitates in a cubic matrix; (d) zirconia-toughened alumina (ZTA), with tetragonal zirconia grains in an Al_2O_3 matrix. Source: Chevalier and Gremillard 2011 [28]. Reprinted with the permission of Elsevier.

able to retransform into the *m* phase when the constraint exerted by the matrix was relieved, i.e. by a crack advancing in the material. The presence of tensile stresses in the vicinity of a crack allows the metastable *t*-ZrO_2 grains to transform into *m*-phase, leading to the formation of a transformation zone. An enhancement in toughness is obtained, because the energy associated with crack propagation is dissipated both in the *t*–*m* transformation and in overcoming the compression stresses due to the volume expansion. Additional contributions to toughness may result from microcracking associated with accommodation of the transformation shape strain and from crack deflection within the transformation zone ahead of the crack [30].

The development of PSZ with such peculiar microstructure can be obtained by adding 8–10 mol% of MgO to ZrO_2 or 4–7 mol% of Y_2O_3 to ZrO_2 [28]. However, in this last system, due to the higher solubility of Y_2O_3 in the ZrO_2 lattice as compared to MgO, it is also possible to retain at room temperature a pure, metastable tetragonal phase. These ceramics are named tetragonal zirconia polycrystals (TZP). In Figure 4.4, a schematic representation of the microstructures of the main types of ZrO_2 ceramics and composites is depicted [28].

TZP has been widely used in biomedical applications. Yttria-stabilized TZP (Y-TZP) ceramics were introduced in the 1980s for use in femoral heads because of their higher fracture toughness compared with Al_2O_3 and low wear rate [24]. In general, Y-TZP refers to ZrO_2 compositions containing 1.5–3.5 mol% Y_2O_3 in solid solution. However, biomedical grade TZP typically contains 3 mol% Y_2O_3 (often referred to as 3Y-TZP). The sintered material commonly consists of a single phase (the metastable *t* phase), fine-grained (0.1–1 µm), fully densified microstructure. With this microstructure and in the absence of strength-limiting flaws, Y-TZP is the strongest and tougher of the ZrO_2-based ceramic materials (see Table 4.4). The fraction of *t*-phase retained at room temperature is dependent on the size of grains and on the Y_2O_3 content. As a consequence, also the

Table 4.4 Typical physical and mechanical properties of load-bearing ceramics for medical devices [20, 24, 25, 31–34].

Property	Al_2O_3	3Y-TZP	ZTA	ATZ
Density (g/cm^3)	3.98	6.08	5.00	5.51
Average grain size (µm)	≤1.8	0.3–0.5	0.4–0.8	0.4
Flexural strength (MPa)	>550	900–1200	900	>1200
Young's modulus (GPa)	380	210	285	n.d.
Fracture toughness, K_{IC} (MPa $\sqrt{m}$)	4–5	6–10	5–7	6.5–8
K_{I0} (MPa $\sqrt{m}$)	2.5	3.2	4.0	/
Hardness (HV)	2200	1000–1300	1500	1530

mechanical properties of TZP ceramics depend on such parameters. In particular, the microstructure plays a pivotal role on the transformation toughening effect in TZP: a critical grain size exists, related to the Y_2O_3 concentration, above which spontaneous *t*–*m* transformation of grains takes place, whereas this transformation would be inhibited in a too fine-grained structure [35]. A schematic representation of this phenomenon is displayed in Figure 4.5 [17].

It has been proved that the wear rate of ZrO_2–ZrO_2 couple is too high to be used in prosthetic joints. Previous studies [36, 37] showed that the wear of this ceramic couple could be up to 5000 times than that of the Al_2O_3–Al_2O_3 one. This behavior was explained taking into account the increase in surface temperature occurring by the sliding of a pair made of low thermal conductivity materials, like ZrO_2. For ZrO_2–ZrO_2 pair, the temperature may rise up to more than 100 °C [38], enhancing the *t*–*m* transformation in the wet environment. This process may lead to several undesired phenomena, such as cracking, pull-out, and catastrophic abrasive wear [24].

It should be mentioned, however, that the recent work of Chevalier et al. [39] opens new perspectives: pin-on-disc tests performed using water as lubricant showed that the wear rate of ZrO_2–ZrO_2 pair was 1 order of magnitude lower than that of the Al_2O_3–Al_2O_3 one.

Despite the excellent fracture strength and fracture toughness of ZrO_2 ceramics, some compositions, such as 3Y-TZP, present a major drawback, since they undergo low-temperature degradation (LTD) in moist atmosphere. This aging phenomenon causes loss of strength and generation of microcracking in presence of water, as discussed in the comprehensive review by Chevalier et al. [39]. LTD consists of a slow transformation of metastable

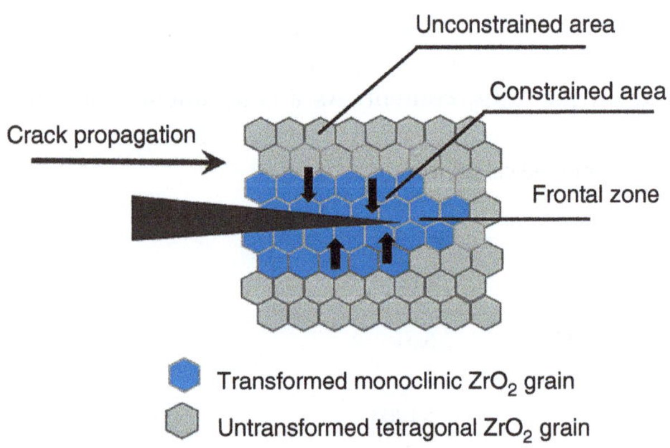

Figure 4.5 Schematic illustration of stress-induced phase transformation toughening, showing transformed *m*-ZrO_2 grains, exerting a compressive stress on an advancing crack. Source: Adapted from Palmero 2015 [17].

t-ZrO_2 to the *m*-phase (without any applied stress) in an important temperature range, typically from room temperature up to around 400 °C, thus including the temperature used for steam sterilization (~140 °C) and the human body temperature (37 °C) [27, 40]. Although LTD has been studied for more than 20 years, the precise mechanism by which moisture catalyzes the phase transformation is still not fully clarified.

Several experimental results show that moisture, in the form of OH^- ions, diffuses into the ZrO_2 lattice during exposure to humid atmosphere. Most probably, the oxygen of environmental water is located on vacancy sites, whereas the hydrogen is placed on adjacent interstitial sites. In any case, irrespective of the mechanism, it is well established that the *t*–*m* transformation starts from the surface of the sample and then proceed in the bulk, inducing surface uplift and microcracks, thus opening the way to water to penetrate below the surface, till the sample interior and finally leading to the development of major cracks. Schubert and Frey [41] showed that the penetration of OH^- leads to a lattice contraction, inducing tensile stresses in the surface of the grains. This destabilizes the *t*-phase and favors its martensitic transformation to the *m*-phase. The mechanism proceeds then in an autocatalytic way since the transformation of one grain leads to a volume increase, stressing up the neighboring grains. A schematic representation of this mechanism is proposed in Figure 4.6 [42].

The oxygen vacancies initially present in ZrO_2 play a major role on water diffusion rate, emphasizing the effect of the stabilizers inside the ZrO_2 lattice. In Y-TZP, many oxygen vacancies are generated by the trivalent cation (Y^{3+}), making the water diffusion rate higher than in other ZrO_2 ceramics stabilized with tetravalent cations, such as CeO_2 (Ce-TZP), in which Ce^{4+} does not induce oxygen vacancies [43].

LTD can have two important consequences for the use of Y-TZP in total hip arthroplasty (THA). First, it leads to roughening and microcracking on the Y-TZP-bearing surface, with a negative impact on the wear behavior. Second, aging generates flaws due to microcracking and transformation. Because Y-TZP is susceptible to SCG (see Figure 4.8), the growth of these flaws with aging can lead to a critical flaw size for SCG to proceed, eventually leading to failure of the bearing. In 1997, the US Food and Drug Administration (FDA) reported on the critical effects of standard steam sterilization procedure (134 °C, 2 bar pressure) on the surface roughness of ZrO_2 implants [28, 43]. In 2001, the Therapeutic Goods Administration in Australia announced a large series of failures (more than 800) in batches of implants processed with a new furnace technology by Saint-Gobain Desmarquest Prozyr® [28, 43]. This event had a catastrophic impact for the use of ZrO_2, and the market sale

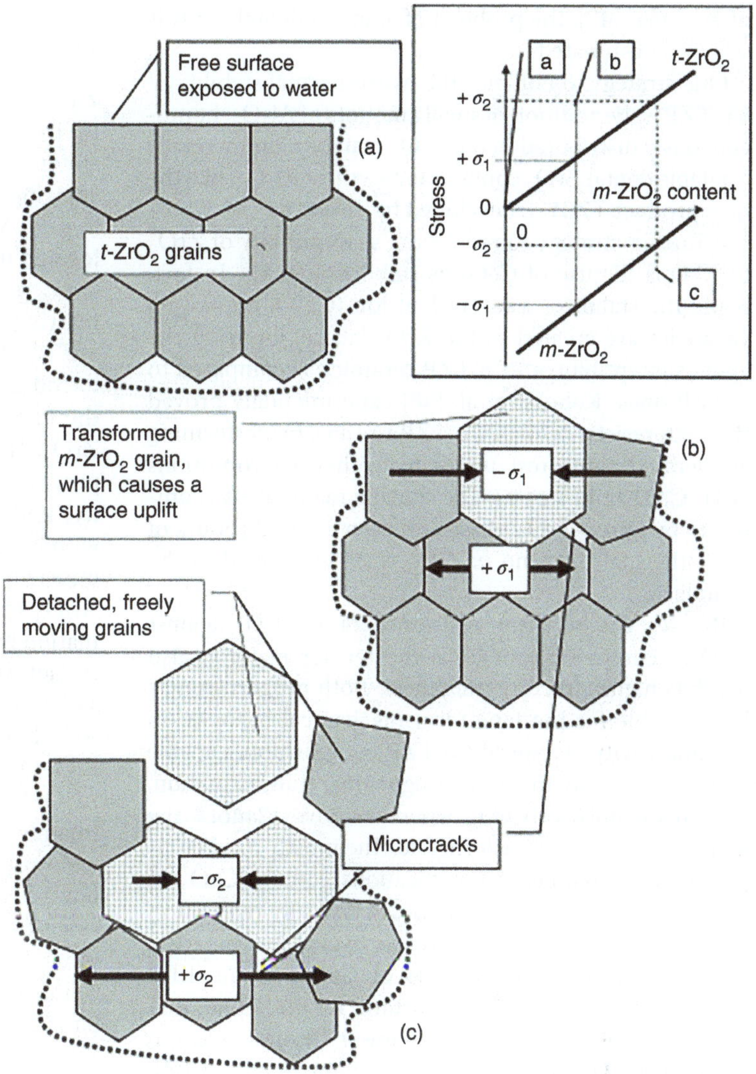

Figure 4.6 Schematic representation of how a partial transformation of *t*-ZrO_2 grains into the m-phase increases the tensile stress in the surrounding *t*-ZrO_2 grains. (a) Sample composed by *t*-ZrO_2 with the top surface exposed to water (liquid or vapor); (b) one grain transforms to monoclinic; on the top surface, it is free to expand, inducing surface uplift. Its expansion, limited by the surrounding untransformed grains, induces a compressive stress ($-\sigma_1$) in the grain and tensile stress ($+\sigma_1$) in the neighboring grains. (c) When more grains transform to monoclinic, they are less constrained and the compressive stress decreases to $-\sigma_2$, whereas they put in larger tensile stress ($+\sigma_2$) on the remaining *t*-ZrO_2 grains. The inset above right reports qualitatively the effect of the m-content on the residual stress in the remnant *m*- and *t*-ZrO_2 as described in Ref. [42]. Source: Lughi and Sergo 2010 [42]. Reprinted with the permission of Elsevier.

decreased of more than 90% between 2001 and 2002, with no evidence of clear renew.

The LTD of Y-TZP can be reduced, but not completely suppressed. Recent work has indicated that a combination of small grain size and high density can ensure a safe window for improving aging resistance [44]. However, the most promising application of ZrO_2 as bearing material appears as reinforcing phase in Al_2O_3 matrix, giving rise to ZTA composites, as reviewed in the following paragraph.

Quite surprisingly, contemporary to the retrieval of the Prozyr® femoral heads form the market, the dental community discovered the use of ZrO_2 [45, 46]. Inlays, onlays, single crowns, and fixed partial dentures have been realized by using ZrO_2 core. Moreover, also implant abutment and implants are today available in ZrO_2 [24]. The success of ZrO_2 in dentistry is imputable to its aesthetic properties, in addition to the mechanical specifications. In fact, 3Y-TZPs are available with translucence of 12–15%, and the color can be adjusted by doping, for example, with iron or rare earth elements, meeting the demand of natural-like restoration [28].

However, all these ZrO_2 dental restorations are exposed in the oral cavity to various factors, which promote degradation. Exposure to saliva, temperature changes, acidification during food intake, and cyclic loading during chewing lead to a decrease of the mechanical stability and possibly to LTD phenomena. However, if aging has been well documented in the orthopedic field, only few studies tackle the aging behavior of Y-TZP dental materials. Even though a few general papers devoted to dental ZrO_2 underline the need to "keep in mind that some forms of ZrO_2 are susceptible to aging and that processing conditions can play a critical role on the LTD of zirconia" [47], the problem of aging in dental ZrO_2 is still underestimated.

One strategy to enhance the hydrothermal stability of 3Y-TZP is the addition of small amounts of Al_2O_3, homogeneously distributed in the ZrO_2 matrix. Commercially available dental ZrO_2 contains 0.25 wt% of Al_2O_3, like the new product TZ3Y-E developed by Tosoh.

A further strategy to reduce the susceptibility of ZrO_2 to LTD is the use of CeO_2 as stabilizing oxide. In fact, being the stabilizer a tetravalent ion (Ce^{4+}), no oxygen vacancies are created in the ZrO_2 lattice, lowering the aging susceptibility of Ce-TZP ceramics as compared to Y-TZP ones. Kohorst et al. [48] experimentally proved the high resistance of 12Ce-TZP to LTD, by performing accelerated aging test under hydrothermal conditions (134 °C, 3 bar, in steam). The starting material was composed by pure *t*-ZrO_2 phase and even after 120 hours of hydrothermal tests, no *m*-ZrO_2 was determined in the samples.

Besides the superior resistance of Ce-TZP against LTD as compared to Y-TZP, the former material also exhibits higher fracture toughness. Both properties may be favorable for the long-term mechanical behavior in the oral cavity. A typical Ce-TZP composition, capable of giving rise to the *t–m* toughening transformation, contains 8 mol% of CeO_2, whereas above 12 mol% the system is no more transformable. The mostly used compositions for biomedical applications contain CeO_2 in the range 10–12 mol% and they are typically referred as to 10Ce-TZP and 12Ce-TZP, respectively.

In spite of the positive role of CeO_2 on the LTD behavior of ZrO_2, it is important to underline that Ce-TZP displays a significantly lower flexural strength (around 500 MPa for 12Ce-TZP) as compared to Y-TZP (1740 MPa for 3Y-TZP) as determined in [48]. This difference was mainly imputed to the larger grain size of the former material as compared to the latter one. In fact, 3Y-TZP was characterized by an average grain size of 0.5 μm, whereas the 12Ce-TZP exhibited larger grain size with an average diameter of 1.8 μm. The larger grain size of Ce-TZP also accounts for its increased transformability and hence fracture toughness. Values up to 10–20 MPa $\sqrt{m}$ were determined for this material [49].

Finally, when dental applications are concerned, it is important to underline that, from an esthetic point of view, Ce-TZP poses more problem than Y-TZP. CeO_2 is yellow and therefore products based on commercial available Ce-TZP powders range from light yellow to almost brownish. A further complication is due to the fact that when Ce^{4+} is reduced to Ce^{3+}, due to reduction conditions – as could happen on the long range in the oral cavity due to food with reducing capabilities – Ce-TZP tends to become dark gray [42].

4.2.3 Inert Ceramics for Biomedical Applications: ZTA Composites

ZTA refers to composite ceramics obtained by adding up to 25% of ZrO_2 to an Al_2O_3 matrix. An example of sintered microstructure is depicted in Figure 4.7 [50], showing a fine dispersion of *t*-ZrO_2 grains in the Al_2O_3 matrix. We can see that the ZrO_2 particles are mainly located in intergranular position, in spite some ultrafine ZrO_2 grains can be also observed within the Al_2O_3 matrix (arrows in Figure 4.7).

ZTA, developed in the second half of the seventies, was introduced in the biomedical field in order to overcome the brittleness of Al_2O_3 and the sensitivity to aging of ZrO_2. This can be the way to get benefits from the Al_2O_3 properties (hardness, stiffness, and thermal conductivity) and ZrO_2 transformation toughening mechanism, without the major drawback associated with its aging under hydrothermal conditions. In fact, the addition of Al_2O_3 to ZrO_2 significantly lowers the ZrO_2 transformation kinetics, allowing the use of ZTA in orthopedics. In fact, starting from June 2000, ZTA became available as femoral head material, commercialized by CeramTec AG (Plochingen, Germany) under the trade name of BIOLOX® *delta*. This material contains 76 wt% of Al_2O_3, 22.5 wt% of Y-TZP, and 1.4 wt% of other oxides (mainly chromium and strontium oxides). However, the widespread use of ZTA in orthopedic surgery started few years later, in 2003, after the FDA approval. Ever since, the use of ZTA in orthopedic surgery continuously increased: in the last 10 years, approximately one million CeramTec ZTA femoral heads and over 700 000 inserts have been implanted worldwide.

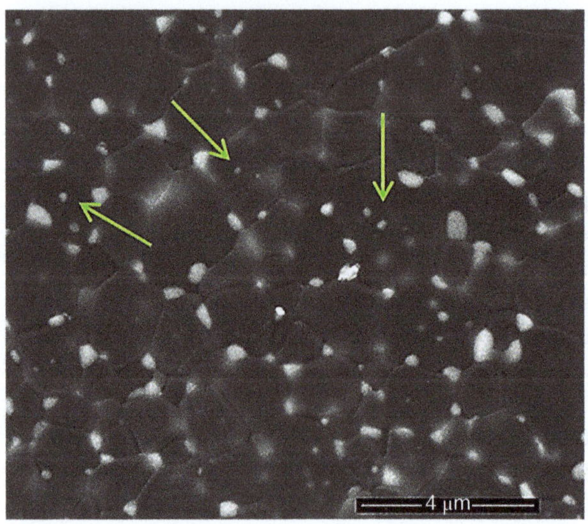

Figure 4.7 Scanning electron microscopy (SEM) micrograph of Al_2O_3–5 vol% ZrO_2 composite sintered at 1600 °C for 1 h. Source: Kern and Palmero 2013 [50]. Adapted with the permission of Elsevier.

In 2011, the Japanese KYOCERA Medical (Osaka, Japan) introduced in the market a second ZTA product named BIOCERAM® AZ209, containing 79 wt% of Al_2O_3, 19 wt% of unstabilized ZrO_2, and 2 wt% of other oxides [51]. Other medical ceramic suppliers are working on developing ZTA biomaterials for hip arthroplasty, but these new materials have not yet been commercialized.

In ZTA, the ZrO_2 particles can exhibit an *m*-phase or a *t*-phase, but the higher mechanical properties (strength and fracture toughness) have been observed in the latter case. Typical properties of ZTA are reported in Table 4.4 and compared to those of monolithic Al_2O_3 and ZrO_2. We can observe a clear increase of mechanical properties, in particular the flexural strength and fracture toughness, of ZTA as compared to monolithic Al_2O_3.

In order to maximize the fracture toughness of ZTA, it is important to optimize the ZrO_2 grains size, by controlling the composition and the processing conditions. In fact, as already reported, the ZrO_2 grain size must range between two critical values: the lowest is the size below which the transformation is completely hindered (even under stresses at the crack tip); the highest is the size for spontaneous transformation to the *m*-phase during cooling [52]. These critical sizes depend on the stiffness of the matrix, on the ZrO_2 amount into the ZTA composite and on the oxide stabilizer nature and content. As an example, ZTA containing 8–15 vol% of unstabilized ZrO_2 [53] showed lowest and highest sizes in the range 0.1–0.4 μm and 0.6–2.0 μm, respectively.

Most important, ZTA shows a higher threshold for subcritical crack propagation (K_{I0}) as compared to both monolithic Al_2O_3 and 3Y-TZP materials, indicating a higher reliability and expected lifetime for the devices based on ZTA [31, 32]. This behavior is shown in Figure 4.8, reporting the crack velocity diagram under static loading for monolithic Al_2O_3 and ZrO_2 and for two types of Al_2O_3–ZrO_2 composites [31]. The so-called microcomposite (Al_2O_3–10 vol% ZrO_2) has the typical microstructure of ZTA, with fine ZrO_2 particles located intergranularly in a fine (micronic or even submicronic) Al_2O_3 matrix (as shown for instance in Figure 4.7). The nanocomposite contains a lower amount of ZrO_2 particles (Al_2O_3–1.7 vol% ZrO_2) having a nanometric size (average diameter of 150 nm) evenly distributed in the Al_2O_3 matrix (average grain size of 5 μm). These ZrO_2 particles were found to be mainly intragranular, with almost a perfect spherical shape. The nanometric size of these ZrO_2 particles makes them almost untransformable.

The V–K_I curves [31] for the four ceramics show the typical three stages of SCG (compare with the scheme of Figure 4.3): by the extrapolation of the curves at very low ($V < 10^{-12}$ m/s) and high ($V > 10^{-2}$ m/s) crack velocities, the threshold K_{I0} (below which no crack propagation occurs) and the toughness K_{IC} values can be determined. K_{I0} and K_{IC} values for monolithic Al_2O_3, Y-TZP, and for the ZTA microcomposite are collected in Table 4.4.

From Figure 4.8, we can see that ZrO_2 exhibits higher K_{I0} and K_{IC} values than Al_2O_3. The difference between the K_{IC} values of these two monolithic materials is remarkable, and the highest value of ZrO_2 is well explained by its *t*–*m* transformation toughening effect ahead of a propagating crack, which leads to an increase in the work of fracture [54]. On the opposite, the lower slope of the segment I of the V–K_{IC} curve of ZrO_2 as compared to Al_2O_3 leads to not too far K_{I0} values. Al_2O_3 seems to have a lower susceptibility to water and thus to stress-assisted corrosion, whereas the ZrO_2 bonds are prone to chemisorption of the polar water molecules, showing a lower fracture energy of this material in presence of water or body fluid.

The ZTA microcomposite shows higher K_{IC} and K_{I0} values than the two monolithic ceramics. In fact, thanks to the Al_2O_3 matrix, this composite shows a low susceptibility to stress-assisted corrosion by water (or body fluid). At the same time, it is reinforced by transformable ZrO_2 particles. Therefore, its V–K_I curve slop is similar to that of Al_2O_3, but shifted towards higher K_I values.

Finally, we can see that the Al_2O_3–ZrO_2 nanocomposite is characterized by a K_{IC} value close to that of ZTA, but a significantly higher K_{I0}. In the nanocomposite, the transformation toughening mechanism has to be ruled out since the *t*–*m* transformation is hindered by the too small size of the *t*-ZrO_2 grains. The behavior of

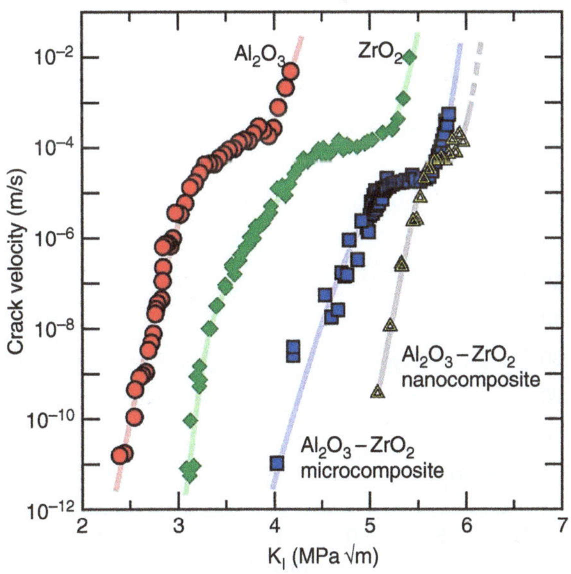

Figure 4.8 Crack velocity versus stress intensity factor (K_I) for biomedical grade Al_2O_3, Y-TZP, ZTA microcomposite, and Al_2O_3–ZrO_2 nanocomposite. Source: Chevalier et al. 2011 [31]. Reprinted with the permission of Elsevier.

nanocomposites was instead attributed to the different coefficient of thermal expansion (CTE) between Al_2O_3 (8×10^{-6} K^{-1}) and ZrO_2 (6×10^{-6} K^{-1}) [24], leading lo large residual stress in the composite with a strong impact on the SCG behavior. It was calculated an important residual compressive stress in the Al_2O_3 matrix, which superimpose to the stress applied by the external stress field, leading to a decrease of the stress intensity factor at the crack tip. A different effect of the residual compressive stress field at low (i.e. around K_{I0}) and high (i.e. at K_{IC}) applied stress intensity factor explains the higher slope of the V–K_I curve of the nanocomposite as compared to traditional ZTA microcomposite.

Because of the t-ZrO_2 particles present within the Al_2O_3 matrix, the strength degradation by hydrothermal aging in ZTA is limited, as compared to monolithic Y-TZP. This is illustrated in Figure 4.9 [31], showing the m-ZrO_2 fraction at various aging time for biomedical grade 3Y-TZP (green line) and for Al_2O_3–ZrO_2 micro- and nanocomposites (blue and yellow symbols). It is clear that both composites do not show any transformation under aging conditions (hydrothermal treatment at 134 °C, 2 bar), whereas 3Y-TZP undergoes rapid surface transformation.

However, remembering that aging occurs by nucleation and growth mechanisms, starting at the surface, the ZrO_2 particles should not form a continuous network in the Al_2O_3 matrix, meaning that their content should be below the percolation limit (~16 vol%) [11, 55]. In this way, the percolative pathway risk is reduced and, consequently, degradation cannot continue deep into the material.

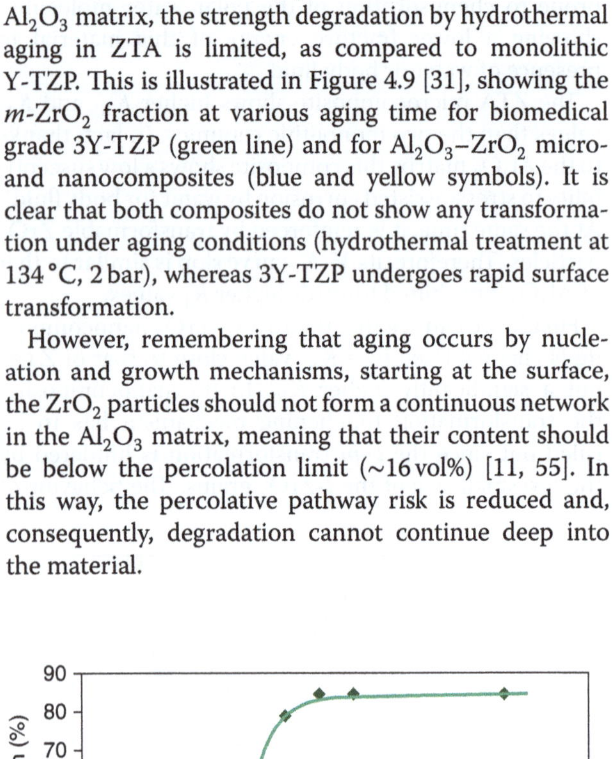

Figure 4.9 Aging kinetics (monoclinic fraction increase versus time at 134 °C, 2 bar) of biomedical grade 3Y-TZP (green line), Al_2O_3–ZrO_2 microcomposite, and nanocomposite. Source: Chevalier et al. 2011 [31]. Reprinted with the permission of Elsevier.

A further strategy to prevent the LTD susceptibility of ZTA is to add unstabilized ZrO_2 particles to the Al_2O_3 matrix, in which the metastabilization of the t-ZrO_2 grains is achieved thanks to their very fine grain size and to the presence of the stiffer Al_2O_3 phase. Therefore, if the addition of yttria is avoided, the formation of oxygen vacancies inside the ZrO_2 lattice is reduced, thus limiting the diffusion of water radicals in the ZrO_2 ceramics and consequent aging. This strategy is the one followed by KYOCERA Medical, which commercializes a ZTA product (Bioceram AZ209 product) containing 19 wt% of unstabilized ZrO_2 grains, as previously described [51].

ZTA also showed an excellent wear behavior. Hip simulator tests indicate that the wear of ZTA-on-ZTA is lower than that of Al_2O_3-on-Al_2O_3. The ZTA/ZTA couple displayed the highest resistance to wear and the lowest amount of surface roughness after five million cycles [51].

However, ZTA containing 14 vol% of Y-TZP particles underwent aging when tested for long time (19 months) in Ringer's solution, promoting the formation of an m-ZrO_2 surface layer, which leads to a significant reduction of the flexural strength [11].

These results demonstrate that, in spite of the advances shown by ZTA composites with respect to monolithic Al_2O_3 and ZrO_2 materials, there is still room for further optimization of the composites.

An example is provided by both BIOLOX *delta* manufactured by CeramTec AG (Plochingen, Germany) and AZ209 manufactured by the Japanese KYOCERA Medical. Both products contain small amount of SrO [51, 56]. During sintering, this additive reacts with Al_2O_3, leading to the *in situ* formation of plate-like aluminates (precisely, strontium hexa-aluminate). This approach, which is becoming increasingly popular [57–59], brings to a fracture toughness increment, since the elongated grains (with high aspect ratios) can induce additional toughening mechanisms by crack deflection and crack bridging [60]. By optimizing the microstructure and the sintering conditions, materials with remarkable mechanical properties are produced, being the flexural strength higher than 1200 MPa, the fracture toughness of 6.5 MPa $\sqrt{m}$, and the Vickers hardness of 1975 HV [11].

4.3 New Approach for Biomedical Grade Ceramics: Zirconia-Based Composites

4.3.1 Y-TZP/Al_2O_3 Composites

Monolithic Y-TZP, containing small amounts of Al_2O_3 (up to 0.25%) is one of the full-ceramic system currently used for dental applications, which is able to replace the traditionally used metals. Owing to their excellent strength, fracture toughness, and damage tolerance, compared with other dental ceramics, they are being used for crowns, bridges, inlays, multiple unit posterior bridges, full-ceramic post-and-core systems, and implant superstructures [61–63].

Kosmač et al. [64] compared the mechanical and aging behavior of standard and biomedical grade Y-TZP samples, the latter containing 0.25% Al_2O_3. Their results showed that, after accelerated aging tests carried out by autoclaving at 140 °C for 24 hours, the standard grade Y-TZP ceramics was characterized by a layer of about 100 μm of thickness on the surface, resulting in an almost 50% strength reduction. A significantly better behavior was determined for the biomedical grade samples since, in this case, a strength reduction after aging of only 10% was observed.

Zhang et al. [65] investigated the role of Al_2O_3 content (from 0.25% to 5%) on the mechanical and aging behaviors of Y-TZP. Their results were consistent with previous investigations confirming that the addition of a small amount of Al_2O_3 could significantly retard the degradation of Y-TZP [63, 66, 67] without compromising the mechanical properties [40, 67]. Accelerated hydrothermal tests were carried out in autoclave at 134 °C for 40 hours. Micro-Raman spectroscopy was carried out on polished cross-sections of 3Y-TZP, in order to determine the m-ZrO_2 phase content as a function of the depth below the surface. We can see from Figure 4.10a [65] that the m-ZrO_2 phase content profiles at the transformation front are the same for the Al_2O_3-free and Al_2O_3-doped 3Y-TZP. However, Al_2O_3 addition significantly decreased the depth of the transformation propagation. After 40 hours of aging, the transformation front penetrated up to a depth of 16 μm in the undoped material, the top of which (around 12 μm) was fully transformed. The transformation front was observed at a depth of about 10 and 12 μm in samples containing 2 and 5 wt% of Al_2O_3, respectively. A different behavior was observed for the sample containing 0.25 wt% of Al_2O_3, since here the m-ZrO_2 saturation plateau was not reached, even after 40 hours of hydrothermal degradation, and the onset of transformation only reached a depth of 4 μm. Cross-sections of the hydrothermally aged samples, at different Al_2O_3 contents, are shown in Figure 4.10b. The hydrothermally degraded regions appeared as a layer with a large amount of intergranular fracture and grain pull-out (Figure 4.10b). The dotted lines allow to better distinguish the degraded region by the pristine one: in fact, in all cases, a distinct border is easily recognized, which can be well correlated with the sharp drop from the m-ZrO_2 saturated plateau to zero, in the depth transformation profiles (Figure 4.10a). The thickness of the degraded zone, as measured by scanning electron microscopy (SEM) after 40 hours of aging, for the 5, 2, 0.25, and 0 wt% Al_2O_3-doped ceramics was 9, 8, 2, and 15 μm, respectively. This confirmed the results obtained by micro-Raman spectroscopy, showing that the addition of Al_2O_3 at 0.25 wt% had the highest degradation retarding effect on 3Y-ZTP.

The behavior shown in Figure 4.10 was explained on the ground of the Al ion segregation at ZrO_2 grain boundaries. In fact, according to Zhang et al. [65], only dissolved and segregated Al^{3+} ions at the ZrO_2 grain boundaries effectively contribute to the improved

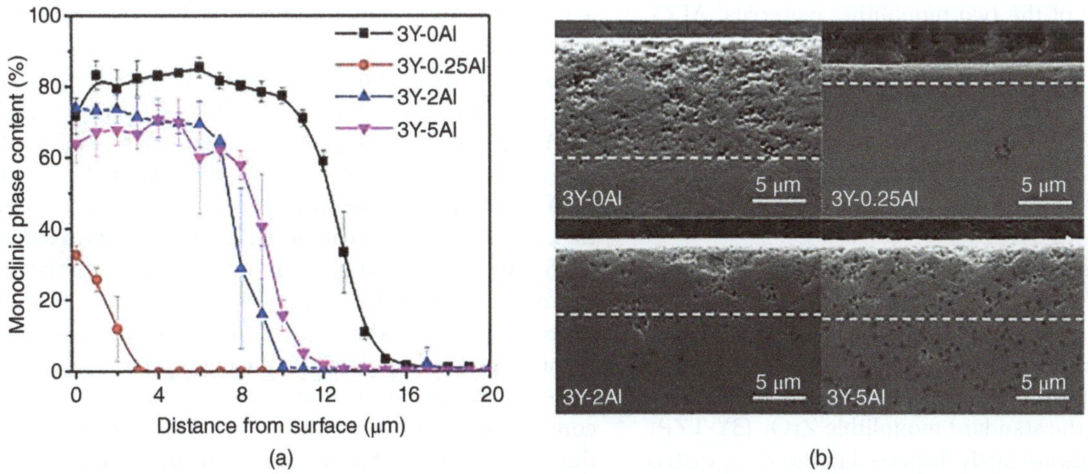

Figure 4.10 (a) Monoclinic ZrO_2 profiles acquired by micro-Raman spectroscopy on cross-sectioned 3Y-TZP samples containing different amounts of Al_2O_3 (0, 2.5, 2, and 5 wt%), sintered for 2 hours at 1550 °C after 40 hours of hydrothermally degradation at 134 °C; (b) the corresponding cross-sectional SEM images. The dotted lines in (b) underline the difference between the degraded zone and the pristine one. Source: Zhang et al. 2015 [65]. Reprinted with the permission of Elsevier.

degradation resistance of Y-TZP ceramics. A previous work demonstrated that the segregated Al^{3+} fundamentally changed the *t–m* transformation from nucleation-driven to growth-driven mechanism [68]. For 3Y-TZP ceramics, this situation is reached at Al_2O_3 content close to 0.25 wt%. On the contrary, in the 2 and 5 wt% Al_2O_3-doped Y-TZPs, the Al_2O_3 solubility limit in ZrO_2 was exceeded and the excess Al_2O_3 precipitated as a secondary phase at grain boundaries or triple points of the ZrO_2 grains. Such precipitated Al_2O_3 secondary phase could induce residual stresses during cooling, owing to CTE and elastic modulus mismatch between the Al_2O_3 and ZrO_2 phases. Since the thermal expansion coefficient of ZrO_2 is higher than for Al_2O_3, the ZrO_2 phase undergoes a net hydrostatic tensile stress, which favors the *t–m* transformation [50], thus explaining the lower degradation resistance of the 2 and 5 wt%-doped ZrO_2 materials as compared to the 0.25 wt%-doped one.

In spite of these achievements, showing increased properties and aging resistance in ZrO_2 samples doped with small amounts of Al_2O_3, it was demonstrated that when the Al_2O_3 content was increased to 25 wt% and the composite was sintered by HIP, the highest strength – over 2000 MPa, was yielded [69]. ZIRALDENT®, manufactured by Metoxit AG and having the above composition, is at the present the strongest biomedical ceramic known [69].

In 2004, Begand et al. [70] presented a new alumina-toughened zirconia (ATZ) material for THA. This material was developed and manufactured by Mathys Orthopädie GmbH (Mörsdorf, Germany) and introduced in the international market in 2010 with brand name Ceramys®. Similarly to the ZTA materials presented by CeramTec GmbH few years earlier, the attempt of Mathys with this new ATZ ceramic was to combine the advantages of the two monolithic materials, Al_2O_3 and ZrO_2, while avoiding their major drawbacks, i.e. the brittleness of Al_2O_3 and the sensitivity to aging of Y-TZP. The properties of the ATZ material proved to be remarkable (see Table 4.4) and in some cases better than those of ZTA, as specified by Mathys. Nevertheless, the ATZ material has up to date not achieved the broad use of its competitor ZTA [20].

The ATZ Ceramys consists of 80 wt% of ZrO_2 and 20 wt% of Al_2O_3. More in detail, Schneider et al. [71] described this product as formed by 61 vol% of *t*-ZrO_2, 17 vol% of *c*-ZrO_2, about 1 vol% *m*-ZrO_2, and Al_2O_3 for the remaining part. The *t*-ZrO_2 is stabilized with 3 mol% of Y_2O_3 as for the standard monolithic ZrO_2 (3Y-TZP). The Al_2O_3 grains are finely dispersed in the ZrO_2 matrix and the average grain size diameter approach is 0.4 μm, both for ZrO_2 and Al_2O_3. Ceramys ATZ was extensively tested in adverse aging conditions to determine its LDT behavior. In spite of the fine grain size of the ZrO_2 grains and the presence of the stiffer Al_2O_3 particles in the composite, the stabilization of ZrO_2 by 3 mol% of Y_2O_3 – the same used in monolithic ZrO_2 materials – put in evidence the wish of slightly overstabilizing the ZrO_2 phase to avoid LTD. Therefore, a certain fraction of *c*-ZrO_2 phase is present in the material, as previously detailed.

Kohorst et al. [48] investigated the microstructural and mechanical features of an ATZ composite, consisting in 20 wt% of Al_2O_3 in a 3Y-TZP matrix and compared them to monolithic 3Y-TZP (containing 0.25 wt% of Al_2O_3) and 12Ce-TZP. In Figure 4.11, the microstructures of these three materials are compared [48]. All samples are characterized by homogeneous microstructures, with average ZrO_2 grain size of 0.5 and 0.3 μm for 3Y-TZP and ATZ, respectively. 12Ce-TZP exhibited a larger grain size of 1.8 μm and, occasionally, showed grain pull-out, as shown by the arrow in Figure 4.11. In Figure 4.12a, the aging behavior of the same three materials is depicted. It can be observed a significant increase of the *m*-ZrO_2 phase content in 3Y-TZP and ATZ due to aging, although this increase was less pronounced in ATZ. In fact, as the transformation of ZrO_2 advances from grain to grain in a nucleation and growth process [40], the Al_2O_3 homogeneous dispersion can retard the progression of the transformation by reducing the contact area between ZrO_2 grains. Furthermore, the addition of Al_2O_3 leads to both an increase in stiffness and a change in elastic strain energy associated with the *t–m* transformation, which is consequently hindered. In the same figure, we can observe that Ce-TZP presents a very low starting amount of *m*-ZrO_2 phase, which does not increase with the aging time.

In Figure 4.12b, we can observe the evolution of the biaxial flexural strength as a function of the aging time for these three materials. First, the samples showed a remarkable difference in the starting value: in fact, average flexural strengths of 1740, 1093, and 495 MPa for 3Y-TZP, ATZ, and Ce-TZP were, respectively, determined. The larger grain size of 12Ce-TZP as compared to the other two samples (see Figure 4.11) accounts for its lower strength. During the maximum aging time of 128 hours, the strength of 3Y-TZP decreased to 1169 MPa, while that of ATZ slightly increased to 1378 MPa. Both changes are statistically significant. In contrast, 12Ce-TZP samples only showed a slight decrease – by less than 3% – after hydrothermal treatment. The gain in strength during aging experienced by ATZ might be attributed to the accumulation of compressive stresses in the near-surface zone, due to the volume increase associated with the *t–m* transformation. These stresses partly compensate for tensile stresses exerted during strength testing, and thus have a reinforcing effect [29, 47, 72]. According to these results, ATZ was recommended as promising alternative

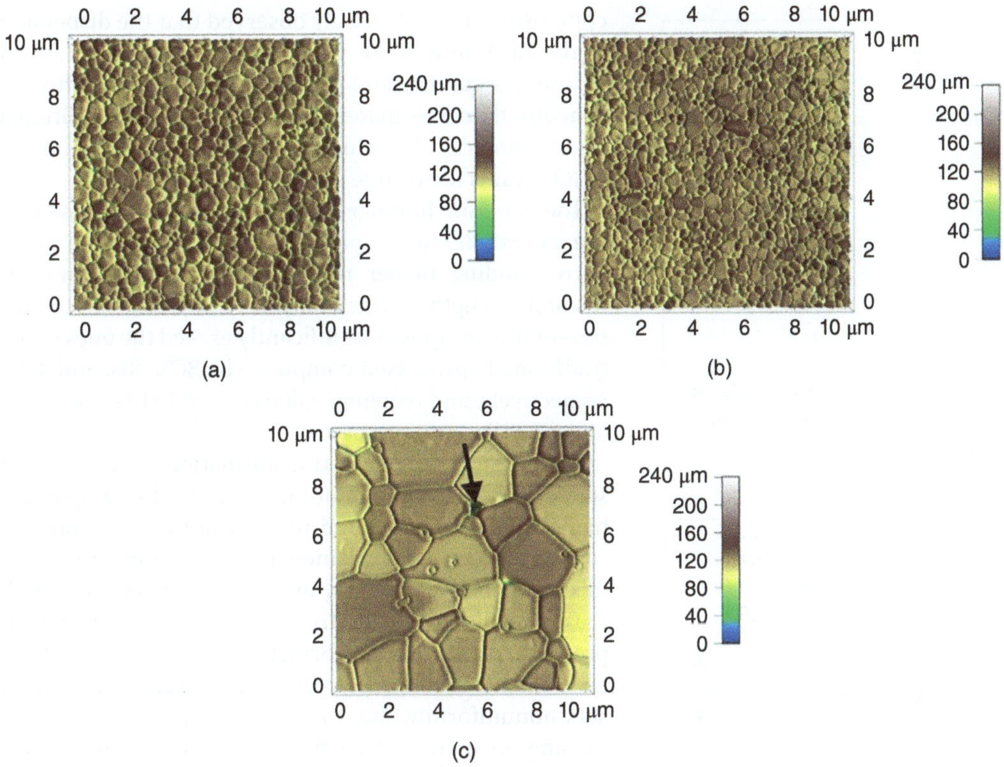

Figure 4.11 Atomic force microscopy (AFM) images of (a) 3Y-TZP, (b) ATZ, and (c) 12Ce-TZP. The arrow in (c) points to a location with a probable pull-out. Source: Kohorst et al. 2012 [48]. Reprinted with the permission of Elsevier.

to Y-TZP for dentistry applications. In fact, the use of ATZ may enhance the clinical long-term performance of ZrO_2-based restorations. Even if its initial strength is lower in comparison to 3Y-TZP, due to its long-term strength characteristics, ATZ is more qualified for the fabrication of restorations which are applied in the hydrothermal environment of the oral cavity.

In general, the mechanical properties as well as the aging behavior of ATZ could be considerably increased by reducing the grain size of the two ceramic phases and – most important – by improving the homogeneity of the phase dispersion.

With this aim, Bartolomé et al. [73] have developed a new synthesis route to prepare ATZ composite powders with an intraparticular phase dispersion, with the final aim of improving the homogeneity of the particle distribution in the sintered material. In this method, the starting material is a homogenous mixture of coarse-grained ceramic raw powders (Al_2O_3, 3Y-TZP, and unstabilized ZrO_2) which are covaporized in the intense focus of a CO_2 laser beam. Subsequent rapid cooling induces the simultaneous gas phase condensation of the components, resulting in the formation of composite nanoparticles characterized by a spherical shape, a narrow size distribution, softly agglomerated by weak van der Waals forces. In addition, the authors suggest that the method allows the formation of a solid solution, in which up to 40 mol% Al_2O_3 was incorporated into a t-ZrO_2 defect crystal structure, giving rise to the composition $Zr_{(1-x)}Al_xO_{(2-x/2)}$ [74, 75]. At higher Al_2O_3 concentrations – 43 mol% in this case – the exceeding Al_2O_3 might form an amorphous shell around these defect crystals. It should be recalled that, under thermodynamic equilibrium conditions, there is no evidence for the formation of a solid solution in the ZrO_2–Al_2O_3 system. However, in gas phase condensation processes, the particle formation occurs within milliseconds, i.e. far from thermodynamic equilibrium, explaining the existence of metastable such solid solution [74, 75]. The $Zr_{(1-x)}Al_xO_{(2-x/2)}$ defect structure seems to remain stable up to a temperature of 900 °C, as seen by its constant domain size. Between 900 and 1100 °C, the ZrO_2 domains start to grow, and the thermal energy is finally used to separate θ-Al_2O_3 and t-ZrO_2 phases. Only a small amount of Al_2O_3 (<3 mol%) remains dissolved in the t-ZrO_2 crystals. Finally, above 1300 °C, θ-Al_2O_3 transforms to α-Al_2O_3. A schematic representation of this process is depicted in Figure 4.13.

As a comparison, ATZ powders were processed by a conventional method, in which the starting mixture

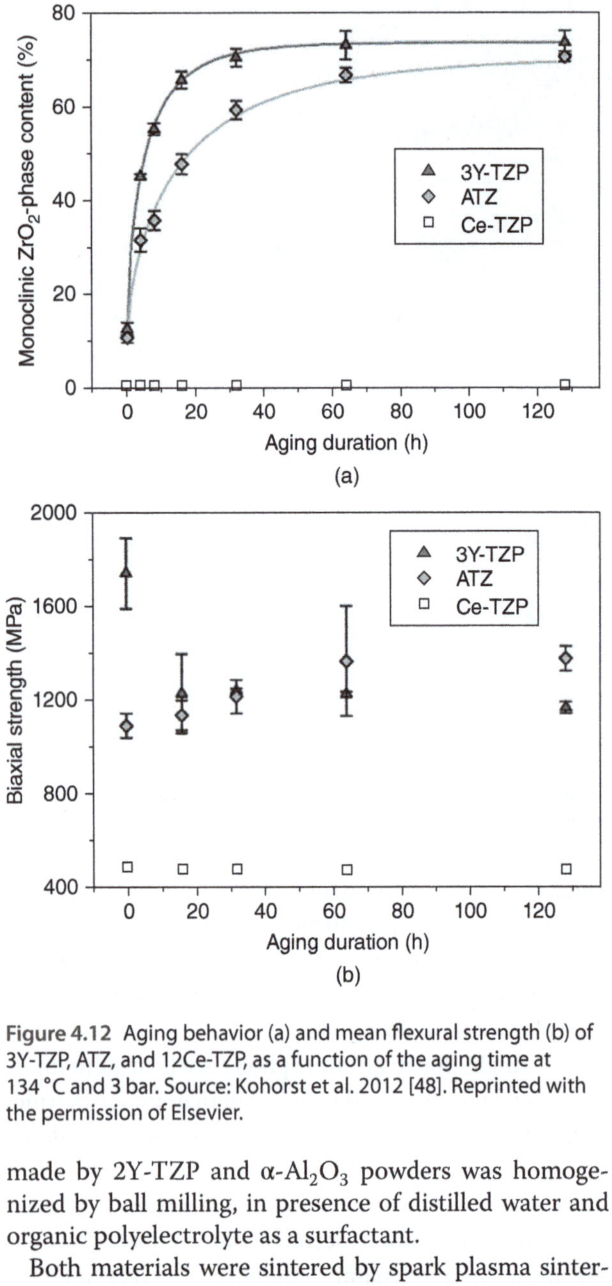

Figure 4.12 Aging behavior (a) and mean flexural strength (b) of 3Y-TZP, ATZ, and 12Ce-TZP, as a function of the aging time at 134 °C and 3 bar. Source: Kohorst et al. 2012 [48]. Reprinted with the permission of Elsevier.

made by 2Y-TZP and α-Al_2O_3 powders was homogenized by ball milling, in presence of distilled water and organic polyelectrolyte as a surfactant.

Both materials were sintered by spark plasma sintering process, carried out at 1400 °C, applying a heating rate of 600 °C/min and an uniaxial pressure of 80 MPa. Figure 4.14 shows the microstructure of the sintered composites. It can be easily observed that the dispersion of the ZrO_2 and Al_2O_3 grains in the composite derived by the gas condensation process is much more homogeneous than the material obtained by the traditional mixing process. Therein, both the ZrO_2 grains and the Al_2O_3 grains form large clusters exceeding 2 μm.

The superior homogeneity of composite obtained by the gas condensation procedure is also reflected in its corresponding higher mechanical properties. In fact, flexural strength, Vickers hardness, and fracture toughness of this composite significantly exceed the ones of the traditionally processed composite by 36%, 8%, and 45%, respectively, and reaching values of 1500 MPa, 14.9 GPa, and 6.8 MPa $\sqrt{m}$, respectively.

Furthermore, the *t–m* transformation under applied stress of the gas-condensation-derived ATZ sample was higher (34%) as compared to the traditional composite (9%). This can be explained by considering the CTE mismatch between Al_2O_3 and ZrO_2, already reported, creating residual tensile stresses in the composite, which promote the *t–m* transformation under stress. However, in the traditionally processed ceramic this stress acts nonuniformly, due to the ZrO_2 aggregated grains, causing an increased partial transformation of *t*-ZrO_2 into *m*-phase during cooling down from the sintering temperature. Consequently, this reduces its transformability during the fracture process compared with the gas-condensation-synthesized ceramics.

Finally, the new composite presented a reduced LTD as compared to the traditional one. This was imputed to the residual Al^{3+} ions dissolved in the ZrO_2 lattice, acting as stabilizers, or even to Al^{3+} ions segregated at ZrO_2 grain boundaries, able to retard the degradation. Finally, the homogeneously distributed Al_2O_3 grains act as an effective constraint to the ZrO_2 grains, retaining the *t*-ZrO_2 in a metastable state and increasing the LTD resistance of the composite as compared to the less homogeneous, traditional material.

4.3.2 Ce-TZP-Based Composites

4.3.2.1 Ce-TZP/Al_2O_3 Composites

The first investigation on Ce-TZP/Al_2O_3 composites belongs to Sato et al. [76] who, in 1989, proved an

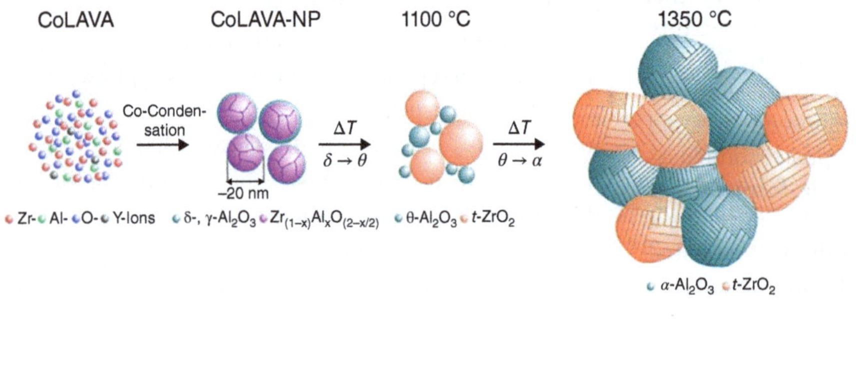

Figure 4.13 Gas phase condensation of Al_2O_3/ZrO_2 hybrid nanoparticles prepared by gas-condensation technique (named CoLAVA process) and their stepwise evolution at increasing sintering temperatures up to 1350 °C. Source: https://www.nature.com/articles/srep20589. Licenced under CC BY 4.0.

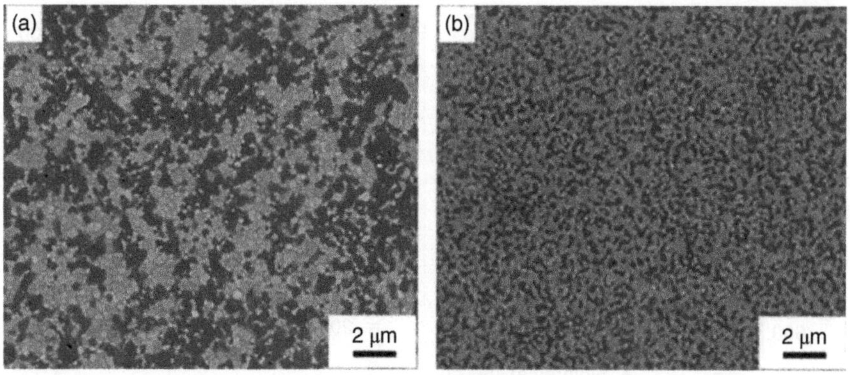

Figure 4.14 SEM micrographs of ATZ-sintered composites derived (a) by the gas condensation process and (b) by the traditional mixing process. Source: https://www.nature.com/articles/srep20589. Licenced under CC BY 4.0.

increase of the hardness and of the Young's modulus of the composite with respect to monolithic Ce-TZP ceramics.

However, the best results were reached by Nawa [49, 77] in 1997, when he developed an intragranular type Ce-TZP/Al_2O_3 composite, in which several nanosized (10–100 nm) Al_2O_3 particles were trapped into ZrO_2 grains. The microstructure of this composite is illustrated in the transmission electron microscopy (TEM) micrograph of Figure 4.15 [49], which relates to 12Ce-TZP/30 vol% Al_2O_3 sintered at 1500 °C for two hours. The black arrows in the figure show the ultrafine Al_2O_3 grains located inside the ZrO_2 grains.

Nawa [77] investigated the role of the Al_2O_3 content (in the range of 0–30 vol%) on the physical, microstructural, and mechanical properties of 12Ce-TZP. The addition of Al_2O_3 particles inhibited the grain growth of the ZrO_2 matrix, at each of the sintering temperature tested (between 1500 and 1650 °C). In samples sintered at 1500 °C, the ZrO_2 average size almost halved (from about 2 to 1 μm) moving from 0 to 30 vol% Al_2O_3.

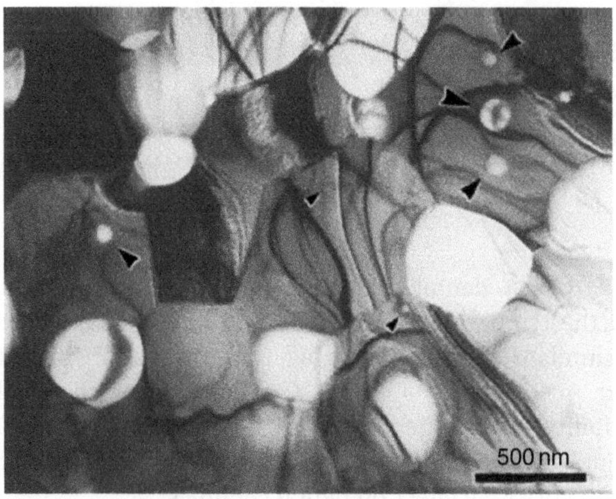

Figure 4.15 TEM micrograph of 12Ce-TZP/30 vol% Al_2O_3 sintered at 1500 °C for two hours. Source: Nawa et al. 1998 [49]. Reprinted with the permission of Elsevier.

Almost the same trend was observed for higher sintering temperatures, precisely at 1550 and 1600 °C. A more remarkable difference was observed in the "oversintered" material at 1650 °C, in which the ZrO_2 average grain size reduced from about 7.5 μm in monolithic 12Ce-TZP to about 2.5 μm in 12Ce-TZP/30 vol% Al_2O_3.

Furthermore, Nawa [77] demonstrated a progressive increase of the fracture strength by increasing the Al_2O_3 content (Figure 4.16a). The highest strength (688 MPa) was achieved with 30 vol% of Al_2O_3 addition, after sintering at 1600 °C. At the same time, the hardness and elastic modulus increased as well, as predicted by the rule of mixture. This strengthening effect was imputed to the flaw size reduction due to microstructural refinement. The same ZrO_2 grain size reduction also favored the retention of the metastable tetragonal phases. That is, reduction of the grain size increased the critical stress for *t*–*m* transformation.

At the same time, a decrease of the fracture toughness was observed, in agreement with the decrease of transformability, which was estimated by the difference between the *m*-ZrO_2 volume fraction in the fractured and polished surfaces (Figure 4.16b).

Thanks to the precise control of the microstructure and composition, the mechanical properties of the Ce-TZP/Al_2O_3 composite were further optimized, giving rise to the commercial product named NANOZR® (Panasonic Electric Works, Tokyo, Japan [21, 78]). This material was characterized by an exceptional fracture strength and fracture toughness of 1500 MPa and 18 MPa $\sqrt{m}$, respectively [79], well superior to those of many other ceramic core materials used in dentistry, as shown in Figure 4.17a. For sake of clarity, the composition of each of the ceramic core material of Figure 4.17a is elucidated in Table 4.5. In Figure 4.17b, the appearance of a three-unit bridge (from the second premolar to the second molar) of the maxilla designed and machined through a computer-aided design (CAD)/cell adhesion molecule (CAM) system from NANOZR (lower) and reference Y-TZP (upper) is shown.

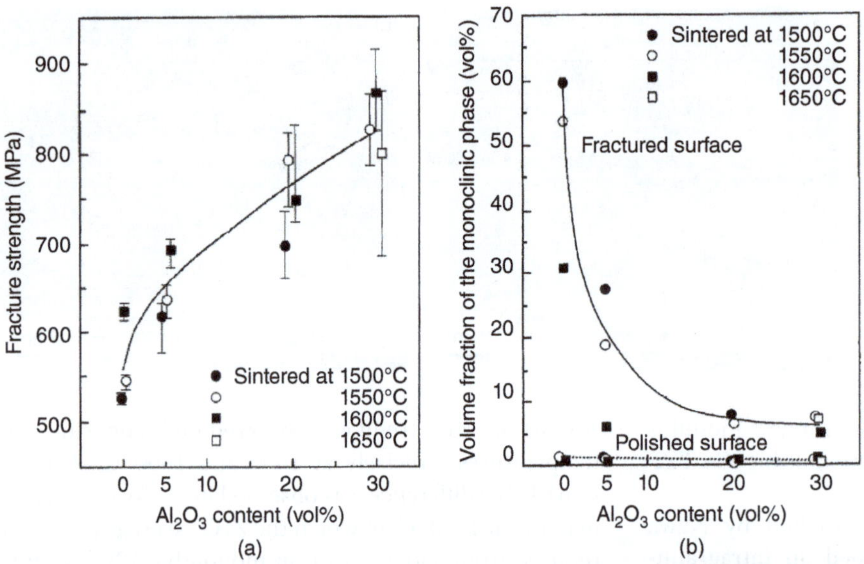

Figure 4.16 Fracture strength (a) and volume fraction of the monoclinic phase on fractured and polished surface (b) of a 12Ce-TZP/Al_2O_3 composites as a function of Al_2O_3 content. Source: Nawa 1998 [77]. Adapted with the permission of Elsevier.

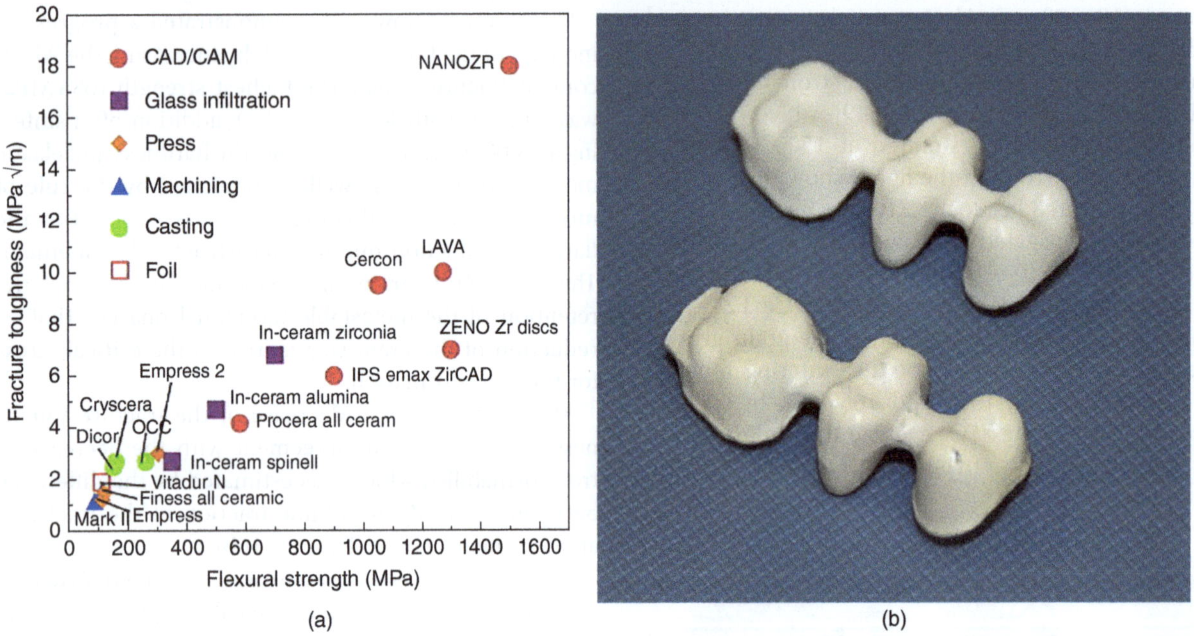

Figure 4.17 Relation between fracture toughness and biaxial flexure strength for many types of ceramic core materials used in dentistry (a); appearance of three-unit bridge core made by NANOZR® (lower) and reference Y-TZP (upper) prepared by a CAD/CAM system. Source: Ban 2008 [79]. Reproduced with the permission of Elsevier.

In view of dental applications, the LDT behavior of NANOZR was investigated under different conditions: (i) physiological saline (0.88% NaCl) at 80 °C for 30 days; (ii) in 4% acetic acid (pH 2.6) at 80 °C for 30 days, and (iii) in an autoclave at 121 °C under 0.20 MPa for 10 days. Before and after exposure to such environments, specimens were subjected to the biaxial flexure test and evaluation of the surface m-ZrO_2 content. The results were compared to those of reference 3Y-TZP [80]. It should be specified that physiological saline is frequently used to test dental materials for chemical corrosion, and the temperature of the solution at 80 °C was used to simulate conditions during the mastication of hot food. Acetic acid in 4% at 80 °C is used for the chemical solubility test, as described in the standard ISO-6872 "Dental Ceramics," since this acid has been reported to have a corrosive effect on dental ceramics.

As shown in Figure 4.18a, both Y-TZP and Ce-TZP/Al_2O_3 have excellent mechanical durability under oral conditions. In fact, no significant decreases occurred

Table 4.5 Core material for the all-ceramic dental restorations shown in Figure 4.17a.

Brand name	Manufacturer	Main composition
NANOZR	Matsushita Electric Works	Ce-TZP/Al_2O_3
LAVA	3M ESPE	Y-TZP
Cercon	DeguDent	Y-TZP
ZENO Zr Discs	Wieland	Y-TZP
In-Ceram Zirconia	Vita	Porous $ZrO_2 \cdot CeO_2 \cdot Al_2O_3$/lanthanide glass
In-Ceram Alumina	Vita	Porous Al_2O_3/lanthanide glass
In-Ceram Spinel	Vita	Porous $MgO \cdot Al_2O_3$/lanthanide glass
IPS emax ZirCAD	Ivoclar	Y-TZP
Procera AllCeram	Nobel Biocare	Al_2O_3
Empress	Ivoclar	Leucite + feldspathic glass
Empress 2	Ivoclar	Leucite + feldspathic glass
OCC	Olympus	Mica/β-spodumene/glass
Crycera	Kyushu Dentceram	β-Metaphosphate calcium/glass
Dicor	Dentsply	Mica/glass
Vitadur N	Vita	Aluminum porcelain
Finesse All-Ceramic	Ceramco	Leucite + feldspathic glass
Mark II	Vita	Feldspar ceramic

Source: Ban 2008 [79]. Reproduced with permission of Elsevier.

in the strength of the two materials before and after soaking in either saline or 4% acetic acid. However, after autoclaving, while Ce-TZP/Al_2O_3 holds its starting strength, a certain decrease occurred in Y-TZP. Figure 4.18b shows the transformed m-ZrO_2 after each treatment. The starting value (4.8% for Ce-TZP/Al_2O_3 and 0.3% for Y-TZP) is imputed to the transformation induced by cutting and grinding operations to which the samples have been submitted prior testing. In Y-TZP, autoclaving induced a significant increase of the starting m-ZrO_2 fraction; on the opposite, it remained stable in Ce-TZP/Al_2O_3, independently on the treatment, showing the excellent durability of the composite in oral conditions and therefore suitable use for dental restorations.

Benzaid et al. [81] investigated the SGC behavior of an ATZ nanocomposite, having a 70 vol% 10Ce-TZP–30 vol% Al_2O_3 composition. As shown in Figure 4.19, the behavior of this composite is compared to those of monolithic Al_2O_3, 3Y-TZP, and 12Ce-TZP. We can observe that the nanocomposite leads to the highest fracture toughness (>8 MPa $\sqrt{m}$) with a threshold (K_{I0}) comparable to that of monolithic 12Ce-TZP. On the other hand, the nanocomposite has a much higher strength than 12Ce-TZP (see Figures 4.16a and 4.18a) and shows an excellent resistance to aging degradation (see Figure 4.18b), thus supporting the use of this material for biomedical applications.

4.3.2.2 Ce-TZP/$MgAl_2O_4$ Composites

Recently, a new type of ZrO_2 composite based on Ce-TZP/magnesium spinel ($MgAl_2O_4$) system was developed [82]. After sintering at 1400 °C for two hours, an almost fully tetragonal matrix (10Ce-TZP), containing a fine and homogeneous dispersion of cubic $MgAl_2O_4$ grains, was obtained. The average size of the ZrO_2 matrix was 500 ± 250 μm, whereas the maximum size of the Al–Mg spinel grains was 200 μm. This material showed a good combination of high strength (about 900 MPa) and toughness (15 MPa $\sqrt{m}$). SGC tests allowed to estimate the threshold stress intensity factor (K_{I0}), below which no significant crack propagation occurs, which is very high (if compared with other biomedical grade ceramics, see values in Table 4.4) and close to 8 MPa $\sqrt{m}$. In addition, the sintered composite showed a high stability under hydrothermal conditions in the time scale for biological application, in agreement with the standard ISO 13356 (i.e. stable after 45 hours of autoclave treatment at 134 °C, which would represent approximately 180 years *in vivo*, based on the extrapolations proposed by Chevalier and Gremillard [43]). Owing to such outstanding properties, this material has been the object of a recent patent, referred to as EP2377506A1.

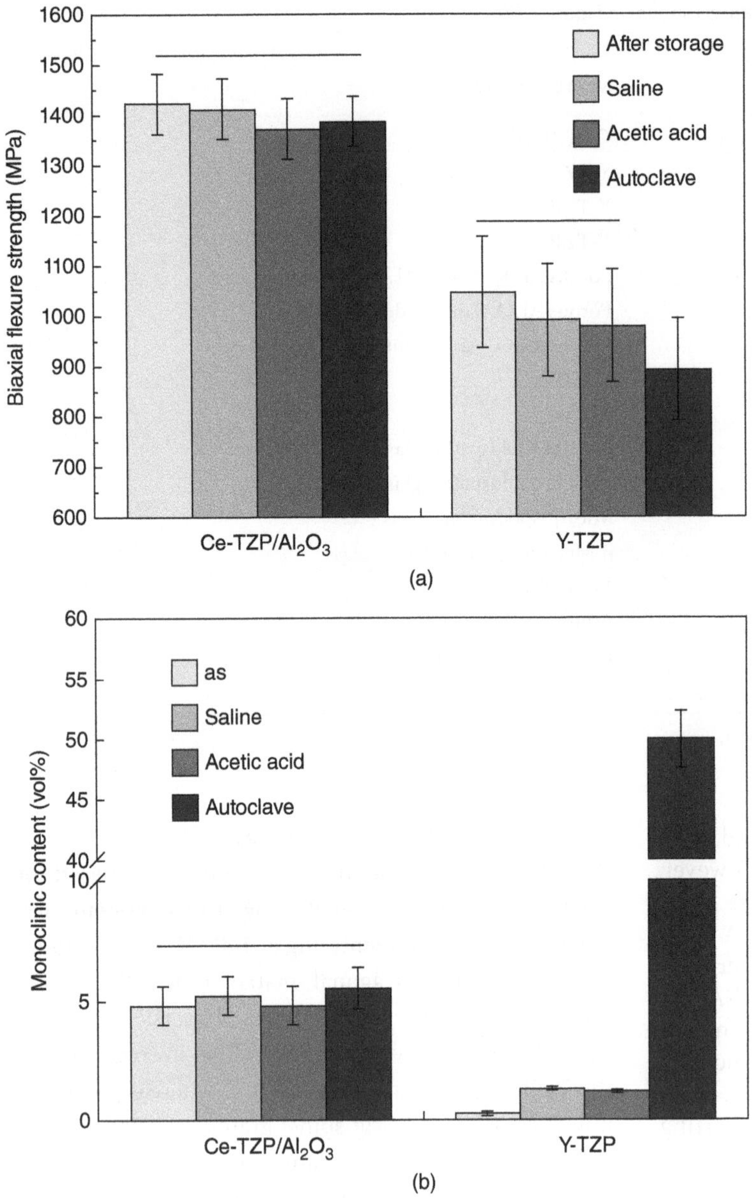

Figure 4.18 Biaxial flexure strength (a) and m-ZrO_2 content (b) of Ce-TZP/Al_2O_3 nanocomposite and of reference Y-TZP before and after storage in various solutions. Horizontal bars indicate no significant difference. Source: Ban et al. 2008 [80]. Adapted with the permission of John Wiley and Sons.

4.3.2.3 Ce-TZP-Based Composites Containing Elongated Grains

The previous paragraphs show that fine, second-phase particles added to a Ce-TZP matrix are necessary to increase the fracture strength of the material: see for instance, Figure 4.16 [77], which clearly shows the progressive increase of the flexural strength of Ce-TZP-based ceramics by increasing the Al_2O_3 amount. In fact, due to the *pinning* effect exerted by the second-phase particles on the Ce-ZrO_2 grain boundaries during sintering, a refinement of the matrix and a consequent strengthening effect is produced.

On the other side, the addition of stiff particles to Ce-TZP matrix could lower the *t*-ZrO_2 transformability and hence the related toughening effect. Therefore, several papers focus on the use of elongated-shaped grains or platelets, embedded in a Ce-TZP matrix, for increasing the toughness of the material by additional bridging/crack deflection mechanisms exerted by such grains.

The first investigations on Ce-TZP reinforced by *in-situ* formed strontium hexa-aluminate ($SrAl_{12}O_{19}$) platelets were carried out by Cutler et al. [83, 84]. In particular, triphasic composites were developed, having the following composition: 12Ce-TZP/Al_2O_3/$SrAl_{12}O_{19}$, in which Al_2O_3 was added in the range of 15–30 vol% and the aluminate phase was obtained by adding $SrZrO_3$ in the range of 0.5–8 wt%, according to the following reaction:

$$SrZrO_3 + 6Al_2O_3 \rightarrow SrAl_{12}O_{19} + ZrO_2 \quad (4.3)$$

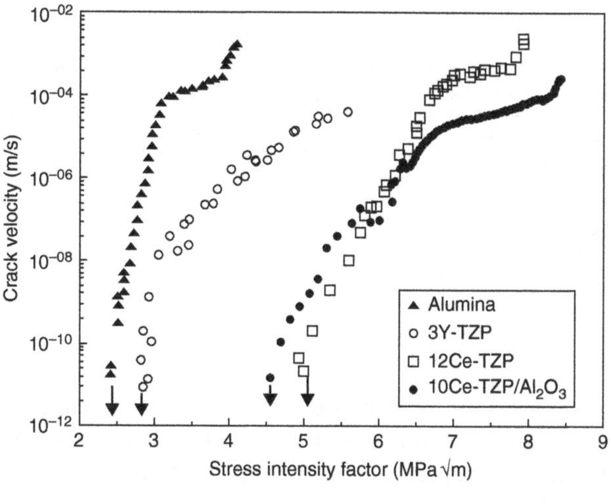

Figure 4.19 V–K_I curves of Ce-TZP/Al_2O_3 nanocomposite as compared to those of monolithic Al_2O_3, 3Y-TZP, and 12Ce-TZP ceramics. Source: Benzaid et al. 2008 [81]. Reprinted with the permission of Elsevier.

The microstructure of this composite consisted of Ce-ZrO_2 grains of 1–3 μm in size, equiaxed Al_2O_3 grains of 0.1–1 μm, and $SrAl_{12}O_{19}$ platelets of 1–3 μm in length. Depending on the composition, fracture strength in the range 500–700 MPa, fracture toughness of 10–15 MPa $\sqrt{m}$, and hardness values of 10–14 GPa were obtained. In particular, a strong relation with the Al_2O_3 content was observed, since the higher the Al_2O_3 amount, the higher the strength and the hardness. The fracture toughness, however, followed the opposite trend. In addition, Cutler et al. showed that the optimal amount of $SrZrO_3$ (then forming $SrAl_{12}O_{19}$ platelets) should be optimized in each different composition: for instance, it is close to 2 wt% for Ce-TZP/15 vol% Al_2O_3 and 4 wt% for Ce-TZP/30 vol% Al_2O_3 composites.

In Figure 4.20, the strength–toughness relationships for the several studied compositions are reported. The figure clearly shows the improvement of both toughness and strength of the three-phasic composites with respect to Ce-TZP and Ce-TZP/Al_2O_3 materials. However, the triphasic composites are characterized by a lower level of transformability as compared to Ce-TZP ceramics, due to the constraining effect exerted by the Al_2O_3 particles. This means that the toughness improvement could be reasonably imputed to crack branching and bridging mechanisms by the elongated phase.

In the following years, several papers reported the use of elongated grains inside ZrO_2-based materials: Ce-TZP composites reinforced by $LaNbO_4$ [85], barium hexa-aluminate ($BaAl_{12}O_{19}$), lanthanum hexa-aluminate ($LaAl_{11}O_{18}$), and cerium hexa-aluminate ($CeAl_{11}O_{18}$) [86–88]. More complex quasi-ternary aluminates, such as $BaMnAl_{11}O_{18}$ and $CeMnAl_{11}O_{19}$ were investigated as well [89, 90]. In the latter case, the hexa-aluminate phase was obtained by simply adding MnO and Al_2O_3 to 12Ce-TZP powders. Thus, the formation of $CeMnAl_{11}O_{19}$ occurred by depletion of CeO_2 from the tetragonal matrix during sintering (from 12 to 10.9 mol%). Furthermore, a cerium reduction from Ce^{4+} to Ce^{3+} was determined.

In order to perfectly control the stoichiometry, the microstructure, and the morphology of the grains in such complex composites, an innovative powder synthesis method was recently developed [12, 91, 92]. Starting from a commercial powder, its surface is coated (or graft) by precursors of the second phase, which crystallizes on the surface of the parent material under proper thermal treatment. The close mixing between the matrix ceramic particles and the precursor is realized at nano/atomic level, assuring an excellent distribution of the second phase in the composite material. In this method, a commercial 10Ce-TZP powder is employed as raw material to develop composite materials having the following composition: 84 vol% Ce-ZrO_2/8 vol% Al_2O_3/8 vol% $SrAl_{12}O_{19}$. Aluminum nitrate and strontium nitrate were used as precursors of the second phases; in addition, in some synthesis cerium ammonium nitrate was also added, in order to precisely tune the ceria amount inside the ZrO_2 lattice (in the range 10.0–11.5 mol%). The nitrate solution was dropwise added to the dispersed ZrO_2 slurry and the suspension was then spray-dried. In this way, ZrO_2 powders were homogeneously coated by the inorganic precursors of the second phases. On thermal treatment, the controlled crystallization of second-phase grains on the ZrO_2 particles was achieved. After sintering, the microstructure was fully dense and highly homogeneous, with optimal distribution of both second phases inside a very fine ZrO_2 matrix. In addition, a fine control of the ceria amount inside ZrO_2 lattice

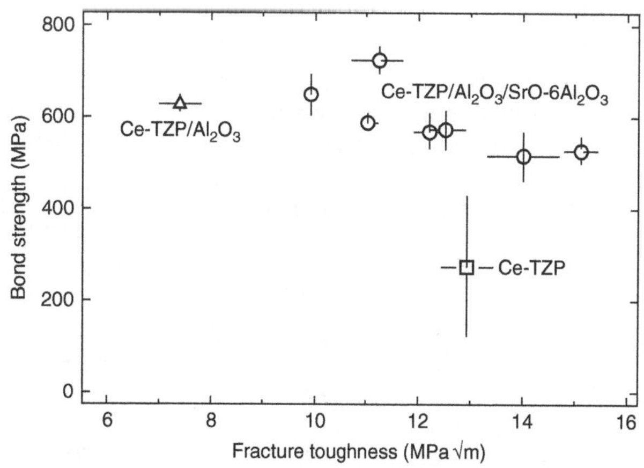

Figure 4.20 Strength–toughness relationships for Ce-TZP (squares), Ce-TZP/Al_2O_3 (triangles), and Ce-TZP/Al_2O_3/$SrAl_{12}O_{19}$ (circles). Source: Cutler et al. 1991 [83]. Reprinted with the permission of John Wiley and Sons.

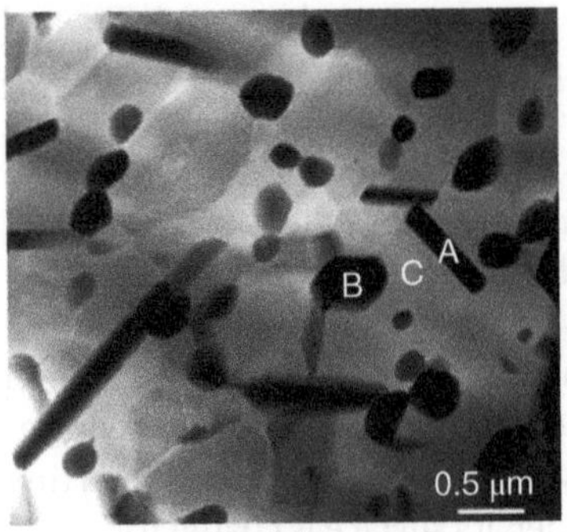

(a)

Grain	Chemical composition			
	Zr (at%)	Ce (at%)	Al (at%)	Sr (at%)
A	6	0	87	6
B	6	0	94	0
C	90	10	0	0

(b)

Figure 4.21 TEM image (a) and chemical composition (at%) on the A, B, and C grains (b) of the 84 vol% Ce-ZrO_2/8 vol% Al_2O_3/8 vol% $SrAl_{12}O_{19}$ sintered sample. Source: Palmero et al. 2015 [91]. Reprinted with the permission of Elsevier.

was obtained. For ceria contents equal or higher than 10.5 mol%, the materials showed a high stability against aging, as verified by *in vitro* hydrothermal tests, thus fully satisfying the stability requirements for medical applications.

The microstructure of a sintered sample is depicted in Figure 4.21, as determined by TEM analysis. Here, grains with three different morphologies can be recognized: bright regular shape, dark elongated shape, and equiaxial shape grains. To define the chemical composition of the particles having different morphologies and phase contrast, energy–dispersive X-ray spectrometry (EDX) nanoprobe was focused on the grains referred to as A, B, and C in Figure 4.21. The corresponding atomic compositions are shown in the table enclosed to the Figure 4.21: even if a low zirconium amount was observed both in A and B grains due to a matrix effect, a quite perfect agreement with their nominal compositions was found. In fact, in the point A (dark elongated grain), an atomic Sr:Al ratio of 6 : 87 (=1 : 14.5) corroborates, within the instrumental error, an aluminate phase composition very close to $SrAl_{12}O_{19}$. At the same time, it was confirmed that the dark equiaxial grain (grain B) was pure Al_2O_3 and the bright phase (grain C) was ceria-stabilized ZrO_2.

In spite of the several publications reporting the use of elongated grains and platelets in Ce-TZP materials, to date their toughening mechanisms by crack bridging was just supposed, but not clearly demonstrated. Available data give some evidence that toughening characteristics of Ce-TZP reinforced *in situ* by hexa-aluminate are strongly dependent on the type and amount of the hexa-aluminate.

In order to investigate the influence of the aluminate structure and composition, in a recent work Kern [93] compared the mechanical properties of a 12Ce-TZP/30 vol% Al_2O_3 composite (referred to as 12Ce-30A) with those of composites reinforced by 30 vol% of $LaAl_{11}O_{18}$ (referred to as 12Ce-30LA6) or 30 vol% of $SrAl_{11}O_{19}$ (referred to as 12Ce-30SA6) phases. 12Ce-30A showed the finest microstructure (ZrO_2 grains in the range 0.3–1 μm), the highest hardness, toughness, and strength. In composites containing hexa-aluminates, Kern observed a slight higher aspect ratio and a broader size distribution of lanthanum aluminate grains as compared to strontium aluminate ones, while the size of 12Ce-TZP matrix was similar in both composites (1–1.5 μm). Both 12Ce-30LA6 and 12Ce-30SA6 materials showed high fracture resistance (in the range 7.5–9 MPa $\sqrt{m}$) and attractive strength (in the range 550–750 MPa), strongly dependent on the sintering temperature. Anyway, 12Ce-30LA6 showed always higher strength and lower fracture resistance as compared to 12Ce-TZP/30 vol% SA6 composites.

A different crack propagation behavior was observed in the three composites (see Figure 4.22). In 12Ce-30A, the crack propagates exclusively in the Ce-TZP matrix:

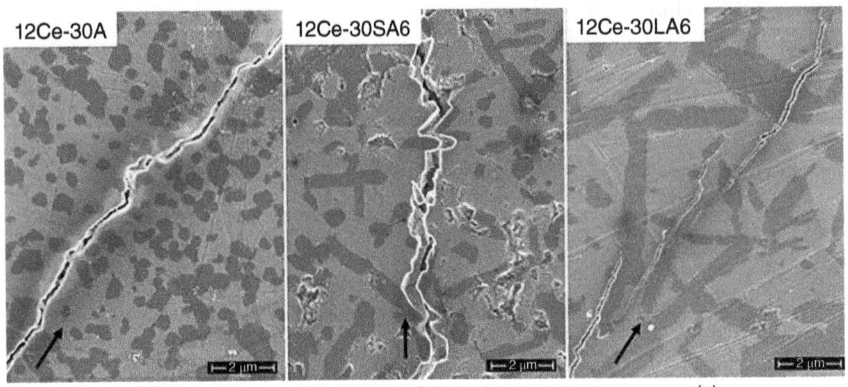

Figure 4.22 Crack propagation in (a) 12Ce-TZP/30 vol% Al_2O_3 (12Ce-30A), (b) 12Ce-TZP/30 vol% $SrAl_{11}O_{19}$ (12Ce-30SA6), and (c) 12Ce-TZP/30 vol% $LaAl_{11}O_{18}$ (12Ce-30LA6). Source: Kern 2014 [93]. Reprinted with the permission of Elsevier.

in fact, cracking through Al_2O_3 grains was not observed, and moderate crack deflection at TZP/Al_2O_3 and presumably at TZP/TZP grain boundaries can be detected. 12Ce-30SA6 shows strong crack deflection at TZP/strontium aluminate grain boundaries. Cracks do not propagate through but rather around the aluminate grains, so that strongly kinked crack paths and grain pull-out are observed. Moreover, a strong transformation toughening and a moderate crack tip toughness were revealed in this type of composite.

In 12Ce-30LA6, a completely different crack propagation behavior is observed. Interfaces between TZP and lanthanum aluminate seem rather strong, so that cracks do propagate through the reinforcement. In addition, cracks running along or onto lanthanum hexa-aluminates stopped after a short distance, where most of the crack energy is absorbed, resulting in interrupted crack paths. The crack tip toughness was high, but the efficiency of the transformation toughening was very low. In summary, this work pointed out the role of the aluminate type and structure on the toughening mechanisms. However, these results show that further efforts are needed to deepen the relationship with transformation toughening proper to Ce-TZP ceramics, also showing that there is still room for further optimizing the compositions and the microstructures, in search of optimal strength and toughness.

4.3.3 ZrO_2/Hydroxyapatite Composites

Some works have investigated the possibility to develop ZrO_2–hydroxyapatite (HA) composites. In fact, the combination of these two phases seems very advantageous for biomedical applications. By one side, ZrO_2 has a very high strength and toughness, as extensively reported in the previous paragraphs. However, as ZrO_2 ceramics are bioinert materials (see Table 4.2), they do not directly bond with natural bone in hip joint replacement or other medical devices. On the other side, HA ceramics, which show a high bioactivity, are characterized by low strength and low fracture toughness which limit their applications to non-load-bearing parts. For this reason, the development of ZrO_2/HA composites, with high mechanical properties and bioactivity, seems particularly convenient.

Based on this strategy, two different approaches were developed, depending on whether an HA-based composite or an HA-added composite is used. The first approach relates to the reinforcement of an HA matrix with different second phases, which could be in the form of powders, platelets, or fibers. In studies involving the use of these materials, the mechanical properties of the HA-based composites were found to be enhanced by a factor of 3. Kong et al. [94] showed that when 15 vol% ZrO_2 and 30 vol% Al_2O_3 was added to HA, the strength and the fracture toughness of the composite moved from 100 MPa and 1 MPa $\sqrt{m}$ to 300 MPa and 3 MPa $\sqrt{m}$, respectively. At the same time, *in vivo* tests ith screw-shaped dental implants showed that HA-based composites were superior to those made with commercially pure Ti [95]. However, further improvements are needed before such materials can be employed for load-bearing applications such as dental/orthopedic implants.

The second strategy involves the improvement of the biocompatibility of load-bearing ceramics (like Al_2O_3, ZrO_2, and their composites) through the incorporation of bioactive materials. In the following, the achievement reached in this field, with ZrO_2 used as matrix material, is reported.

Kong et al. [96] developed ZrO_2–20 wt% Al_2O_3 composite (ZA), to which different amounts of HA (up to 40 vol%) were added. The addition of HA induced a significant microstructural evolution in the composite: in fact, while ZA showed a fine and homogeneous microstructure, on addition of HA, the grains of Al_2O_3 became coarser, assuming an acicular shape at the highest HA content. At the same time, HA with plate-like shape were observed. In addition, during sintering, a reaction between HA and ZrO_2 occurred, inducing the formation of TCP. In spite of the flexural strength decreased by increasing the HA amount, the composite still presented satisfying values (>400 MPa at the highest HA content). From *in vitro* test with osteoblastic cell lines, the proliferation and the differentiation of cells on the composites gradually increased, as the amount of HA increased. From the mechanical and biological evaluations, the composition in which 30 vol% of HA was added to ZA was found to be optimal for load-bearing biological applications.

In the field, important results were achieved by Matsumoto and coworkers [97] who developed 3D porous ZrO_2/HA composite scaffolds, at increasing amounts of HA. Porous scaffolds were fabricated by impregnating the struts of a polyurethane sponge by immersion in ZrO_2/HA slurries. The impregnated sponges were then dried at 70 °C for one hour, heated at 700 °C for three hours to burn out the sponge block and the binder and then sintered at 1500 °C for five hours.

A representative image of a prepared scaffold is shown in Figure 4.23 [97]. The porous structure of the synthesized scaffold was related to the dipping time of the polymer sponge in the ceramic slurry containing the ceramic powders (Figure 4.23b–d). The scaffold with the highest porosity (~91%) also showed interconnected pores, thus suitable for application as bone substitute. The compressive strength of the scaffolds increased from 0.3 ± 0.01 MPa to 13.8 ± 0.94 MPa as the ZrO_2 content

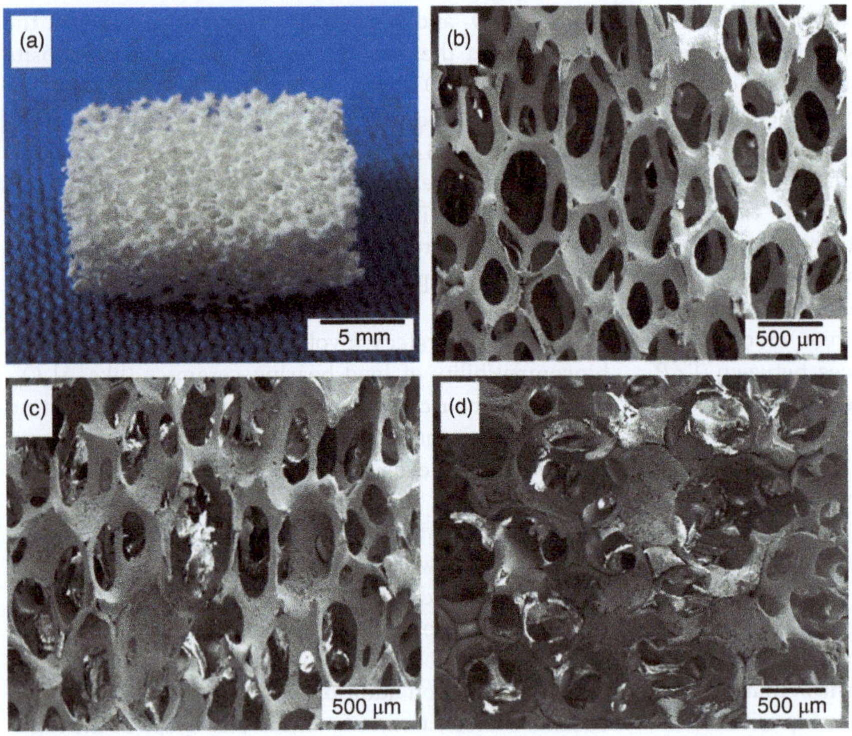

Figure 4.23 (a) Synthesized porous ZrO_2/HA scaffold with 91 ± 2.8% porosity. (b–d) SEM images of porous scaffolds; (b) 91.2 ± 2.8%, (c) 80.8 ± 4.3%, (d) 71.4 ± 2.5%. Data are shown as the mean ± SD ($n = 5$). Source: An et al. 2012 [97]. Reprinted with the permission of Elsevier.

increased from 0% to 100% in the scaffold. In particular, the highest strength was achieved for the composition 70 : 30 ZrO_2/HA. This was imputed to the significantly increased cubic phase, due to partial transformation of ZrO_2/HA into TCP and/or calcium zirconium oxide ($CaZrO_3$) during high temperature sintering [98, 99].

SEM images of osteoblasts cultured in the ZrO_2/HA scaffolds with two different ZrO_2/HA compositions (ZrO_2/HA 50/50 and 80/20) are shown in Figure 4.24 [97]. Scaffolds containing more than 80% of ZrO_2 showed less affinity to cells as compared to materials with less ZrO_2. In fact, at day 3 of the culture, the cells on the surface of a scaffold composed of 50/50 showed a well-spread morphology, whereas the cells on the surface of a scaffold composed of 80/20 ZrO_2/HA were less attached, showing spindle shape (Figure 4.24a–d). At day 5 of culture, a large number of cells had adhered and proliferated to the 50/50 surface, whereas the cell proliferation was still minimal on the 80/20 surface (Figure 4.24e–h). A plot of cell number against culture period showed that cell proliferation was significantly higher in the scaffolds containing less than 80% ZrO_2 (Figure 4.23i). The attenuation of cell adhesion and proliferation on the ZrO_2-rich scaffold might be caused by the low affinity of ZrO_2 for proteins [7, 100].

In addition, porous ZrO_2/HA scaffolds containing bone-marrow-derived stromal cells (BMSCs) were implanted into critical size bone defects for six weeks, in order to evaluate the bone tissue reconstruction with this material. The results of this *in vivo* study showed that a BMSC-loaded ZrO_2/HA scaffold provided a suitable 3D environment for BMSC survival and enhanced bone regeneration around the implanted material.

In summary, this work demonstrated that porous ZrO_2/HA composite scaffold has excellent mechanical properties and cellular/tissue compatibility and would be a promising substrate to achieve both bone reconstruction and regeneration needed in the treatment of large bone defects.

Finally, ZrO_2/HA composite coatings were used on orthopedic implants in the past decade [101–103]. These composite coatings possessed better mechanical properties and biocompatibility as compared to pristine ZrO_2 or HA. Wang et al. [103] in 2010 fabricated nanocomposite coatings on titanium via electrodeposition method. These coatings comprised fluorinated HA and ZrO_2 and exhibited high bonding strength, low dissolution rate, and good *in vitro* bioactivity [103].

4.4 Conclusion

ZrO_2 holds unique and reliable combination of physicochemical and mechanical properties, which enable its use in biomedical applications, especially in the field of hard tissue surgery. In fact, yttria-stabilized TZP (Y-TZP) ceramics were introduced in the 1980s for use in femoral heads because of their higher fracture toughness and strength as compared to the previously

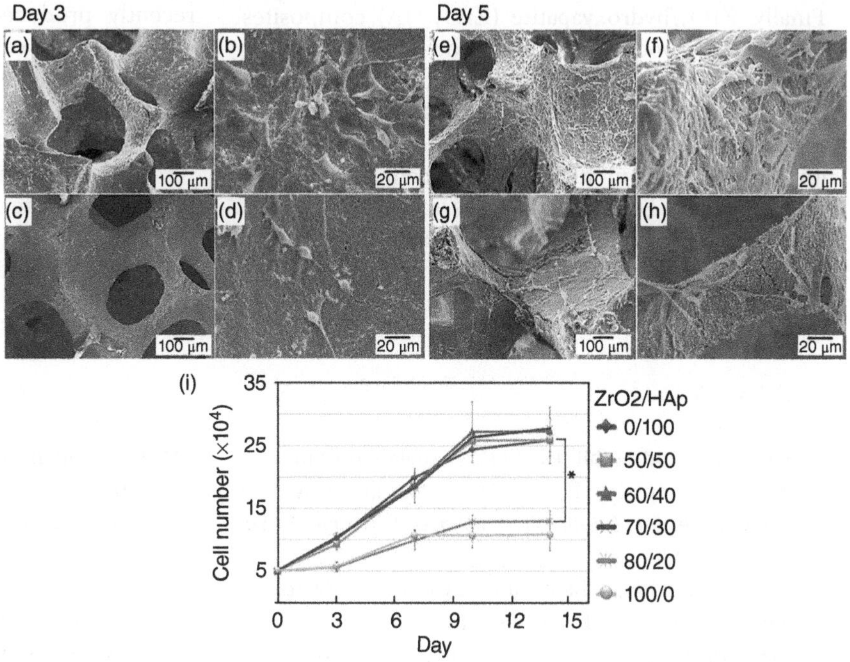

Figure 4.24 SEM images of adhered cells on scaffold. Three days after cell seeding: (a) 50/50, (b) high magnification of 50/50, (c) 80/20, (d) high magnification of 80/20. Five days after cell seeding: (e) 50/50, (f) high magnification of 50/50, (g) 80/20, (h) high magnification of 80/20. (i) Cell proliferation on the ZrO_2/HA composite scaffolds (with different ZrO_2/HA ratio) at day 3, 7, 10, and 14. Data are shown as the mean ± SD ($n = 4$). Source: An et al. 2012 [97]. Reprinted with the permission of Elsevier.

used biomedical grade Al_2O_3. These outstanding properties are the consequence of phase transformation (from tetragonal to monoclinic ZrO_2 phase) toughening, which increases the resistance to crack propagation and makes the material flaw tolerant.

On the other hand, because of this ability to transform, some ZrO_2 compositions used in medicine (such as 3Y-TZP) present a major drawback, since they can undergo degradation at low temperature and in presence of moist atmosphere. These conditions correspond to those of standard steam sterilization procedure (134 °C, 2 bar of pressure) and of *in vivo* environment to which the orthopedic devices are exposed. Due to such aging phenomenon, in the late 1990s the catastrophic failure of many (more than 800) ZrO_2 ceramic femoral heads processed with a new furnace technology by Saint-Gobain Desmarquest Prozyr® occurred. This event had a catastrophic impact for the use of ZrO_2 in the biomedical field, with a strong market sale decrease between 2001 and 2002, without any renew in the following years.

Such issue pushed the development of new load-bearing bioceramics, by following two alternative approaches.

The first implies the use of ZrO_2 as reinforcing phase in Al_2O_3, giving rise to the well-known ZTA composites. ZTA was identified as a practical alternative to monolithic ZrO_2, able to reduce the long-term effects of aging. It was demonstrated that sintered ZTA were biocompatible and did not exhibit inflammation and wear debris during *in vivo* histological examinations, which makes them favorable for clinical applications. Today, ZTA is a widely used material for femoral heads, commercialized by two major companies, CeramTec AG (Plochingen, Germany) and the Japanese KYOCERA Medical (Osaka, Japan) under the trade name of BIOLOX *delta* and BIOCERAM AZ209, respectively.

The second approach relates to the development of aging-free ZrO_2 ceramics, which could be the way to fully exploit the outstanding properties of ZrO_2 without the major drawback associated with its degradation under *in vivo* conditions. This could be realized by using tetravalent ions, such as Ce^{4+}, as ZrO_2 stabilizers, which lowers the aging susceptibility as compared to Y-TZP. The major drawback of Ce-TZP ceramics is the low fracture strength: addition of proper second phase to increase strength, hardness, and wear resistance is therefore required. Ce-TZP-based composites are today produced as promising candidates for use in the biomedical field. Al_2O_3, Mg–Al spinel, and other platelets/elongated grains (used or further increasing the toughness of the material by additional bridging/crack deflection mechanisms) have been developed. Within these strategies, ZrO_2 ceramics are fully qualified to have a strong potential as biomaterials. An example is provided by the commercial dental product NANOZR (Panasonic Electric Works, Tokyo, Japan), which shows an exceptional fracture strength and fracture toughness, well superior to those of many other ceramic core materials used in dentistry. In any case, although the good results achieved, there is still room for further optimization of the microstructure, composition, and ZrO_2 stabilization strategies in order to achieve excellent reliability in the biomedical devices.

Finally, ZrO_2/hydroxyapatite (ZrO_2/HA) composites have been developed as well, being the most challenging between the ZrO_2-based developed compositions. The combination between inert (ZrO_2) and active (HA) oxides could be the way to increase the bonding ability with natural bone in hip joint replacement or other medical devices. For these reasons, in the past decade composite ZrO_2/HA coating for orthopedic implants have been developed. Also, innovative 3D scaffolds, based on ZrO_2/HA composite materials, have been recently produced: due to the excellent mechanical properties and cellular/tissue compatibility, they would be a promising substrate to achieve both bone reconstruction and regeneration needed in the treatment of large bone defects. In any case, in future, further research on studying the effects of aging, fatigue life, and long-term phase stability of ZrO_2 ceramics should be carried out to confirm the enduring significance of ZrO_2 as bone repair and/or replacement material.

References

1 Patel, N.R. and Gohil, P.P. (2012). Review on biomaterials: scope, applications & human anatomy significance. *Int. J. Emerging Technol. Adv. Eng.* **2** (4): 91–101.

2 Hench, L.L. (1991). Bioceramics: from concept to clinic. *J. Am. Soc.* **74** (7): 1487–1510.

3 Thamaraiselvi, T.V. and Rajeswari, S. (2004). Biological evaluation of bioceramic materials – a review. *Trends Biomater. Artif. Organs* **18** (1): 9–17.

4 Koch, K., Brave, D., and Nasseh, A.A. (2012). A review of bioceramic technology in endodontics. *Roots – Int. Mag. Endod.* **4**: 6–12.

5 López, J.P. (2014). Alumina, zirconia, and other non-oxide inert bioceramics. In: *Bio-Ceramics with Clinical Applications* (ed. M. Vallet-Regí). Chichester, UK: Wiley https://doi.org/10.1002/9781118406748.ch6.

6 Kohon, D.H. (2004). Bioceramics. In: *Standard Handbook of Biomedical Engineering and Design.* New York, NY: McGraw-Hill.

7 Cao, W. and Hench, L.L. (1996). Bioactive materials. *Ceram. Int.* **22**: 493–507.

8 Thomas, M.V. and Puleo, D.A. (2009). Calcium sulfate: properties and clinical applications. *J. Biomed. Mater. Res. Part B* **88** (2): 597–610.

9 Best, S.M., Porter, A.E., Thian, E.S., and Huang, J. (2008). Bioceramics: past, present and for the future. *J. Eur. Ceram. Soc.* **28**: 1319–1327.

10 Ohtsuki, C., Kamitakahara, M., and Miyazaki, T. (2009). Bioactive ceramic-based materials with designed reactivity for bone tissue regeneration. *J. R. Soc. Interface* **6**: S349–S360.

11 Rahaman, M.N., Yao, A., Bal, B.S. et al. (2007). Ceramics for prosthetic hip and knee joint replacement. *J. Am. Ceram. Soc.* **90**: 1965–1988.

12 Palmero, P., Montanaro, L., Reveron, H., and Chevalier, J. (2014). Surface coating of oxide powders: a new synthesis method to process biomedical grade nano-composites. *Materials* **7**: 5012–5037.

13 Jenabzadeh, A.R., Pearce, J.S., and Walter, W.L. (2012). Total hip replacement: ceramic-on-ceramic. *Semin. Arthroplasty* **23** (4): 232–240.

14 Willmann, G. (2003). Ceramic femoral head retrieval data. *Clin. Orthop. Relat. Res.* **417**: 19–26.

15 Pezzotti, G. and Yamamoto, K. (2014). Artificial hip joints: the biomaterials challenge. *J. Mech. Behav. Biomed. Mater.* **31**: 3–20.

16 Evans, A.G. (1978). Microfracture from thermal expansion anisotropy – I. Single phase systems. *Acta Metall.* **26**: 1845–1853.

17 Palmero, P. (2015). Structural ceramic nanocomposites: a review of properties and powders' synthesis methods. *Nanomaterials* **5**: 656–696.

18 Seidel, J. and Rödel, J. (1997). Measurement of crack tip toughness in alumina as a function of grain size. *J. Am. Ceram. Soc.* **80**: 433–438.

19 Piconi, C. (2011). Alumina. In: *Comprehensive Biomaterials*, vol. **1** (ed. P. Ducheyne, K.E. Healey, D.W. Hutmacher, et al.), 73–94. Amsterdam: Elsevier.

20 Piconi, C. and Porporati, A.A. (2016). Bioinert ceramics: zirconia and alumina. In: *Handbook of Bioceramics and Biocomposites.* Switzerland: Springer International Publishing.

21 Piconi, C., Condo, S.C., and Kosmač, T. (2014). Chapter 11. Alumina and zirconia-based ceramics for load-bearing applications. In: *Advanced Ceramic for Dentistry* (ed. J. Shen and T. Kosmač), 219–253. Wathmann, MA: Butterworth-Heinemann (Elsevier).

22 Helmer, J.D. and Driskell, T.D. (1969). Research on bioceramics. In: *Symposium on Use of Ceramics in Surgical Implants.* South Carolina: Clemson University.

23 Rieger, W. (2001). Ceramics in orthopedics. 30 years of evolution and experience. In: *World Tribology Forum in Arthoplasty* (ed. C. Rieker, S. Oberjolzer and U. Wyss), 1–13. Bern, Germany: Verlag Hans Huber.

24 Piconi, C. and Maccauro, G. (1999). Zirconia as a ceramic biomaterial. *Biomaterials* **20**: 1–25.

25 Maccauro, G., Rossi Iommetti, P., Raffaelli, L., and Manicone, P.F. (2011). Alumina and zirconia ceramic for orthopaedic and dental devices. In: *Biomaterials Applications for Nanomedicine* (ed. R. Pignatello), 299–309. InTech.

26 Garvie, R.C. and Swain, M.V. (1985). Thermodynamics of the tetragonal to monoclinic phase transformation in constrained zirconia microcrystals – Part 1 In the absence of an applied stress field. *J. Mater. Sci.* **20** (4): 1193–1200.

27 Marshall, D.B. and Ritter, J.E. (1987). Reliability of advanced structural ceramics and ceramic matrix composites. A review. *Ceram. Bull.* **66**: 309–317.

28 Chevalier, J. and Gremillard, L. (2011). Zirconia as a biomaterial. In: *Comprehensive Biomaterials*, vol. **1** (ed. P. Ducheyne, K.E. Healey, D.W. Hutmacher, et al.), 95–108. Amsterdam: Elsevier.

29 Garvie, R.C., Hannink, R.H., and Pascoe, R.T. (1975). Ceramic steel? *Nature* **258**: 703–704.

30 Kelly, J.R. and Denry, I. (2008). Stabilized zirconia as a structural ceramic: an overview. *Dent. Mater.* **24**: 289–298.

31 Chevalier, J., Taddei, P., Gremillard, L. et al. (2011). Reliability assessment in advanced nanocomposite materials for orthopaedic applications. *J. Mech. Behav. Biomed. Mater.* **4**: 303–314.

32 Kirsten, A., Begand, S., Oberbach, T. et al. (2010). Subcritical crack growth behavior of dispersion oxide ceramics. *J. Biomed. Mater. Res. Part B* **95** (1): 202–206.

33 Nevarez-Rascon, A., Aguilar-Elguezabal, A., Orrantia, E., and Bocanegra-Bernal, M.H. (2011). Compressive strength, hardness and fracture toughness of Al_2O_3 whiskers reinforced ZTA and ATZ nanocomposites: Weibull analysis. *Int. J. Refract. Met. Hard Mater.* **29**: 333–340.

34 Daguano, J.K.M.F., Santos, C., Souza, R.C. et al. (2007). Properties of ZrO_2–Al_2O_3 composite as a function of isothermal holding time. *Int. J. Refract. Met. Hard Mater.* **25**: 374–379.

35 Theunissen, G.S.A.M., Bouma, J.S., Winnbust, A.J.A., and Burggraaf, A.J. (1992). Mechanical properties of ultra-fine grained zirconia ceramics. *J. Mater. Sci.* **27**: 4429–4438.

36 Ratner, B.D., Hoffmann, A.S., Schoen, F.J., and Lemons, J.E. (2004). *Biomaterials Science: An Introduction to Biomaterials in Medicine*, 2e. New York: Elsevier.

37 Watanabe, M., Iio, S., and Fukuura, I. (1984). Aging behavior of Y-TZP. *Adv. Ceram.* **12**: 391–398.

38 Amin, K.E. and Nag, D. (1995). Tribological characteristics of zirconia-yttria ceramics. *Ceram. Bull.* **74** (5): 80–84.

39 Chevalier, J., Calés, B., Drouin, J.M., and Stefani, Y. (1997). Ceramic-ceramic bearing systems compared on different testing configurations. In: *Bioceramics 10* (ed. L. Sedel and C. Rey), 271–274. Amsterdam: Elsevier.

40 Lawson, S. (1995). Environmental degradation of zirconia ceramics. *J. Eur. Ceram. Soc.* **15**: 485–502.

41 Schubert, H. and Frey, F. (2005). Stability of Y-TZP during hydrothermal treatment: neutron experiments and stability considerations. *J. Eur. Ceram. Soc.* **25**: 1597–1602.

42 Lughi, V. and Sergo, V. (2010). Low temperature degradation -aging- of zirconia: a critical review of the relevant aspects in dentistry. *Dent. Mater.* **26** (8): 807–820.

43 Chevalier, J. and Gremillard, L. (2009). Ceramics for medical applications: a picture for the next 20 years. *J. Eur. Ceram. Soc.* **29**: 1245–1255.

44 Muñoz-Saldaña, J., Balmori-Ramírez, H., Jaramillo-Vigueras, D. et al. (2003). Mechanical properties and low-temperature aging of tetragonal zirconia polycrystals processed by hot isostatic pressing. *J. Mater. Res.* **18** (10): 2415–2426.

45 Guazzato, M., Albakry, M., Ringer, S.P., and Swain, M.V. (2004). Strength, fracture toughness and microstructure of a selection of all-ceramic materials. Part II. Zirconia-based dental ceramics. *Dent. Mater.* **20**: 449–456.

46 Denry, I. and Holloway, J.A. (2010). Ceramics for dental applications: a review. *Materials* **3**: 351–368.

47 Denry, I. and Kelly, J.R. (2008). State of art of zirconia for dental applications. *Dent. Mater.* **24**: 299–307.

48 Kohorst, P., Borchers, L., Strempel, J. et al. (2012). Low-temperature degradation of different zirconia ceramics for dental applications. *Acta Biomater.* **8**: 1213–1220.

49 Nawa, M., Nakamoto, S., Sekino, T., and Niihara, K. (1998). Tough and strong Ce-TZP/alumina nanocomposites doped with titania. *Ceram. Int.* **24**: 497–506.

50 Kern, F. and Palmero, P. (2013). Microstructure and mechanical properties of alumina 5vol% zirconia nanocomposites prepared by powder coating and powder mixing routes. *Ceram. Int.* **39** (1): 673–682.

51 Kurtz, S.M., Kocagöz, S., Arnholt, C. et al. (2014). Advances in zirconia toughened alumina biomaterials for total joint replacement. *J. Mech. Behav. Biomed. Mater.* **31**: 107–116.

52 Evans, A.G., Burlingame, N., Drory, M., and Kriven, W.M. (1981). Martensitic transformations in zirconia-particle size effects and toughening. *Acta Metall.* **29**: 447–456.

53 Heuer, A.H., Claussen, N., Kriven, W.M., and Rühle, M. (1982). Stability of tetragonal ZrO_2 particles in ceramic matrices. *J. Am. Ceram. Soc.* **65**: 642–650.

54 Evans, A.G. and Heuer, A.H. (1980). Review-transformation toughening in ceramics: martensitic transformations in crack-tip stress fields. *J. Am. Ceram. Soc.* **63**: 241–248.

55 Pecharroman, C., Bartolomé, J.F., Requena, J. et al. (2003). Percolative mechanism of ageing in zirconia containing ceramics for medical applications. *Adv. Mater.* **15**: 507–511.

56 Stewart, T.D., Tipper, J.L., Insley, G. et al. (2003). Long-term wear of ceramic matrix composite materials for hip prostheses under severe swing phase microseparation. *J. Biomed. Mater. Res. Part B* **66B**: 567–573.

57 Guo, R., Guo, D., Chen, Y. et al. (2001). In situ formation of $LaAl_{11}O_{18}$ rodlike particles in ZTA ceramics and effect on the mechanical properties. *Ceram. Int.* **28**: 699–704.

58 Liu, X.Q. and Chen, X.M. (2002). Effects of $Sr_2Nb_2O_7$ additive on microstructure and mechanical properties of 3Y-TZP/Al_2O_3 ceramics. *Ceram. Int.* **28**: 209–215.

59 Jin, X. and Gao, L. (2004). Effects of powder preparation method on the microstructure and mechanical performance of ZTA/$LaAl_{11}O_{18}$ composites. *J. Eur. Ceram. Soc.* **24**: 653–659.

60 Chen, Z., Chawla, K.K., and Koopman, M. (2004). Microstructure and mechanical properties of in situ synthesized alumina/Ba-β-alumina/zirconia composites. *Mater. Sci. Eng., B* **367**: 24–32.

61 Hondrum, S.O. (1992). A review of strength properties of dental ceramics. *J. Prosthet. Dent.* **67**: 859–855.

62 Seghi, R.R., Denry, I.L., and Rosenstiel, S.F. (1995). Relative fracture toughness and hardness of new dental ceramics. *J. Prosthet. Dent.* **74**: 145–150.

63 Tinschert, J., Zwez, D., Marx, R., and Anusavice, K.J. (2000). Structural reliability of alumina-, feldspar-, leucite-, mica-, and zirconia-based ceramics. *J. Dent.* **28**: 529–535.

64 Kosmač, T., Dakskobler, A., Oblak, C., and Jevnikar, P. (2007). The strength and hydrothermal stability of Y-TZP ceramics for dental applications. *Int. J. Appl. Ceram. Technol.* **4** (2): 164–174.

65 Zhang, F., Vanmeensel, K., Inokoshi, M. et al. (2015). Critical influence of alumina content on the low temperature degradation of 2–3 mol% yttria-stabilized TZP for dental restorations. *J. Eur. Ceram. Soc.* **35**: 741–750.

66 Jones, D.W. and Sutow, E.J. (1987). Stress corrosion failure of dental porcelain. *Br. Ceram. Trans.* **86**: 40–43.

67 Luo, J. and Stevens, R. (1999). Porosity-dependence of elastic moduli and hardness of 3Y-TZP ceramics. *Ceram. Int.* **25**: 281–286.

68 Nogiwa-Valdez, A.A., Rainforth, W.M., Zeng, P., and Ross, I.M. (2013). Deceleration of hydrothermal degradation of 3Y-TZP by alumina and lanthana co-doping. *Acta Biomater.* **9** (4): 6226–6235.

69 Rieger, W., Kobel, S., and Weber, W. (2008). Processing and properties of zirconia ceramics for dental applications. *Spectrum Dialogue*, Reprint, March 2008. Available online: http://www.lastruttura.it/ Contents/Documents/3%20Premium%20HT/Letteratura%20zirconia%20dentale.pdf (accessed May 2016).

70 Begand, S., Oberbach, T., and Glien, W. (2005). ATZ: a new material with a high potential in joint replacement. *Key Eng. Mater.* **284–286**: 983–986.

71 Schneider, J., Begand, S., Kriegel, R. et al. (2008). Low temperature aging of alumina toughened zirconia. *J. Am. Ceram. Soc.* **91**: 3613–3618.

72 Kosmac, T., Oblak, C., Jevnikar, P. et al. (2000). Strength and reliability of surface treated Y-TZP dental ceramics. *J. Biomed. Mater. Res.* **53**: 304–313.

73 Bartolomé, J.F., Smirnov, A., Kurland, H.D. et al. (2016). New ZrO_2/Al_2O_3 nanocomposite fabricated from hybrid nanoparticles prepared by CO_2 laser co-vaporization. *Sci. Rep.* **6**: 20589. https://doi.org/10.1038/srep20589.

74 Balmer, M.L., Lange, F.F., and Levi, C.G. (1994). Metastable phase selection and partitioning for $Zr_{(1-x)}Al_xO_{(2-x/2)}$ materials synthesized with liquid precursors. *J. Am. Ceram. Soc.* **77**: 2069–2075.

75 Inamura, S., Miyamoto, H., Imaida, Y. et al. (1994). Formation and hot isostatic pressing of ZrO_2 solid solution in the system ZrO_2-Al_2O_3. *J. Mater. Sci.* **29**: 4913–4917.

76 Sato, T., Endo, T., and Shimada, M. (1989). Postsintering hot isostatic pressing of ceria-doped tetragonal zirconia/alumina composites in an argon oxygen gas atmosphere. *J. Am. Ceram. Soc.* **1989** (72): 761–764.

77 Nawa, M. (1998). The effect of TiO_2 addition on strength and toughening in intragranular type 12Ce-TZP/Al_2O_3 nanocomposites. *J. Eur. Ceram. Soc.* **18**: 209–219.

78 Panasonic Biomedical. http://www.die-modellmacher.de/wp-content/uploads/Nano-ZR-brochure.pdf (accessed May 2016).

79 Ban, S. (2008). Reliability and properties of core materials for all-ceramic dental restorations. *Jpn. Dent. Sci. Rev.* **44**: 3–21.

80 Ban, S., Sato, H., Suehiro, Y. et al. (2008). Biaxial flexure strength and low temperature degradation of Ce-TZP/Al_2O_3 nanocomposite and Y-TZP as dental restoratives. *J. Biomed. Mater. Res. Part B* **87B** (2): 492–498.

81 Benzaid, R., Chevalier, J., Saâdaoui, M. et al. (2008). Fracture toughness, strength and slow crack growth in a ceria stabilized zirconia–alumina nanocomposite for medical applications. *Biomaterials* **29**: 3636–3641.

82 Apel, E., Ritzberger, C., Courtois, N. et al. (2012). Introduction to a tough, strong and stable Ce-TZP/$MgAl_2O_4$ composite for biomedical applications. *J. Eur. Ceram. Soc.* **32**: 2697–2703.

83 Cutler, R.A., Mayhew, R.J., Prettyman, K.M., and Virkar, A.V. (1991). High-toughness Ce-TZP/Al_2O_3 ceramics with improved hardness and strength. *J. Am. Ceram. Soc.* **74** (1): 179–186.

84 Cutler, R.A., Lindemann, J.M., Ulvensoen, J.H., and Lange, H.I. (1994). Damage-resistant SrO-doped Ce-TZP/Al_2O_3 composites. *Mater. Des.* **15** (3): 123–133.

85 Maschio, S., Pezzotti, G., and Sbaizero, O. (1998). Effect of $LaNb0_4$ addition on the mechanical properties of ceria-tetragonal zirconia polycrystal matrices. *J. Eur. Ceram. Soc.* **18**: 1779–1785.

86 Ori, S., Kojima, T., Hara, T. et al. (2012). Fabrication of Ce-TZP/β-hexaaluminate composites using amorphous precursor of the second phase. *J. Ceram. Soc. Jpn.* **120** (3): 111–115.

87 Miura, M., Hongoh, H., Yogo, T. et al. (1994). Formation of plate-like lanthanum-β-aluminate crystal in Ce-TZP matrix. *J. Mater. Sci.* **29** (1): 262–268.

88 Tsukuma, K. and Takahata, T. (1986). Mechanical property and microstructure of TZP and TZP/Al_2O_3 composites. *Adv. Struct. Ceram. Symp., Mater. Res. Soc.* **78**: 123–135.

89 Yamaguchi, T., Sakamoto, W., Yogo, T. et al. (1999). In situ formation of Ce-TZP/Ba-hexaaluminate composites. *J. Ceram. Soc. Jpn.* **107** (9): 814–916.

90 Tsai, O.F., Chon, U., Ramachandran, N., and Shetty, D.K. (1992). Transformation plasticity and toughening in CeO_2-partially-stabilized zirconia–alumina (Ce-TZP/Al_2O_3) composites doped with MnO. *J. Am. Ceram. Soc.* **75** (5): 1229–1238.

91 Palmero, P., Fornabaio, M., Montanaro, L. et al. (2015). Towards long lasting zirconia-based composites for dental implants. Part I: Innovative synthesis, microstructural characterization and in vitro stability. *Biomaterials* **50**: 38–46.

92 Fornabaio, M., Palmero, P., Traverso, R. et al. (2015). Zirconia-based composites for biomedical applications: role of second phases on composition, microstructure and zirconia transformability. *J. Eur. Ceram. Soc.* **35**: 4039–4049.

93 Kern, F. (2014). A comparison of microstructure and mechanical properties of 12Ce-TZP reinforced with alumina and in situ formed strontium- or lanthanum-hexaaluminate precipitates. *J. Eur. Ceram. Soc.* **34** (2): 413–423.

94 Kong, Y.M., Kim, S., Kim, H.E., and Lee, I.S. (1999). Reinforcement of hydroxyapatite bioceramic by addition of ZrO_2 coated with Al_2O_3. *J. Eur. Ceram. Soc.* **82** (11): 2963–2968.

95 MacDonald, D.E., Betts, F., Stranick, M. et al. (2001). Physicochemical study of plasma-sprayed hydroxyapatite-coated implants in humans. *J. Biomed. Mater. Res.* **1** (54): 480–490.

96 Kong, Y.M., Bae, C.Y., Lee, S.H. et al. (2005). Improvement in biocompatibility of ZrO_2–Al_2O_3 nano-composite by addition of HA. *Biomaterials* **26**: 509–517.

97 An, S.H., Matsumoto, T., Miyajima, H. et al. (2012). Porous zirconia/hydroxyapatite scaffolds for bone reconstruction. *Dent. Mater.* **28**: 1221–1231.

98 Himann, R.B. and Vu, T.A. (1997). Effect of CaO on thermal decomposition during sintering of composite hydroxyapatite–zirconia mixtures for monolithic ceramic implants. *J. Mater. Sci. Lett.* **16**: 437–439.

99 Matsuno, T., Watanabe, K., Ono, K., and Koishi, M. (2000). Microstructure and mechanical properties of sintered body of zirconia coated hydroxyapatite particles. *J. Mater. Sci. Lett.* **19**: 573–576.

100 Kawahara, H. (1987). Bioceramics for hard tissue replacements. *Clin. Mater.* **2**: 181–206.

101 Balamurugan, A., Balossier, G., Kannan, S. et al. (2007). Electrochemical and structural characterisation of zirconia reinforced hydroxyapatite bioceramic sol–gel coatings on surgical grade 316L SS for biomedical applications. *Ceram. Int.* **33**: 605–614.

102 Jelínek, M., Dostálová, T., Teuberová, Z. et al. (2007). Study of laser created ZrO_2 and hydroxyapatite/ZrO_2 films for implantology. *Biomol. Eng.* **24**: 103–106.

103 Wang, J., Huang, C., Wan, Q. et al. (2010). Characterization of fluoridated hydroxyapatite/zirconia nano-composite coating deposited by a modified electrocodeposition technique. *Surf. Coat.* **204**: 2576–2582.

5

Bioceramics Derived from Marble and Sea Shells as Potential Bone Substitution Materials

Miculescu Florin[1], Mocanu A. Cătălina[1], Stan E. George[2], Maidaniuc Andreea[1], Miculescu Marian[1], Voicu S. Ioan[3], and Iulian Antoniac[1]

[1] *Department of Metallic Materials Science, Physical Metallurgy, Faculty of Material Science and Engineering, Politehnica University of Bucharest, Bucharest, Romania*
[2] *Laboratory of Multifunctional Materials and Structures, National Institute of Materials Physics, Măgurele-Bucharest, Romania*
[3] *Department of Analytical Chemistry and Environmental Engineering, Faculty of Applied Chemistry and Material Science, Politehnica University of Bucharest, Bucharest, Romania*

5.1 Introduction

One of the most interesting and promising areas of materials science research is constituted by the materials for biomedical application, especially those used in the orthopedic and dentistry surgery. In the last decades, significant progresses have been recorded in the domain of biomaterials device, among the most important being found in the field of ceramic materials for bone regeneration. The biomaterials of this class are often named bioceramics. The notable increasing number of publications and patents on the topic is leading step by step to their wide use in current clinical applications.

Due to the growing demand for biomaterials used for bone substitution, in the last five decades, complex research were made in order to produce them synthetically, with low costs and in large quantities. The materials used to produce synthetic bone grafts, especially the bioceramics, were introduced as an alternative to traditional bone substitutes (autografts). Among them, the ceramics of calcium phosphate (CaP), such as hydroxyapatite (HAP, $Ca_{10}(PO_4)_6(OH)_2$), are the most suitable materials, with excellent biological properties [1, 2].

From a historical perspective, the oldest ceramic materials were synthetic and their evolution in medical practice can be traced back to antiquity. The discovery of dental restorations inside ancient Egyptian sarcophagi, as well as artificial teeth, was followed by dental implantation and transplantation at the end of eighteenth century. According to an 1892 report, the next important evolutionary step was the use of plaster bone void filler [3, 4]. Three decades later, Albee [5] published the first reports on the replacement of plaster with tricalcium phosphate (TCP, $Ca_3(PO_4)_2$). However, research on the application of ceramic as a material for bone substitution started in 1960 [6–8]. The osteoceramic (ceramic composite consisting of TCP and $MgAl_2O_4$) was one of the first ceramics proposed for use after *in vivo* testing in animal model (i.e. dogs) [6]. Because of the compelling experimental results in terms of biocompatibility (both *in vitro* and *in vivo*), further studies [9–19] advanced the use of substituents based on HAP and TCP as a main option.

One of the foremost reasons for the intense study of HAP is determined by its chemical composition and its structural similarity with natural bone mineral phase [20, 21]. Bone is in fact a unique composite, comprising a matrix of mainly collagen hydrogel fibers, inorganic constituents, mostly HAP (a multi-doped carbonated HAP), and other salts such as calcium carbonate ($CaCO_3$) or calcium citrate. In terms of volume, bone is made up of about 35–45% mineral apatite, 30–45% of organic substances, and 15–25% of water [22, 23].

Thus, one way to address the problems of hard tissue reconstruction is to synthesize materials that elicit properties similar to those of the natural bone. Given this goal, properties such as bioactivity, osteoconductivity, and the non-inflammatory and non-immunogenic behavior, make synthetic HAP the most versatile bioactive ceramic used in various medical applications, especially in those focused on bone reconstruction [2, 22].

Among CaPs, HAP is known to be the less soluble and the most stable compound in aqueous solutions, $pH \geq 4.2$ [24]. Due to its bioactive nature, the HAP helps bone growth without inducing fracturing or dissolution phenomena. It is a stable compound which decomposes at temperatures generally in the range of 800–1200 °C, depending on stoichiometry.

The classical or the alternative synthesis methods, as well as the extension of the application range of

Bioceramics and Biocomposites: From Research to Clinical Practice, First Edition. Edited by Iulian Antoniac.

HAP are subjects of numerous research studies [1, 9–11, 21, 25–44]. Nowadays, HAP-derived products are used in the form of powders, porous blocks, or granules for filling bone defects or gaps [2]. An alternative view is the preparation of HAP from sustainable biological resources. In this respect, the natural origin precursors can be divided into two categories:

- hard tissue (such as human, cattle, sheep, chicken, and fish bones or other dental structures),
- natural structures of calcite/aragonite (corals, sea and land shells, cuttlefish bone, marble, and eggshells).

Starting from these precursors [45], several approaches to the synthesis of HAP biomaterials are possible: hydrothermal methods [9–11, 28, 39, 43, 46], mechano-chemical synthesis [42, 47, 48], electrochemical deposition techniques, sol–gel method [21, 25–27, 31, 49], and methods based on chemical precipitation from aqueous solutions [1, 29, 30, 34, 36, 37, 40, 41, 50, 51]. The quality, thermal stability, dissolution speed, fusibility capacity, and mechanical properties of these HAP particles depend on several parameters. The most important are: (i) Ca/P molar ratio of the precursors and final product, (ii) the resulted morphology, and (iii) the crystallinity of HAP [29].

Although the mentioned materials have been extensively studied [12, 33, 34, 36, 38, 52–57], materials and new approaches in the realm of production of substitutes based on HAP for bone treatment continue to be developed and investigated. This chapter attempts to summarize the progresses to date, being focused primarily on the materials science perspective regarding the research of bone substitute precursors, such as marble and various types of sea shells.

5.2 Biomimetic Approaches for Biomaterials Design

Bones fracture as a result of trauma or because of the natural aging process is a typical failure for this type of tissue. The treatment usually involves surgery for implanting a temporary or permanent prosthesis, which is still a challenge in orthopedics, especially in the case of extended bone defects [58]. In the past decade, the ability to understand the processes involved in biomineralization has improved significantly, leading to the development of biomimetic synthesis methods and the production of a new generation of materials [57, 59].

The word *biomimetic* was used for the first time in the dictionary of Webster in 1974 having the following definition: "the study of the formation, structure, or function of biologically produced substances and materials (as enzymes or silk) and biological mechanisms and processes (as protein synthesis or photosynthesis) especially for the purpose of synthesizing similar products by artificial mechanisms which mimic natural ones" [60].

Natural bones can be considered a nanocomposite made out of mineral fractions including small crystals of apatite and non-stoichiometric CaP, and organic fractions that together confer mechanical strength. The strategies for mimicking bone's structure and function include both the study of separated bone's components (included within the study fields of polymers or ceramics) and their composites.

The polymers are usually categorized into synthetic polymers – such as polylactic acid (PLA) and polyglycolic acid (PGA) – and copolymers derived from polymers of polysaccharide origin (e.g. starch, alginate, chitin/chitosan, gelatin, cellulose, hyaluronic acid derivatives), proteins (soy, collagen, fibrin, silk), and the existing variety of biofibers (e.g. lignocellulose natural fibers) [58, 60]. Other classifications divide polymers into two basic categories: (i) resorbable or biodegradable and (ii) non-absorbable (polyethylene, polymethyl methacrylate [PMMA], cellulose). Since synthetic polymers are produced under controlled conditions, they exhibit reproducible mechanical and physical properties and predictable tensile strength, modulus of elasticity, and degradation rate [58].

There are many materials made out of cellulose, in the fiber form, that can be considered biomimetic, since the early used fibers were of silk, sinew, and vegetable nature [60]. The first biomimetic synthetic fiber was nylon. Since nylon is not a reconstructed natural material, its classification in this category and the recognition of its usefulness come from its resemblance to natural fibers, especially silk [61].

A study on the design and manufacture of elastin analogous to Dan Urry synthesis methods has shown that it offers a wide range of controllable mechanical properties, thus presenting many opportunities for biomimetic materials and molecular machines in this class. The elasticity of elastin derives from the chain of five hydrophobic amino acids: valine–proline–glycine–valine–glycine being produced in the form of fibers in order to develop scaffolds for skin grafts and arterials [62]. On the other hand, the protein similar to the one existing in the spider silk was synthesized from mammalian cells and was successfully transformed into fibers. The purpose of this process is the production of significant amounts of artificial silk for clinical development of synthetic ligaments and suture thread [63].

The polymers used in orthopedic purpose falls within the class of polyanhydrides. Due to rapid degradation and well-defined surface, they are intended to stimulate bone growth or bone replacement, given that they may be *in situ* light cured. In order to ensure the desired mechanical properties, they are copolymerized with amides. The other class of materials, the bioceramics, can be grouped according to their bioactivity and resorption after implantation in the body into three categories: bioinert ceramics (e.g. alumina, zirconia), bioactive (e.g. HAP), and bioresorbable (e.g. tricalcium phosphate) [64].

In terms of energy consumption, the most economical way to strengthen the hard biological tissues is the use of crystalline or semicrystalline $CaCO_3$ in polymorphic form of aragonite, calcite, dolomite, and some other salts. They are all found under the generic name of *ceramics*. Moreover, from the desired characteristic point of view, in addition to the biocompatibility and mechanical (viscoelastic behavior included) properties, biomimetic ceramic materials should elicit a chemical composition and the porous surface able to provide rapid osseointegration [58].

5.2.1 Apatites

Apatite term refers to a group of several minerals that are of interest in interdisciplinary research and with applications in areas such as mineralogy, geology, energy, depollution, or medicine. Apatite is widespread as auxiliary mineral in volcanic rocks. It is also found in small amounts within metamorphic rocks. Its structural geometry is dominated by complexes of anions and cations that fill in the blanks of irregularly shaped polyhedrons.

Apatite have the general formula given by $Ca_{10}(PO_4)_6X_2$, where X is usually F (fluorapatite, FAP), OH (HAP), or Cl (chlorapatite, ClAP) [65, 66]. In the apatite lattice, Ca can be replaced with ½CO_3 or ½O given its tolerance to substitutions or formation of solid solutions [67]. From the mineralogical point of view, the FAP ($Ca_5[(PO_4)_3F]$) and ClAP ($Ca_5[(PO_4)_3Cl]$) appear as hexagonal-based prism crystals, well defined, but often in the form of granular compacts, finely crystallized. Under the long action of atmospheric agents (CO_2, H_2O), the fluor and ClAP are converted to phosphorites, which are heterogeneous mixtures of HAP ($Ca_5[(PO_4)_3OH]$) and carbonated apatite ($Ca_{10}[(PO_4)_6CO_3]\cdot H_2O$). In the apatite crystal lattices, there are PO_4^{3-} ions, along with F^-, Cl^-, HO^-, or CO_3^{2-} ions [66, 68].

HAP is an important material based on calcium phosphate that is similar to the mineral component of natural bone and teeth [21, 69]. Pure HAP with Ca/P ratio of 1.67 has exceptional biocompatibility and bioactivity properties, making possible its application as a bone substitute material and dental implants for over 50 years [53]. High temperature decomposition of HAP leads to the formation of β-TCP and α-TCP phases, having superior solubility in aqueous media, and thus being absorbed much faster *in vivo* [2, 58, 69]. In addition, CaPs containing small amounts of sodium, magnesium, carbon (in the form of carbonates), and occasionally fluoride ions have been shown to be more suitable for the bone implants manufacture compared to the pure chemicals that were used until recently [70].

Biological apatite is another apatite form, comprising the mineral phases of calcified tissues (enamel, dentine, bone) [24, 46, 71]. The bone and tooth mineral are impure forms of HAP. The most important composition differences arise because of the Ca/P ratio variation (1.6–1.7), and also the percentage of $CaCO_3$ and the quantity of water.

The biological apatite has a microcrystalline structure, with crystals of 400 Å length and 150 Å width in bones and dentin, and a 400 Å width and 100 nm to 5 μm length in the enamel [67, 72]. The cation sublattice in biological apatite always includes small amounts of sodium, potassium, magnesium, and other elementary ions, while the anion sublattice includes carbonates, sulfates, fluorides, and other ions, the total content of these additional elements not exceeding 5% [73].

Biological apatite nanocrystals (of approximately 50 nm long) are aligned parallel to the collagen fibers, orientation which otherwise is considered as the source of the remarkable mechanical strength of bone [58].

Nanocrystalline biomimetic apatite, analogous to bone minerals, is used for various medical applications due to its biological properties: it has been shown that a similar material is formed at the interface between the bone and bioactive materials, and its formation is considered critical in the implant osseointegration. Because of this, nanometric apatites are used as material for the coating of orthopedic metallic prostheses, for mineral bioresorbable cements, and for bioresorbable mineral–polymer composites.

The nanocrystalline apatite materials are considered biomimetic materials due to the low-temperature formation conditions, physiological pH, and physico-mechanical characteristics (e.g. non-stoichiometry, crystal size, presence of non-apatitic species, hardness, elasticity modulus) [54, 69, 74]. Biomaterials based on calcium phosphate have the Ca/P molar ratio in the range of 0.5–2 and are most sought for the reconstruction of various bone defects, especially in dentistry, orthopedic surgery, and trauma [53, 67, 73].

5.2.2 Calcium Carbonates

Calcium carbonate is one of the most abundant substances in nature, being found in the form of calcite, aragonite, marble, as well as limestone, chalk, dolomite, and other variations [75, 76]. $CaCO_3$ occurs in nature in two crystalline forms: calcite (trigonal crystal system) and aragonite (orthorhombic crystal system) [66]. Natural calcite crystals appear as trigonal crystals, colorless, or colored by impurities. In large transparent crystals the phenomenon of birefringence (double refraction of light) was observed, especially in the calcite from Iceland ("Iceland Spar") [76]. The aragonite consists of rhombic prism crystals, white, or colored due to impurities. It is harder than calcite and is stable at low temperatures [66].

The compact forms of $CaCO_3$, such as limestone, naturally found in nature as sedimentary rocks, are the result of partial dissolving and reprecipitating of skeletal fragments and shells of sea molluscs, coral, or animals during the past geological ages [68, 77]. Limestone is widespread in the Earth's crust, and it is usually mixed with other minerals, e.g. magnesium carbonate and is called dolomite, or mixed with clay and becomes shale. Marble is the result of metamorphism and recrystallization of limestone or dolomite rocks. Chalk is a white calcium carbonate, fine-grained, and very crumbly, being made up of remnants of fossilized animals [76].

5.3 Biogenic Precursors for Hydroxyapatite

Research on biologically derived transplants indicates the imperfection of these solutions, mainly because of the limited quantity of donor tissue, the morbidity rates, and the potential risks of an immunological incompatibility and to disease transmission. From this perspective, alloplastic materials are preferred as a reasonable option because they can be processed and modified to meet the specific requirements of a particular application. Moreover, they are unproblematic in terms of potential infections or immunological incompatibility [14, 58, 78].

Therefore, one of the key subjects of biomaterials research for clinical applications is the investigation on the development of new materials for the reconstruction of bone tissue. In this respect, consistent efforts were dedicated to the development of efficient and cost-effective methods for producing calcium phosphate with apatitic structure from natural biogenic resources [64].

From the moment (1974) Roy and Linnehan successfully obtained HAP from coral [79], began the worldwide intensive study of hydrothermal alteration of biogenetic calcium carbonate ($CaCO_3$) in calcium phosphate–based ceramics [9]. Biological systems can produce inorganic materials (such as $CaCO_3$) with different structure, morphology, and polymorphism. Such biological systems are seen in many marine organisms, such as mussels, snails, sea urchins, and molluscs with nacreous shell [9]. In all these cases, the main components are $CaCO_3$ shells and other organic components, such as anionic protein and glycoprotein [36, 38, 51, 80]. Similarly, marble is a widespread natural resource and it is used as precursor to obtain HAP due to the high content of $CaCO_3$ and small concentrations of other elements (e.g. Mg, Si). Raw natural materials are first processed for the removal of impurities. After that, the pure $CaCO_3$ or CaO are used for the synthesis of calcium phosphates, especially HAP [36, 40].

HAP synthesized from these resources presents a tissue response that is superior to synthetically produced HAP, due to porosity, chemical, and structural similarity to the bone mineral phase and osseointegration ability [51, 80]. The physical properties, such as phase composition, thermal stability, and particle size are important parameters for each material used as a precursor for the synthesis of high-purity and high-performance HAP [13, 59].

The following review of literature is based primarily on data on HAP obtaining from potential precursors of marble and marine shell types (different sea shells), where the major component $CaCO_3$ is present in various polymorphic forms. They are differentiated at the crystallographic and compositional level: calcite (trigonal), aragonite (orthorhombic), and dolomite ($CaCO_3{\cdot}MgCO_3$) [76]. Table 5.1 presents the types and species of natural precursors used for the synthesis of HAP.

5.3.1 Marble

The marble is a crystalline variety of $CaCO_3$, which is extracted from quarries, which may look like white crystal sockets that resembles sugar – hence the name sugar marble – colored pink, yellow, green, or black due to different impurities that infiltrates into the mass of $CaCO_3$ (ferritic oxides, quartz) [76, 83].

Marble is available in the form of calcite or dolomite (Table 5.1), it shows different textures, some strong, others weak, and a variation of grain size in the range of 75 μm to 1.75 mm [84]. In the case of the marble with resistant texture, high values of the coefficients of thermal expansion are registered, in contrast to the low value of the maximum tensile stress and deformation energy density, both parameters involved in the material cracking during the calcination process. From this point of view, the marble with weak resistance texture show isotropic thermal expansion behavior, exposed to cracking due to higher values of deformation stress and strain energy. The structural and mechanical properties of marble, under different conditions of pressure and temperature, depend on the systematic layout of calcite/dolomite grains [83, 84].

Table 5.1 Biogenic precursors used for the synthesis of hydroxyapatite.

Chemical compound	Polymorphic form	Crystallographic system	Natural species
Marble			
$CaCO_3$	Calcite	Trigonal	—
$CaCO_3{\cdot}MgCO_3$	Dolomite		
Sea shells			
$CaCO_3$	Calcite	Trigonal	• *Crassostrea angulata* [9] • *Paphia undulata* [1] • *Mytilus galloprovincialis* (brown mussel) [2, 81] • *Crassostrea gigas* [53, 59]
	Aragonite	Orthorhombic	• *Anadara granosa* [32, 34, 38, 82] • *Strombus gigas* [10] • *Tridacna gigas* [10] • *Muricopsis* sp. [12] • *Helix* sp. [12] • *Nacres* (Mother of pearl) [33]
$CaCO_3{\cdot}MgCO_3$	Dolomite	Trigonal	• *Heterocentrotus mammillatus* [11] • *Heterocentrotus trigonarius* [11]

The dissociation of the marble with a high content of $CaCO_3$ (calcite) takes place at temperatures in the 800–900 °C range under normal pressure. When dolomite is the prominent phase, the temperatures change according to the $MgCO_3/CaCO_3$ ratio. While pure magnesium carbonate decomposes at temperatures of 400–480 °C, dolomitic marble dissociates at higher temperatures: above 500 °C in the case of fine and dense crystalline structures, and above 600 °C for highly crystalline structures [85].

The size of marble plates influences the calcination process time. Thus, the calcination completion of large pieces will be made in a longer time compared to the small pieces, because the reaction starts on the outside and propagates inwards [85].

5.3.2 Sea Shells

Huge amounts of marine shellfish (clams, snails, and other shells) are widely spread along coastlines, these materials being of high availability. Besides their applications as building materials or biological aerated filter holders, shells have recently aroused particular interest for biomedical applications [9, 59] due to their low cost, high accessibility, and good biological properties.

Shells are predominantly composed of a mineral phase (~96 wt% calcium carbonate in different polymorphic forms or even dolomite), 4 wt% organic materials, and rare impurities (SiO_2, MgO, Al_2O_3, SrO, P_2O_5, Na_2O, SO_3, and alkaline salts) [33, 59, 86, 87].

Among the calcite-based shells present, the Portuguese oyster (*Crassostrea angulata*) is currently studied [9, 53, 59] for bone regeneration. The availability of *C. angulata* is explained by its use in food industry. In terms of quantity, this species has supported European production of oysters for nearly a century, recording an annual production of 100 000 tonnes.

The oyster's shell morphology is influenced by several factors, such as the type of substrate on which they grow on, the degree of population agglomeration, and environmental conditions [88–90]. At a structural level, the shell consists of four distinct layers: periostracum (highly insoluble coat protein), prismatic layer, calcitostracum, and hipostracum. The calcitostracum, also known as pearl substrate, constitutes the bulk of the shell. The layer consists mainly of spreadsheets disposed between the thin conchiolin membranes. The latter is a compositional scleroprotein that has 6.5% H, 50.7% C, and 16.7% N. Each prism of the prismatic layer consists of an aggregate of calcite crystals set in a matrix of conchiolin that even after dissolving the mineral constituents retain their overall prismatic configuration [89].

Aragonite crystal form is one of the least abundant and it is found in the shell of a bivalve marine mollusc species, *Anadara granosa*, often met in dry areas covered by the sea at high tide [33, 82]. The shells are microlayered composites of minerals and polymers generally containing 95–99 wt% $CaCO_3$ and 1–5% organic macromolecules. It presents an exceptional nano arrangement and a resistance of 3000 times higher than that of mineral crystals themselves [10, 11]. In some organisms, $CaCO_3$ can be simultaneously found into two polymorphs, but separated into different layers. A typical example is the mussels' shell (*Mytilus* sp.) that consists of two layers: a pearly layer at the interior that is based on aragonite crystals and an outer prismatic layer with lattice structures resembling a honeycomb-shaped prism made out of calcite crystals [12].

During the growth of pearls (*Nacres*), the prismatic layer is firstly formed, and then the shimmer layer adds as the shell thickness increases in time. The pearly layer can be compared to a laminated film of 0.5 μm thickness composed of aragonite polygonal crystals and small amounts of protein polymer between them [33]. The polymeric matrix, which is soft, moist, and deformable contributes to the ultimate fracture strength when the material is tested in shear conditions. These cross-lamellar morphologies can be also detected among gastropods: shells of the *Muricopsis* sp. and snails of the *Helix* sp. [12, 60].

In contrast to the above-mentioned structures, in the echinoids spines (*Heterocentrotus mammillatus*) and slate pencil urchin (*Heterocentrotus trigonarius*) species, calcium carbonate is found in a less-prevalent marine form, namely dolomite. In structural terms, this form of calcium carbonate is made of smooth and continuously curved single Mg-enriched calcite crystals ($(Ca,Mg)CO_3$) [91]. Due to the Mg presence in the composition, after calcination, the tricalcium magnesium phosphate (β-TCMP) that stabilizes the structure of β-TCP *in vivo*, occurs [11].

5.4 Synthesis Routes

5.4.1 Preparation of Precursors

All routes used for the synthesis of HAP from marble or sea shells comprise two preliminary preparation steps of the raw material: cleaning foreign particles coming from the natural environment (sand, dirt) and deproteinization (for shell-type precursors) [1, 32–36, 41].

The cleaning step is made using brushes in dry or wet state (under douche of distilled water). Cleaning agents are not recommended in order to prevent the chemical reactions with marble/sea shells. After wet cleaning, the material is dried in mild conditions (sun or at room temperature [RT]).

Following the drying step, the marble can be processed directly without any intermediate steps. In the case of shells, the preliminary cleaning process is followed by deproteinization, performed by boiling the shells in stainless steel containers or ovens, for at least 30 minutes, until the crust detaches completely from the organic matter. The same result is obtained by immersion for 24 hours in a solution of 50% concentration hydrogen peroxide dissolved in water. After the removal of organic matter, the shells are dried in the oven at 60 °C. In a 1000 ml lab glass cylinder, a solution of dilute sulfuric acid is prepared (15% acid and 85% distilled water), with which the stains remaining on the shells surface are removed. A second drying in oven at 60 °C for three days, follows [35].

After the preparation step, $CaCO_3$ that is found in both types of materials can be processed by employing two main routes in the presence of various acids and variable working conditions: (i) thermal decomposition of $CaCO_3$ into CaO and its treatment with acidic substances (see Figures 5.1 and 5.2) or (ii) direct treatment with acids.

5.4.2 Basic Techniques for Hydroxyapatite Synthesis

Properties such as bioactivity, solubility, sintering, pourability, tensile strength, and proteins and bone growth factors adsorption can be tailored by controlling the composition (the ionic substitution into the lattice), the size, and the morphology of HAP particles. A very important aspect is the development of cheap HAP synthesis methods, which can also allow a very precise control of the mentioned features. From this point of view, low temperature techniques seem to be particularly well suited to achieve this objective [92].

Different methods for the synthesis of HAP from natural precursors are described in detail in the literature [1, 29, 30, 34, 36, 37, 40, 41, 50, 51]. These include precipitation in colloidal aqueous solutions, the sol–gel methods [21, 25–27, 31, 49], the solid-state technique, hydrothermal technique [9–11, 28, 39, 43, 46], and the microemulsion by high-pressure homogenization (HPH) and mechano-chemical approaches [21, 42, 47, 48, 51].

5.4.2.1 Wet Precipitation

The methods based on the precipitation of aqueous solutions are widely used in the synthesis of CaP and particularly of HAP. The advantages of wet routes are that the probability of contamination is very low during processing. Possible disadvantages are related to the possible alteration of the final product composition, which can vary even with the smallest differences in the reaction conditions. The duration of obtaining a stoichiometric HAP is of the order of days, which is the most unfavorable part when working on an industrial scale [28, 36].

The difficulty with respect to the most used conventional precipitation methods is the synthesis of well-defined and reproducible calcium orthophosphates. Problems can arise due to the imprecise control of the factors governing the precipitation, such as pH, temperature, and the Ca/P molar ratio of reagents. All this can lead to the synthesis of products with different stoichiometry and morphology, which in turn consequents to different *in vitro/in vivo* behaviors.

The wet chemical precipitation of CaP from solution is based on the methods proposed by Rathje in 1939

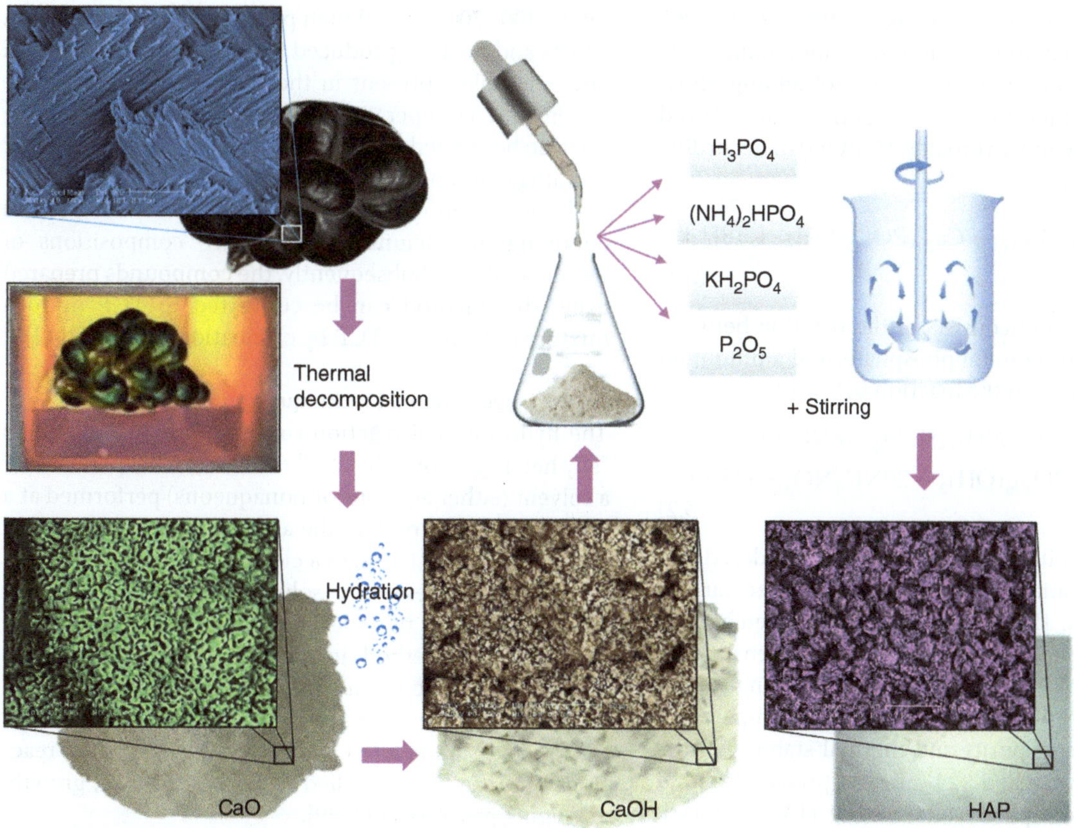

Figure 5.1 Processing steps for hydroxyapatite synthesis by thermal decomposition of sea shells precursors (i–iv).

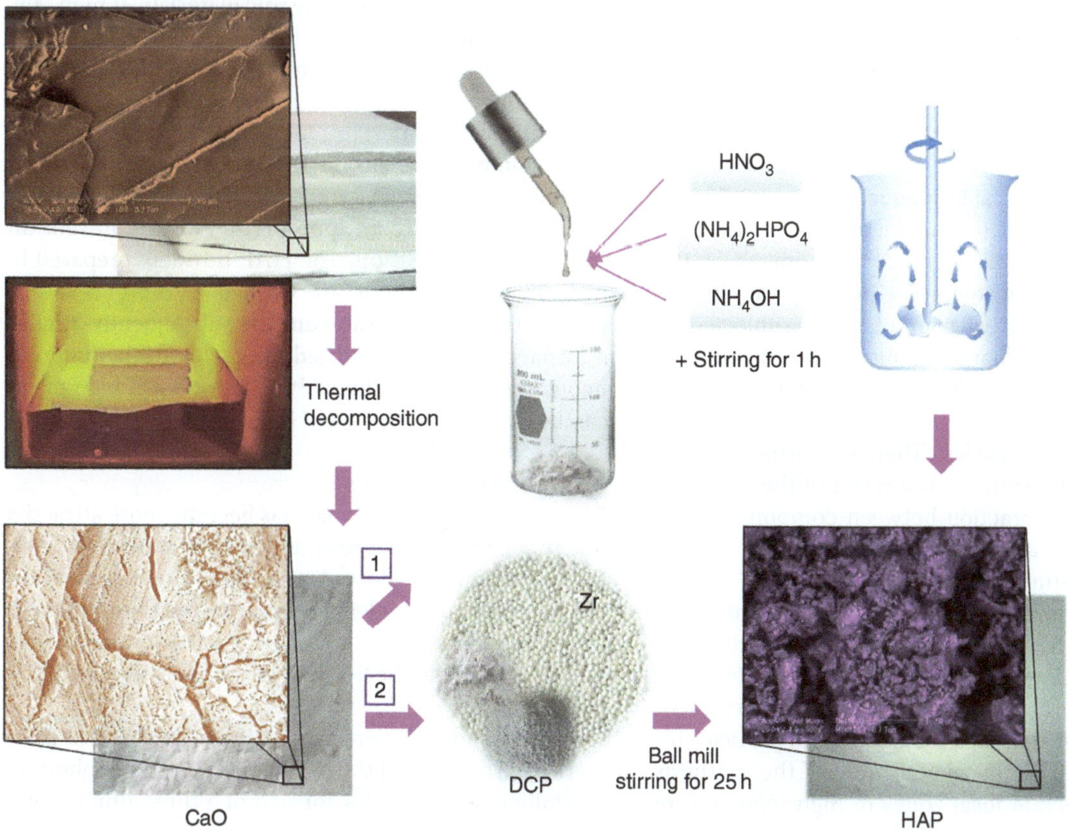

Figure 5.2 Processing steps for hydroxyapatite synthesis by thermal decomposition of marble precursors (1: v–vii, 2: viii).

[93–95] and by Hayek and Newesely in 1963 [93, 94, 96] and involves the chemical reaction of inorganic oxide solutions. The Rathje method consists of adding phosphoric acid by pipetting in a continuously stirred suspension of calcium hydroxide ($Ca(OH)_2$), according to the reaction below:

$$10Ca(OH)_2 + 6H_3PO_4 \rightarrow Ca_{10}(PO_4)_6(OH)_2 + 18H_2O \quad (5.1)$$

Hayek et al. method consists of the reaction between calcium nitrate, ammonium phosphate, and ammonium hydroxide, according to the reaction below [96]:

$$10Ca(NO_3)_2 + 6(NH_4)_2HPO_4 + 8NH_4OH \rightarrow Ca_{10}(PO_4)_6(OH)_2 + 20NH_4NO_3 + 6H_2O \quad (5.2)$$

Chemical precipitation technique is considered the most economical and the easiest way to prepare various HAP biomaterials. The obtained HAP was tested both in neutral and high alkaline solutions in order to ensure the thermal stability of the phase formed by sintering at high temperatures (1100–1300 °C). Once this temperature exceeded, the phasic purity and thermal stability of the HAP powder is reached [24]. By co-precipitation in alkaline solutions, biphasic mixtures of HAP and TCP can be obtained [71].

Although wet chemical methods are highly popular due to their economic benefits and versatility, the effects of sintering temperature, reaction time, concentration of calcium ions, calcination, and the use of different reagents on the morphological properties of HAP particles are not yet fully understood [97].

5.4.2.2 Mechano-Chemical Technique

The mechano-chemical technique represents the coupling of mechanical and chemical phenomena at the molecular scale and involves the mechanical disruption and the chemical behavior of solids subjected to mechanical stress. Mechano-chemical synthesis route is a simple and accessible method used to obtain inorganic compounds. However, it is not commonly used due to the monodispersed particles. They are formed during mechano-chemical synthesis as a result of the reactants spraying and the interaction between components (i.e. the synthesis material and the aqueous solution used as the reaction medium).

The reaction product particles are formed as two-dimensional nuclei in the points of contact of the reactants, so that, in time, the volume will increase. Varying the temperature and duration of the heat treatment applied to the activated mixture can control particle size [48]. The mechano-chemical activation of the synthesis products can generate local zones of high temperature (up to 400–700 °C) and high pressure due to the friction effects and the heat produced by the adiabatic expansion of gas bubbles (present in the slurry), while the whole system is at a temperature close to the ambient. Pressure can also be applied at ambient temperature using specific grinding equipment (e.g. low-energy ball mill) [92].

The mechano-chemical processes usually lead to the obtaining of calcium-deficient HAP compositions of low crystallinity. Subsequently, the compounds prepared using this method can be converted to TCP or to a mixture of HAP and TCP by calcination at 700 °C [42].

5.4.2.3 Hydrothermal Technique

The hydrothermal reaction can explicitly be defined as "any heterogeneous chemical reaction, in the presence of a solvent (either aqueous or nonaqueous) performed at a higher temperature than the ambient one and at a pressure greater than 1 atm, in a closed system" [98].

Aqueous suspensions, solutions, and gels may be converted into the desired crystalline phases by hydrothermal method in a single-stage process, taking place at temperatures below 350 °C and pressures under 150 atm. It has been stated that particle size and morphology are favored by the solution-mediated reactions and can be controlled during nucleation, growth, and aging processes [92, 99].

The crystal growth under hydrothermal conditions is carried out in an autoclave resistant to corrosive salts used for the synthesis of inorganic materials, at high temperature and high pressure for a few hours. As solvent for the solutions preparation is used the distilled water; the acetone and ethanol being used for the washing of the synthesized materials [98].

The temperature inside the autoclave is monitored by thermocouples inserted into special sheaths. The stirring rate is set to an appropriate value to prevent the material sedimentation. The HAP powders prepared by hydrothermal methods are washed in the end several times into deionized water and are subsequently dried in a furnace or are freeze-dried [92]. Chemically homogeneous and well-crystallized HAP powders of high purity can be obtained in this way [100].

5.4.2.4 Sol–Gel Technique

Recently, sol–gel technology has become more attractive due to the remarkable advantages it offers in the fabrication of ceramic powders. Among these one can mention: the homogeneous molecular mixture, the low processing temperature, the ability to generate particles of nanometer dimensions, or the flexibility to obtain nanocrystalline powders [21, 25].

A *sol* is a stable dispersion of colloidal particles or polymers in a solvent and the particles may be amorphous or crystalline, while a *gel* is formed of a three-dimensional

(3D) continuous lattice, which comprises a liquid phase.

In the first stage of the sol–gel process, the hydrolysis and polycondensation reactions lead to the formation of a colloidal solution of hydroxide particles, whose size do not exceed a few tens of nanometers. Increasing the apparent concentration of the dispersed phase or other external condition changes (pH, solvent substitution) lead to the formation of intense contacts between particles and a monolithic gel, in which the solvent molecules are enclosed in a flexible but stable enough manner. The 3D formed lattice consists of hydroxide particles.

However, current studies on HAP produced by sol–gel synthesis indicate that the final product is always accompanied by a secondary phase of calcium oxide (CaO). Since this affects the biocompatibility, a direct method for the removal of CaO has been attempted by washing the calcined powders with dilute hydrochloric acid (HCl) or other acids [26].

5.4.2.5 Microemulsion by High-Pressure Homogenization (HPH)

Most of the research is lately directed toward microemulsion method for the synthesis of different types of nanoparticles, including those of HAP. Microemulsions consist of thermodynamically stable dispersions, optically transparent and isotropic, of two immiscible liquids. The microemulsion or the microreactor of the system is made up of maximum 100 nm sized particles.

The advantage of this method consists of increasing the homogeneity of chemical decomposition at the nanometer level, facilitating the preparation of nanocrystals with relatively equal sizes. In respect to the synthesis of HAP nanoparticles, this is made by microemulsion of oil in water (O/W), using a system of HPH [38, 44, 101]. This system is provided with a small valve in the center through which fluid passes, creating intense shear and turbulence conditions. The impact along with the pressure drop leads to particle disintegration and dispersions. Particle size uniformity depends on several parameters such as operating pressure and number of cycles [38].

5.4.3 Synthesis of Hydroxyapatite by Thermal Treatment of Marble and Shells

One of the most popular routes is the conversion by calcination of $CaCO_3$, present in the marble or marine shells, into CaO. After the dissociation reaction, the resulting CaO is converted by accurate methods into HAP powder.

The temperature of $CaCO_3$ dissociation varies depending on the type of polymorph, furthermore being strongly influenced by the chemical purity and physical characteristics of the precursor material [85, 102]. The calcination reaction is endothermic and is favored by high temperatures [34, 103]:

$$CaCO_3 \xrightarrow{t^{\circ}} CaO + CO_2 \tag{5.3}$$

5.4.3.1 Calcination of the Raw Material

The thermal decomposition of $CaCO_3$ is based on the chemical reaction at elevated temperature that produces carbon dioxide (CO_2) release and CaO formation [34, 103–105].

The observed reaction rate depends on: (i) the heat transfer (heat must firstly be dispersed on the material surface and then through the outer layer of the formed CaO and subsequently in the next reaction zone) and (ii) the mass transfer (calcium dioxide should be released through the outer oxide layer formed. Therefore, the pressure in the reaction zone must be much higher than that from the outside). Maintaining the decomposition requires increasing the pressure and therefore the temperature in the reaction zone [34]. Empirically, it has been shown that the decomposition reaction starts at around 600 °C, but in the literature studies the temperatures up to 1200 °C are reported [34, 40, 106]. The calcination can be achieved in electric furnace muffles or tubular furnaces under nitrogen flow (the minimum temperature of 800 °C being required) [36, 40].

The raw material can be treated either in its natural state (after various preparatory operations) or as transformed into micrometer size powder. The powder is obtained by crushing the materials in a mortar [34, 59] and milling using a ball mill or a shredder with balls and bowls of zirconia or alumina [56]. At temperatures above 900 °C, the CaO crystals have characteristic dimensions of the hundreds of nanometers [51, 56].

5.4.3.2 Calcium Oxide Conversion into Hydroxyapatite

This step is performed mainly by wet (chemical precipitation) and mechano-chemical methods. The preparation of HAP by chemical precipitation is done by treating the obtained CaO powder with a wide range of acids of different concentrations. An optional step, but rather common, is the hydration with a specific amount of distilled water, depending on the amount of the powder and the desired concentration. The reaction between CaO and water is an exothermic one. The released heat becomes apparent when a whistling steam appears from the mixture after the addition of water drops over the CaO powder. $Ca(OH)_2$ is obtained from the reaction:

$$CaO + H_2O \rightarrow Ca(OH)_2 \tag{5.4}$$

$Ca(OH)_2$ has a low solubility in water at ambient temperature (<0.2 g/100 ml), thus its filtering on filter paper leads to the retaining of almost the entire amount of $Ca(OH)_2$ [1].

In 1977, for the first time, Jarcho et al. [107] obtained ultrafine HAP powder from the reaction between $Ca(OH)_2$ and phosphoric acid at RT. Increasing the concentration of raw materials leads to the formation of needle-like HAP particles. After the aging process, their crystallite size is reduced and so greater specific surface area [51]. Since then, several synthesis methods have been advanced, which can be classified based on the $Ca(OH)_2$ (i–iv)/CaO (v–viii) concentration and described as follows:

(i) Reaction of calcium hydroxide with phosphoric acid

0.15 M phosphoric acid (prepared by dissolving 1.7 ml of phosphoric acid in 200 ml of distilled water) was added dropwise to the $Ca(OH)_2$ of 0.25 M concentration (prepared by dissolving 2.8 g of CaO in 200 ml of distilled water) [51]. The acid was gradually added, 1 ml/min, in order to preserve the reaction at a pH of 9–10, and at a temperature of 25–60 °C. The substances are stirred constantly with a magnetic stirrer [25]. The reaction proceeds according to the following equation:

$$10Ca(OH)_2 + 6H_3PO_4 \rightarrow Ca_{10}(PO_4)_6(OH)_2 + 18H_2O \quad (5.5)$$

After completion of the reaction, a gelatinous precipitate is obtained, of whose pH is maintained by the pipetted addition of a solution of ammonia. The resulting solution is allowed to age for 24 hours, after which the precipitate separated by filtration is washed with distilled water in order to remove the residual hydroxide and then is dried in an oven at 80 °C for eight hours.

Increasing the temperature leads to a highly crystalline HAP, while decreasing the pH results in obtaining a calcium-deficient HAP [25, 41]. Ca/P molar ratio of the derived reagents is 1.67. This process has been also applied with 0.6 M phosphoric acid and a solution of 1.0 M $Ca(OH)_2$ [41].

(ii) Reaction of calcium hydroxide with ammonium phosphate

$Ca(OH)_2$ is mixed with 100 ml of distilled water and converted into a slurry with a solution with a concentration of 0.3 M. One hundred milliliters of diammonium hydrogen phosphate ($(NH_4)_2HPO_4$) of 0.3 M concentration is pipetted, which will react with the suspension at 40 °C (see Eq. (5.6)).

$$10Ca(OH)_2 + 6(NH_4)_2HPO_4 \rightarrow Ca_{10}(PO_4)_6(OH)_2 + 12NH_4OH + 6H_2O \quad (5.6)$$

The resulting solution is stirred for 2–5 hours, and it precipitates overnight or in 24 hours at RT. The precipitate is filtered with filter paper (Whatman®, grade 40) and is dried at 110 °C for five hours [37].

(iii) Reaction of calcium hydroxide with potassium dihydrogen phosphate

0.1 M $Ca(OH)_2$ is prepared by dissolving overnight the CaO powder in deionized water in a sealed reactor. A solution of 0.06 M phosphate is prepared by dissolving the potassium dihydrogen phosphate (KH_2PO_4) in deionized water and then is added to the reactor via a peristaltic pump at a rate of 22 ml/min (depending on the amount of HAP to be produced; the actual mass of reactants is also determined). The mixture was stirred for five hours under a nitrogen atmosphere in order to obtain a milky white suspension containing the HAP precipitate (Eq. (5.7)). The powder is separated from the solution by centrifugation and drying at 110 °C [36, 50].

$$10Ca(OH) + 6KH_2PO_4 \rightarrow Ca_{10}(PO_4)_6(OH)_2 + 6KOH + 12H_2O \quad (5.7)$$

(iv) Reactions of calcium hydroxide with phosphorus pentoxide

Two powder mixtures containing two or three reagents in solid state can be obtained:

$$10Ca(OH)_2 + P_2O_5 \rightarrow Ca_{10}(PO_4)_6(OH)_2 + 9H_2O \quad (5.8)$$

$$9CaO + Ca(OH)_2 + 3P_2O_5 \rightarrow Ca_{10}(PO_4)_6(OH)_2 \quad (5.9)$$

The mixtures are obtained in a ball mill at a rotational speed of 790 rpm for up to two hours. In both cases, the synthesis reactions occur mainly by acid–base solid-state reaction between the activated solids either on surface or by dry milling [47].

The major difference between these two variants consists of the presence of free water, which is released when the mixture is completely converted to HAP. Phosphorous pentoxide easily reacts with water from the $Ca(OH)_2$, leading to the formation of phosphoric acid (Eq. (5.10)). Simultaneously, calcium hydrogen phosphate ($CaHPO_4$) is formed by acid–base reaction, as an intermediate stage (according to the Eq. (5.11)). Equation (5.8) is, therefore, a chain of intermediate reactions obtained by grinding for 30 minutes, leading in the end to obtaining of HAP:

$$10Ca(OH)_2 + P_2O_5 \rightarrow 6H_3PO_4 + 9CaO + Ca(OH)_2 \quad (5.10)$$

$$6H_3PO_4 + 9CaO + Ca(OH)_2 \rightarrow 6CaHPO_4 + 4Ca(OH)_2 + 3H_2O \quad (5.11)$$

$$6CaHPO_4 + 4Ca(OH)_2 + 3H_2O \rightarrow Ca_{10}(PO_4)_6(OH)_2 + 9H_2O \quad (5.12)$$

(v) Reaction of calcium oxide with nitric acid and diammonium hydrogen phosphate

CaO powder is firstly converted according to the reaction of calcium nitrate with a solution of 25% nitric acid (by continuous stirring):

$$CaO + 2HNO_3 \rightarrow Ca(NO_3)_2 + H_2O \tag{5.13}$$

A solution of diammonium hydrogen phosphate (phosphate was prepared by dissolving 12.73 g in 30 ml of distilled water) is pipetted in calcium nitrate solution kept at room temperature. The solution of ammonium hydroxide is added in order to maintain the pH in the range 8–10 and to ensure the formation of a stoichiometric HAP [40]:

$$10Ca(NO_3)_2 + 6(NH_4)_2HPO_4 + 8NH_4OH \rightarrow Ca_{10}(PO_4)_6(OH)_2 + 20NH_4NO_3 + 6H_2O \tag{5.14}$$

The mixture is stirred for one hour to ensure a complete reaction and was subjected to an aging treatment for 24 hours. The precipitated HAP is kept in the centrifuge tube at 24 °C for 24 hours, and then freeze-dried. Freezing takes place at temperatures below −52 °C for 48–72 hours. After water vaporization, the HAP is obtained in the form of a powder conglomerate [30, 40].

(vi) Reaction of calcium oxide with diammonium hydrogen phosphate

This method provides good control of Ca/P ratio of the obtained HAP. The method was applied [34] for obtaining various Ca/P ratios. Pipetted phosphate in 600 ml of distilled water was mixed with the CaO powder, and all the suspensions are heated at 70, 80, 90 °C and continuously stirred at 300 rpm until a paste is formed. The slurry is dried at 120 °C for 15 hours, and then calcined at 900 °C for 4 hours.

(vii) Reaction of calcium oxide with ammonium dihydrogen orthophosphate and sucrose

2.8 g of CaO are dissolved in 100 ml of 0.05 M concentration sucrose, to which is added by pipetting 100 ml of 0.03 M concentrated ammonium dihydrogen orthophosphate solution. The mixture is stirred for 24 hours, and then heated at 10–95 °C for 2 hours. The formed HAP powder is separated by centrifugation and washed with distilled water to remove impurities. Drying is done in a vacuum oven for 12 hours [29]. The reaction depends on the used amount of saccharides, the content of the obtained HAP powder decreasing with the sucrose content in the precipitation solution. During calcination, the oxidation of carbonaceous materials formed from the sucrose degradation produces heat, a phenomenon that leads to the dehydration of HAP, and the formation of β-TCP [108].

Mechanically, the synthesis of HAP can be achieved either by direct acid treatment of CaO powder or by hydration of a powder part (Eq. (5.4)), combining it with CaO and subsequently treating the mixture with acid. The methods are based on:

(viii) Reaction of calcium oxide with anhydrous calcium phosphate

CaO powder can be mixed with anhydrous calcium hydrogen phosphate (DCPA), in designed amounts so that their molar ratio is 3 : 2. Their mixing can be made in a conventional ball mill, the grinding medium being made of zirconia balls and ethanol. The rotation speed and the milling time is usually set at 370 rpm for 15 hours [42, 48, 109].

$$4CaO + 6CaHPO_4\ Ca_{10}(PO_4)_6(OH)_2 + 2H_2O \tag{5.15}$$

The powder mixture is loaded into the ball mill, and the mechanical activation of the mixture is made using high speeds for 25 hours.

5.4.4 Synthesis of Hydroxyapatite by Chemical Treatment of Marble and Shells

5.4.4.1 Hydrothermal Methods

Hydrothermally, the synthesis of the HAP is possible by conducting the following reactions:

(i) Reaction of calcium carbonate with diammonium hydrogen phosphate and water

The raw material ($CaCO_3$) crushed into small-millimeter-sized pieces is added to the autoclave filled with solution of diammonium hydrogen phosphate having a concentration between 0.12 and 0.6 g/ml [10, 39]. The hydrothermal treatment is carried out at temperatures between 180 and 240 °C and a pressure of 15 atm for ~9 hours [10, 46].

For an optimum conversion of the $CaCO_3$ the following parameters are preferred: diammonium hydrogen phosphate concentration of 0.2 g/ml and temperature of 180 °C for eight hours. The reaction of hydrothermal transformation occurs according to the Eq. (5.16) [11]:

$$10CaCO_3 + 6(NH_4)2HPO_4 + 2H_2O \rightarrow Ca_{10}(PO_4)_6(OH)_2 + 4H_2CO_3 \tag{5.16}$$

In the powder form, the $CaCO_3$ with a solution of diammonium hydrogen phosphate (Ca/P ratio = 5/6) are mixed homogeneously in a Teflon bottle filled with deionized water. After appropriate stirring, the bottle is sealed in an autoclave and heated at 220 °C for six hours [9, 46].

(ii) Reaction of calcium carbonate with calcium pyrophosphate

The mixture is made at a molar ratio of 3 : 4, corresponding to the Ca/P ratio of HAP composition (i.e. 1.67). The grinding is made at a speed of 170 rpm, for two to eight hours in a polyethylene bottle half filled with zirconia beads [28, 69]. The resultant powder (see Eq. (5.17)), together with distilled water maintained at a pH = 7 are placed in a Teflon bottle, which is properly stirred. In the autoclave, the Teflon glass is heated to 120 or 180 °C:

$$4CaCO_3 + 3Ca_2O_7P_2 + H_2O \rightarrow Ca_{10}(PO_4)_6(OH)_2 + 4CO_2 \quad (5.17)$$

(iii) Reaction of calcium carbonate with phosphoric acid

When calcium pyrophosphate is replaced with phosphoric acid, the Teflon glass will contain a suspension of 0.2 g powdered $CaCO_3$ in 40 ml of various concentration acid and distilled water maintained at the same pH using an ammonium solution with concentration of 28% [43]. The synthesis reaction, in this case, takes place according to the equation:

$$10CaCO_3 + 6H_3PO_4\ Ca_{10}(PO_4)_6(OH)_2 + 10CO_2 + 8H_2O \quad (5.18)$$

In the last two cases (ii and iii), the autoclave is allowed to cool to room temperature and the obtained suspension is filtered and dried in an oven at a temperature of 60–150 °C for one day. Subsequently, the obtained powder is thermally treated at a temperature of 1100 °C for one hour [28, 43, 46].

5.4.4.2 Sol–Gel Methods

The key factors are the additive types used in this method and the drying process conditions. The processing on the sol–gel route requires an optimum value of pH or a high temperature. By mixing the precursors at molecular level, an enhancement of the final product homogeneity is obtained, while by adjusting the Ca/P ratio the degree of crystallinity can be controlled [25, 27].

$CaCO_3$ powder is mixed with orthophosphoric acid (H_3PO_4) in a molar ratio of 5 : 3. The solution is kept in the alkaline ammonia for 24 hours, and then an aging treatment can be applied in an oil bath at 80–90 °C for 16 hours [26, 49]. The transformation reaction takes place according to the Eq. (5.18).

The obtained apatitic gel is filtered and dried in an oven at 120 °C for 15 hours [21]. In order to remove remaining organic traces, the submicrometer-sized HAP powder is calcined at 400 °C and then sintered at a temperature of at least 1000 °C (starting at 600 °C with a heating rate of 100 °C/h) [21, 26]. Due to the agglomerated shape resulting after the calcination, the sintering time may be extended up to 24 hours. The final size of HAP particle diameters varies between 4 and 11 μm [25, 31].

5.4.4.3 Microemulsion by High-Pressure Homogenization (HPH)

Obtaining uniform particles of $CaCO_3$ by double emulsion technique is made in four main steps. This method itself may be considered as a previous step for any of the methods described above, so that, in the end, the obtained powder must be treated with a phosphorus-based acid in order to obtain the desired product, the HAP.

Initially, the precursors are transformed to a fine powder, which is sorted with a 90 μm stainless steel sieve. Screened powder is dissolved in an organic microemulsion (O/W), which was stirred moderately at a speed of 100 rpm for five minutes to form the $CaCO_3$ suspension. The resulting slurry is passed through the inlet of the HPH for preshredding at a moderate pressure of 300–500 bar, for three cycles, each followed by a second pass at high pressure of 1500 bar for 25 cycles. The resulting transparent suspension is filtered and dried in oven at 80–100 °C for a day and then sintered at 650 °C for six hours [38, 110].

This method leads to a significantly uniformization of particle size, due to cavitation, the collision between particles, and shear forces. The size of the particles can be controlled by the number of processing cycles and on the working pressure of HPH [38, 44, 101].

5.5 Processing of Marble and Shells-Derived Hydroxyapatite

Whatever the followed synthesis process, the obtained products are powdery, their grain size being in nanometer range. As implantable products that can be further obtained from these powders one can mention scaffolds and pellets (see Figure 6.1). Due to the multilayered structure of human bone, the latter must present structures that mimic the biological form, because their function is to become a matrix for the subsequent tissue in-growth [35, 111]. If the particle size of HAP is not uniform, a size sorting is done, so that the finished products will be composed only of particles of approximately equal diameter.

5.5.1 Thermal Processing of the Hydroxyapatite Powder

The heat treatments applied according to conventional methods take place in electric furnaces, in air or nitrogen atmosphere, at a heating rate appropriately selected according to the maximum sintering temperature

[42, 47]. For the temperature range of 500–800 °C, the required time is ~4–5 hours [36, 37], and when the temperature exceeds 900 °C the time can be reduced to 1–2 hours. The resulting powder is called *heat-treated hydroxyapatite* [40].

The heat treatment performed at higher temperatures (not exceeding the melting temperature of the material), applied to HAP suspensions or powders for the production of porous materials and densification of the microstructure is defined as sintering [112]. Sintering may be carried out both by conventional methods or by using microwaves. In this case, the product is called *sintered hydroxyapatite.*

Microwave sintering of ceramics was first proposed in 1954. Its use was motivated by the fast transformation, the short time (15–30 minutes [113]), and the lower sintering temperatures (950–1200 °C) [114] required for the apatite powder densification.

The difference between the conventional process and the microwave sintering is that the material heated through the microwave absorbs electromagnetic energy in all its volume and converts it into heat from the interior to the exterior, against the transfer of heat from the outside to the inside made by conduction, radiation, or convection, as the case of the conventional process. HAP's ability to absorb microwaves is quite low, but increases with the temperature. The advantage of this type of sintering is due to the fact that the maximum needed temperature does not exceed 900 °C, which is important given that this reduces the risk of its decomposition [115, 116].

5.5.2 Dense Products (Pellets)

HAP powder compression can be made by cold or hot pressing, the latter involving high temperatures and long sintering time, leading to a coarser grain size and to the decomposition of the materials, as well as the deterioration of the mechanical properties of the resulting product [113].

Therefore, studies are focused on obtaining pellets by cold pressing, using manual hydraulic presses [117]. Further, the powder is mechanically mixed with physiologic serum, cellular polystyrene, or polyvinyl alcohol (PVA) in a high-shear mill. Samples are uniaxially pressed at 23–390 MPa [6, 118]. The resulting pellets (see Figure 5.3) are dried in the sun or at ambient temperature for seven days. After drying, the material is treated in the oven in order to remove the residual water. Slow drying process ensures the stability of samples at the molecular level, before being subjected to sintering. If the drying speed is too high, the pellets may crack under the residual contraction stress, unevenly distributed [1].

Various sintering routes were proposed, depending on the desired mechanical characteristics. Examples of regimes dedicated for sintering of marble and shells-derived HAP include:

- microwave sintering at a temperature of 900–1200 °C, for 15 minutes at a heating rate of 20 °C/min [113];
- conventional sintering in oven at a temperature of 650–750 °C for three hours [1];
- conventional sintering in oven at a temperature of 800–1000 °C for two to three hours [113, 118];
- humid atmosphere sintering at 1200 °C for two hours [119].

Depending on the mold dimensions, the height and diameter of the obtained cylinders ranges from 3 to 10 mm, and 8 to 15 mm, respectively. The required amount of powder and binder (e.g. distilled water, saline solution) varies according to the desired mass concentration [118].

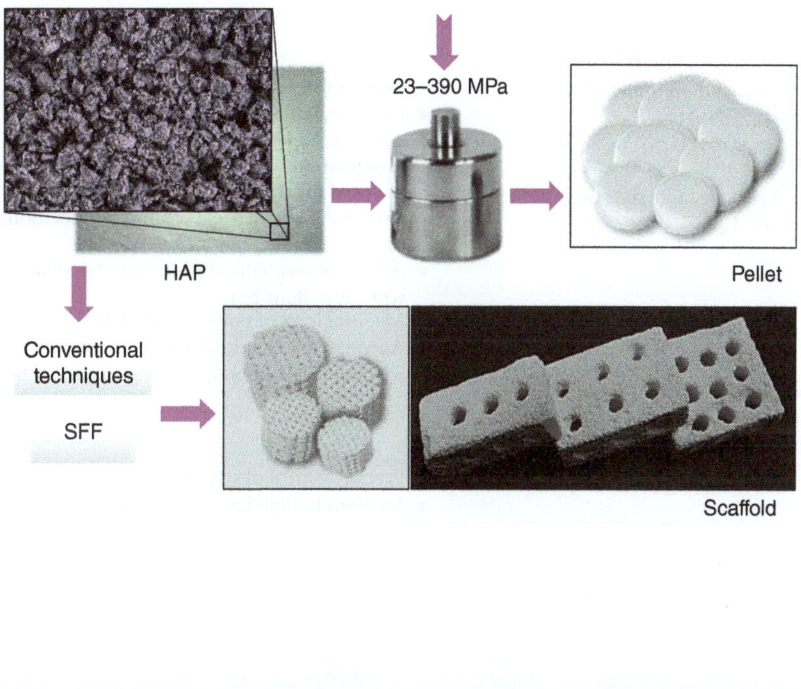

Figure 5.3 Derived hydroxyapatite processed by cold pressing and scaffolding techniques.

5.5.3 Porous Products (Scaffolds)

At the bone tissue level, the cells and the extracellular matrix (ECM) are organized as 3D structures. The tissue engineering technologies propose bone equivalent porous structures, called "scaffolds," which play a role in cell accommodating, growth, and subsequent tissue regeneration. The bone structure varies with the location within the body, thus shaping of the biomaterial will depend on the anatomy of the reconstruction zone and the mechanical loads will bear [120, 121].

The scaffold matrix should have high porosity and a pore size suitable for cell migration, for the growth of newly formed tissues, and for the appropriate distribution of nutrients. Bone regeneration requires pore sizes between 100 and 150 μm, while the vascularization and ossification requires pore diameter of at least 300 μm [121]. Secondly, the anatomical shape of the matrix must be compatible with the orientation of the formed bone tissue. A fine matching of the scaffold degradation with bone's healing rate also needs to be accomplished [15, 16, 122].

Scaffolds are mainly fabricated of highly resistant biocompatible and bioactive materials with chemical and phase composition similar to the natural bone mineral. For this reason, HAP and TCP are among the most recommended biomaterials for scaffold type applications. Compared to the TCP, which elicit a high degradation rate, HAP induces a more rapid bone growth [111].

The need for such products has led to the development of numerous methods for manufacturing 3D scaffolds, classified into two categories: (i) conventional manufacturing methods and (ii) SFF techniques or "rapid prototyping" (RP). Each of these methods generates different properties and characteristics of the internal architecture, such as the size and structure of the pores (see Figure 5.3, Table 5.2), interconnectivity, or mechanical properties [16, 135].

Table 5.2 Scaffold fabrication techniques.

Technique (References)	Advantages	Disadvantages
Conventional techniques		
Solvent casting/salt leaching [16, 123, 124]	• Controllable porosity and pore size • Medium level of porosity (20–50%) • Partial interconnectivity	• Toxic solvents • Poor mechanical properties (compared to cancellous bone)
Freeze-drying [12, 16, 125, 126]	• High level of porosity (≥90%) • Good interconnectivity	• Poor mechanical properties (for load-bearing applications) • Long-time sublimation of solvents
Thermally induced phase separation (TIPS) [16, 127]	• Controllable pore size • Good interconnectivity • Adequate substrate for cell attachment and migration	• Residual solvents trapped in final products
Gas foaming [16, 128]	• No need for toxic solvents usage • Controllable pore size (30–700 μm)	• Poor mechanical properties (for load-bearing applications)
Polymer sponge [9, 12, 129–132]	• High level of porosity (≥90%) • Controllable pore size (100–400 μm) • Microporosity (1–10 μm) in the pore walls	• Poor mechanical properties (compared to cancellous bone)
Solid free-form fabrication techniques		
Stereolithography (SLA) [14, 16, 121]	• Complex internal structures • High level of porosity 70–90% porosity • Adequate substrate for cell attachment and proliferation	• Applicable only for photopolymers
Selective laser sintering (SLS) [16, 121]	• No need for structure postprocessing • Does not influence cell viability or metabolic processes • Adequate mechanical properties (similar with cancellous bone)	• Trapped powder inside the small pores (which can lead to cell growth blockage) • Resolution depends on laser beam size
Three-dimensional printing (3DP) [16, 52, 123]	• Medium level of porosity (45–60%) • Adequate mechanical properties (similar with cancellous bone)	• Pore dimension depends on powder particle size • Mechanical properties depend on bonding capacity of powdered layers • Trapped powder inside the small pores (which can lead to cell growth blockage)
Robocasting [133, 134]	• Precise control of structure's thickness • Medium to high level of porosity (55–75%)	• Mechanical properties depend on mixture composition

5.5.3.1 Conventional Processing Methods

Conventional methods are generally classified by the method of removal of the pore-forming agents, in (i) heating-based methods and (ii) dissolution-based methods. Pore-forming agents from the class of polymers (such as naphthalene, starch, cellulose, or PMMA) can be removed by heating, while sugars and salts are usually removed by dissolution.

Casting methods are applied to obtain cements or suspensions. The process requires the dispersion of the ceramic material in a liquid phase, followed by drying in order to obtain a porous preform and ends with a sintering program for achieving the required mechanical properties [136].

Different aspects, methods of preparation and processing of scaffold type structures are proposed in dedicated reviews [14–16, 121, 123, 129, 137], further being presented only those compatible to ceramic materials, especially apatitic ones.

(i) Solvent casting/salt leaching

This method consists of dissolving the polymer and the mixture of ceramic powder in an organic solvent and casting the resulting solution into a 3D predefined mold. Evaporation of the solvent yields the scaffold. By addition to the mixture of pore-forming agents, such as salt or sugar particles, porous scaffolds can be obtained. In this case, the proportion polymer–pore-forming agent controls the pore size and porosity of the final product. The added particles are removed by immersion in water or other suitable solvent. The simple preparation process and the low-cost equipment are among the most important advantages. The main disadvantages are the impossibility to obtain complex shapes and the possible residual solvents that can damage the cells and biological tissues through protein denaturation.

The method was used for obtaining porous scaffolds by dissolving HAP powder in acetic acid with concentration of ≥99.5% (mass ratio 1 : 3) and vigorous stirring at 70 °C for four hours. Salt, with a pore size in the range of 200–500 μm, was added to the obtained homogeneous suspension, followed by constant stirring for 10–15 minutes. Further, the solution was poured into a cylindrical Teflon mold and sonicated for 15 minutes. After the complete solidification, and removal from the mold, the products were immersed in distilled water for at least five days in order to eliminate the acetic acid salt. At the end of the process, the samples were washed with deionized water for 24 hours to ensure a complete removal of the acetic acid. Finally, the material was dried at 100 °C for 24 hours [124].

(ii) Lyophilization (freeze-drying)

The freeze-drying uses organic solvents or water for the production of porous structures in the absence of pore-forming agents. One of the benefits of this method lies in the ability to realize scaffolds without the use of high temperatures. The size and morphology of the pores of such a structure are dependent on the specific processing parameters: freezing rate, temperature, and concentrations of organics. However, the obtained products have low and irregular pore sizes, typically in the range of 15–35 μm [125].

Porous HAP scaffolds were obtained following this method after the preparation of ceramic slurries by ball milling the HAP powder in camphene ($C_{10}H_{16}$) hot liquid in containers of high-density polyethylene. The procedure continued with heating in an oven at 55 °C for 20 hours, in order to obtain a stable dispersed suspension. Liquid camphene has a vapor pressure at 55 °C similar to that of water at 18 °C, but it evaporates quicker. The resulting hot solution was then poured into molds made of polyurethane; at room temperature, the solidification occurred almost immediately. Within three minutes the solidification was complete, a green body was obtained, and it was frozen at temperatures of about −40 °C. After removal from the mold, the bodies were placed in the ambient atmosphere with an air-flow rate of 0.01–0.05 m/s for the sublimation of frozen camphene, for 24 hours. Subsequently, the samples were sintered at temperatures of 1600 °C for four hours, without the need for special processes of binder combustion [125, 126].

(iii) Thermally induced phase separation (TIPS)

This method uses a volatile organic solvent with a low melting point in order to dissolve the mixture of polymer and ceramic particles (e.g. HAP). Initially, the polymer solution is rapidly cooled in order to induce the phase separation. This leads to the solidification of the solvent, the dissolved polymer being forced to occupy the interstitial spaces, and thereby a porous scaffold is obtained. By tailoring a number of variables, such as the type of polymer and solvent, the polymer concentration and the phase separation temperature, a variety of scaffolds with different architectures can be generated. The main advantage of this method is the possibility to obtain a high porosity by the facile adjustment of the process parameters. It has been proven that the TIPS method followed by cool drying can produce structures with a porosity of 95% [16].

Some studies report obtaining scaffolds starting from a nanosized HAP powder and polylactic glycolic acid (PLGA). Initially the powder was dispersed by sonication in water, and after the complete dispersion, the polymer was added. The resulting compound of PLGA/HAP was heated in the sonicator at a temperature of 65 °C until the mixture turned into a homogeneous suspension. The suspension was heated at 15 °C above the crystallization temperature. The resulting solid was immersed in a bath maintained at a constant desired annealing temperature for a maximum of eight hours. The annealed sample was placed in liquid nitrogen for quick freezing. Finally, the material was dried at 60 °C for two days in order to remove the solvent and obtain the porous scaffold [127].

(iv) Gas foaming

This technique involves the use of a gas as pore-forming agent in order to create interconnected pores. It was developed in order to remove the organic solvents from the manufacturing process, residues that may lead to postimplantation inflammatory reactions. CO_2 is one of the most widely used gases for supercritical fluid processing. Initially, a polymer is placed in a chamber saturated with CO_2 at high pressure. As the pressure is rapidly decreased, the pore nucleation and formation processes appear due to the thermodynamic instability in the gas-polymer system.

The morphology and the resulting structure pore size are influenced by the manufacturing parameters: temperature, pressure, saturation degree, and depressurization time. The obtained scaffold has a sponge-like structure, with pores in the range of 30–700 μm and a porosity of up to 85% [16].

HAP-based scaffolds were obtained by the addition of a bioresorbable polymer, namely PLA. Both materials were vacuum dried before processing, in order to prevent the polymer degradation by hydrolysis. CO_2 had 99.99% purity. The homogeneous dispersion of the particles, without causing significant degradation of the polymer, was performed by hot extrusion. PLA tablets and ceramic particles were firstly mixed in the dry state and subsequently extruded with a micro-compounder, equipped with two bevel rotating screws of reduced capacity. In order to limit the polymer degradation, the mixing was carried out under nitrogen flow at a preset temperature of 200 °C, using a screw rotation speed of 100 rpm and for a total time of four minutes.

The extruded rods were inserted into cylindrical molds and placed in the pressure vessel at 150–250 bar and 195 °C (above the melting point of the PLA). CO_2 diffuses slowly at near ambient temperature in a semicrystalline polymer. Its melting accelerates the diffusion and increases the dioxide solubility. The polymer saturation with CO_2 occurred after about 10 minutes, which resulted in a solution of melted polymer gas. By the rapid gas release, the nucleation by supersaturation was induced and growth of these nuclei generated the porous scaffold's structure [128].

(v) Electrocentrifugation

The electrocentrifugation is a versatile process, which involves the use of an electrical charge to create non-woven scaffolds from a polymer solution. By this technique, different high-porosity models of fibers can be produced. The fiber diameter and its morphology are controlled by several variables: the solution viscosity, charge density, molecular weight of the polymer, and electric intensity. The major advantage of this method is the production of highly porous scaffold with interconnected pores. The disadvantage is represented by the need of organic solvents.

The method was adapted for HAP nanoparticles, which were mixed with cellulose acetate and subsequently dissolved in a solvent containing acetone and acetic acid in a 50 : 50 volume ratio. The solution was sonicated for one hour to prevent the precipitation of the cellulose acetate [69]. The subsequent processing is similar to that described for salt leaching (i).

(vi) Polymer sponge

The polymer sponge method consists of coating a substrate composed of polymer foams with layer of ceramic slurry [130, 138]. The method allows the manufacture of ceramic scaffolds with the highest possible degree of porosity (99 vol%) [9, 131].

For HAP, the slurry was obtained by mixing the ceramic powder with monomers (acrylamide and methylenebisacrylamide), a dispersing agent, a surfactant, and deionized water. The suspension was de-agglomerated by grinding it in ball mill for 24 hours and de-aerated under vacuum until no more air bubbles issuing from the sample are observed.

Polymerization of the monomers was achieved by adding ammonium persulfate as a catalyst and tetramethylethylenediamine as an initiator. The suspension was filled by immersion of pieces of polyurethane foam in the vacuum to force the ceramic particles to migrate into the pores. The foams were then removed from the suspension and placed in a chamber with nitrogen to avoid contamination with oxygen that may inhibit the polymerization. After drying, the polymerized samples were heated at 600 °C for one hour (the heating ensures the combustion of the polyurethane foam). The final product was obtained by sintering at 1350 °C for two hours [132].

Another ceramic paste can be obtained by mixing a water-based HAP suspension with an organic polymer, such as PMMA. The insertion of the PMMA pore-forming agent in this case is limited by a series of requirements. The pore-forming agent should be stable; in powder form, it should not dissolve in methyl methacrylate monomers (MMA); and should not react with the HAP counterpart. Pore formation process should begin only when the polymer interacts with the ceramic suspension [120].

5.5.3.2 Solid Free-Form (SFF) Techniques

Scaffold's porous architecture can be precisely controlled via several SFF techniques, which rely on computer-aided design (CAD) for the device custom manufacturing. In these techniques, the complex architecture is obtained via layer-by-layer deposition of the additive material.

Most of the conventional methods for scaffold manufacturing do not allow the fabrication of customized and complex internal architecture of the pores. The advantage of the SFF, in this regard, is the possibility of thereof execution for a given defect, starting from an image obtained by X-ray computed tomography techniques [15]. In addition, SFF techniques have advantages (Table 5.2) in terms of reproducibility of the designed scaffold and the precise control on the 3D architecture (internal structure, geometry, spatial distribution, and pore size), so that both the biological and mechanical performance can be improved [139].

The most used methods to achieve ceramic scaffold are the stereolithography (SLA), selective laser sintering (SLS), 3D printing (3DP), and robocasting.

(i) Stereolithography (SLA)

One of the oldest SFF technologies, the SLA, was developed in 1986 by the Chuck Hull company [140]. Since then, it has been extensively used, including in biomedical engineering. From the construction point of view, SLA system consists of a tank with photosensitive liquid resin, a built in mobile platform, a UV laser to irradiate the resin, and a dynamic system of mirrors.

The process uses the UV laser to build a layer-by-layer 3D scaffold based on photosensitive liquid resin. When a layer is completely solidified, the platform is lowered vertically, at a short distance, in the resin basin. Then a quantity of liquid resin covers the previously solidified layer, forming a layer. These steps are repeated until the complete formation of the desired 3D structure. Finally, untreated resin is washed and the scaffold undergoes a UV irradiation processing in order to be fully treated [14].

The same principle can be applied in the case of ceramic scaffolds, noting that the binder must be a photosensitive polymer. A suspension of HAP is mixed with a low viscosity acrylic resin (resin content in the ceramic suspension is 20–50%). The resin is then burned and resulted in a ceramic scaffold having a porosity of ~50%.

An indirect method of manufacturing bioceramic scaffolds involves combining the SLA method with the casting type one. By SLA, an epoxy resin mold is obtained, into which a suspension of ceramic acrylate is poured (HAP mixed with acrylic resin). The matrix is removed by heat treatment and a 3D scaffold with the reverse shape of the mold is obtained [16].

3D microstructures with enhanced resolution can be achieved using micro-stereolithography (μSLA). This process involves the use of a single photon beam that can be focused more precisely by minimizing the spot size of the laser. The process of manufacturing the complex 3D microstructures is determined by the overlapping of layers having thicknesses lower than 10 μm. The material is prepared in the form of a suspension of HAP powder and 20% volume proportion of photosensitive resin. After obtaining the 3D structure, this is subjected to the sintering process, after which the scaffold presents a completely interconnected porous structure, with a pore size of ~300 μm [16].

(ii) Selective laser sintering (SLS)

This technique was developed at the University of Texas in 1986 [140, 141] and entered the market only in 1992 [16]. The manufacturing principle consists in the use of a CO_2 laser beam to fuse or sinter the desired region of the powder surface, on the powder bed, thus forming a layer of material. Along with the sintering of the first layer, the powder bed is lowered to a height equal to the thickness of a single layer. The process is repeated until the desired structure is obtained from the solid powder, and the amount of residual powder is removed [14].

The manufacturing of bioceramic scaffolds proved to be challenging by SLS, the difficulty of applying this technique emerges from the heating and cooling rates associated with the use of a high-energy laser. Such an indirect method seems more feasible for achieving porous ceramic scaffolds. The method involves coating the apatite powder particles with a polymeric binder. During the indirect SLS process, the binder layer is melted, and the particles stick to each other. The subsequently applied sintering removes the binder by combustion and the 3D structure is sintered.

(iii) 3D Printing (3DP)

3D printing is one of the techniques of printing that uses an inkjet binder, developed at Massachusetts Institute of Technology (MIT) in 1989 [142] and dedicated to the obtaining of 3D solid objects with complex structures. The manufacturing process involves spraying a liquid binder onto the surface of a powder bed, joining the particles and forming a solid layer. The powder bed is then lowered, so that a new layer of powder is spread on the above surface layer using a cylinder. This process is repeated until the designed object is obtained embedded inside the non-fused powder. A bulk powder removal step is required to obtain the finished product [14, 143].

The technique can also be applied in the case of porous scaffolds based on HAP powder. In this case, in order to obtain high density and satisfactory mechanical properties, postprocessing is required by applying heat treatments to the finished products. This is similar to the SLS method described above. Porous HAP-based products are thereby obtained, with internal channels of sizes ranging between 450 and 570 mm, and properties similar to those of the human bone [144].

(iv) Robocasting

Also known as *assembly by direct printing* or *micro-robotic deposition*, the robocasting is a method that involves depositing a robotic water-based colloidal suspension with high solid load and minimum organic content (1 wt%). The resulting structure is capable of supporting entirety its own weight during assembly, due to the viscoelasticity properties and composition. The deposition is usually made in oil bath in order to prevent uneven drying during assembly.

A ceramic slurry was prepared with 40–50% HAP powder dispersed in distilled water. The mixture was milled with zirconia balls for one hour in order to improve its homogeneity and stability. Adding an amount of hydroxypropyl methylcellulose previously dissolved provided the viscosity of the mixture, and the gelation was produced by adding an appropriate amount of polyethyleneimine (PEI) as a flocculant. The viscosity of the final mixture was corrected to the desired composition by adjusting the pH with HNO_3 or NH_4OH. Stirring for one hour in the same stirrer was followed after each addition. The quality of the final blend was evaluated according to the printability – the minimum diameter of the tip from which the mixture extraction is possible without clogging – and stability – the ability to maintain the shape during drying and sintering of the assembled structures [15, 145, 146].

5.6 Material Characterization

Material characterization represents a preliminary stage in evaluating the performance of a medical device. In the case of a material derived from shells or marble, complex characterization techniques are employed to track various material features after each stage of processing.

Physical changes due to calcination and sintering (color change or transition from compact state into powder) can be assessed using optical microscopy. Morphological aspects relevant to the use of these materials as bone substitutes are commonly analyzed by scanning electron microscopy (SEM), which may highlight the shape, size, and distribution of the particles and the pores in the microstructure. Coupling SEM with energy dispersive spectroscopy (EDS) provides a good estimation of the elemental chemical composition of materials and products. Based on these results, the Ca/P molar ratio can be calculated, this being considered one of the decisive indicators for the identification of calcium phosphates and the future performance of the products they form. The structural aspects are frequently analyzed by X-ray diffraction (XRD), which unveils the phase composition and crystallinity, and by Fourier transform infrared (FTIR) spectroscopy, which assesses the bonding architecture and type of functional groups within the material.

Depending on the material destination, many other characterization techniques can be applied to assess the physico-chemical, mechanical, or surface properties. This section concludes with information on the thermal stability of materials after precursor decomposition, oxidation, and subsequent dehydration, the data highly relevant to the design of the thermal processing programs [7, 22, 147].

5.6.1 Chemical Composition

Compositional analysis of marble and shells-derived ceramics showed that such materials contain mainly calcium (Ca), phosphorus (P), oxygen (O), carbon (C), as well as other elements present in low concentrations. For example, in the case of powders obtained by precipitation with potassium dihydrogen phosphate, EDS spectra indicates, besides the characteristic peaks of CaPs, also the presence of a significant peak corresponding to potassium [36]. This impurity is generally removed by subsequent heat treatment [36]. The presence of toxic metals, resulting from various synthesis processes, must be strictly controlled. The maximum levels of toxic metals recorded in the HAP for surgical applications are currently stated by the ASTM F1185-03 (2014) and ISO 13779-2:2008 standards [13, 147].

HAP derived from marble and shells differs from the biomimetic apatite grown in simulated body fluid (SBF) by the content of carbonate ions, their levels being much lower in the former [24].

Identification of materials derived from marble and sea shells is possible by the evaluation of the Ca/P molar ratio [148]. Theoretically, the thermal decomposition maintains the materials' Ca/P molar ratio around 1.67, a value corresponding to the stoichiometric HAP [31]. However, there are numerous synthetic procedures, which owned to the necessary processing/sintering temperature (e.g. Ca/P is 2.04 at 600 °C, 1.99 at 900 °C, and 1.94 at 1200 °C [147] and/or the variability of precursors, lead to materials with different compositions from that of stoichiometric HAP. Specifically, the Ca/P molar ratio of ceramics derived from marble and shells is found in the range of 1.65–2.04. Results closer to the targeted Ca/P value of 1.67 are obtained with synthesis methods based on alkaline hydrolysis [13, 147].

5.6.2 Structure

The crystallographic structure of HAP, firstly identified in 1930, comprises units of Ca^{2+}, $(PO_4)^{3-}$, and OH^-. HAP crystallizes in the hexagonal crystal system and have space group of $P6_3/m$ [81]. In marble or sea shells-derived HAP, the evaluation of crystal purity and identification of the material phases is usually made by XRD. On the other hand, the identification and assessment of existing functional groups in HAP structure can be made only indirectly by XRD, the most appropriate method of analysis being the FTIR spectroscopy [25].

5.6.2.1 X-Ray Diffraction (XRD) Studies

The structural analysis can be used to track the course of synthesis reaction of HAP derived from marble and shells. Structural analysis of the precursors allowed for the identification of $CaCO_3$ type of phase (i.e. aragonite or calcite) [13, 147].

Further, structural analysis of HAP obtained by microemulsion and calcination at various temperatures indicates that at 25 °C the samples are amorphous and sharp peaks being recorded once the temperature reaches 650 °C. At 750 °C, pure HAP is obtained, presenting a high crystallinity degree. Residual or decomposition phases such as CaO or β-TCP are not identifiable up to 1200 °C [101, 110].

In the case of dry mechano-chemical method, the evolution of the reaction between phosphorus pentoxide and $Ca(OH)_2$ was evaluated by XRD at several reaction stages [47]. After 15 minutes of milling, the peaks corresponding to $Ca(OH)_2$ degrade significantly and most of the raw material is converted to amorphous phases. The presence and the amount of water that resulted in the reaction accelerate its progress. The occurrence of very weak peaks demonstrated the formation of HAP in the grounded mixture, and their intensity has slightly increased after another 15 minutes of grinding. The synthesis reaction was completed after about 30 minutes of continuous grinding. The complete conversion is related to the close contact between particles and their shear during milling process [42, 47].

Compared to the commercial HAP, the marble and shells-derived HAP shows diffraction patterns with broader peaks, which indicate their lower degree of structuring. The presence of low quantities of residual phases in either amorphous or crystalline has also been signaled in few situations. In order to obtain a pure phase of HAP with similar structural features to those of human bone apatite, some sintering programs can be applied [13, 36].

After the sintering at high temperatures, the structural XRD analyses revealed the characteristic HAP diffraction lines as high and sharp peaks due to the complete degradation of the organic components involved on some synthesis routes. The influence of processing temperature on the structure of the resulted material is easy to be discerned by XRD: with the increase of temperature, the augment of intensity of diffraction maxima is observed, accompanied by their width reduction [147].

While some results suggest that the HAP decomposes forming (i) β-TCP and CaO at a temperature of 600–700 °C [118] and (ii) α-TCP and β-TCP at temperatures in the range of 1180–1250 °C [118] in the case of the synthesis of HAP by $Ca(OH)_2$ treatment with phosphoric acid and its sintering at temperatures up to 1300 °C, no secondary phases were revealed by XRD [41, 51]. Other analysis suggested that the HAP derived from marble and shells is structurally stable up to at least 1000 °C [147].

The transformation of HAP into β-TCP was observed after the powder derived from marble and shells was hot pressed at 1000 °C for one hour, and the resulting pellets were sintered at 1200 °C for two hour. At temperatures higher than 1300 °C, a partial conversion of the β-TCP into α-TCP was observed [118]. It has also been shown that the decomposition of HAP at temperatures over 1300 °C leads to the formation of tetracalcium phosphate (TTCP). Because TTCP is metastable, the obtaining of a single-phase pellet requires rapid quenching or the absence of moisture in order to prevent the decomposition of the TTCP into HAP and CaO [2, 149].

The sintering method is also influencing the structure of marble and shells-derived HAP: compared to processing in the furnace, by microwave sintering (at any temperature) the HAP powder maintains its thermal stability and the sharp peaks observed in the XRD analysis indicating a high crystallinity degree [2, 40, 41]. The diffractograms obtained on the pellets microwave sintered at 900–1200 °C showed HAP as the predominant crystalline phase. In similar conditions, the sintering of pellets made from Ca-deficient HAP led to the emergence of bi-phasic materials HAP/β-TCP. Between 1100 and 1200 °C, the conversion of β-TCP into α-TCP was observed, where the HAP corresponding peaks remaining unchanged [113].

The discrepancy between the assumptions regarding marble and sea shells-derived HAP thermal degradation is mainly due to the variability of the chemical composition of the precursors (this is also specific to other ceramic products derived from natural precursors) [150]. When Ca/P = 1.50, the beginning of the HAP degradation was observed after the powder was pressed and sintered at 600 °C, by the appearance of β-TCP as minor phase. In some areas of the XRD diagram of this material, the HAP peaks were poorly defined suggesting its incomplete crystallization. The increase of the sintering temperature (up to 1200 °C) and of the holding time (up to four hours) resulted in the synthesis of a single HAP phase material [118].

5.6.2.2 Fourier Transformed Infrared (FT-IR) Spectroscopy Analyses

The short-range order of a CaP compound can be easily assessed by FT-IR spectroscopy. The FT-IR spectrum of HAP is studied in the 400–4000 cm^{-1} wavelength range, where functional groups such as phosphate (PO_4^{3-}), hydroxyl (OH^-), hydrogen phosphate (HPO_4^{2-}), or carbonate (CO_3^{2-}) elicit their characteristic vibration bands [34]. The corresponding orthophosphate bands are the prominent ones. They appear at different positions in the range of 400–1200 cm^{-1} [13, 21, 34, 47, 151, 152]: the bands in the region of 950–1100 cm^{-1} correspond to the ν_1 symmetric and triply degenerated ν_3 asymmetric stretching modes, and those in the 565–603 cm^{-1} range correspond to the ν_4 doubly degenerated bending modes, while around 470 cm^{-1} the signature ν_2 bending mode of O—P—O bonds peaks. For Ca/P = 0.67, the PO_4^{3-} group corresponding bands can be found at 953, 1027, and 1067 cm^{-1} wave numbers; for Ca/P = 1.67, they are located at 962, 1023, and 1087 cm^{-1} [34], and for Ca/P = 2.67, they are located at 963, 1024, and 1086 cm^{-1} [13, 34].

The characteristic bands of structural OH^- groups can be identified at ~630 (librational mode) and ~3600 (stretching mode) cm^{-1} [21, 26, 34]: for Ca/P = 0.67, the presence of hydroxyl ions is observed at 612 cm^{-1}; for Ca/P = 1.67, the OH^- bands are located at 628, 3642, 3572 cm^{-1} and for the Ca/P = 2.67 the recorded wave numbers are located at 630 and 3643 cm^{-1}. The sharpness of the librational mode of hydroxyl and ν_4 doubly degenerated bending modes of orthophosphate serves as an indicator of the crystalline quality of HAP.

Various transformations in the structure of materials can be observed function of the synthesis route. The powder obtained by precipitation shows low-intensity bands at 1406–1478 cm^{-1}, corresponding to the presence of CO_3^{2-} groups (ν_3 stretching modes) within the samples. They are accompanied by a low-intensity ν_2 CO_3^{2-} band (usually one-fifth of sister ν_3 carbonate band intensity), located at ~872 cm^{-1}. Sometimes, this band obscures the presence of non-apatitic domains (namely, HPO_4^{2-} groups) [151].

The positions of the ν_3 CO_3^{2-} bands can designate the type of HAP carbonatation. "B-type" carbonatation (carbonate replaces phosphate in the HAP structure) is indicated by the 1410 and 1450 cm^{-1} positions, while the "A-type" carbonatation (carbonate replaces hydroxyl in the HAP structure) is pointed out by the 1455 and 1540 cm^{-1} positions [151, 153].

The adsorbed water band can also be identified for some CaP products: bending mode (~1640 cm^{-1}) and stretching mode (2500–3600 cm^{-1}) [151]. This can be absorbed from the atmosphere and replace the PO_4^{3-} or OH^- groups during the synthesis process [13, 22, 147].

By thermal processing at 1000–1300 °C, the loss of CO_3^{2-} groups occurs. The sintered powder FT-IR spectrum can be therefore very different from that of commercial HAP, the OH^- and PO_4^{3-} characteristic band distributions being similar [31]. The absence of other functional groups indicates a phasic purity and thus FTIR spectroscopy can serve as complementary investigation tool to XRD.

5.6.3 Morphology

Current strategies for obtaining ceramic biomaterials are focused on a careful control of the morphological characteristics in order to ensure the best possible similarity to the bone tissue. The mineral component of bone tissue is organized in HAP microcrystals with widths of 10–15 nm and lengths of several micrometers [148]. Starting from the submicrometer level down to the nanometric one, the HAP size, shape, and particle agglomeration trends are influencing the material sintering ability. The morphology also influences the behavior in biological environment: nano-HAP shows far superior bioactivity compared to the one with coarser crystallites [86]. Also, there is a consensus that the 3D scaffolds for bone reconstruction must have a porosity of 40–60% in order to promote rapid diffusion of nutrients and cell migration and the recommended pore size for bone regeneration ranges from 50 to 1000 μm. The size of connections is still under debate, but nowadays varies between 15 and 50 μm [72].

5.6.3.1 Morphology of Powders

The granular size of ceramics derived from marble and sea shells ranges from 100 nm to 0.3–1.0 μm, depending on the fabrication method [34, 147]. After synthesis, the heat treatment of powders at temperatures between 70 and 90 °C allows the obtaining of the dense particles grouped in crystals with dimensions of tens of nanometers. The temperature increase leads to elevated thermal vibration energy, enhanced atoms diffusion at the crystal boundaries, and expansion. The agglomeration of rod-like crystals of HAP powder is similar to the morphology of commercial products, the grain size distribution being narrowed to diameters of 15–20 nm, and lengths of ~30–70 nm. The phenomenon is even more enhanced if the resulting powder is obtained by mechano-chemical route, where the particles' agglomeration may occur before the drying process [31, 118]. Oven dried powders show crystallite sizes in the range of 7–34 nm, as confirmed by the XRD analyses [2].

The synthesis methods commonly end with sintering programs at high temperatures, due to the positive influence on morphology (the sintering improves the particle size growth, their uniformity, and the microstructure densification) [34, 147].

The sintering at 900 °C of HAP powder derived from marble and sea shells leads to an increase of the grain size from tens of nanometers up to hundreds of nanometers. Sintered powders present differentiated areas of coarse grains of about 100 nm and fine grains with dimensions of ~20 nm. Once the temperature is raised to 1000 °C, this distribution is reduced and the size of the grains is found in the range of 150–200 nm. However, once the threshold of 1000–1100 °C is surpassed, the grain size increases to approximately 1 μm and the microstructure densification begins. Further, the sintering at 1200 °C leads to the increase of the grain size up to 2–5 mm and the formation of a dense microstructure in 98% of the volume. After sintering at 1300 °C, the thermal degradation of HAP derived from marble or shells occurs, and morphological changes of the secondary phases can be observed (mostly β-TCP, having with grains of about 100 nm) [42, 118].

5.6.3.2 Morphology of Dense Products (Pellets)

As in the case of powders, the sintering of ceramic products derived from marble and shells induces significant changes of the morphological characteristics. For the HAP pellets with a Ca/P molar ratio of 1.50, the sintering at 800 °C generates particles with sizes in the range of 250–500 nm. When the sintering temperature is increased to 1000 °C, the particles size raises to 0.6–2.0 μm, and the appearance of residual pores and secondary phases (CaO) is induced [118, 120]. For HAP pellets with Ca/P = 1.62, an accentuated variation of the average particle size is observed: compared to the pellets sintered at 900 °C, for the ones sintered at 1000 °C, the average particle size increases sharply from 100 to ~500 nm. After further sintering at 1200 °C, the average grain size increases almost three times. For HAP pellets with Ca/P = 1.67, the cross-sectional SEM analysis of specimens sintered at temperatures of 800–1200 °C for 15 minutes showed a microstructure with dense and uniform grains whose size increased from 130 nm to 1.59 μm when the temperature raised from 900 to 1200 °C [113, 154].

5.6.3.3 Morphology of Porous Products (Scaffolds)

If in case of powders, the morphological aspects are highlighted especially by electron microscopy techniques, and the porous structure of the products obtained from these powders can be observed by stereomicroscopy. The method involves the prior cutting of the pellet using a diamond saw and the cross-section surface polishing by grinding with silicon carbide paper. The sample preparation continues with cleaning, drying, and cross-sectional staining. The images obtained after coloring are used to measure the pore size distribution by analyzing the intersection lengths from the cross-section. The total porosity can be determined by comparison (between the density of the bulk pellet and the theoretical density of HAP, i.e. 3.156 g/cm^3). The difference between the micro- and macro-porosity can rarely be emphasized by this technique [120]. Oven drying can also induce porous morphologies with interconnected pores, applicable in bone tissue engineering [13, 34]. At 600 °C (and four hours holding time), a density of 2.38 g/cm^3 is obtained. At 800 °C, a one minute sintering time results in a density of 2.07 g/cm^3 (65.5% of the theoretical density of HAP). The value increases up to 2.77 g/cm^3 when the holding time in the oven reaches four hours. When the holding time exceeds four hours (the maximum reported time was 24 hours), a gradual decrease of the density is recorded, down to 2.10 g/cm^3 [118].

Increasing the sintering temperature to 1100 °C results in a density improvement up to 2.9 g/cm^3 (91.77% of the theoretical density) [118]. Further, the sintering at 1200–1400 °C leads to a density decrease, from 2.85 to 2.05 g/cm^3, due to the partial decomposition of HAP into α-TCP and TTCP [118, 155, 156].

The technologies for tissue substitution currently encountered a limitation due to their inability to create synthetic vascular systems. Natural tissues are supplied with nutrients and oxygen by means of intricately branched blood vessels and capillaries. The maximum distance between these capillaries is about 200 μm, a value related to the limit of the oxygen diffusion [157, 158]. For this reason, the size and interconnectivity of pores play an important role, especially if the scaffold is designed for tissue regeneration applications. Due to the difficulty of obtaining full 3D information from 2D images, the interconnectivity of the porous HAP structures can be experimentally determined by immersing the scaffold in black pigment solution, followed by centrifugation. The sample is then sectioned, dried, and photographed. The black colored pores indicate the liquid accessibility, either directly or through the neighboring pores [120, 159].

A different level of porosity yielded within the same product is still difficult, although this represents a necessary requirement: the bone tissue has a dense outer structure (with a porosity of less than 10%), which becomes porous inside (porosity >50%). Mimicking this structure, even by modern methods of SFF fabrication type, still remains a challenge [121].

5.6.4 Mechanical Properties

The mechanical properties of some types of marble and species of sea shells are comparable to those of human bones, being one of the main reasons for their use as a source for bone substitute materials. The *Tridacna gigas* and *Lobatus gigas* species shells represent a good example, their dense structure providing excellent mechanical properties. In the case of the shells partially transformed into HAP, their fracture strength is around 137–218 MPa, and for the fully transformed ones the value decreases to 70–150 MPa, a value similar to the one of the human compact bone [10]. The compression strength values for such marine species are found in a wide range, from 50 to 300 MPa [11], of which only the minimum values are preserved and are suitable for materials with application in bone reconstruction. In the case of powders obtained from *T. gigas* and *L. gigas* clams species, the tensile strength is comparable to that of the human bone [10, 11, 147].

Despite a chemical composition that is common to all species, the microstructure of sea shells has a really increased tenacity compared to the non-biogenic $CaCO_3$. All these properties are also found in the case of HAP powder derived from this type of sea shells (oyster, *Muricopsis* sp., and *Helix* sp. shells) [12].

Similarly, the architectural organization and structural properties of the mother of pearl (Nacres) play an important role in terms of mechanical properties observed for bone substitute products made from fine HAP powder resulting after their processing [12, 33]. Table 5.3 summarizes some of the mechanical properties of this products.

- *The overall mechanical strength* of products derived from marble and shells [10, 11, 25] varies inversely with the Ca/P molar ratio value until it reaches 1.67. After the Ca/P ratio value exceeds 1.67, a sudden decrease of mechanical strength is recorded. In addition, the resistance decreases almost exponentially with the increase of porosity [159]. Ceramic materials derived from marble and shells are, like any other ceramic material, fragile. Their fragility derives from the presence of the ionic bonds in the material. Due to the material organization, the breaking is not preceded by any plastic deformation, so that any crack propagation will not be inhibited by deformation (as in ductile materials) but will continue to spread until failure [1, 137, 159]. The fragility of these materials is a serious challenge for porous scaffold structures whose purpose is to replace natural bone without any transient loss of the required mechanical support [137]. The high porosity degree contributes to the decrease of scaffold mechanical resistance [161] and also to their difficult handling. The improvement of mechanical properties may be achieved by sintering at high temperatures, to the detriment of microporosity. But limiting the microporosity reduces on one hand the degree of resorption and on the other hand the bioactive processes that contribute to the bone regeneration [161]. The sintering temperature, phase purity, porosity, and size of the HAP grains affect the mechanical properties of ceramics [154]. The products used for bone substitution should not show mechanical properties superior to those of the human bone, because the phenomenon of *stress shielding* may appear. During this process, the very rigid implant prevents the uniform distribution of loads along the bone and ultimately leads to the atrophy of the cortical bone. Moreover, due to the regular movements of the natural bone, any implanted HAP structure must be able to effectively transmit the tensile loads; lack on this property will prevent bone regeneration and remodeling [25].
- *The compression strength* of ceramics obtained after synthesis is directly influenced by the manufacturing

Table 5.3 Mechanical properties of HAP products [1, 11, 16, 17, 111, 124, 125, 127, 128, 132, 137, 145, 159, 160].

Fabrication method	Mechanical properties (MPa)		
	Compression strength	Modulus of elasticity	Bending strength
Pellet			
Cold pressing (manual hydraulic press)	7–160	—	—
Scaffold			
Solvent casting	8–10	0.15–150	—
Freeze-drying	12–30	20	—
Thermally induced phase separation (TIPS)	0.7–2.5	—	—
Polymer sponge	0.3–22	4000–8000	—
Stereolithography (SLA)	57	—	—
Selective laser sintering (SLS)	31	20–60	16
Three-dimensional printing (3DP)	0.7–21	—	0.69
Robocasting	10–20	—	—

method. Generally, the bioceramics that consist of a single phase (calcium-deficient HAP) present higher compression strength values than materials composed of HAP and β-TCP. The sintering at 750 °C results in a compression strength of 7.05 MPa [1, 119]. Higher compression strength is obtained for scaffolds produced by 3D printing (i.e. 21 MPa), value found between the similar mechanical properties of the cortical and the cancellous bone, respectively. However, scaffolds are not suitable for the large load-bearing regions of the human skeleton [16, 123, 162]. In the case of products obtained by SLS, the compression strength values range between 41 MPa (scaffolds) and 157 MPa (pellets) [16].

- *The hardness* is influenced by the porosity and the average grain size of sintered HAP. The hardness starts to decrease once the maximum grain size limit is reached, despite its high density [8]. The hardness testing of HAP pellets showed an improvement from 3.45 to 4.85 GPa with the increase of the sintering temperature from 900 to 1200 °C [113]. In the case of biphasic HAP/TCP ceramics, a comparative study showed a maximum hardness of 4.28 GPa for a sintering temperature of 1000 °C. At temperatures of 1000–1400 °C, the hardness decreases due to the conversion of β-TCP into α-TCP. This phase transformation induces residual stresses in the densified material, which may be the main reason for the slightly lower hardness values [113]. A similar behavior can be observed for hardness testing of pellets [154]: Vickers microhardness increased from ~0.9 to ~4 GPa when the sintering temperature rose from 600 to 900 °C, and then sharply decreased to ~1.5 GPa when treated at 1400 °C. The variation of the pellets hardness with the sintering temperature is similar to that observed in the case of density, indicating that the hardness is not controlled only by the bonding between the product particles but also by other factors such as particle size or the appearance of secondary phases during the sintering process [7, 163].
- *The fracture strength* varies with the sintering temperature and decreases with the increase of the porosity, not exceeding 1.2 MPa. Thus, pellets sintered at 900 °C recorded a value of 0.56 MPa and with the temperature increase to 1000 °C this value raise to 0.75 MPa. At temperatures over 1200 °C, the fracture strength of biphasic HAP/TCP pellets increases to 0.92 MPa, while the density tends to decrease [113, 159].
- *The modulus of elasticity* is another property highly influenced by porosity. The obtained experimental values are found between 35 and 120 GPa, being more or less close to those of the natural hard tissue components: dental enamel – 74 GPa, dentin – 21 GPa, and compact bone – 18–22 GPa. The bending modulus of elasticity is in the range of 44–88 GPa. At temperatures of 1000–1100 °C, HAP-dense bioceramics have a superplastic behavior, with wear resistance and friction coefficient comparable to those of dental enamel [159].

5.6.5 Thermal Stability

5.6.5.1 Dimensional Stability

The dimensional stability of HAP is evaluated during the sintering process because it can be associated with the contraction phenomena unevenly distributed in the sample volume. The unevenness can lead to excessive cracking of the sintered ceramic product, so to its uselessness. In the case of porous structures, the avoidance of this phenomenon is a challenge from the manufacturing point of view. At 650–750 °C, depending on the HAP pellet purity, length and diameter shrinkages are recorded in the range of 2.88–13% and 1.29–8.4%, respectively [1].

The material shrinkage that occurs during the heat treatments performed for the densification and optimization of microstructure affects the mechanical properties and the dimensional accuracy of the SFF fabrication products. Designing dimensional additions can solve this issue, but the contraction evolution during postprocessing must be known before the dimensional compensation [164].

5.6.5.2 Mass Stability

In the case of ceramics derived from marble and shells, independent of the synthesis method or temperature, the obtained thermogravimetric analysis curves did not show peaks corresponding to the decomposition of any organic components [13, 42, 147]. However, the thermal behavior of this type of material strongly depends on the synthesis method.

The thermal gravimetric analysis (TGA) curve of the HAP obtained by calcination has no inflection up to the temperature of 365 °C. Lack of mass loss is explained by the lack of collagen and organic fragments within the sample derived from natural resources [13]. A slight deflection is recorded in the early stage of the alkaline hydrolysis synthesis methods [147].

After the drying heat treatment, the analysis of HAP samples indicates a mass loss of up to 8.5%. The dry powder presents a higher weight loss in the temperature range of 25–400 °C (about 5%).

The rapid loss is recorded due to the strong endothermic behavior induced by the physicochemical removal of water from HAP. Between 250 and 400 °C, water is completely removed from the HAP lattice. Up to 650 °C, no noticeable weight loss is recorded, but, in the 650–1000 °C range, the material lose is about 3% of its mass due to dehydroxylation and its conversion into β-TCP [13]. After sintering at 1000 °C, the marble and shells-derived materials can lose up to 4.5% by mass (while commercial HAP would lose about 6.5%).

In the case of HAP powder obtained by mechanical methods, the TGA curve shows no fluctuations up to 550 °C, due to the loss of moisture since the step of HAP forming by mechano-chemical activation. Therefore, the lack of any other prominent endothermic reactions and weight losses at the studied temperatures of reaction suggests that the reaction between the precursor and the anhydrous calcium hydrogen phosphate is largely completed after 25 hours of mechanical activation at room temperature [42].

5.7 *In vitro* Behavior

The biological response of implanted products is influenced by numerous factors, such as surface chemistry, size, shape, place, and time of implantation. *In vitro* testing allows a better understanding of the interaction between the implanted material, cells, and tissues. The interrelated aspects can be highlighted using *in vitro* tests in solutions, which simulate the internal intercellular medium or in various human or animal cell cultures. The bone itself is a dynamic tissue, which can be reabsorbed or remodeled [165].

The obtaining of edifying results depends mainly on the properties of the product: porosity, pore size, and surface properties [18, 27]. The material should allow the vascularization and cell transport through the pores and the growth factors that facilitate the proliferation and differentiation of cells.

Furthermore, the implanted material must be chemically stable, with open fully interconnected porosity, and a suitable pore size, in order to allow in-growth of cells and cellular migration along the porous structure [123, 133]. Thus, the interconnection degree and size of pores model the inner cell growth and decisively influence the osteoconductive properties [52, 55, 166].

The pore size is a material feature of high importance: if the pores are too small, the occlusion appears and, therefore, the cellular penetration and the neovascularization will not be accomplished. An average pore size of 200–900 μm is admitted [123]. Conversely, some researchers report that the bone reconstruction can be achieved only through a temporary 3D matrix with a macroporous structure and pore sizes in the range of 1.2–2.0 mm. This concept has both advantages and disadvantages: due to the high surface/volume ratio it promotes the growth of cells, tissues, and blood vessels, but to the detriment of mechanical properties [123, 167]. In this respect, the use of such products is indicated only in areas with low mechanical loads [133].

The microporosity must be adequate to the implanted area in order to ensure the neovascularization and capillary growth. The pores of less than 10 μm inhibit the cell growth, those between 15 and 50 μm facilitate the fibrovascular colonization, while those between 50 and 150 μm induce the osteoid growth. A dimension larger than 150 μm supports the internal formation of mineralized bone [12, 52]. The porosity and the interconnectivity are also important for an accurate diffusion of nutrients and for the removal of metabolic wastes resulting from the activity of the subsequently grown cells [123, 133].

From the surface point of view, both the chemical and the topographical characteristics can control and affect the cell adhesion and proliferation. The chemical properties are closely related to the ability of cells to adhere to the material surface and of the proteins interaction with those. The topography plays an important role in ensuring the osteoconductivity [123].

5.7.1 Biocompatibility

The *in vitro* cytotoxic response of biomaterials can be made on various cell lines, of both animal or human origin, such as embryonic and adult stem cells, stromal cells from bone marrow, muscle-derived stem cells, osteoblasts, and osteoclasts [14, 123, 160, 165].

Recently, the acidic phospholipids proved to be responsible for the precipitation of the HAP from metastable CaP solutions, playing an important role in the mineralization process. After an incubation time of five days at a temperature of 25 °C, the formation of the following compounds was observed: HAP crystals, Ca–phospholipid–PO_4 complexes, and lipids isolated from bone. In the case of Ca–phospholipid–PO_4 complexes, calcium is bound to its hydrophilic groups (phosphate, hydroxyl, or carboxyl group), which is advantageous for the germination of HAP. Bone matrix vesicles, reported to be those that initiate the tissue mineralization, are rich in acidic phospholipids. In the early stages of mineralization, these are calcium rich before increasing the inorganic phosphate level [168].

Some studies have focused on the use of osteoblast and osteoclast cultures in order to evaluate the *in vitro* biological performances of scaffold, according to the methodology described in Ref. [[122]]. The effect of HAP on cell proliferation is usually estimated by flow cytometry or MTT assays [169], as stipulated in the International Standard ISO-10993-part 1: Biological Evaluation of Medical Devices Part 1: Evaluation and Testing. The morphology of cells can be visualized by fluorescence and SEM microscopy techniques.

The results should show that there are no signs of toxicity or morphological changes, i.e. the cells proliferating and spreading on the material's surface [46, 69, 166].

Nano-HAP is known to promote osteoblast cell adhesion and differentiation, the cells that grow around the material showing clear signs of phagocytosis [58]. The colonization of the cells on the scaffold surface indicates the ECM synthesis, usually taking place after seven days. The SEM analysis can highlight the intercellular matrix formation, which contains fibers on the HAP scaffold [166].

Regarding the results on osteoclast cell cultures, SEM examinations indicate that they produce gaps of various shapes and depths, with different magnitude depending on the type of scaffold. The degradation areas are harder to discern in the case of scaffold fabrication of pure HAP with respect to the biphasic calcium phosphate (BCP) ones, regardless of type of cells. In the case of BCP scaffolds, the areas of resorption are more clearly defined, the degradation gaps being deeper and showing numerous well-defined lobules [165].

ISO 10993-1 standard stipulates that the cellular death induced by a given biomaterial can be quantified with a lactate dehydrogenase (LDH) experiment. LDH is an intracellular enzyme found in all types of cells. When a cell dies, this active enzyme is released and thus the LDH activity can be considered proportional to the number of dead cells [170].

A comparison between the results obtained by various microscopy techniques indicated that the cells tend to follow the surface model – irregular, fluted – of the scaffold. By fluorescence microscopy technique, the cell nucleus appears in blue color and the actin cytoskeleton in red, highlighting an area that is completely covered with cells; thus, demonstrating the scaffold capacity to promote cell adhesion, proliferation, and colonization of the entire structure without influences from the obtaining methods on the induced cytotoxic effect of the cell lines [14–16].

5.8 Degradation in Biological Environment

Several authors have reported on the evaluation of CaPs' behavior in various artificial physiological media solutions, such as distilled water, Michaelis buffer solution, Ringer's solution, or SBF [12, 171–173].

HAP presence within the implanted material is a key factor for the *in vitro* biomineralization, so that, independent of the scaffold manufacturing method, it must not allow the fully conversion of HAP into more soluble phases. HAP biodegradation in physiological medium is not sufficient in order to achieve the optimal bone formation. The presence of β-TCP phase leads to a faster release of Ca^{2+} and PO_4^{3-} ions, but drastically reduces the available area for bone cell proliferation: it was found that the dense scaffolds manufactured from HAP powder partially converted into β-TCP degrades after about 60 days of immersion, being observed a preferential solubilization of β-TCP grains [173].

The optimal bioresorbability is achieved when the two phases (i.e. HAP and β-TCP) are properly mixed, and finally a BCP is obtained. The biological performance of the BCP mixtures is controlled by their gradual dissolution profile, by the release of ions, and by the biomineralization capacity. The material remnant after the dissolution acts as a template for the new bone formed. Bone-like apatite formation in SBF is favored by the much lower values of the solubility of β-TCP and HAP products [173].

Variations of the Ca/P molar ratio between 1.5 and 2.0 suggest the presence of different CaPs (HAP, TTCP, and TCP) within the materials derived from marble and sea shells, and led to differences in degradation speeds. Currently, it is considered that the materials with high contents of TCP facilitate an extensive bone remodeling around the implant, while TTCP and HAP develops a strong interface with the host tissue [174, 175].

According to the solubility diagram for the CaO–P system, at a pH in the range of 4.2–8.0, HAP is the least soluble of the CaPs and dissolves more slowly than the TCP. More specifically, TCP is dissolved 12.3 times faster than HAP in acid environment and 22.3 times faster in an alkaline environment [176].

The SBF solution, having an ionic concentration similar to the human blood plasma, was used, for the first time, by Kokubo et al., in order to emphasize the similarity between the *in vitro* and the *in vivo* behavior of different ceramic types [177, 178]. An ISO standard is now dedicated to such bioactivity tests – ISO/FDIS 23317: 2014 (Implants for surgery – *In vitro* evaluation for apatite-forming ability of implant materials). The SBF soaking can also be used for chemical growth of biomimetic carbonated HAP materials. Preliminary bioactivity testing of HAP products or the synthesis of HAP using SBF as a medium for precipitation are carried out in quasi-homeostatic conditions at a temperature of 37 °C and pH = 7.4 [7, 71, 179, 180].

In the case of BCP scaffolds, the pH evolution in SBF solution shows a slight decrease from 7.4 to 7.17 within the first 15 days of immersion, after which the pH tends to increase to 7.24 after 60 days of immersion, due to the leaching of the more soluble β-TCP phase. The changes of ion concentration and pH of the solution are due to the scaffold's surface absorption of Ca^{2+} and PO_4^{3-} ions, which will gradually crystallize to form the biomimetic apatite layer [167]. It can be noted that the high solubility of the β-TCP maintains a sufficiently high concentration of ions on the surface of the material, which favors the nucleation of the apatite [134, 167]. As the immersion time is prolonged, the apatite formation within the scaffold is increased. The resulted biomimetic apatitic layer consists of spheroidal particles, relatively small, suggesting a high rate of germination [80, 124].

In the case of the products in which the conversion of β-TCP into α-TCP occurred, it is noted an improvement in the rate of Ca and P ions release, as well as a significantly higher initial dissolution of α-TCP [181]. But the highest initial dissolution rate was recorded for TTCP monophasic products [181]. The rapid increase in Ca and P concentration of the solution was followed by a decrease of the P, and then Ca content, indicating a saturation of the solution with respect to one of the calcium phosphate metastable [181, 182].

A different *in vitro* study demonstrates that the rate of TCP dissolution in the lactose buffer is three times higher than that recorded for HAP [176]. The addition of these particles has initially a low effect on the alkaline pH of the buffer solution, leading in time to its severe decrease. Dissolution rate of calcium and phosphorus ions is naturally higher in a solution of pH = 6.2 compared to the one with pH 7.2 [175].

The *in vitro* scaffold degradation was studied by immersion in physiological fluid, present within the blood plasma and tissue fluids, demonstrating the growing trend of Ca^{2+} concentration with immersion time [183]. Also, it is highlighted that the samples start dissolving from the 14th day of immersion, with a dissolution rate of 0.014–0.019 wt%/d. The replacement of the physiological fluid with synthetic blood plasma or sea water does not facilitate the dissolution in the first 30 days of immersion [80]. On the other hand, the microwave-sintered scaffolds lead to high Ca^{2+} release, compared to the ones conventionally sintered at the same temperature. Thus, after 12 days of immersion, the concentration of calcium release ions in the case of microwave scaffold sintered at 1200 °C is about 6 ppm, while in the case of those conventionally sintered at the same temperature is only about 4 ppm. When the sintering is performed at 1000 °C, the recorded rates of calcium dissolution are similar for both type of scaffolds (being situated around 10–11 ppm). The degradation mechanism of HAP products is mainly determined by the phenomenon of dissolution, which easily occurs at the pores and the grain boundaries. The fine grains obtained after the microwave sintering increase the grain boundaries exposed to the solution, and thus leaching of more calcium ions from the scaffolds occurs. Such behavior may be beneficial for bone growth [183].

The mentioned studies also highlighted that the dissolution and re-precipitation of biomimetic apatite crystallites promote the osseointegration, the biomimetic HAP bonding to the living bone through a collagen-rich layer. The thickness of the chemically grown apatite layer and the shape (e.g. porous, acicular, or nodular) of the crystallites is composed of, depends on the initial product characteristics: the chemical composition of the raw powder, the surface integrity, and the co-association of other phases [174]. The porous apatite formation is beneficial to the proliferation of cells from the neighboring bone tissue, since the blood flow can be realized easily through such porous structures.

SEM analyses reveal that products made from pure HAP does not undergo extensive dissolution even after 28 days of immersion in different solutions, the corresponding pH having a fairly constant value of 7.2 [174].

5.9 *In vivo* Performance Evaluation

Once the results of the *in vitro* tests are confirmed, animal testing is a necessity in order to obtain a monitored assessment of the obtained material behavior in intended applications. It is especially targeted its ability to induce osseointegration, osteoconduction, osteoinduction, and osteogenesis.

Based on the product geometry and surface properties, the *in vivo* studies conclude that any occurred damage influence the proliferation and cellular adhesion, essential properties for bone regeneration [15, 78]. In the same time, the internal architecture, by means of size, shape, and pore interconnection pattern is a key in order to provide suitable *in vivo* mechanical performances. Such morphological properties also control the degree and direction of bone regeneration, making them optimal for the reconstruction of various defects [184].

Within the bone tissue a pore matrix with orientation from the outside to the inside ensures the surface, space, and route of cell migration from the periosteum toward the interior of the implant. This matrix also enables proper cell adhesion and formation of blood vessels that support and reshape newly formed bone [17, 159].

Therefore, ensuring a micro- and macro-sized porosity to the scaffolds of HAP is crucial for the bone integration rate and quality. Dense products with high mechanical strength are indicated for defects in highly loaded areas [11, 17].

Studies show that the increase of the surface area and pore volume can accelerate the *in vivo* deposition of apatite layers, enhancing the bone regeneration [159]. However, a scaffold with such properties could present also few major disadvantages. Firstly, these scaffolds present a high fragility correlated with low mechanical properties, which prevents their use in the regeneration of large bone defects. Secondly, one can mention their unpredictable rate of degradation. If the dissolution will occur too quickly, the mechanical stability of the product will be compromised, a property that is already questionable. Furthermore, the dramatic increase of Ca and P concentration into the surrounding implant medium can induce local cellular death [123].

Moreover, currently, a balance between the rate of resorption, remodeling, and formation of new bone tissue is assiduous looked for. The resorption of powder products based on CaPs (i.e. HAP, β-TCP, α-TCP) is achieved due to two different mechanisms: (i) by chemical dissolution due to the continuous flow of biological fluids and (ii) by degradation of macrophages or osteoclasts cells [185]. Bone growth and regeneration process must be fast, and the quality of the new bone needs to be comparable or superior with respect to the host bone tissue. This ensures a positive response to physiological and biological changes generated by the osseointegration of the implant material and its controlled degradation in non-toxic products, which can be metabolized or excreted via normal physiological mechanisms [78].

In the case of the BCP products, the HAP acts as a bioinert agent, while TCP is bioresorbable counterpart. Implants fabricated from powders exhibiting phase transformations should ensure uniform and homogeneous obtaining of the desired porosity degree after implantation, in *in vivo* conditions. The bioresorbable phase is expected to undergo extensive resorption within the body, in a certain period of time, ensuring a uniform porosity of the "aged" implant [186].

Reported clinical trials, made in order to assess the efficacy of HAP products derived from marbles and shells were mostly performed on rats [10, 11] and rabbits [15, 185, 187] but also on a number of large animal models – pigs, dogs, or goats [17, 188, 189]. The defects were induced both in areas with high mechanical loads (e.g. the femoral distal bone [10, 11, 185], tibia [15], or mandible [17]), but also in areas with low mechanical loads (e.g. the trepanation defects from the skull [187] or the radius bone [189]). Defects sizes vary with the study case and with the implantation location. In the mandible and skull cases, the defects are circular with diameters from 8 to 11 mm, while in the case of long bones the resections are rectangular with sizes of $3 \times 3\,mm^2$ or $10 \times 5\,mm^2$ [10, 187].

Different outcomes for the *in vivo* behavior of the materials were reported as described below; these are influenced by the chemical composition of the product obtained by sintering (pure HAP, BCP (HAP/β-TCP) or β-TCP). Also, the place of implantation in the test animal offers complementary information regarding *in vivo* behavior of calcium phosphates.

The *in vivo* testing on rats involved implantation of HAP rectangular scaffolds (derived from sea shells) or β-TCMP (derived from sea urchin spines) in the distal femur [10, 11]. Six weeks after the implantation, micro-CT images did not indicate the migration or movement of the implant, and no resorption phenomena. Electron microscopy clearly evidenced the bone regeneration around implants and the interconnection between them and the host tissue. Also, the migration of newly formed bone tissue through the marginal pores is observed [11]. Histological examination of sectioned implants indicates a direct apposition of bone within the implant, and the absence of the fibrous tissue around it. This demonstrates the biocompatibility, osseointegration, and good fixation of the implant [10, 137].

In the *in vivo* testing on rabbit model, the reconstitution of trepanation defects by implanting certain HAP-based scaffolds is reported [15, 187]. Also, BCP material is used to repair the defects induced in long bones (e.g. tibia and femur) [185].

In the first case, the tibia, the micro-CT images obtained after 8 and 16 weeks of implantation, total healing, or bone in-growth are observed in all the explanted scaffolds. The bone healing progresses by the rapid growth of new trabeculae from the outside toward the inside of the implant, along the HAP scaffolds. Most of the new bone is derived from the periosteal and endosteal surfaces of the bone that is adjacent to the defect.

At higher magnification, scaffold's cross-sections indicate the HAP particles' coverage with a new bone that radially increases in time. Mature bone is composed of soft tissue, bone marrow, and blood vessels and is located on the defect periphery [15, 187].

After both periods, the bone attachment directly to the implant surface is observed, indicating the osteoconduction and also bone tissue advances inward the scaffold toward its center. Only after 16 weeks it can be affirmed that the bone is mature and has a lamellar structure [187].

In the second case, the femur, the analysis made by SEM microscopy on the implants surface, highlighted a partial degradation of the BCP implant material, after eight weeks of implantation. This indicates the partial healing of defects in the absence of toxic or inflammatory reactions, suggesting the need for longer periods of implantation for the total resorption of the addition material [185].

The *in vivo* tests made on dog model [176, 188] were carried out by the implantation of BCP scaffolds in periodontal defects. Explantation after six months indicates, according to the micro-CT analysis, that newly formed bone was well mineralized and perfectly attached to the ceramic implant surface. The relative abundance of needle microcrystals in the immediate vicinity of HAP and β-TCP is dependent on β-TCP/HAP ratio of the BCP product before implantation. The higher this ratio is, the more abundant the newly formed microcrystals are. The formation of such crystals can be explained by precipitation of Ca and P ions released from TCP phase of the implant [176].

Electron microscopy and EDS analyses highlight the similarity between the Ca/P ratio and the particle size (length, width, and thickness) of newly formed microcrystal and the apatite crystal of pre-existing bone. The large crystals associated with the newly formed calcified layers have been shown to be similar from compositional and crystallographic points of view with bone apatite [188].

The microcrystal properties are somehow independent of the existing β-TCP/HAP ratio before implantation. After six months, there was a significant increase in the implant microporosity, due to the preferential dissolution of the large crystals of β-TCP. Regardless of the β-TCP/HAP ratio value, the *in vitro* tests indicated that particles of HAP remnant in the implant are more numerous than the β-TCP ones, confirming the higher dissolution rate of β-TCP than the latter.

As it has been shown in the *in vitro* tests, the formation of the apatite microcrystals is caused by dissolution/reprecipitation processes. Thus, the partial solubilization of the implant, either HAP or β-TCP, induce a local increase of calcium and phosphate ion concentrations, and thereby the increase of the degree of saturation in the surrounding environment. This results in the precipitation of apatite microcrystals that can incorporate also other ions (e.g. $CaCO_3$, Mg) and organic molecules from biological fluids [188].

In mandibular periodontal defects [190], pure HAP implants were explanted at five and nine weeks from pigs. It was noted, however, that after both periods of implantation normal bone tissue was formed by direct apposition to the HAP implant. At five weeks, the bone growth average was 14%, compared to 23% after nine weeks. In this period, it is recognized that newly formed bone penetrates and fills the scaffold's channels [17].

In addition to the periodontal defects, HAP or β-TCP porous blocks were implanted into the intramedullary channel of the radius bone in goats. The SEM micrographs of the explants revealed the presence of osteoblasts and collagen fibers at the implant–host tissue interface. Collagen fibers are attached to the HAP surface either by direct connection or by globular deposits. The histology tests demonstrated the normal and complete ossification by the development of haversian channels and osteoblastic cells, well-defined on the implant periphery. Also, the blood vessels are normally developed within the haversian channels and marrow spaces; at the moment of the explantation, a small amount of formed bone marrow can already be observed [16, 189].

In the case of β-TCP, SEM results show the formation of new bone tissue at the interface region. In this case, the discontinuity degree at the interface is reduced with respect to HAP blocks, which suggests a faster bone growth. It also shows reticular formation of collagen structures and trabecular bone within the mineralization process. Histological analysis shows the haversian channels and the bone marrow spaces formation, which emphasizes the angiogenesis by the bone marrow development within the center of the unresorbed material. The periosteum appears slightly thickened and the bone marrow contains some fat cells and a large number of blood vessels [189].

In all the *in vivo* results presented above, the presence of osteoblasts and the direct apposition to implant of the newly formed bone tissue are excellent indicators of the biocompatibility and the osteoconductivity [17] of the implants from CaP materials derived from marble and shells. Moreover, their feasibility in the reconstruction of large bone defects, as well as those present in areas with variable mechanical loads, is demonstrated [10, 107, 187, 191].

5.10 Conclusions

It took almost five decades of progressive research in bioceramics field, since the idea of HAP-based bone substituents was born, to an achievable, proofed resolution nowadays. We refer here to the one brought by the deep spread resources in the form of marine shellfish on one side and calcitic/dolomitic marble on the other side. In both cases, it goes down to the calcium carbonate composition and the possibility of facile conversion to a bone-like apatite.

Both the synthesis methods and product processing techniques tend to escalate to a higher technology, but the marble and shells-derived ceramics are still encountering some limitations. Based on our findings on the synthesis processes, regardless the followed route, the reaction between raw materials and acids is usually incomplete, and so materials' biocompatibility may be restrained by the residual calcium oxide that is present in the final apatite powder. Moreover, it is of high importance to fully assure the elimination of cytotoxic acids from the material after the heat treatment of synthesized HAP.

The HAP powder processing is currently narrowed down by specific disadvantages of each method, the most important of them being the incapacity of fully reproducing the porosity of natural bone tissue. Conventional methods on one side are difficult to control for a multisized pore structure. We found that microporosity is still a heavy task also for SFF techniques, due to the lack of fully suitable binders and the compromise between powder particles' size and equipment's limitations. Moreover, the compromise between porosity and mechanical properties of these products is still required until densification mechanisms are properly controlled.

Despite these constrains, studies show us that such raw material used as HAP precursors can be an attractive low-cost alternative to the traditional bone reconstruction approaches. Therefore, we are in depth of more research work on that matter.

Acknowledgment

This work was supported by a grant of the Romanian National Authority for Scientific Research and Innovation, CNCS-UEFISCDI, project number PN-III-P2-2.1-PED-2016-0892.

References

1 Mohammad, N.F., Muhammed, M.H., Zakaria, Z. et al. (eds.) (2012). Characterization of calcium phosphate bioceramic from *Paphia undulata* shells. In: *2012 International Conference on Biomedical Engineering (ICoBE)*, 114–116. IEEE.

2 Santhosh, S. and Prabu, S.B. (2012). Characterization of nano-hydroxyapatite synthesized from sea shells through wet chemical method. *Int. J. Nanosci.* **11** (05): 1250031.

3 Dressmann, H. (1892). Ueber knochenplombierung bei hohlenformigen defekten des knochens. *Beitr. Klin. Chir.* **9**: 804–810.

4 Peltier, L.F. (1961). The use of plaster of Paris to fill defects in bone. *Clin. Orthop.* **21**: 1–31.

5 Albee, F.H. (1920). Studies in bone growth: triple calcium phosphate as a stimulus to osteogenesis. *Ann. Surg.* **71** (1): 32.

6 Tas, A.C., Korkusuz, F., Timucin, M., and Akkas, N. (1997). An investigation of the chemical synthesis and high-temperature sintering behaviour of calcium hydroxyapatite (HA) and tricalcium phosphate (TCP) bioceramics. *J. Mater. Sci. Mater. Med.* **8** (2): 91–96.

7 Gibson, I.R. and Bonfield, W. (2002). Novel synthesis and characterization of an AB-type carbonate-substituted hydroxyapatite. *J. Biomed. Mater. Res.* **59** (4): 697–708.

8 Dorozhkin, S.V. (2010). Bioceramics of calcium orthophosphates. *Biomaterials* **31** (7): 1465–1485.

9 Yang, Y., Yao, Q., Pu, X. et al. (2011). Biphasic calcium phosphate macroporous scaffolds derived from oyster shells for bone tissue engineering. *Chem. Eng. J.* **173** (3): 837–845.

10 Vecchio, K.S., Zhang, X., Massie, J.B. et al. (2007). Conversion of bulk seashells to biocompatible hydroxyapatite for bone implants. *Acta Biomater.* **3** (6): 910–918.

11 Zhang, X. and Vecchio, K.S. (2013). Conversion of natural marine skeletons as scaffolds for bone tissue engineering. *Front. Mater. Sci.* **7** (2): 103–117.

12 Luz, G.M. and Mano, J.F. (2010). Mineralized structures in nature: examples and inspirations for the design of new composite materials and biomaterials. *Compos. Sci. Technol.* **70** (13): 1777–1788.

13 Shavandi, A., Bekhit, A.E.-D.A., Ali, A., and Sun, Z. (2015). Synthesis of nano-hydroxyapatite (nHA) from waste mussel shells using a rapid microwave method. *Mater. Chem. Phys.* **149–150**: 607–616.

14 Stevens, B., Yang, Y., Mohandas, A. et al. (2008). A review of materials, fabrication methods, and strategies used to enhance bone regeneration in engineered bone tissues. *J. Biomed. Mater. Res. Part B* **85** (2): 573–582.

15 Abarrategi, A., Moreno-Vicente, C., Martínez-Vázquez, F.J. et al. (2012). Biological properties of solid free form designed ceramic scaffolds with BMP-2: in vitro and in vivo evaluation. *PLoS ONE* **7** (3): e34117.

16 Thavornyutikarn, B., Chantarapanich, N., Sitthiseripratip, K. et al. (2014). Bone tissue engineering scaffolding: computer-aided scaffolding techniques. *Prog. Biomater.* **3** (2–4): 61–102.

17 Chu, T.M.G., Orton, D.G., Hollister, S.J. et al. (2002). Mechanical and in vivo performance of hydroxyapatite implants with controlled architectures. *Biomaterials* **23** (5): 1283–1293.

18 Lobo, S.E. and Livingston Arinzeh, T. (2010). Biphasic calcium phosphate ceramics for bone regeneration and tissue engineering applications. *Materials* **3** (2): 815–826.

19 Gunduz, O., Sahin, Y., Agathopoulos, S. et al. (2014). A new method for fabrication of nanohydroxyapatite and TCP from the sea snail *Cerithium vulgatum*. *J. Nanomater.* **2014**: 1.

20 Hsieh, M.F., Chin, T.S., Perng, L.H., and Perng, H.G. (2001). Gel-to-ceramic conversion during

hydroxyapatite synthesis. *J. Am. Ceram. Soc.* **84** (9): 2123–2125.

21 Wijesinghe, W.P.S.L., Mantilaka, M.M.M.G.P.G., Premalal, E.V.A. et al. (2014). Facile synthesis of both needle-like and spherical hydroxyapatite nanoparticles: effect of synthetic temperature and calcination on morphology, crystallite size and crystallinity. *Mater. Sci. Eng., C* **42**: 83–90.

22 Jevtic, M., Mitric, M., Skapin, S. et al. (2008). Crystal structure of hydroxyapatite nanorods synthesized by sonochemical homogeneous precipitation. *Cryst. Growth Des.* **8** (7): 2217–2222.

23 Mantripragada, V.P., Lecka-Czernik, B., Ebraheim, N.A., and Jayasuriya, A.C. (2013). An overview of recent advances in designing orthopedic and craniofacial implants. *J. Biomed. Mater. Res. Part A* **101** (11): 3349–3364.

24 Bayraktar, D. and Tas, A.C. (1999). Chemical preparation of carbonated calcium hydroxyapatite powders at 37 C in urea-containing synthetic body fluids. *J. Eur. Ceram. Soc.* **19** (13): 2573–2579.

25 Shavandi, A., AE-DA, B., Sun, Z.F., and Ali, A. (2015). A review of synthesis methods, properties and use of hydroxyapatite as a substitute of bone. *J. Biomimetics Biomater. Biomed. Eng.* **25**: 98–117.

26 Hsieh, M.-F., Perng, L.-H., Chin, T.-S., and Perng, H.-G. (2001). Phase purity of sol-gel-derived hydroxyapatite ceramic. *Biomaterials* **22** (19): 2601–2607.

27 Layrolle, P., Ito, A., and Tateishi, T. (1998). Sol-gel synthesis of amorphous calcium phosphate and sintering into microporous hydroxyapatite bioceramics. *J. Am. Ceram. Soc.* **81** (6): 1421–1428.

28 Rhee, S.-H. (2002). Synthesis of hydroxyapatite via mechanochemical treatment. *Biomaterials* **23** (4): 1147–1152.

29 Kim, I.-S. and Kumta, P.N. (2004). Sol–gel synthesis and characterization of nanostructured hydroxyapatite powder. *Mater. Sci. Eng., B* **111** (2–3): 232–236.

30 Zainuddin, N.M., AMM, J., Anwar, R., and Hassan, O.H. (2015). Hydroxyapatite material study for synthetic skull design construction for slip casting method. In: *Proceedings of the International Symposium on Research of Arts, Design and Humanities (ISRADH 2014)*, 221–227. Springer.

31 Mustaffa, R., Yusof, M., Reusmaazran, M., and Abdullah, Y. (2015). A novelty of synthetic hydroxyapatite from cockle shell and characterization. *Adv. Mater. Res.* **1087**: 429–433.

32 Mohammad, N.F., Zahid, M.A., Awang, S.A. et al. (2010). Synthesis and characterization of bioceramic from Malaysian cockle shell. In: *IEEE Symposium on Industrial Electronics & Applications (ISIEA)*, 2010, 413–416.

33 Lemos, A.F., Rocha, J.H.G., Quaresma, S.S.F. et al. (2006). Hydroxyapatite nano-powders produced hydrothermally from nacreous material. *J. Eur. Ceram. Soc.* **26** (16): 3639–3646.

34 Fadli, A., Akbar, F., Putri, P. et al. (2014). Hydroxyapatite powder prepared by low temperature hydrothermal method from sea shells. *Sci. Eng.* **1**: 4–5.

35 Hoque, M.E., Shehryar, M., and Islam, K.M.N. (2014). Processing and characterization of cockle shell calcium carbonate ($CaCO_3$) bioceramic for potential application in bone tissue engineering. *J. Mater. Sci. Eng.* **2** (4): 132.

36 Jones, M.I., Barakat, H., and Patterson, D.A. (2011). Production of hydroxyapatite from waste mussel shells. *IOP Conf. Ser. Mater. Sci. Eng.* **18**: 192002.

37 Raya, I., Mayasari, E., Yahya, A. et al. (2015). Shynthesis and characterizations of calcium hydroxyapatite derived from crabs shells (*Portunus pelagicus*) and its potency in safeguard against to dental demineralizations. *Int. J. Biomater.* **2015**. https://doi.org/10.1155/2015/469176.

38 Kamba, A.S., Ismail, M., Ibrahim, T.A.T., and Zakaria, Z.A.B. (2013). Synthesis and characterisation of calcium carbonate aragonite nanocrystals from cockle shell powder (*Anadara granosa*). *J. Nanomater.* **2013**: 5.

39 Koonawoot, R., Thiansem, S., Punyanitya, S. et al. (2011). Synthesis of hydroxyapatite powder from mollusc shell. *Adv. Mater. Res.* **311–313**: 1621–1624.

40 Rujitanapanich, S., Kumpapan, P., and Wanjanoi, P. (2014). Synthesis of hydroxyapatite from oyster shell via precipitation. *Energy Procedia* **56**: 112–117.

41 Santhosh, S. and Balasivanandha Prabu, S. (2013). Thermal stability of nano hydroxyapatite synthesized from sea shells through wet chemical synthesis. *Mater. Lett.* **97**: 121–124.

42 Yeong, K.C.B., Wang, J., and Ng, S.C. (2001). Mechanochemical synthesis of nanocrystalline hydroxyapatite from CaO and $CaHPO_4$. *Biomaterials* **22** (20): 2705–2712.

43 Yoshimura, M., Sujaridworakun, P., Koh, F. et al. (2004). Hydrothermal conversion of calcite crystals to hydroxyapatite. *Mater. Sci. Eng., C* **24** (4): 521–525.

44 Maleki Dizaj, S., Barzegar-Jalali, M., Zarrintan, M.H. et al. (2015). Calcium carbonate nanoparticles as cancer drug delivery system. *Expert Opin. Drug Delivery* **12** (10): 1649–1660.

45 Gunduz, O. (2014). A simple method of producing hydroxyapatite and tri calcium phosphate from coral

(*Pocillopora verrucosa*). *J. Aust. Ceram. Soc.* **50** (2): 52–58.

46 Montazeri, L., Javadpour, J., Shokrgozar, M.A. et al. (2010). Hydrothermal synthesis and characterization of hydroxyapatite and fluorhydroxyapatite nano-size powders. *Biomed. Mater.* **5** (4): 045004.

47 Kim, W., Zhang, Q., and Saito, F. (2000). Mechanochemical synthesis of hydroxyapatite from $Ca(OH)_2$-P_2O_5 and CaO-$Ca(OH)_2$-P_2O_5 mixtures. *J. Mater. Sci.* **35** (21): 5401–5405.

48 Avvakumov, E. and Karakchiev, L. (2004). Mechanochemical synthesis as a method for the preparation of nanodisperse particles of oxide materials. *Chem. Sustainable Dev.* **12**: 287–291.

49 Anitha, P. and Pandya, H.M. (2013). Comprehensive review of preparation methodologies of nano hydroxyapatite. *J. Environ. Nano Technol.* **3** (1): 101–121.

50 Shariffuddin, J.H., Jones, M.I., and Patterson, D.A. (2013). Greener photocatalysts: hydroxyapatite derived from waste mussel shells for the photocatalytic degradation of a model azo dye wastewater. *Chem. Eng. Res. Des.* **91** (9): 1693–1704.

51 Santhosh, S. and Prabu, S.B. (2012). Synthesis and characterisation of nanocrystalline hydroxyapatite from sea shells. *Int. J. Biomed. Nanosci. Nanotechnol.* **2** (3–4): 276–283.

52 Abdulrahman, I., Tijani, H.I., Mohammed, B.A. et al. (2014). From garbage to biomaterials: an overview on egg shell based hydroxyapatite. *J. Mater.* **2014**: 1–6.

53 Akram, M., Ahmed, R., Shakir, I. et al. (2014). Extracting hydroxyapatite and its precursors from natural resources. *J. Mater. Sci.* **49** (4): 1461–1475.

54 Brzezińska-Miecznik, J., Haberko, K., Sitarz, M. et al. (2015). Hydroxyapatite from animal bones – extraction and properties. *Ceram. Int.* **41** (3, Part B): 4841–4846.

55 Clarke, S.A., Walsh, P., Maggs, C.A., and Buchanan, F. (2011). Designs from the deep: marine organisms for bone tissue engineering. *Biotechnol. Adv.* **29** (6): 610–617.

56 Gergely, G., Wéber, F., Lukács, I. et al. (2010). Nano-hydroxyapatite preparation from biogenic raw materials. *Cent. Eur. J. Chem.* **8** (2): 375–381.

57 Orlić, S., Ivanković, H., and Tkalčec, E. (2006). Preparation of highly porous hydroxyapatite ceramics from cuttlefish bones. *Matrib* **2006**: 162–167.

58 Dorozhkin, S.V. (2009). Calcium orthophosphate-based biocomposites and hybrid biomaterials. *J. Mater. Sci.* **44** (9): 2343–2387.

59 Wu, S.-C., Hsu, H.-C., Wu, Y.-N., and Ho, W.-F. (2011). Hydroxyapatite synthesized from oyster shell powders by ball milling and heat treatment. *Mater. Charact.* **62** (12): 1180–1187.

60 Vincent, J.F. (2009). Biomimetics—a review. *Proc. Inst. Mech. Eng, Part H* **223** (8): 919–939.

61 Mossman, S.T. and Morris, P.J. (1994). *The Development of Plastics*. Royal Society of Chemistry.

62 Huang, L., McMillan, R.A., Apkarian, R.P. et al. (2000). Generation of synthetic elastin-mimetic small diameter fibers and fiber networks. *Macromolecules* **33** (8): 2989–2997.

63 Lazaris, A., Arcidiacono, S., Huang, Y. et al. (2002). Spider silk fibers spun from soluble recombinant silk produced in mammalian cells. *Science* **295** (5554): 472–476.

64 Macha, I.J., Ozyegin, L., Oktar, F.N., and Ben-Nissan, B. (2015). Conversion of ostrich eggshells (*Struthio camelus*) to calcium phosphates. *J. Aust. Ceram. Soc.* **51**: 125–133.

65 Gordon, L.M., Tran, L., and Joester, D. (2012). Atom probe tomography of apatites and bone-type mineralized tissues. *ACS Nano* **6** (12): 10667–10675.

66 Spacu, P., Stan, M., Gheorghiu, C., and Brezeanu, M. (1978). *Tratat de chimie organica*. Bucuresti: Ed. Tehnica.

67 Elliott, J., Wilson, R., and Dowker, S. (2002). Apatite structures. *Adv. X-Ray Anal.* **45**: 172–181.

68 Nenitescu, C.D. (1979). *Chimie Generala*. Bucuresti: Ed. Didactica si Pedagogica.

69 Gouma, P., Ramachandran, K., Firat, M. et al. (2010). Novel bioceramics for bone implants. In: *Advances in Bioceramics and Porous Ceramics II*, 35–44. Wiley.

70 Dorozhkin, S. (2008). A novel, environmentally friendly process for the fabrication of calcium phosphate bioceramics. *Inorg. Mater.* **44** (2): 207–210.

71 Tas, A.C. (2000). Combustion synthesis of calcium phosphate bioceramic powders. *J. Eur. Ceram. Soc.* **20** (14–15): 2389–2394.

72 Ślósarczyk, A., Paszkiewicz, Z., and Paluszkiewicz, C. (2005). FTIR and XRD evaluation of carbonated hydroxyapatite powders synthesized by wet methods. *J. Mol. Struct.* **744–747**: 657–661.

73 Ivanchenko, L.A. and Pinchuk, N.D. (2003). Making calcium phosphate biomaterials. *Powder Metall. Met. Ceram.* **42** (7–8): 357–371.

74 Hattori, T. and Lwadate, Y. (1990). Hydrothermal preparation of calcium hydroxyapatite powders. *J. Am. Ceram. Soc.* **73** (6): 1803–1805.

75 Wieczorek-Ciurowa, K., Paulik, J., and Paulik, F. (1980). Influence of foreign materials upon the thermal decomposition of dolomite, calcite and magnesite part I. Influence of sodium chloride. *Thermochim. Acta* **38** (2): 157–164.

76 Beral, E. and Zapan, M. (1977). *Chimie Anorganica*. Bucuresti: Ed. Tehnica.

77 Herz, N. and Waelkens, M. (1988). *Classical Marble: Geochemistry, Technology, Trade*. Brill Archive.

78 Park, S.H., Tofighi, A., Wang, X. et al. (2011). Calcium phosphate combination biomaterials as human mesenchymal stem cell delivery vehicles for bone repair. *J. Biomed. Mater. Res. Part B* **97** (2): 235–244.

79 Roy, D.M. and Linnehan, S.K. (1974). Hydroxyapatite formed from coral skeletal carbonate by hydrothermal exchange. **247**: 220–222.

80 Sych, E., Pinchuk, N., Tovstonog, A. et al. (2014). The structure and properties of calcium phosphate ceramics produced from monetite and biogenic hydroxyapatite. *Powder Metall. Met. Ceram.* **53** (7–8): 423–430.

81 Lu, X., Qian, J., Zhou, H. et al. (2011). In vitro cytotoxicity and induction of apoptosis by silica nanoparticles in human $HepG_2$ hepatoma cells. *Int. J. Nanomed.* **6**: 1889–1901.

82 Sirisoam, T., Saelee, C., Thiansem, S. and Punyanitya, S. Preparation and characterization of high purity calcium oxide from cockleshells for using in bioceramic synthesis.

83 Plevová, E., Kožušníková, A., Vaculíková, L., and Martynková, G.S. (2010). Thermal behavior of selected Czech marble samples. *J. Therm. Anal. Calorim.* **101** (2): 657–664.

84 Shushakova, V., Fuller, E.R. Jr.,, Heidelbach, F. et al. (2013). Marble decay induced by thermal strains: simulations and experiments. *Environ. Earth Sci.* **69** (4): 1281–1297.

85 Toprak, G. (2007). *Characteristics of Limes Produced from Marbles and Limestones*. Citeseer.

86 Santhosh, S. (2014). A novel structure for implant surfaces based on a natural precursor microwave and electrospinning technologies.

87 Trinkūnaitė-Felsen, J., Žalga, A., and Kareiva, A. (2012). Characterization of naturally derived calcium compounds used in food industry. *Chemija* **23** (2): 76–85.

88 Batista, F.M., Ben-Hamadou, R., Fonseca, V.G. et al. (2008). Comparative study of shell shape and muscle scar pigmentation in the closely related cupped oysters *Crassostrea angulata, C. gigas* and their reciprocal hybrids. *Aquat. Living Resour.* **21** (01): 31–38.

89 Galtsoff, P.S. (1964). *The American Oyster Crassostrea Virginica Gmelin*. Unites States Department of the Interior, Fish and Wildlife Service, Bureau of Commercial Fisheries.

90 Quayle, D.B. (1988). *Pacific Oyster Culture in British Columbia*. Department of Fisheries and Oceans.

91 Su, X., Kamat, S., and Heuer, A. (2000). The structure of sea urchin spines, large biogenic single crystals of calcite. *J. Mater. Sci.* **35** (22): 5545–5551.

92 Riman, R.E., Suchanek, W.L., Byrappa, K. et al. (2002). Solution synthesis of hydroxyapatite designer particulates. *Solid State Ionics* **151** (1–4): 393–402.

93 Salma, K., Berzina-Cimdina, L., and Borodajenko, N. (2010). Calcium phosphate bioceramics prepared from wet chemically precipitated powders. *Process. Appl. Ceram.* **4** (1): 45–51.

94 Hench, L.L. and Wilson, J. (1993). *An Introduction to Bioceramics*. World Scientific.

95 Rathje, W. (1939). Zur Kenntnis der Phosphate I: Über Hydroxylapatit. *Bodenkd. Pflanzenernährung* **12** (1–2): 121–128.

96 Hayek, E., Newesely, H., and Rumpel, M.L. (2007). Pentacalcium monohydroxyorthophosphate. *Inorg. Synth.* **7**: 63–65.

97 Loo, S.C.J., Siew, Y.E., Ho, S. et al. (2008). Synthesis and hydrothermal treatment of nanostructured hydroxyapatite of controllable sizes. *J. Mater. Sci. Mater. Med.* **19** (3): 1389–1397.

98 Byrappa, K. and Yoshimura, M. (2012). *Handbook of Hydrothermal Technology*. William Andrew.

99 H-B, Z., K-C, Z., Li, Z.-Y. et al. (2009). Morphologies of hydroxyapatite nanoparticles adjusted by organic additives in hydrothermal synthesis. *J. Cent. South Univ. Technol.* **16** (6): 871–875.

100 Azis, Y., Jamarun, N., Arief, S., and Nur, H. (2015). Facile synthesis of hydroxyapatite particles from cockle shells (*Anadaragranosa*) by hydrothermal method. *Orient. J. Chem.* **31** (2): 1099–1105.

101 Koumoulidis, G.C., Katsoulidis, A.P., Ladavos, A.K. et al. (2003). Preparation of hydroxyapatite via microemulsion route. *J. Colloid Interface Sci.* **259** (2): 254–260.

102 McIntosh, R., Sharp, J., and Wilburn, F. (1990). The thermal decomposition of dolomite. *Thermochim. Acta* **165** (2): 281–296.

103 Stanmore, B. and Gilot, P. (2005). Review—calcination and carbonation of limestone during thermal cycling for CO_2 sequestration. *Fuel Process. Technol.* **86** (16): 1707–1743.

104 Khinast, J., Krammer, G.F., Brunner, C., and Staudinger, G. (1996). Decomposition of limestone: the influence of CO_2 and particle size on the reaction rate. *Chem. Eng. Sci.* **51** (4): 623–634.

105 Satterfield, C.N. and Feakes, F. (1959). Kinetics of the thermal decomposition of calcium carbonate. *AlChE J.* **5** (1): 115–122.

106 Rodriguez-Navarro, C., Ruiz-Agudo, E., Luque, A. et al. (2009). Thermal decomposition of calcite: mechanisms of formation and textural evolution of CaO nanocrystals. *Am. Mineral.* **94** (4): 578–593.

107 Jarcho, M., Kay, J.F., Gumaer, K.I. et al. (1977). Tissue, cellular and subcellular events at a bone-ceramic hydroxylapatite interface. *J. Bioeng.* **1** (2): 79–92.

108 Bose, S. and Saha, S.K. (2003). Synthesis of hydroxyapatite nanopowders via sucrose-templated sol–gel method. *J. Am. Ceram. Soc.* **86** (6): 1055–1057.

109 Yang, X. and Wang, Z. (1998). Synthesis of biphasic ceramics of hydroxyapatite and β-tricalcium phosphate with controlled phase content and porosity. *J. Mater. Chem.* **8** (10): 2233–2237.

110 Guo, G., Sun, Y., Wang, Z., and Guo, H. (2005). Preparation of hydroxyapatite nanoparticles by reverse microemulsion. *Ceram. Int.* **31** (6): 869–872.

111 Toibah, A.R., Fatimah, M., Siti Sainillah, S. et al. (2012). Calcium phosphate ceramics prepared from natural waste materials.

112 Champion, E. (2013). Sintering of calcium phosphate bioceramics. *Acta Biomater.* **9** (4): 5855–5875.

113 Veljović, D., Zalite, I., Palcevskis, E. et al. (2010). Microwave sintering of fine grained HAP and HAP/TCP bioceramics. *Ceram. Int.* **36** (2): 595–603.

114 Menezes, R.R., Souto, P.M., and Kiminami, R.H. (2012). *Microwave Fast Sintering of Ceramic Materials.* INTECH Open Access Publisher.

115 Agrawal, D. (2006). Microwave sintering of ceramics, composites and metallic materials, and melting of glasses. *Trans. Indian Ceram. Soc.* **65** (3): 129–144.

116 Ehsani, N., Sorrell, C., and Ruys, A. (2013). Microwave hybrid processing of hydroxyapatite. *J. Biomimetics Biomater. Tissue Eng.* **18** (108): 2.

117 Merry, J., Gibson, I., Best, S., and Bonfield, W. (1998). Synthesis and characterization of carbonate hydroxyapatite. *J. Mater. Sci. - Mater. Med.* **9** (12): 779–783.

118 Hung, I., Shih, W.-J., Hon, M.-H., and Wang, M.-C. (2012). The properties of sintered calcium phosphate with [Ca]/[P] = 1.50. *Int. J. Mol. Sci.* **13** (10): 13569–13586.

119 Zyman, Z., Tkachenko, N., and Polevodin, D. (2007). Biphasic (HA/β TCP) calcium phosphate ceramics. *Funct. Mater.* **14** (4): 586–589.

120 Li, S.H., De Wijn, J.R., Layrolle, P., and De Groot, K. (2002). Synthesis of macroporous hydroxyapatite scaffolds for bone tissue engineering. *J. Biomed. Mater. Res.* **61** (1): 109–120.

121 Bose, S., Vahabzadeh, S., and Bandyopadhyay, A. (2013). Bone tissue engineering using 3D printing. *Mater. Today* **16** (12): 496–504.

122 Rocha, J., Lemos, A., Agathopoulos, S. et al. (2006). Hydrothermal growth of hydroxyapatite scaffolds from aragonitic cuttlefish bones. *J. Biomed. Mater. Res. Part A* **77** (1): 160–168.

123 Salgado, A.J., Coutinho, O.P., and Reis, R.L. (2004). Bone tissue engineering: state of the art and future trends. *Macromol. Biosci.* **4** (8): 743–765.

124 Mehrabanian, M. and Nasr-Esfahani, M. (2011). HA/nylon 6, 6 porous scaffolds fabricated by salt-leaching/solvent casting technique: effect of nano-sized filler content on scaffold properties. *Int. J. Nanomed.* **6**: 1651–1659.

125 Araki, K. and Halloran, J.W. (2005). Porous ceramic bodies with interconnected pore channels by a novel freeze casting technique. *J. Am. Ceram. Soc.* **88** (5): 1108–1114.

126 Chen, G., Ushida, T., and Tateishi, T. (2001). Development of biodegradable porous scaffolds for tissue engineering. *Mater. Sci. Eng., C* **17** (1–2): 63–69.

127 Huang, Y., Ren, J., Chen, C. et al. (2007). Preparation and properties of poly(lactide-co-glycolide)(PLGA)/nano-hydroxyapatite (NHA) scaffolds by thermally induced phase separation and rabbit MSCs culture on scaffolds. *J. Biomater. Appl.* **22**: 409–432.

128 Mathieu, L.M., Mueller, T.L., Bourban, P.-E. et al. (2006). Architecture and properties of anisotropic polymer composite scaffolds for bone tissue engineering. *Biomaterials* **27** (6): 905–916.

129 Teixeira, S., Rodriguez, M.A., Pena, P. et al. (2009). Physical characterization of hydroxyapatite porous scaffolds for tissue engineering. *Mater. Sci. Eng., C* **29** (5): 1510–1514.

130 Jo, I.-H., Shin, K.-H., Soon, Y.-M. et al. (2009). Highly porous hydroxyapatite scaffolds with elongated pores using stretched polymeric sponges as novel template. *Mater. Lett.* **63** (20): 1702–1704.

131 Jach, K., Pietrzak, K., Kalinski, D., and Chmielewski, M. Influence of binder on porous ceramic properties prepared by polymeric sponge method. *Adv. Sci. Technol.* **2011**, **22** (5): 409–432.

132 Ramay, H.R. and Zhang, M. (2003). Preparation of porous hydroxyapatite scaffolds by combination of the gel-casting and polymer sponge methods. *Biomaterials* **24** (19): 3293–3302.

133 Schumacher, M., Deisinger, U., Detsch, R., and Ziegler, G. (2010). Indirect rapid prototyping of biphasic calcium phosphate scaffolds as bone substitutes: influence of phase composition, macroporosity and pore geometry on mechanical properties. *J. Mater. Sci. - Mater. Med.* **21** (12): 3119–3127.

134 Russias, J., Saiz, E., Deville, S. et al. (2007). Fabrication and in vitro characterization of three-dimensional organic/inorganic scaffolds by robocasting. *J. Biomed. Mater. Res. Part A* **83** (2): 434–445.

135 Bernardo, J.R. (2010). *Indirect Tissue Scaffold Fabrication via Additive Manufacturing and Biomimetic*

Mineralization, vol. **63**, 164–169. Virginia Polytechnic Institute and State University.
136 Chevalier, E., Chulia, D., Pouget, C., and Viana, M. (2008). Fabrication of porous substrates: a review of processes using pore forming agents in the biomaterial field. *J. Pharm. Sci.* **97** (3): 1135–1154.
137 Gao, C., Deng, Y., Feng, P. et al. (2014). Current progress in bioactive ceramic scaffolds for bone repair and regeneration. *Int. J. Mol. Sci.* **15** (3): 4714–4732.
138 Appleford, M.R., Oh, S., Cole, J.A. et al. (2007). Ultrasound effect on osteoblast precursor cells in trabecular calcium phosphate scaffolds. *Biomaterials* **28** (32): 4788–4794.
139 Lohfeld, S., Barron, V., and McHugh, P. (2005). Biomodels of bone: a review. *Ann. Biomed. Eng.* **33** (10): 1295–1311.
140 Hull, C.W. (1986). *Apparatus for Production of Three-Dimensional Objects by Stereolithography*. Google Patents.
141 Beaman, J.J. and Deckard, C.R. (1990). *Selective Laser Sintering with Assisted Powder Handling*. Google Patents.
142 Sachs, E.M., Haggerty, J.S., Cima, M.J., and Williams, P.A. (1994). *Three-Dimensional Printing Techniques*. Google Patents.
143 Wätjen, A.M., Gingter, P., Kramer, M., and Telle, R. (2014). Novel prospects and possibilities in additive manufacturing of ceramics by means of direct inkjet printing. *Adv. Mech. Eng.* **6**: 141346.
144 Sa, M.-W. and Kim, J.Y. (2013). Design of multi-scaffold fabrication system for various 3D scaffolds. *J. Mech. Sci. Technol.* **27** (10): 2961–2966.
145 Miranda, P., Saiz, E., Gryn, K., and Tomsia, A.P. (2006). Sintering and robocasting of β-tricalcium phosphate scaffolds for orthopaedic applications. *Acta Biomater.* **2** (4): 457–466.
146 Eqtesadi, S., Motealleh, A., Miranda, P. et al. (2014). Robocasting of 45S5 bioactive glass scaffolds for bone tissue engineering. *J. Eur. Ceram. Soc.* **34** (1): 107–118.
147 Kim, S.-K. (2013). *Marine Biomaterials: Characterization, Isolation and Applications*. CRC Press.
148 Dorozhkin, S.V. and Epple, M. (2002). Biological and medical significance of calcium phosphates. *Angew. Chem. Int. Ed.* **41** (17): 3130–3146.
149 Wang, P.E. and Chaki, T. (1993). Sintering behaviour and mechanical properties of hydroxyapatite and dicalcium phosphate. *J. Mater. Sci. Mater. Med.* **4** (2): 150–158.
150 Mkukuma, L., Skakle, J., Gibson, I. et al. (2004). Effect of the proportion of organic material in bone on thermal decomposition of bone mineral: an investigation of a variety of bones from different species using thermogravimetric analysis coupled to mass spectrometry, high-temperature X-ray diffraction, and Fourier transform infrared spectroscopy. *Calcif. Tissue Int.* **75** (4): 321–328.
151 Markovic, M., Fowler, B.O., and Tung, M.S. (2004). Preparation and comprehensive characterization of a calcium hydroxyapatite reference material. *J. Res. Nat. Inst. Stand. Technol.* **109** (6): 553–568.
152 Sima, L.E., Stan, G.E., Morosanu, C.O. et al. (2010). Differentiation of mesenchymal stem cells onto highly adherent radio frequency-sputtered carbonated hydroxylapatite thin films. *J. Biomed. Mater. Res. Part A* **95** (4): 1203–1214.
153 Elliott, J.C. (1964). The crystallographic structure of dental enamel and related apatites.
154 Asif, M., Wang, W., Wang, H. et al. (2014). Fluoridation and sintering of hydroxyapatite material and their mechanical properties. *J. Wuhan Univ. Technol. Mater. Sci. Ed.* **29** (1): 190–196.
155 Ramesh, S., Tan, C., Bhaduri, S. et al. (2008). Densification behaviour of nanocrystalline hydroxyapatite bioceramics. *J. Mater. Process. Technol.* **206** (1): 221–230.
156 Lin, F.-H., Chun-Jen, L., Ko-Shao, C., and Jui-Sheng, S. (2000). Thermal reconstruction behavior of the quenched hydroxyapatite powder during reheating in air. *Mater. Sci. Eng., C* **13** (1): 97–104.
157 Lovett, M., Lee, K., Edwards, A., and Kaplan, D.L. (2009). Vascularization strategies for tissue engineering. *Tissue Eng. Part B: Rev.* **15** (3): 353–370.
158 Rouwkema, J., Rivron, N.C., and van Blitterswijk, C.A. (2008). Vascularization in tissue engineering. *Trends Biotechnol.* **26** (8): 434–441.
159 Dorozhkin, S.V. (2013). Calcium orthophosphate-based bioceramics. *Materials* **6** (9): 3840–3942.
160 Soon, Y.-M., Shin, K.-H., Koh, Y.-H. et al. (2011). Fabrication and compressive strength of porous hydroxyapatite scaffolds with a functionally graded core/shell structure. *J. Eur. Ceram. Soc.* **31** (1–2): 13–18.
161 Daculsi, G. and Miramond, T. (2013). Calcium phosphate–derived biomaterials. In: *Encyclopedia of Biophysics* (ed. G.C.K. Roberts), 206–211. Springer.
162 Bermudez, O., Boltong, M., Driessens, F., and Planell, J. (1993). Compressive strength and diametral tensile strength of some calcium-orthophosphate cements: a pilot study. *J. Mater. Sci. Mater. Med.* **4** (4): 389–393.
163 Cao, H., Zhang, L., Zheng, H., and Wang, Z. (2010). Hydroxyapatite nanocrystals for biomedical applications. *J. Phys. Chem. C* **114** (43): 18352–18357.

164 Tian, X., Li, D., and Heinrich, J.G. (2011). *Net-Shaping of Ceramic Components by Using Rapid Prototyping Technologies*. INTECH Open Access Publisher.

165 Monchau, F., Lefèvre, A., Descamps, M. et al. (2002). In vitro studies of human and rat osteoclast activity on hydroxyapatite, β-tricalcium phosphate, calcium carbonate. *Biomol. Eng.* **19** (2–6): 143–152.

166 Cerroni, L., Filocamo, R., Fabbri, M. et al. (2002). Growth of osteoblast-like cells on porous hydroxyapatite ceramics: an in vitro study. *Biomol. Eng.* **19** (2–6): 119–124.

167 Sánchez-Salcedo, S., Balas, F., Izquierdo-Barba, I., and Vallet-Regí, M. (2009). In vitro structural changes in porous HA/β-TCP scaffolds in simulated body fluid. *Acta Biomater.* **5** (7): 2738–2751.

168 Boskey, A. and Posner, A. (1976). In vitro nucleation of hydroxyapatite by a bone calcium-phospholipid-phosphate complex. *Calc. Tissue Int.* **22**: 197–201.

169 Alliot-Licht, B., Gregoire, M., Orly, I., and Menanteau, J. (1991). Cellular activity of osteoblasts in the presence of hydroxyapatite: an in vitro experiment. *Biomaterials* **12** (8): 752–756.

170 Duta, L., Stan, G.E., Popa, A.C. et al. (2016). Thickness influence on in vitro biocompatibility of titanium nitride thin films synthesized by pulsed laser deposition. *Materials* **9** (1): 38.

171 Wu, C. and Xiao, Y. (2009). Evaluation of the in vitro bioactivity of bioceramics. *Bone Tissue Regener. Insights* **2**: 25.

172 Mohamed, K.R., El-Rashidy, Z.M., and Salama, A.A. (2011). In vitro properties of nano-hydroxyapatite/chitosan biocomposites. *Ceram. Int.* **37** (8): 3265–3271.

173 Bohner, M. and Lemaitre, J. (2009). Can bioactivity be tested in vitro with SBF solution? *Biomaterials* **30** (12): 2175–2179.

174 Priya, A., Nath, S., Biswas, K., and Basu, B. (2010). In vitro dissolution of calcium phosphate-mullite composite in simulated body fluid. *J. Mater. Sci. Mater. Med.* **21** (6): 1817–1828.

175 Klein, C.P., de Blieck-Hogemrst, J., Wolket, J., and De Groot, K. (1990). Studies of the solubility of different calcium phosphate ceramic particles in vitro. *Biomaterials* **11** (7): 509–512.

176 Kohri, M., Miki, K., Waite, D.E. et al. (1993). In vitro stability of biphasic calcium phosphate ceramics. *Biomaterials* **14** (4): 299–304.

177 Cüneyt Tas, A. (2000). Synthesis of biomimetic Ca-hydroxyapatite powders at 37°C in synthetic body fluids. *Biomaterials* **21** (14): 1429–1438.

178 Kokubo, T., Kushitani, H., Sakka, S. et al. (1990). Solutions able to reproduce in vivo surface-structure changes in bioactive glass-ceramic A-W3. *J. Biomed. Mater. Res.* **24** (6): 721–734.

179 Mateescu, M., Rguitti, E., Ponche, A. et al. (2012). Biomimetic evaluation of β tricalcium phosphate prepared by hot isostatic pressing. *Biomatter* **2** (3): 103–113.

180 Yun, H., Park, E.K., and Lim, J.W. (2014). Novel process to fabricate 3D porous calcium phosphate scaffolds at room temperature. *Biomater. Res.* **18** (1): 1–7.

181 Ducheyne, P., Radin, S., and King, L. (1993). The effect of calcium phosphate ceramic composition and structure on in vitro behavior. I. Dissolution. *J. Biomed. Mater. Res.* **27** (1): 25–34.

182 Radin, S. and Ducheyne, P. (1993). The effect of calcium phosphate ceramic composition and structure on in vitro behavior. II. Precipitation. *J. Biomed. Mater. Res.* **27** (1): 35–45.

183 Wu, Q., Zhang, X., Wu, B., and Huang, W. (2013). Effects of microwave sintering on the properties of porous hydroxyapatite scaffolds. *Ceram. Int.* **39** (3): 2389–2395.

184 Lee, J.T., Chow, K.L., Wang, K., and Tsang, W.-H. (2011). Is macroporosity absolutely required for preliminary in vitro bone biomaterial study? A comparison between porous materials and flat materials. *J. Funct. Biomater.* **2** (4): 308–337.

185 Gauthier, O., Bouler, J.-M., Aguado, E. et al. (1999). Elaboration conditions influence physicochemical properties and in vivo bioactivity of macroporous biphasic calcium phosphate ceramics. *J. Mater. Sci. Mater. Med.* **10** (4): 199–204.

186 Kivrak, N. and Taş, A.C. (1998). Synthesis of calcium hydroxyapatite-tricalcium phosphate (HA-TCP) composite bioceramic powders and their sintering behavior. *J. Am. Ceram. Soc.* **81** (9): 2245–2252.

187 Simon, J.L., Michna, S., Lewis, J.A. et al. (2007). In vivo bone response to 3D periodic hydroxyapatite scaffolds assembled by direct ink writing. *J. Biomed. Mater. Res. Part A* **83** (3): 747–758.

188 Daculsi, G., LeGeros, R., Nery, E. et al. (1989). Transformation of biphasic calcium phosphate ceramics in vivo: ultrastructural and physicochemical characterization. *J. Biomed. Mater. Res.* **23** (8): 883–894.

189 Ghosh, S.K., Nandi, S.K., Kundu, B. et al. (2008). In vivo response of porous hydroxyapatite and β-tricalcium phosphate prepared by aqueous solution combustion method and comparison with bioglass scaffolds. *J. Biomed. Mater. Res. Part B* **86** (1): 217–227.

190 Ratner, B.D. (2015). The biocompatibility of implant materials. In: *Host Response to Biomaterials: The*

Impact of Host Response on Biomaterial Selection (ed. S.F. Badylak), 37. Elsevier.

191 Osborn, J. (1991). *The Biological Profile of Hydroxyapatite Ceramic With Respect to the Cellular Dynamics of Animal and Human Soft Tissue and Mineralized Tissue Under Unloaded and Loaded Conditions. (Retroactive Coverage)*, 185–225. Elsevier Science Publishers B V, Biomaterials Degradation: Fundamental Aspects and Related Clinical Phenomena (The Netherlands).

6

Bioglasses and Glass-Ceramics in the Na_2O–CaO–MgO–SiO_2–P_2O_5–CaF_2 System

Simeon Agathopoulos[1] *and Dilhan U. Tulyaganov*[2]

[1] *Materials Science and Engineering Department, University of Ioannina, Ioannina, Greece*
[2] *Turin Polytechnic University in Tashkent, Niyazova, Uzbekistan*

6.1 Introduction

Various bioactive and biocompatible glasses have been developed as bone replacement materials owing to their ability to develop direct chemical bond not only to bones but also to soft tissues via a combination of cellular mechanism and chemical dissolution leading to bone regeneration and to control gene transcription through glass dissolution products. Although more than four decades have passed and remarkable advancements have been made, the 45S5 Bioglass® discovered by Hench still acts as a paradigm for designing most of the bioactive glass compositions.

It is globally accepted that the pioneer studies of Hench opened new perspectives for glasses. The first bioactive glass, 45S5 Bioglass, showed that when it was implanted in the bone, strong bonding to bone was developed. Postoperation examination showed that a zone of carbonated partially substituted hydroxyapatite (HCA) layer, similar to the mineral part of bones, was spontaneously grown on the surface of the glass. That was an unexpected result since it was discovered a glass which, instead of regular corrosion, in the environment of body fluids undergoes a spontaneous modification resulting in a HCA. The mechanism of hydroxyapatite (HA) formation on silicate bioactive glasses has been thoroughly investigated both *in vitro* and *in vivo*. It is generally accepted that it involves dissolution of Ca2+ ions from the surface of bioactive glasses that increases the supersaturation in the surrounding liquid, with respect to HA components, and enables precipitation of HA on the surface of the glasses, which has been already transformed (due to leaching effect) into a layer with features of silica gel. In particular, the dissolution of the silicate chains in the glass results in the formation of silanol groups on material's surface, which are essential nucleation sites for HA formation. Thus, HA chemically precipitates in the silica gel. Note that the pK_a of silicate acid is strongly alkaline, which favors the precipitation of HA. In general, HA forms more rapidly onto the surfaces of glasses and other amorphous phases, which favor easy and rapid release of Ca ions, than onto crystalline materials.

However, it was soon realized that bioactive glasses cannot be used in load-bearing applications due to their pronounced brittleness. Glasses propagate easily a crack since there is no element to act as a crack arrester in their bulk. Moreover, the crystallization of the already known highly bioactive glasses, such as 45S5 Bioglass, resulted in multiphase ceramics which were very brittle. A multiphase ceramic easily breaks due to the different coefficient of thermal expansion (CTE) of the different crystalline phases. Thus, the idea for developing glass-ceramics which can combine the high bioactivity of the glasses and the good mechanical properties of the ceramics was rapidly emerged. The main approach was to have, in the same material, the features of HA, whether existing in the material itself or be spontaneously produced when the material was in contact with the body environment, according to the principles of the mechanism for the induced bioactivity of the bioglasses. During this endeavor over all these decades since 1970s, it was realized that the developed glass-ceramics had also very good mechanical properties and aesthetics, which are very attractive features especially for dental prosthetic materials.

As happened in several technological milestones, which changed even our daily life, including, as mentioned above, the discovery of bioactive glass by Hench in the late 1960s, glass-ceramics is also a result of an accident. It was in the 1950s when an oven forgotten in turned-on mode allowed Stokey to discover the first

Bioceramics and Biocomposites: From Research to Clinical Practice, First Edition. Edited by Iulian Antoniac.

glass-ceramic in this oven, instead of a complete molten and destroyed overfired glass. Thus, the development of glass-ceramics, used in a wide range of applications, goes hand-by-hand with the development of glass-ceramics in dentistry and biomedicine in general.

Nowadays glass-ceramics are proposed for any possible applications where ceramics and glasses can be proposed, from household uses to thermal, chemical, energy, electronics, dielectric, environmental, biological, medical, space, etc. This is because glass-ceramics provide great possibilities to tune their properties, such as transparency, strength, resistance to abrasion, CTE through the control of the composition, extent of crystallization, crystal morphology, crystal size, and aspect ratio. The development of nanostructures, which can provide extraordinary values for electronic properties and ultra high mechanical strength, is a novel challenge that opens for the glass-ceramics. A specific challenge for glass-ceramics is that they would imitate the complex naturally occurred structures and result in even machineable or nonfragile ceramics. We all know that Mother Nature knows to endow with extraordinary properties in all her creations. We address the reader to the excellent book of W. Hoeland and G.H. Beall, "Glass-ceramics technology," for further information and details in many systems of glass-ceramics and to discover the magnificent world of glass-ceramics.

Accordingly, glass-ceramics can be considered as very flexible materials since the features of the glass and the ceramics can be apparently combined suitably together in a proportion which is demanded by the producer. This is a very attractive approach because, in general, ceramics are mechanically strong materials with good chemical durability and high melting point, compared to glasses. However, only few ceramics can reach absolute densification during sintering. Thus, the grain boundaries and the triple junctions among the grains can be completed by a glassy phase resulted in completely dense materials. Moreover, it is not easy to produce ceramics with very fine microstructure via conventional power technology techniques, in terms of the similarity of grains in their shape and size. However, careful and controlled crystallization of glasses may result in such fine microstructures of ceramics.

With regard to the design of new chemical compositions for biomaterials, the chemical composition of the already very popular bioactive materials, such as Bioglass, Ceravital®, and A-W glass-ceramics, which all contain CaO and SiO_2, fit well to the above concepts and approaches. Under the umbrella of this general approach and aspect, in this chapter, we describe a new Na_2O–CaO–MgO–SiO_2–P_2O_5–CaF_2 system for bioglass and glass-ceramics.

6.2 General Technical Aspects

The synthesis of the parent glass is an important step for the development of the final glass-ceramic material because, as stressed above, the chemical nature and the proportion of the principal components in the parent glass determine the crystalline phases precipitated from the glass reservoir in the resultant glass-ceramic. Under this perspective, the incorporation of additives in the basic glass composition is also a very important factor because it can considerably influence the process and the properties of the final product. The results of this process endow the resultant glass-ceramic with the desired properties. On this assumption, before analyzing the particular system, in this paragraph, we briefly present the most important technical features of the process to produce the glass-ceramic materials.

In the laboratory conditions homogeneously blended glass batch is thoroughly melted in, preferably, Pt crucibles (e.g. Pt–Rh) which safely sustain at high temperatures (up to 1600 °C), compared to the crucibles made of porcelain, or alumina, where an uptake of elements from the crucible (which can cause a noncontrolled contamination of the glass) inevitably occurs, along with a high risk to break the crucible during melting, handling, or casting. To avoid extended foaming of the glass batch (if it contains low-temperature volatile compounds such as carbonates, ammonium salts, etc.), preheating (at the temperature range 800–1100 °C) is recommended. If the glass is not apparently homogenous or if the glass has not enough low viscosity to allow easy casting, higher temperatures should be tried, or, when this is not possible (because of furnace or crucible limitations), longer melting time is suggested. It must be mentioned that the glasses are amorphous materials; thus, they do not have melting point, like the crystalline solids. Thus, the aforementioned state of the liquid glasses actually means a temperature range where the glasses obtain the typical features of a regular viscous liquid.

After melting, the glass is poured rapidly in a cold environment. Spontaneous crystallization of the glass during casting must be necessarily avoided. The ability of a glass to be crystallized in this casting stage depends on its composition. There are glasses which are highly prone for spontaneous devitrification, while there are glasses which are very stable. A high amount of glass modifiers (such as alkalis and alkaline earths) results in glasses which are highly prone for rapid spontaneous crystallization. These glasses have usually poor glass features and exhibit low chemical stability (chemical durability) in moisture and water environment. The glasses with high amount of glass formers (e.g. SiO_2, P_2O_5) are usually more stable during casting process.

Rapid reduction of temperature during casting results in glass-frits. This can be done by pouring the glass-melt into cold water, or between metallic plates (splat cooling), or even between metallic rollers for even faster cooling. The resultant glass-frits can be ground and sieved, to be sintered afterwards as regular ceramic powders. To obtain the glass in a block form, the molten glass is poured rapidly on preheated metallic (e.g. from bronze) mold, with a temperature about the T_g of the glass. Then, the metallic mold is rapidly (and carefully, for not altering the shape of the glass) placed in another furnace with a temperature close to the T_g of the glass. The furnace remains at this temperature for about an hour and then the sample cools down to room temperature naturally. Any attempt for an earlier removal of the glass from the furnace can cause an immediate spontaneous break of the glass block. This heat treatment (annealing) is necessary when we produce glass blocks because it removes the residual stresses from the glass occurred due to the rapid cooling from the temperature of the melting regime to the T_g. The glasses with no annealing at T_g can break at any time at room temperature, even after many months after their production, because these residual stresses have not been removed.

The glass, either as a compressed green-sample of glass-frit (produced with conventional powder technology methods) or as a glass-block sample (after annealing), is heat treated at temperatures higher than the T_g but lower than the softening point (T_s) to produce the glass-ceramic material. Thermal analysis is very important for the whole process, since it allows the determination of the T_g and the T_s of the glasses, as well as the crystallization temperatures (T_c) of the crystallized phases which can crystallize from this glass. The T_g of the glass and the T_c of the crystallized phases can be determined by the differential thermal analysis (DTA or DSC), and the T_g and T_s from dilatometry measurements. These results, which can be combined with microstructure observations and crystallographic analyses, allow the design of the correct heat treatment process to obtain the desired glass-ceramics, in terms of their crystallographic regime and microstructure. The addition of nucleation agents, which are usually oxides that affect the heterogeneous crystallization of the glass, strongly affects this process (and the temperatures referred above). It is also noteworthy that the thermal analysis allows to determine the mechanism of crystallization (surface or bulk crystallization) of the glass and to calculate the activation energy (E_a) of crystallization. For the former, DTA (or DSC) is realized with powders of glass-frit with different grain size; if the crystallization peaks shift with the change of the grain size, then the glass is prone to surface crystallization mechanism, whereas bulk crystallization mechanism occurs when the crystallization peaks are stable regardless of the particle size of the powder. To calculate the E_a of crystallization, the DTA is carried out at different heating rates.

To obtain dense glass-ceramic materials with a fine crystalline structure, in the samples produced with powder techniques, sintering must ideally occur and be completed before crystallization starts. In the bulk glasses, bulk crystallization must preferably occurred in the whole bulk of the block, rather than surface crystallization, since the latter mechanism usually results in long elongated crystals which form from the surface of the glass block toward the center of the sample. The correct design of the composition, including the addition of nucleation agents in the raw materials, aims to satisfy the above requirements. Moreover, the heat treatment of the glass must be designed in such a way as to favor the ideal nucleation and crystal growth. Obviously, the ideal glass-ceramics must be dense with small (even at nanoscale) and well-interlocked, one to the other, grains. Since ceramics have usually higher density than the corresponding glasses with the same composition, this difference in densities between the glass and the resulting ceramics must be small; if the difference is big, then defects in the form of holes, voids, etc. are expected to form in the bulk of the glass-ceramic materials.

6.3 Design of Compositions

6.3.1 CaO–MgO–SiO_2 System

Glasses and glass-ceramics in the ternary CaO–MgO–SiO_2 system have attracted considerable technological interest because of their good mechanical and chemical properties. In particular, glass-ceramics of diopside ($CaMgSi_2O_6$), wollastonite ($CaSiO_3$), and melilite (mainly solid solutions of gehlenite [$Ca_2Al_2SiO_7$] and akermanite [$Ca_2MgSi_2O_7$]) have been thoroughly investigated because of their interesting set of properties. Glass-ceramics of this ternary system have been indicated for wear resistance, thermomechanical, biomedical, and ceramic-coating applications, due to their attractive mechanical and chemical properties. Nevertheless, the wide application of this family of materials is limited due to the relatively elevated processing temperatures needed for glass melting and/or devitrification. Furthermore, high energy consumption opposes the current global trends related to environmental and economic issues.

Provided that appropriate nucleating agents are incorporated in suitable amounts, crystallization of diopside- and wollastonite-based glass-ceramics takes place via bulk crystallization mechanism. In the CaO–MgO–SiO_2

system, the first stage of crystallization occurs via separation of phases, rich in divalent metal oxides and having relatively simple crystal structures, primarily diopside-type solid solutions.

The effect of crystallization-stimulating additions can result from several mechanisms. For example, Cr_2O_3 remarkably increases the crystallization rate only for Fe-containing compositions as the corresponding mechanism includes formation of spinels, which, in turn, actively catalyze the formation of pyroxene phases. The catalytic effect of fluorides in pyroxene-based systems is due to the intensification of phase separation in the liquid phase, associated with an enrichment of the segregated zones with the pyroxene component. As a result, diopside-type solid solutions are formed in the fluoride-containing compositions at the first stage of crystallization. The stimulating effect of titania additions in pyroxene systems was found insufficient. In the case of melilite and wollastonite glass-ceramics, it has been found that sulfides of Fe, Mn, and Zn as well as fluorides might promote successful bulk crystallization.

6.3.2 Na_2O–CaO–SiO_2 System

In the Na_2O–CaO–SiO_2 ternary system, a wide bioactive composition region is known. This region overlaps the bioactivity region of the P_2O_5-containing Na_2O–CaO–SiO_2 system, being, however, somewhat curtailed in the SiO_2 poor region, but more extended toward the Na_2O–SiO_2 and the CaO–SiO_2 regions. The kinetics of HA formation seemingly depends on Na_2O/CaO ratio. Little differences in apatite formation rates have been reported between the P_2O_5-containing 45S5 Bioglass and the corresponding P_2O_5-free Na_2O–CaO–SiO_2 glass. The bone-bonding ability that characterizes the CaO–SiO_2 region in the Na_2O–CaO–SiO_2 ternary system features great interest for developing new bioactive compositions. Several amorphous and crystalline phases of $CaSiO_3$ (CS) have been proposed as candidate bioactive materials since they induce fast formation of HA layer while soaked in simulated body fluid (SBF). Among them, α-CS ceramics with CaO/SiO_2 molar ratios 0.76 and 1 have been thoroughly investigated. The dissolution (i.e. Ca2+ leaching) of amorphous CS was faster than crystalline α-CS and β-CS, resulting in faster increase of pH of SBF and hence faster formation of HA.

6.3.3 Modifications: Addition of B_2O_3, P_2O_5, CaF_2, and Na_2O to CaO–MgO–SiO_2 System

In the modern applications of biomaterials, it is widely accepted that there are specific bone restoration and regeneration needs, including scaffolds for bone tissue engineering, which require controllable bioactivity and gradual resorption of implants (i.e. not very intensive or very fast, respectively) to enable concurrent replacement by newly formed bone. It must be also mentioned that degradation products of bioactive glasses can suitably activate gene expression of osteoblasts, stimulate production of growth factors, and favor cell proliferation. The bioactivity and biocompatibility is experimentally assessed through immersion tests in SBF, *in vitro* osteoblasts' cell cultures, and *in vivo* implantations, to evaluate biomaterials' potential for further consideration and experimentation in biomedical applications and clinical testing and applications. Under the modern perspectives of biomaterials science and technology, it is widely accepted that the relationship between the biological behavior of the glass-ceramic materials and the properties (and thus the structure, determined by IR and Raman spectroscopy) of the glasses as well as their devitrification behavior after heat treatment is of a great importance. This is the only way to be able to tune the biological performance of the produced glass-ceramics.

In this regard, certain glass compositions in the CaO–MgO–SiO_2 system can be modified by adding oxides, such as B_2O_3, P_2O_5, CaF_2, and Na_2O which are body-friendly and their presence has been implicated in the expression of bioactivity performance. In simple, *in vitro* experiments carried out with immersion of the produced glasses and glass-ceramics in SBF at 37 °C, these features should involve recording of dissolution phenomena and formation of microcrystallites of HA, which can be accounted for structural modifications taking place at the surface of the glasses and glass-ceramics from the very beginning of immersion in SBF. Formation of both silica gel and HA at the surface of those materials after two to three weeks in SBF should occur. The influence of the structural features of those glasses and glass-ceramics on bioactivity performance is of great importance. An interesting feature is also the effect of the amount of phosphates (P_2O_5) on favoring the deposition of carbonated HA, α or β-type (i.e. the carbonate substitution occurs at hydroxyl or phosphate sites, respectively).

The role of B in bioactivity of glasses is a subject of open debate. Na_2O usually facilitates the melting of the glasses to occur at lower temperatures. Finally, the presence of F in HA improves mechanical properties. The influence of Al_2O_3 in this system was also investigated, because alumina is a well-known inert bioceramic which, when added in bioglasses, provides better mechanical properties but it jeopardizes bioactivity (at high amounts, higher than 3% or 5%). To allow the reader to understand the behavior of these materials to a maximum extent and therefore to assess them for applications, a wide range of features and properties of the produced materials is presented.

The determination of the structural features of the glasses, using experimental results of Raman and infrared (IR) spectroscopy, as well as to shed light in the possible influence of these features on the crystalline phases formed after heat treatment, registered at X-ray diffractograms, is also of a great interest. It is also interesting to analyze the influence of the production route, whether processed via glass powder compacts or crystallization of bulk materials, on these features. Earlier studies have shown that doping with B_2O_3, P_2O_5, and CaF_2 favors densification of glass powder compacts with similar chemical compositions.

According to the studies in the above systems mentioned above, a composition with the formula $Na_2O{\cdot}B_2O_3{\cdot}3MgO{\cdot}7CaO{\cdot}9SiO_2{\cdot}0.60P_2O_5{\cdot}CaF_2$ can adequately represent a bioactive system in the investigated system. The following section is specifically dedicated to describe the precise details for the design of this and other relevant compositions.

The basic composition of the parent glass was set within the narrow ranges of 51–52% SiO_2, 37–39% CaO, and 9–12% MgO (in this paper, all the compositions are referred to wt%, unless it is otherwise stated). This composition is located in the primary field of the pseudowollastonite crystallization in the $CaO–MgO–SiO_2$ ternary system and it is close to the composition of the liquid in the invariant equilibrium of the transition type (51.4% SiO_2, 36.8% CaO, 11.8% MgO).

$$\text{liquid} + \text{pseudowollastonite} \leftrightarrows \text{akermanite } (Ca_2Mg[Si_2O_7]) + \text{wollastonite} \quad (6.1)$$

and of the eutectic type (51.6% SiO_2, 35.6% CaO, 12.8% MgO)

$$\text{liquid} \leftrightarrows \text{wollastonite} + \text{diopside} + \text{akermanite} \quad (6.2)$$

Table 6.1 summarizes the batch compositions of the eight investigated glasses. The first G-Al compositions were designed to comprise 1.94 wt% Al_2O_3. It is well established that alumina inhibits glass dissolution and retards its bioactivity. With regard to bioactivity, the amount of alumina that is tolerated depends on glass compositions but is in the order of 1.0–1.5 wt%. G-Al seemingly exceeds recommended threshold for alumina and therefore its behavior could be compared to the compositions G-1, G1-a, G-1b, G-2, and G-3, where Al_2O_3 was substituted by B_2O_3. The relevant features of the investigated compositions are as follows:

(a) The CaO/SiO_2 molar ratio was maintained between 0.77 and 0.82.
(b) B_2O_3, Na_2O, and CaF_2 were incorporated in equimolecular basis.
(c) The compositions G-1a and G-1b derived from the composition 1, by gradually increasing the amount of P_2O_5 in the order G-1 < G-1a < G-1b.
(d) The amounts of CaO and SiO_2 increased in the order G-1 < G-2 < G-3.

The glasses G-1d and G-1e were designed to be boron free. With respect to the molecular formula of glass G-1b ($Na_2O{\cdot}B_2O_3{\cdot}3MgO{\cdot}7CaO{\cdot}9SiO_2{\cdot}0.60P_2O_5{\cdot}CaF_2$), B_2O_3 – substitution takes place in the glass G-1d according to the scheme

$$2B^{3+} \rightarrow 1.5Si^{4+}$$

and in the second glass, designated as G-1e,

$$2B^{3+} \rightarrow Si^{4+} + 0.2P^{5+} + 0.5Ca^{2+}$$

Accordingly, glass G-1d is slightly richer in Si^{4+} and poorer in Ca^{2+} and P^{5+} than the glass G-1e.

6.4 Materials and Methods

6.4.1 Synthesis

The glasses can be produced via conventional melting. For the glasses listed in Table 6.1, fine powders of technical grade of SiO_2 (purity >99.5%) and $CaCO_3$ (>99.5%), and reagent grade of H_3BO_3, $4MgCO_3{\cdot}Mg(OH)_2{\cdot}5H_2O$, Na_2CO_3, CaF_2, Al_2O_3, and $NH_4H_2PO_4$ were used.

Homogeneous mixtures of batches (~100 g), obtained by ball milling, were preheated at 1000 °C for one hour for decarbonization. Complete melting was done in Pt crucibles at 1400–1550 °C (according to each particular composition) for one hour in air. Both bulk and powder frit-glasses were produced. Blocks of bulk transparent and colorless glasses with no crystalline inclusions (confirmed by X-ray and Scanning electron microscopy [SEM] analyses afterwards) were produced by easy casting of melts on preheated bronze molds and subsequent immediate annealing at 600 °C (i.e. close to the transformation temperature T_g) for one hour. Glass-frits were obtained by quenching whereby the molten glass was rapidly poured into cold water. To obtain fine powders, the frits were dried and then grounded in a high-speed porcelain mill.

Glass-ceramics were produced by controlled heat treatment of the glasses in air. The ramp of the heat treatment was decided according to the results of the thermal analysis of the glasses, as presented in the Section 6.5 for each composition. In the case of the samples with powder compacts (from glass-frit), conventional powder metallurgy techniques were employed; thus, along with crystallization, sintering – which must occur before

Table 6.1 Chemical compositions of experimental glasses.

Glass		SiO_2	Al_2O_3	B_2O_3	CaO	MgO	P_2O_5	Na_2O	CaF_2
G-Al	wt%	41.13	1.94	3.97	29.86	9.20	3.24	4.72	5.94
	mol%	40.36	1.12	3.36	31.40	13.45	1.35	4.48	4.48
G-1	wt%	41.39	—	5.33	30.05	9.25	3.26	4.74	5.98
	mol%	40.36	—	4.48	31.40	13.45	1.35	4.48	4.48
G-1a	wt%	40.73	—	5.24	29.57	9.10	4.81	4.67	5.88
	mol%	40.10	—	4.45	31.18	13.37	2.00	4.45	4.45
G-1b	wt%	40.08	—	5.16	29.10	8.96	6.32	4.59	5.79
	mol%	39.82	—	4.43	30.97	13.27	2.65	4.43	4.43
G-2	wt%	42.23	—	4.89	31.54	8.50	2.99	4.36	5.49
	mol%	41.15	—	4.12	32.92	12.34	1.23	4.12	4.12
G-3	wt%	42.95	—	4.52	32.80	7.86	2.77	4.03	5.07
	mol%	41.82	—	3.80	34.22	11.41	1.15	3.80	3.80
G-1d	wt%	46.06	—	—	28.66	8.83	6.22	4.53	5.70
	mol%	45.45	—	—	30.30	12.99	2.60	4.33	4.33
G-1e	wt%	43.48	—	—	30.44	8.75	7.19	4.49	5.65
	mol%	43.10	—	—	32.33	12.93	3.02	4.31	4.31

crystallization – was also studied. The samples were produced as follows. Fine powder of glass-frit was granulated by mixing in a 5 vol% polyvinyl alcohol solution (PVA) (wt% proportion frit/PVA = 97.5/2.5). Parallelepiped bars ($4 \times 5 \times 50\ mm^3$) were prepared by uniaxial pressing (200 MPa). After debinding at 450 °C for two hours, the bars of glass-powder compacts were sintered at several temperatures (between 650 and 920 °C) for one hour at a slow heating rate (2–3 °C/min) to avoid deformation. In some cases, production of coatings (thickness ~100 μm) was also attempted as follows. Glass-frit, granulated with PVA, was applied on pellets of several polished substrates (i.e. zirconia, Ti, and hydroxyapatite) and crystallized similarly to the glass compacts at 800 °C for one hour.

6.4.2 Characterization Techniques

When powders were involved in the experiments, their mean particle size, calculated by the particle size distribution curves, are obtained by light scattering technique (Coulter LS 230, UK, Fraunhofer optical model). The powders of glass-frits (after milling) had an average particle size of about 11–14 μm and their specific surface area, measured by BET technique (Micromeritics, Gemini II 2370, USA), was between 0.3 and 0.7 m^2/g.

The structural analysis of the produced glasses was done at the surface of bulk glasses by Raman spectroscopy (micro-Raman system; Renishaw 1000, UK) using the 532 nm line of a solid state laser at 60 mW for excitation. Raman scatter was collected by means of a microscope (Leica, UK) equipped with lenses 50× and 100×. Infrared reflectance spectra were measured with a Fourier-transform IR spectrometer (Perkin Elmer Spectrum GX) equipped with a 30° off-normal reflectance attachment and the appropriate source and detector. All spectra were measured at room temperature with 2 cm^{-1} resolution against a high-reflectivity aluminum mirror and represent the average of 64 scans. These spectroscopic techniques have also used to study the *in vitro* mineralization process of hydroxyapatite formation on the glass surfaces after their immersion in SBF.

Thermal analysis comprised measurements with differential thermal analysis (DTA; Labsys Setaram TG-DTA/DSC, France; heating rate 5 °C/min, in air) and dilatometry (Bahr Thermo Analyse DIL 801 L, Germany; heating rate 3 °C/min). Crystallographic analysis was done by X-ray diffraction (XRD; Rigaku Geigerflex D/Mac, C Series, Cu K_α radiation, Japan). Microstructure observations were done by field-emission scanning electron microscopy (FE-SEM Hitachi S-4100, Japan; 25 kV acceleration voltage, beam current 10 μA) under secondary electron mode. Energy-dispersive spectroscopy (EDS) was employed for chemical analysis. The Archimedes method was used to measure the apparent density of the glass and glass-ceramic blocks (immersion in ethyleneglycol). Vickers microhardness was estimated from 10 indentations for each sample (Shimadzu microhardness tester type M, Japan; load of 9.8 N). Weibull statistics were employed to evaluate the mechanical reliability of materials (i.e. three-point flexural strength of parallelepiped bars, $3 \times 4 \times 40\,mm^3$; Shimadzu Autograph AG 25 TA, 0.5 mm/min displacement). Water absorption was measured according to the ISO standard 10545-3, 1995 (i.e. weight gain of dried bulk samples after immersion into boiling water for two hours, cooling for three hours, and sweeping of their surface with a wet towel). The linear shrinkage during sintering was also calculated from the dimensions of the green and the resulting sintered samples.

The experimental procedure to evaluate the *in vitro* bioactivity (by immersion experiments in SBF), the *in vitro* biocompatibility with cell culture studies, and the clinical trials are described in the Chapters 6, 7, and 8, respectively.

6.5 Structural Features of Glasses, Devitrification, and Materials' Properties

Glass-ceramics are produced via controlled crystallization of the parent glass, where the crystalline phases are precipitated from the reservoir of the glass. The extent of crystallization depends on heat treatment, i.e. the temperature, the heating rate, the stages of heating, and the dwell at each temperature. Thus, before presenting the properties of glass-ceramics, we focus in the results of the thermal analysis of the parent glasses, since this is a decisive information for setting the parameters of heat treatment of the glasses. Moreover, the crystallized phases are direct results of the structure of the parent glass. Thus, in this chapter we emphasize in the results related to the glass-structural features and in their relationship to the crystalline phases developed in the glass-ceramics. In the Section 6.5.1 we present the features of the B- and Al-containing glasses and glass-ceramics, in the Section 6.5.2 the B-containing and Al-free glasses and glass-ceramics, and in the Section 6.5.3 the B-free (and Al-free) glasses and glass-ceramics.

6.5.1 B- and Al-Containing Glasses and Glass-Ceramics

The thermal analysis of the glass G-A1 (Figure 6.1) provides the necessary information for setting up the optimum crystallization schedule. In particular, the dilatometry measurements show that the transition temperature (T_g) was at ~625 °C and the softening point at ~670 °C. T_g was detected by DTA at a slightly higher temperature (~640 °C). The DTA showed a single exothermic peak for crystallization with maximum at 797 °C. The decomposition of PVA was also detected at ~400 °C (endothermic peak). Accordingly, after debinding (450 °C, two hours), sintering of bars of glass-powder compacts was carried out starting at 650 °C, i.e. slightly lower than the dilatometric softening point. Then, sintering of these samples was conducted at different temperatures, specifically 700, 750, 800, 825, 850, 900, and 920 °C.

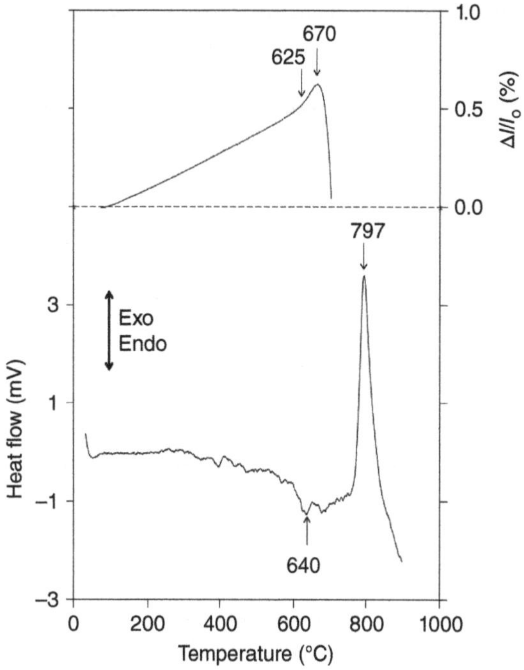

Figure 6.1 Thermal analysis (dilatometry top curves and DTA bottom curves) of G-A1 glass.

The influence of sintering temperature on density and linear shrinkage of the resulting glass-ceramics is presented in Table 6.2. Densification safely occurred until 800 °C, reaching a maximum of density ($2.89\,g/cm^3$) and shrinkage (13.8%) at 750 °C. Linear shrinkage values were remarkably constant over the investigated temperature range. At 650 °C, powdered frit achieved higher density than that of bulk glasses, whose density was measured as $2.80\,g/cm^3$. The dramatic decrease of density occurs for the glass-ceramics sintered at temperatures ≥800 °C. It is worthy to note that this composition features a broad sintering span of about 150°, since remarkable consistency in the values of the properties were recorded for the materials sintered between 650 and 800 °C.

Figure 6.2 shows that at 650 °C the material is amorphous. Crystallization occurs at ≥700 °C, resulting in formation of a single phase, akermanite. A single phase formation was correctly anticipated from the single exothermic peak of DTA (Figure 6.1). It should be mentioned that in this type of systems, heating rate often affects the temperature of crystallization onset (i.e. lower heating rate favors evolution of crystalline phases at lower temperatures).

The glass-ceramics sintered at 800 °C (one hour) have homogeneous white color throughout the entire

Table 6.2 Density and linear shrinkage of compacts made of the glass powders G-A1 sintered at different temperatures.

	Sintering temperature (°C)							
Property	**650**	**700**	**750**	**800**	**825**	**850**	**900**	**920**
Density (g/cm^3)	2.83	2.88	2.89	2.86	2.78	2.67	2.50	2.09
Linear shrinkage (%)	13.6	13.6	13.8	13.6			13.5	13.3

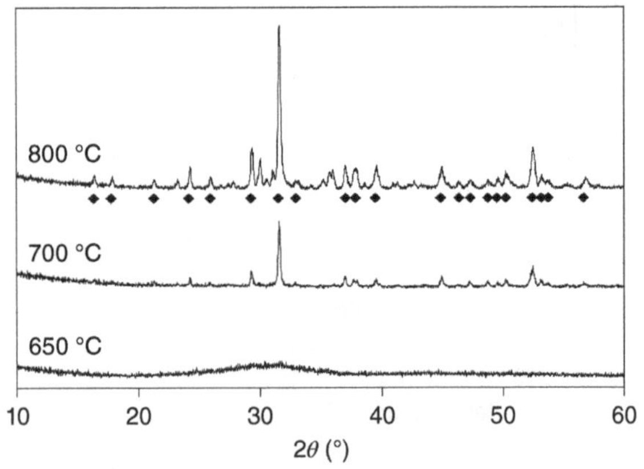

Figure 6.2 Akermanite predominantly forms at ≥700 °C (JCPDS card of akermanite-synthetic no. 87-0052).

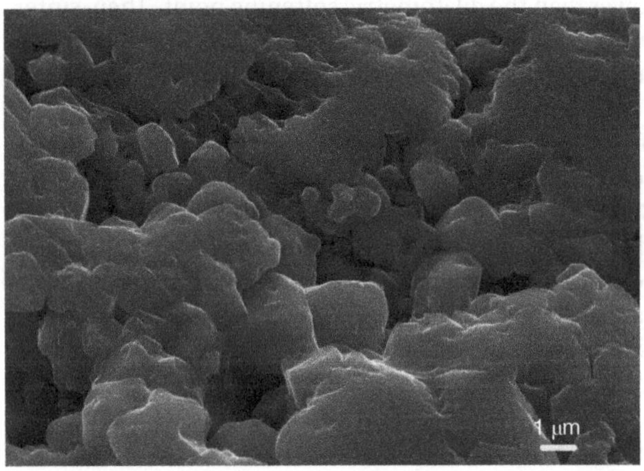

Figure 6.3 Characteristic microstructure of G-A1 glass-ceramics after heat treatment at 800 °C for one hour observed at fracture surfaces of bulk samples.

bulk and the surface. Their microstructure is shown in Figure 6.3. It is observed that a dense and highly crystallized structure which comprises a network of interlocking elongated and prismatic crystals of akermanite embedded in a glassy phase. There is no evidence of porosity. This dense microstructure is attributed to glassy phase which likely forms due to the doping oxides (e.g. P_2O_5, etc.) in the main ternary system. Consequently, in the investigated composition, sintering starts at temperatures close to the glass transition point. A liquid phase forms and wets the surface of the grains. Heating at temperatures close to the softening point causes lowering of viscosity of the liquid and densification advances via viscous coalescence. This is an important feature of the investigated system because in several glass-ceramic systems, crystallization process has an inhibition effect on densification occurring via viscous flow.

With regards to the mechanical properties, Vickers microhardness is 4.43 (±0.66) GPa and the average flexural strength is ~110 MPa (for the samples sintered at 800 °C, complete Weibull statistical analysis is shown in Figure 6.4), which matches well to enamel. Water absorption is 0.16%. Furthermore, the linear CTE is 9.9×10^{-6} K^{-1} (70–500 °C), which matches well to the CTE of other materials used in biomedicine, such as t-ZrO_2 (TZP) and Ti. Typical microstructures of interfaces developed between G-A1 glass-ceramic and the three substrates TZP, Ti, and HA after one hour heating at 800 °C are shown in Figure 6.5. A continuous interface, free of cracks or gaps was observed in the case of TZP. A reaction zone of TiO_2 (with an ambiguous fragile nature) forms in the case of Ti substrate. An ideal joining was obtained between HA and G-A1, where the two phases diffused one to another and no interface can be observed.

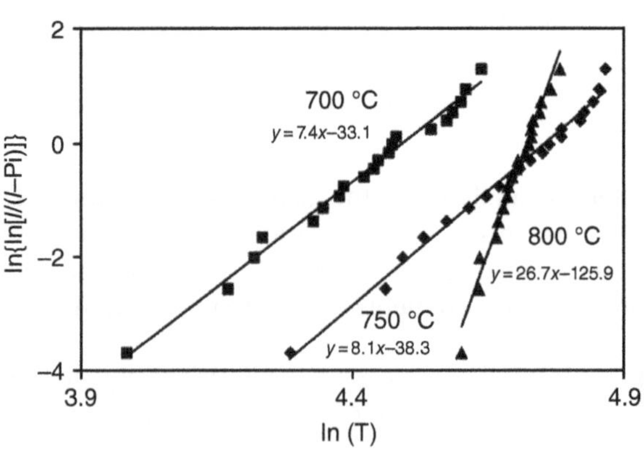

Figure 6.4 Weibull statistics of flexural strength (three-point bending) of glass-ceramics obtained from G-A1 glass at different temperatures (T, bending strength; P, fracture probability).

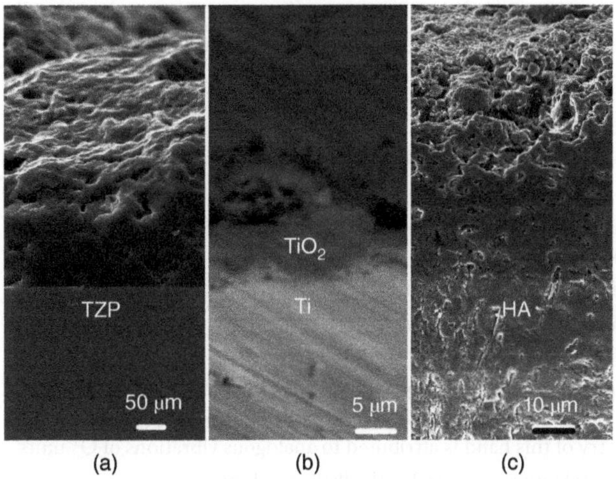

Figure 6.5 Microstructure of interfaces developed between G-A1 glass-ceramic (upper part of the images) and (a) zirconia (TZP), (b) Ti, and (c) hydroxyapatite (HA) after crystallization at 800 °C, one hour.

6.5.2 B-Containing Glasses and Glass-Ceramics (Al-Free)

6.5.2.1 Glasses

The five compositions G-1, G-1a, G-1b, G-2, and G-3 were completely melted at 1400 °C after one hour and the melts were easily cast, resulting in transparent and colorless glasses with no visible crystalline inclusions, as was also confirmed by X-ray and SEM analyses afterwards.

Their microstructure (after annealing at 600 °C) was similar and showed clear evidences of liquid–liquid phase separation (Figure 6.6), where droplets of segregated liquid phase, seemingly sorted in two groups of bigger (oval shaped) and smaller droplets (like tiny spots), are seeing to be homogeneously distributed in the glass matrix.

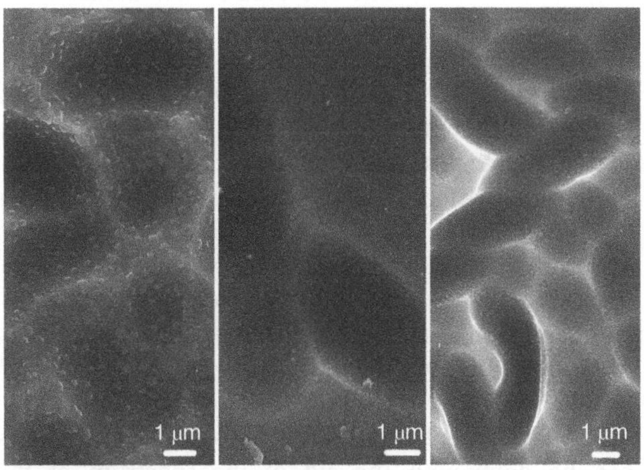

Figure 6.6 Phase separation occurred in the investigated annealed bulk glasses (observed by SEM after etching of polished surfaces with 2% HF solution).

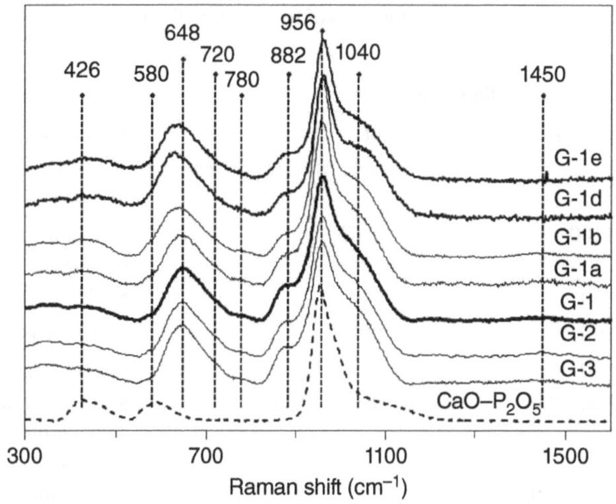

Figure 6.7 Raman spectra of the investigated glasses, obtained from the surface of bulk samples, together with the spectrum of the binary $0.72CaO·0.28P_2O_5$ glass. (The plots have been arbitrarily shifted vertically for clarity.)

The Raman spectra of all the Al-free glasses are shown in Figure 6.7. For comparison purposes, the spectrum of the binary $0.72CaO·0.28P_2O_5$ glass is also plotted. The spectra of the five glasses (G-1, G-1a, G-1b, G-2, and G-3) exhibited similar spectral features. There was a dominant band at about 956 cm^{-1}, a shoulder at its high frequency side at c. 1040 cm^{-1}, bands at 648 cm^{-1} and 882 cm^{-1}, a broad band envelope double peaking at 340 and 420 cm^{-1}, and a number of bands of weak intensities at 580, 780, and 1450 cm^{-1}. Along the order of the glasses whose P_2O_5 content increases (i.e. G-1, G-1a, G-1b), the intensity of the peak at 956 cm^{-1} increased but the intensity of the 882 cm^{-1} band decreased, the peak of the 648 cm^{-1} band envelope downshifted in frequency, whereas the shoulder at 1040 cm^{-1} upshifted, and the two peaks at 420 and 580 cm^{-1} became progressively more evident.

Table 6.3 summarizes the assignment of peaks and bands of Raman spectra. According to previous Raman studies on alkali and alkaline earth silicate glasses, bands in the 800–1300 cm^{-1} region have been assigned to the asymmetric vibration of SiO_4 tetrahedra, where the precise peak wavenumber depends on the number of nonbridging oxygens (NBOs) constituting the tetrahedron. In particular, the bands near 1100 cm^{-1} have been attributed to the stretching of a single NBO on a SiO_4 tetrahedron ($SiØ_3O^-$: Q^3), resulting from the presence of network-modifying cations. Similar bands near 950 cm^{-1} have been assigned to $Si–O^-$ stretching in silicate tetrahedral units with two NBOs ($SiØ_2O_2^{2-}$: Q^2), while the similar band near 900 cm^{-1} has been assigned to the

Table 6.3 General assignments of Raman and IR bands.

Band (cm^{-1})		
Raman	**IR**	**Assignment**
		Silicates
1100	1075	Stretching of a single NBO on a SiO_4 tetrahedron ($SiØ_3O^-$: Q^3) resulting from the presence of network-modifying cations
950	950	Si–O^- stretching in silicate tetrahedral units with two NBOs ($SiØ_2O_2^{2-}$: Q^2)
900	900	Si–O^- stretching in silicate tetrahedral units with three NBOs ($SiØO_3^{3-}$: Q^1)
850		Stretching vibrations of monomer SiO_4^{4-} unit (Q^0)
550–750	400–550, 780	Si–O–Si bending motions in Q^2 units (Raman at 650 cm^{-1}, IR at 780 cm^{-1}); in IR, rocking motion of Si–O–Si bridges is at 400–550 cm^{-1}. In Raman, the high frequency asymmetry of this band is attributed to analogous vibrations of Q^1 units
1020–1050		Vibrations in structural units associated with alkali metal cations
		or
		Si–O^0 from bridging oxygen in structural units that contain NBOs (Q^3, Q^2, and Q^1)
		Phosphates
950–980	1400–400	Vibrations of the Q^2, Q^1, and Q^0 phosphate units: P–O^- bonds and O—P—O bridges in PO_4^{3-} units
590		Symmetric stretching of the P—O^- bonds
425		O–P–O bending of orthophosphate PO_4^{3-} unit (Q^0)
		Borates
	1200–1450	B–O stretching of BO_3 units
	850–1200	B–Ø stretching of $BØ_4$ units
	~700	B–Ø–B linkages of the borate network
	1430, 1245	Vibrations of metaborate triangles
1300–1500	1050, ~1400	Stretching of B–O^- dangling bonds in trigonal $BØ_2O^-$ units
780	1010–1050	Vibrations of $BØ_4^-$ units

analogous vibrations in silicate tetrahedral units with three NBOs ($SiØO_3^{3-}$: Q^1). Bands near 850 cm^{-1} have been assigned to the stretching vibrations of monomer SiO_4^{4-} unit (Q^0). The existence of these units in the glass network is witnessed by the bands between 550 and 750 cm^{-1}, registered in the spectra. The bands between 1020 and 1050 cm^{-1} have been assigned to Si–O^0 from bridging oxygen in structural units that contain NBOs (Q^3, Q^2, and Q^1). A second interpretation has assigned them to vibrations in structural units associated with alkali metal cations.

Accordingly, the structure of the investigated glasses should have the following features. The bands at 956 and 882 cm^{-1} can be assigned to Si—O^- stretching in silicate units with two and three NBOs (Q^2 and Q^1), respectively. The observable abrupt profile of the 882 cm^{-1} band is probably due to Raman scattering contributions from vibrations of SiO_4^{4-} units (Q^0). The shoulder at 1030 cm^{-1} suggests the coexistence of Q^2, Q^1, and Q^3 units in the silicate network, probably with a small concentration of Q^3 units, since the Q^3 Si–O^- stretching vibrations, that occur at about 1100 cm^{-1}, appear to have very weak intensity. The observed Raman bands in the low frequency region of 550–750 cm^{-1} further support these assignments. In particular, earlier studies have attributed the band at ~650 cm^{-1} to Si–O–Si bending motions in Q^2 units and the high frequency asymmetry of this band to analogous vibrations of Q^1 units.

The very weak bands at 780 and 1450 cm^{-1} can be attributed to vibrations in borate units. According to earlier studies on alkali and alkaline earth borate glasses, the bands in the 1300–1500 cm^{-1} region should originate from the stretching of the B–O^- dangling bonds in trigonal ($BØ_2O^-$) units, while the bands at 780 cm^{-1} should be correlated with vibrations of $BØ_4^-$ units.

The assignment of bands associated to phosphates can be done with the aid of the spectrum of the $0.72CaO{\cdot}0.28P_2O_5$ glass, which exhibits one strong band at 952 cm^{-1} and two broad bands at 590 and 425 cm^{-1}. The latter two bands have been assigned to the symmetric stretching of the P—O$^-$ bonds and the O—P—O bending modes of the orthophosphate PO_4^{3-} unit (Q^0), respectively. Accordingly, the bands at 580 and 420 cm^{-1} in the spectra of the investigated glasses can be assigned to analogous vibrations of PO_4^{3-} units. The P—O$^-$ stretching vibrations should also contribute at increasing intensity of the 956 cm^{-1} band of the vibrations of Q^2 silicate units. The observed high degree of modification of the phosphate units can be interpreted on the basis of an acid–base concept. The optical basicity of the glass former oxides increases in the order of $P_2O_5 < B_2O_3 < SiO_2$. Increasing basicity of modifier oxides (Na_2O, MgO, CaO) causes an increase of the tendency for reaction with strong acid, such as P_2O_5. Hence, in the investigated glasses, CaO should react first with P_2O_5, resulting in isolated PO_4^{3-} units. This assumption agrees fairly well with the changes observed in the spectra over increasing P_2O_5 content. Hence, the changes of the bands at 956, 420, and 580 cm^{-1} can be assigned to the vibrations of PO_4^{3-} units. Evidently, in the presence of alkali and alkali earth cations, the phosphate tetrahedra were totally modified to highly charged PO_4^{3-} units. The decrease of the 882 cm^{-1} band intensity can be attributed to a smaller number of Q^1 units in the silicate network. The frequency downshift of the 648 cm^{-1} band envelope and the upshift of the 1040 cm^{-1} shoulder are attributed to increasing number of Q^n units containing less NBOs. This trend is rather expected because increasing amount of P_2O_5 in the glass network causes a decrease of the total number of the available modifier cations for silicate and borate units.

The infrared (IR) absorption spectra of the Al-free glasses are shown in Figure 6.8, together with the spectrum of tricalcium phosphate (TCP), for comparison

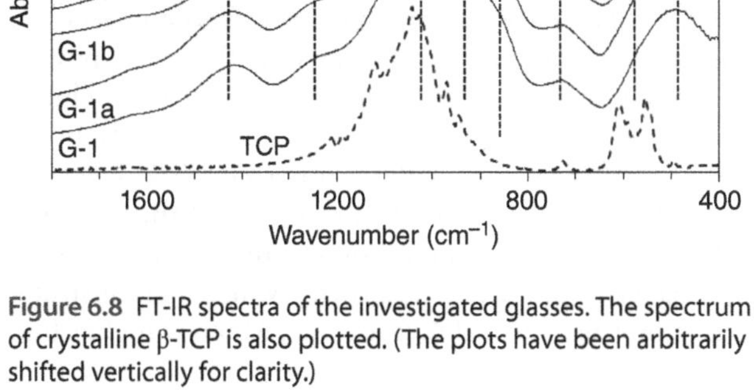

Figure 6.8 FT-IR spectra of the investigated glasses. The spectrum of crystalline β-TCP is also plotted. (The plots have been arbitrarily shifted vertically for clarity.)

purposes. There is a broad absorption band with two peak maxima at 1024 and 932 cm^{-1}, and two shoulders at the low (900 cm^{-1}) and another one at the high frequency side (1250 cm^{-1}). The spectra also show two broad bands at lower frequencies, one at 485 cm^{-1} and another one weak at 732 cm^{-1}.

Table 6.3 summarizes the assignment of peaks and bands of IR spectra. In earlier studies on silicate glasses, absorption peaks at 1075 cm^{-1} have been attributed to asymmetric stretch vibrations of Si—O$^-$ bonds in Q^3 tetrahedral units, and bands near 950 and 900 cm^{-1} have been assigned to analogous vibrations of Q^2 and Q^1 units, respectively. Generally, the absorption band envelope in the 800–1200 cm^{-1} frequency region is well defined at lower frequencies on the depolymerization of silicate network. Accordingly, the observed shoulder at 860 cm^{-1} can be attributed to the vibrations of Q^0 units while the absorption peak at around 932 cm^{-1} can be attributed to the vibrations of Q^1 and Q^2 units. Absorption bands between 400 and 550 cm^{-1} have been attributed to rocking motion of Si—O—Si bridges and at about 780 cm^{-1} to bending vibrations of the same units. These bands shift to lower frequencies as the concentration of the modifier oxide in the glass increases. Therefore, the absorption peaks at 485 and 732 cm^{-1} can be attributed to the vibrations of various Q^n silicate units containing NBOs, suggesting of a high modification degree of the silicate network. Consequently, the IR spectra indicate the presence of Q^0 (880 cm^{-1}) and the coexistence of various Q^2 (ii) and Q^3 (i) species (1024 cm^{-1}).

The presence of B_2O_3 in the structure of the B-containing glasses (G-1, G-1a, G-1b, G-2, and G-3) is evident in the infrared spectra. In general, there are three distinguished absorption regions in the infrared spectra of borate glasses: 1200–1450 cm^{-1} (B—O stretching of BO_3 units), 850–1200 cm^{-1} (B–Ø stretching of $BØ_4$ units), and a region around 700 cm^{-1}, attributed to the bending of B–Ø–B linkages of the borate network. The IR spectra exhibited peaks at 1430 and 1245 cm^{-1}, which denote the existence of triangular borate units. According to earlier studies on alkali and alkaline earth borate glasses, peaks at these frequencies are assigned to the vibrations of metaborate triangles. In addition, the band at ~730 cm^{-1} is in the region of deformation modes of the above units. Simultaneous observation of Raman and IR spectra suggests $BØ_2O^-$ units. Nevertheless, the existence of pyroborate $BØO_2^-$ and $BØ_4^-$ units cannot be securely concluded from the IR spectra. The reason is that vibrations due to $BØO_2^-$ and $BØ_4^-$ units can be observed between 850 and 1200 cm^{-1} ($BØ_4^-$: 1010–1050 cm^{-1}, $BØO_2^-$: 1050 and ~1400 cm^{-1}), where the Si–O and P–O vibrations are also IR active. For instance, the phosphate glasses exhibit absorption bands in the frequency range between 1400 and $400\,cm^{-1}$, which, according to previous studies, can be attributed to vibrations of Q^2, Q^1, and Q^0 phosphate units.

More specifically, the vibrations of phosphate tetrahedral with four NBOs (PO_4^{3-}) also occur at about $1030\,cm^{-1}$ (asymmetric stretching vibrations) and $570\,cm^{-1}$ (bending vibrations), as the comparison with the IR spectrum of crystalline β-TCP reveals. It is well known that β-TCP crystallizes in the rhombohedral space group $R3c$ and its unit cell contains 21 $[Ca_3(PO_4)_2]$ formula units, or more specifically, three types of crystallographically nonequivalent PO_4^{3-} groups located at general points of the crystal. Hence, its infrared spectrum could be used as indicative for the possible absorption peaks of the internal modes of the PO_4^{3-} tetrahedra in glasses. Accordingly, the absorption between 1200 and $750\,cm^{-1}$ in the IR spectra of glasses might be attributed to the superimposition of the P–O asymmetric stretch modes of PO_4^{3-} units, the Si–O vibrations of various Q^n silica species, and the vibrations of $BØ_4^-$ units.

The dilatation curves (Figure 6.9) shows that the transition point (T_g) of the glasses G-1, G-2, and G-3 ranged between 585 and 590 °C and their softening point (T_s) between 625 and 640 °C. From the slope of the linear part of these plots between 100 and 500 °C, the CTE of the glasses G-1, G-2, and G-3 were calculated as $10.3\times10^{-6}\,K^{-1}$, $10.7\times10^{-6}\,K^{-1}$, and $9.18\times10^{-6}\,K^{-1}$, respectively. A single strong exothermic peak, attributed to crystallization, was registered in the DTA of these three glasses, which was slightly shifted toward higher temperatures from the glass G-1 to the glass G-3 (Figure 6.9). Finally, the density of the annealed (at 600 °C) glasses was $2.87\,g/cm^3$ for all the investigated five glasses.

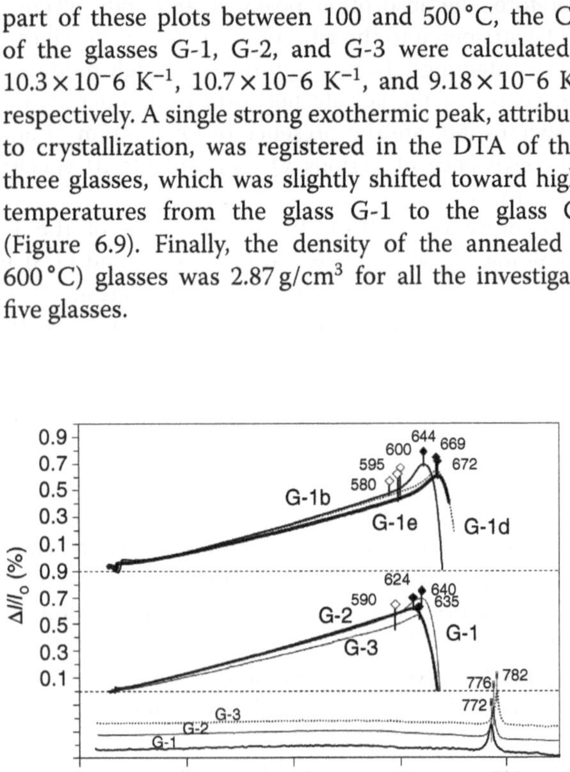

Figure 6.9 Thermal analysis of Al-free glasses G-1, G-2, G-3, and G-1b, and the Al- and B-free G-1d and G-1e glasses: dilatation curves of bulk annealed and DTA curves of glass powders.

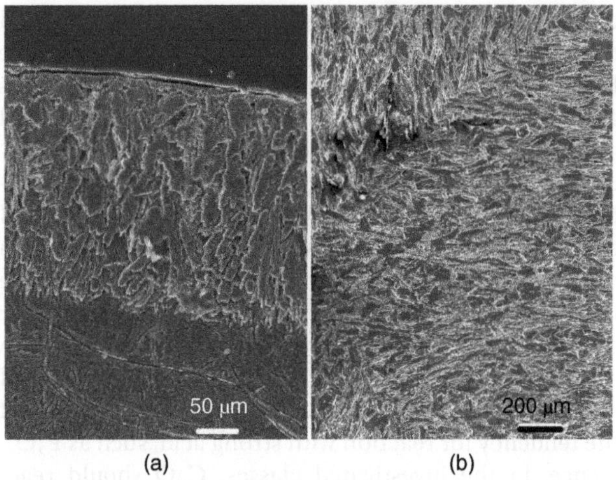

Figure 6.10 Evolution of the microstructure of the annealed bulk glass G-1 after one hour heat treatment at 800 °C (a; the outer surface of the sample is at the top of the image) and 900 °C (b), observed by SEM at secondary electron mode after etching of polished surfaces with 2% HF solution. Similar microstructures were observed in all the investigated glasses.

6.5.2.2 Crystallization of Bulk Glasses

After heat treatment at 700 °C, the effect of phase separation was still obvious in the bulk glasses (similar to Figure 6.6) but more pronounced since the bigger droplets were obviously dispersed in the glass matrix; however, there was still no evidence of crystallization. The microstructure of the bulk glasses heat treated at 800 °C (Figure 6.10a) unequivocally suggests that the glasses are prone to surface crystallization. Crystal growth advanced toward the core of the bulk glass and after heat treatment at 900 °C the crystallization process was completed (Figure 6.10b). Element analysis (by EDS) assigned the acicular shaped crystals to wollastonite and the dendritic ones to pyroxene. There were no striking differences among the microstructures of the five investigated bulk glasses (G-1, G-1a, G-1b, G-2, and G-3). Both surface crystallization and the big crystals formed suggested that glass-ceramics from these compositions must be prepared via powder metallurgy processing of glass-powder compacts, which is presented in the following section.

6.5.2.3 Glass-Ceramics from Glass-Powders Compacts

The crystallization temperatures of the glass-powder compacts (i.e. 700, 750, 800, 850 °C) were chosen considering the temperatures of glass transition (i.e. 585–590 °C, Figure 6.9), the exothermic peak of crystallization (i.e. 772–782 °C, Figure 6.9), and the results of dilatometry measurements of as-pressed glass-powder compacts (plots are not shown), which demonstrated that sintering starts at 620–625 °C, which is higher than T_g.

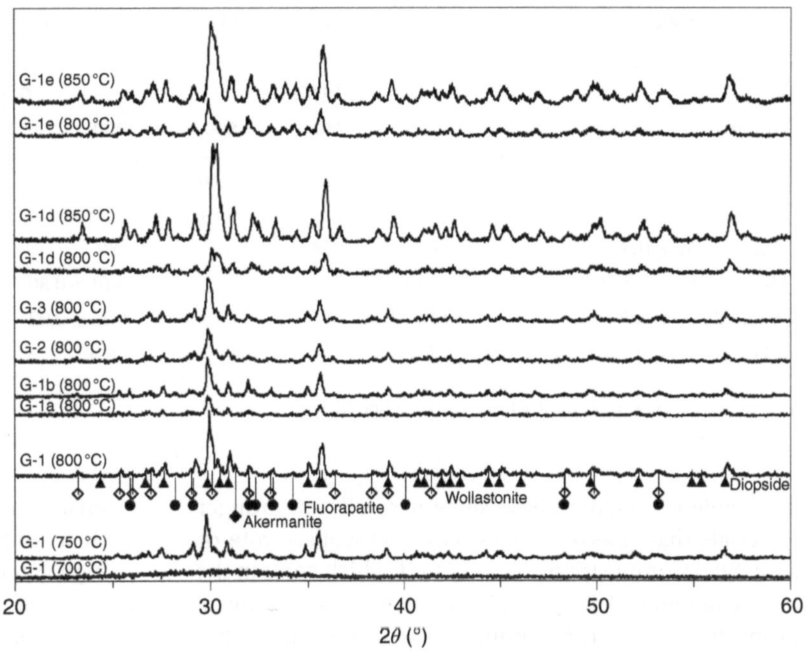

Figure 6.11 X-ray diffractograms of the glass-powder compacts from the Al-free compositions heat treated for one hour in air. (Diopside, $CaMgSi_2O_6$, ICDD card: 01-071-1067; Fluorapatite, $Ca_5(PO_4)_3F$, ICDD card: 01-071-0880; Wollastonite, $CaSiO_3$, ICDD card: 00-042-0550; Akermanite, $Ca_2MgSi_2O_7$, ICDD card: 35-0592; the diffractograms have not been normalized; full-scale of intensity axis: 7.500 cps).

Completely dense samples of dark gray color but of amorphous nature were obtained at 700 °C, indicating that sintering should precede crystallization. Devitrification starts at higher temperatures (750 °C). White color and high degree of densification characterized the samples G-1, G-1a, G-1b, G-2, and G-3 heat treated at 750 and 800 °C. These results agree with the X-ray diffractograms of these compositions shown in Figure 6.11, where the influence of the temperature of heat treatment on the crystallinity of the composition G-1, as well as the crystalline phases formed in the Al-free glasses at 800 °C is presented. Heat treatment of the powder compacts of G-1, G-1a, G-1b, G-2, and G-3 at 850 °C caused development of visible bubbles underneath the surface of the samples and a general decay of the properties of the produced glass-ceramics. Thus, the optimum temperature span for the heat treatment of these compositions was between 750 and 800 °C.

Diopside, wollastonite, together with akermanite and fluorapatite as minor phases, were identified in the X-ray diffractograms after heat treatment at 750 and 800 °C (Figure 6.11). The microstructure of the glass-ceramics with compositions G-1, G-2, and G-3 heat treated at 800 °C is shown in Figure 6.12. Well-defined big prismatic crystals and smaller acicular ones were embedded in glassy matrix. The prismatic crystals were highly packed and significantly bigger in the glass-ceramics G-2 and G-3 than in G-1. Elemental EDS analyses assigned the big crystals to diopside and the small ones to wollastonite (marked with d and w in Figure 6.12, respectively). However, with respect to stoichiometric diopside and wollastonite, the crystals assigned to diopside featured

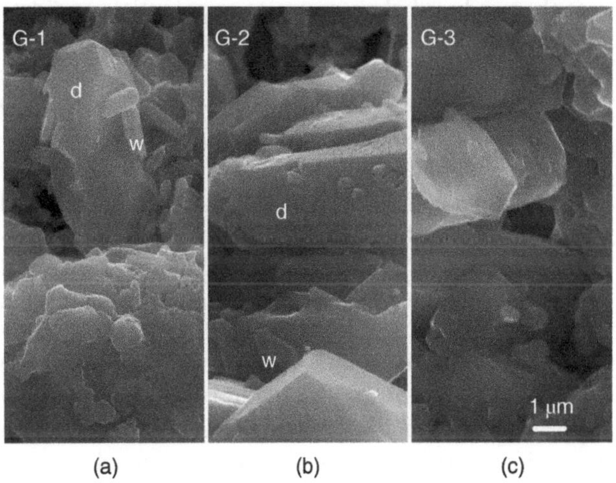

Figure 6.12 Typical microstructures of glass-powder compacts made of the compositions (a) G-1, (b) G-2, and (c) G-3 heat treated at 800 °C for one hour, observed by SEM at secondary electron mode after etching of polished surfaces with 2% HF solution (d, diopside; w, wollastonite).

a slight excess in Ca, while the crystals assigned to wollastonite featured a slight deficiency of Si. The above deviations from stoichiometry might suggest formation of solid solutions.

The properties of the powder compacts of the composition G-1, G-2, and G3 heat treated at different temperatures are listed in Table 6.4. The values of three-point bending strength are relatively higher than the values reported for powder-compacts made of glasses of other similar compositions, which are usually lower than 100 MPa. It has been proposed that diopside is a

Table 6.4 Properties of glass-powder compacts of G-1, G-2, and G-3 heat treated at different temperatures for one hour.

	G-1 (°C)			G-2 (°C)			G-3 (°C)		
Property	**700**	**750**	**800**	**700**	**750**	**800**	**700**	**750**	**800**
Shrinkage (%)	14.1	14.5	13.6	13.9	13.5	13.4	13.8	13.6	13.6
Density (g/cm^3)	2.87	2.85	2.84	2.82	2.93	2.90	2.81	2.88	2.86
Bending strength (MPa)	90	108	116	80	134	141	78	138	139
Microhardness[a)] (GPa)	4.53 ± 0.35			4.61 ± 0.30			4.65 ± 0.40		
Water absorption[a)] (%)	0.16 ± 0.02			0.15 ± 0.02			0.17 ± 0.02		
CTE[a)] 100–500 °C (10^{-6} K^{-1})	9.4			10.8			10.3		

a) They correspond to samples heat treated at 800 °C.

preferable crystalline phase since it results in stronger materials than glass-ceramics based on wollastonite or anorthite. Compositions G-2 and G-3, which contain the lowest amount of fluxes, exhibit the better mechanical properties than G-1. According to the analysis in Section 6.5.1, the values of Vickers microhardness and CTE indicate the produced glass-ceramics as potential candidate materials for biomedical applications.

An important feature to produce dense glass-ceramics is the difference between the density of the glass and the corresponding crystallized phase. In the investigated systems, there is relatively big difference between the density of glass with a composition of diopside (2.75 g/cm^3) and the crystallized diopside (3.27 g/cm^3), but a negligible difference in the case of wollastonite (2.87 and 2.92 g/cm^3 for the glass and the crystals, respectively). The experimental results showed that the processing of glass-ceramics using glass-powder compacts and the addition of B_2O_3, P_2O_5, Na_2O, and CaF_2 considerably suppressed the effect of this deleterious phenomenon and uniform crystallization seemingly occurred over the entire bulk of the glass-powder compacts.

At this point, two important issues should be addressed:

(a) *The role of B_2O_3, Na_2O, P_2O_5, and CaF_2 on sintering*: The experimental results demonstrated that in these compositions, the production of good-quality glass-ceramics has to be done via glass-powder compacts, since the added B_2O_3, Na_2O, P_2O_5, and CaF_2 in the quantities used act as efficient fluxes, resulting in dense products but do not favor bulk crystallization. Densification of glass-powder compacts starts at 620–625 °C, it advances at higher temperatures, likely by viscous flow sintering, and it is almost completed at 700 °C. Evidently, these additions considerably influence the diffusion process of the components, increase the stability of the glass against crystallization at the temperature of sintering onset, lower the melting point of glasses, enhance their sintering ability, shift crystallization toward higher temperatures, and broaden the temperature range of densification. Indeed, the produced materials were melted and crystallized at temperatures lower than those applied in other similar materials, reported in literature. Moreover, beyond the effect of viscosity, the choice of the composition of the basic glass in the CaO–MgO–SiO_2 system and the overall effect of B_2O_3, P_2O_5, Na_2O, and CaF_2, as they were used in the present study, probably result in a multicomponent system whose excess of free energy, related to chemical gradient, favors diffusion and enhances sintering.

(b) *Correlation between glass structure and crystalline phases:* Thermodynamic calculations of the isothermal section of the sub-solidus CaO–MgO–SiO_2 phase diagram at 800 °C, using the database of Huang et al. (and by neglecting B_2O_3, P_2O_5, Na_2O, and CaF_2), shows that the assemblage of the thermodynamically stable phases comprises wollastonite, diopside, and akermanite. The agreement between thermodynamic calculations and the XRD analyses suggests that there is no influence of these fluxes on the products of crystallization of the investigated parent glasses within the range of the amounts used.

Liquid–liquid phase separation, extensively observed in the microstructure of the glasses, stimulates the devitrification process during heat treatment at 750–800 °C, resulting in predominant crystallization of diopside, wollastonite, together with akermanite and fluorapatite, as minor phases. The structural units of glass network define these crystallized phases formed. According to the results of Raman and IR spectroscopy, the most important features of the structure of the as-cast annealed glasses are summarized as follows. There is evidence of coexistence of, Q^1, Q^2, and the Q^0 units in the silicate network. The presence of orthophosphate PO_4^{3-} units resulted in characteristic bands of symmetric stretching of the P—O$^-$ bonds and O—P—O bending modes in the Raman and IR spectra of the glasses. Simultaneous observation of Raman and IR spectra indicated the existence of $BØ_2O^-$ and Q^0 silicate units. Accordingly, it is suggested that $[Si_2O_7]^{6-}$ dimmers (i.e. Q^1 units) resulted in sorosilicates, such as akermanite, while single chains with general formula of $[SiO_3]^{2-}$ (i.e. Q^2 units) constituted the main structural units of pyroxene (diopside) and pyroxenoids (wollastonite). Orthophosphate PO_4^{3-} units of the glass structure should result in fluorapatite precipitation, particularly in the compositions with relatively high P_2O_5 content. Boron and sodium should predominantly accumulate in the glassy phase of the produced glass-ceramics.

6.5.3 B-Free (and Al-Free) Glasses and Glass-Ceramics

The two investigated B- and Al-free glasses G-1d and G-1e were completely melted after one hour at 1400 °C and easily cast, resulting in transparent and colorless blocks with no crystalline inclusions, as confirmed by X-ray and SEM analyses.

The Raman spectra of them are shown in the upper part of Figure 6.7. It is clearly seen that they are quite similar. A novel mathematic way was developed to precisely determine the structural differences among them by subtracting their Raman spectra. According to this method, the difference between the two spectra was calculated by minimizing the function $|RDS(\nu)|^2$, summed for all ν (ν = frequency) within the region where comparison has physical reason to be made. To subtract the Raman spectrum of glass G-1d by the spectrum of glass G-1e, this function is $RDS_{de}(\nu) = D(\nu) - [C_1E(\nu) + C_2 + C_3\nu]$, where $D(\nu)$ is the frequency function of the glass G-1d and $E(\nu)$ that of glass G-1e. The parameters C_1, C_2, C_3 have the physical meaning of scaling and creating a baseline for each spectrum. The resultant spectrum "(G-1d)-(G-1e)" is plotted in Figure 6.13.

According to Table 6.3, the Raman and IR spectra of Figures 6.7 and 6.8 suggest that the glasses G-1d and G-1e are typical silicate glasses, built up with silica tetrahedra and similar phosphates units. Hence, the broad positive band of Figure 6.13 around 1050 cm^{-1} indicates an increasing concentration of Si—O^0 bonds from bridging oxygens in Q^3, Q^2, and Q^1 structural units, which contain NBOs in glass G-1d than in G-1e. The weak negative band between 790 and 980 cm^{-1} indicates a decrease in the formation of silicate units with bigger number of NBOs than Q^3, such as Q^2, Q^1, and Q^0. The difference in the distribution of silicate tetrahedral units in the network of these two glasses can be attributed to the slightly lower concentration of SiO_2 and higher concentration of Ca^{2+} ions

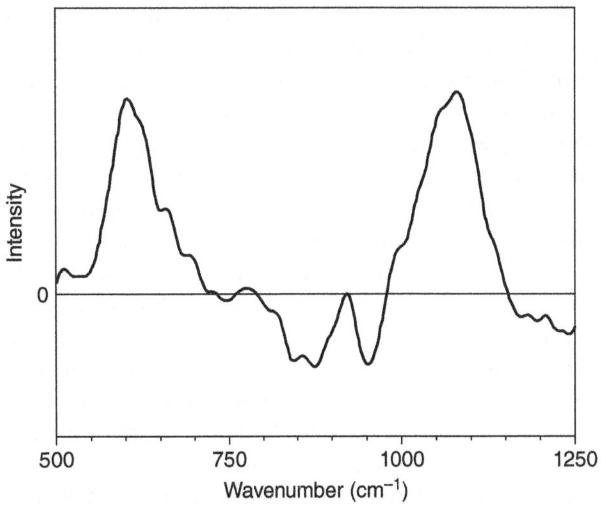

Figure 6.13 Calculated spectrum "(G-1d)-(G-1e)" yielded by the mathematical subtraction of the Raman spectrum of intact glass G-1d by the relevant spectrum of glass G-1e, shown in Figure 6.7. (The spectra of glasses G-1d and G-1e have been normalized. For better resolution, the spectrum "(G-1d)-(G-1e)" has been smoothened.)

(~2 mol% Table 6.1) in glass G-1e than G-1d. Hence, the silicate network of glass G-1e seems to exhibit a higher degree of depolymerization. It is well known that smaller silicate units, such as Q^1 and Q^0, form when the concentration of modifier cations increases and that of formers decreases. Furthermore, the divalent Ca^{2+} cations, which have larger field strength than monovalent Na^+, prefer smaller silicate units with higher negative charge for charge neutralization.

From the dilatation curves plotted in Figure 6.9 (the curve of the parent glass G-1b is also plotted for comparison purposes), the T_g was 595 and 600 °C and T_s was 669 and 672 °C for G-1d and G-1e, respectively, while the CTE values (for 200–400 °C) were generally high in the level of ~10×10^{-6} K^{-1} but the CTE of glass G-1e was slightly smaller than G-1d. These thermal properties are directly related to the network connectivity of the glasses. Accordingly, the higher T_g and T_s and the lower CTE of the investigated glasses G-1d and G-1e than the B-containing parent glass G-1b can be attributed to the change of the B_2O_3/SiO_2 ratio in the glasses due to the substitution of B in the network of the glass structure via the schemes $2B^{3+} \rightarrow 1.5Si^{4+}$ (glass G-1d) and $2B^{3+} \rightarrow Si^{4+} + 0.2P^{5+} + 0.5Ca^{2+}$ (glass G-1e).

Heat treatment of the glass-powder compacts at 700 °C (i.e. above T_g) showed that the samples maintained their amorphous nature but were completely dense indicating that sintering precedes crystallization in these systems. Devitrification occurred after heat treatment at higher temperatures. The X-ray diffractograms for the two compositions after heat treatment at 800 and 850 °C are shown in Figure 6.11. Pyroxene phase of diopside was predominantly formed. There was evidence of formation of wollastonite and fluorapatite as well. The same assemblage of phases, but with a significant increase in intensity, was registered in the diffractograms of samples heat treated at 850 °C. This means that the B-free glass-ceramics G-1d and G-1e had a simpler phase assemblage (diopside, wollastonite, and fluorapatite) than the B-containing glass-ceramics, e.g. G-1b, etc. (diopside, wollastonite, akermanite, and fluorapatite).

The absence of B in the compositions G-1d and G-1e did not significantly affect sintering and devitrification behavior, which was similar to analogous B-containing glasses, resulting in completely dense samples of white color and attractive appearance with no-cracks or visible open porosity after heat treatment at 800 and 850 °C. However, it should be noted that in the case of the parent glass G-1b and the other B-containing compositions, heat treatment at 850 °C caused the development of visible bubbles underneath the surface of the samples and a general properties decrease of the glass-ceramics. The differences observed might be due to an expected increase of the activation energy for viscous flow (E_{vf}) as a result of increasing both SiO_2 content and network connectivity in the B-free glasses. The E_{vf} values for SiO_2 (1100–1400 °C) and for B_2O_3 (26–1300 °C) are 710 kJ/mol, and 347 kJ/mol, respectively.

6.6 *In vitro* Biomineralization Ability (SBF Tests and HA Formation)

The *in vitro* bioactivity is reflected in materials' capability to induce HA formation onto their surfaces. In this study, this was investigated by immersion of either powders or glass blocks (with mirror-polished surfaces, i.e. final polishing with 1 μm diamond paste and then cleaning by ultrasonic agitation) in SBF at 37 °C (±0.5 K). The SBF has an ionic concentration of Na^+ 142.0, K^+ 5.0, Ca^{2+} 2.5, Mg^{2+} 1.5, Cl^- 147.8, HCO_3^- 4.2, HPO_4^{2-} 1.0, SO_4^{2-} 0.5 (in mM), buffered at pH = 7.25 by tris(hydroxymethyl)aminomethane (Tris, 50 mM) and hydrochloric acid. The SBF was either not changing at all during the entire time of the experiments or renewing daily. In case of powders, which had 0.3–0.7 m^2/g surface area (measured by the BET method), we used a ratio of either 0.2 g powder/ml SBF or 0.002 g powder/ml SBF (to enhance, in the latter case, the formation of HA). The analysis of the supernatant liquid comprised pH measurements and determination of the concentration of Ca^{2+}, Mg^{2+}, B^{3+}, P^{5+}, Si^{4+}, Na^+, and Al^{3+} by inductively coupled plasma – optical emission spectroscopy (ICP-OES, Jobin Yvon, JY 70 plus, France). The solid samples were analyzed with XRD, IR and Raman spectroscopy, and SEM/EDS.

Typical curves of the ionic concentrations in the liquid over immersion time of glass-powders for all the investigated compositions powders are shown in Figure 6.14. Dissolution spontaneously took place immediately, even after one hour. In all cases, alkaline reaction occurred attributed to the exchange of Na^+/H^+ ions, similarly to the 45S5 Bioglass (Figure 6.14a). The concentration of Ca2+ continuously increased even after one month of immersion in SBF (Figure 6.14b). Phosphorous concentration rapidly decreased, indicating the active role of P on the transformation of glasses' surface during immersion in SBF. The concentration of Si reached a plateau, descending afterwards. In the alumina containing G-A1, the concentration of Al3+ was always very low in the liquid. ICP measurements showed no considerable changes in the concentrations of Mg2+ and B3+ over immersion time. These curves strongly resemble the behavior of oxides containing CaO–SiO_2. Thus, the investigated glasses should follow the biomineralization mechanism proposed by Kokubo: (i) Ca2+ ions are exchanged with H^+ resulting in a pH increase, (ii) a silica gel layer forms and provides favorable nucleation sites for apatite, and (iii) apatite layer forms and thickens on them.

The formation of calcium phosphates onto the surfaces of the glasses and glass-ceramics was observed in SEM analysis (Figure 6.15). The Al-containing glass and glass-ceramics with the composition G-A1 favored the formation of submicron precipitates, enriched in Ca and P (found by EDS), which was more enhanced in the glass than in the glass-ceramics (left-hand side and right-hand side in Figure 6.15a, respectively).

In all the Al-free glasses, their surfaces were completely covered by HA submicron particles after immersion for one, two, three (Figure 6.15b), and four weeks (Figure 6.15c) in SBF, suggesting their high *in vitro* bioactivity. The nature of these particles (i.e. they are HA) was confirmed by XRD, IR, and Raman spectroscopy as well as by EDS analysis (where the Ca/P ratio was determined as 1.67). Prolong immersion caused development of the size of the calcium-P precipitates. Moreover, increasing amount of CaO and SiO_2 (i.e. the glasses G-2 and G-3) apparently caused faster mineralization kinetics. Similar images have been reported in earlier studies on amorphous and crystalline phases of $CaSiO_3$.These results suggest that the surface of the Al-free glasses undergo suitable modifications resulting in a layer which acts as nucleation center of Ca–P precipitates, according to the aforementioned mineralization mechanism. From such SEM images it was suggested that there is an incubation time of ~7 days for the formation of the first calcium-phosphate precipitates. Kokubo has mentioned 10 days of incubation time for the $20Na_2O$–$80SiO_2$

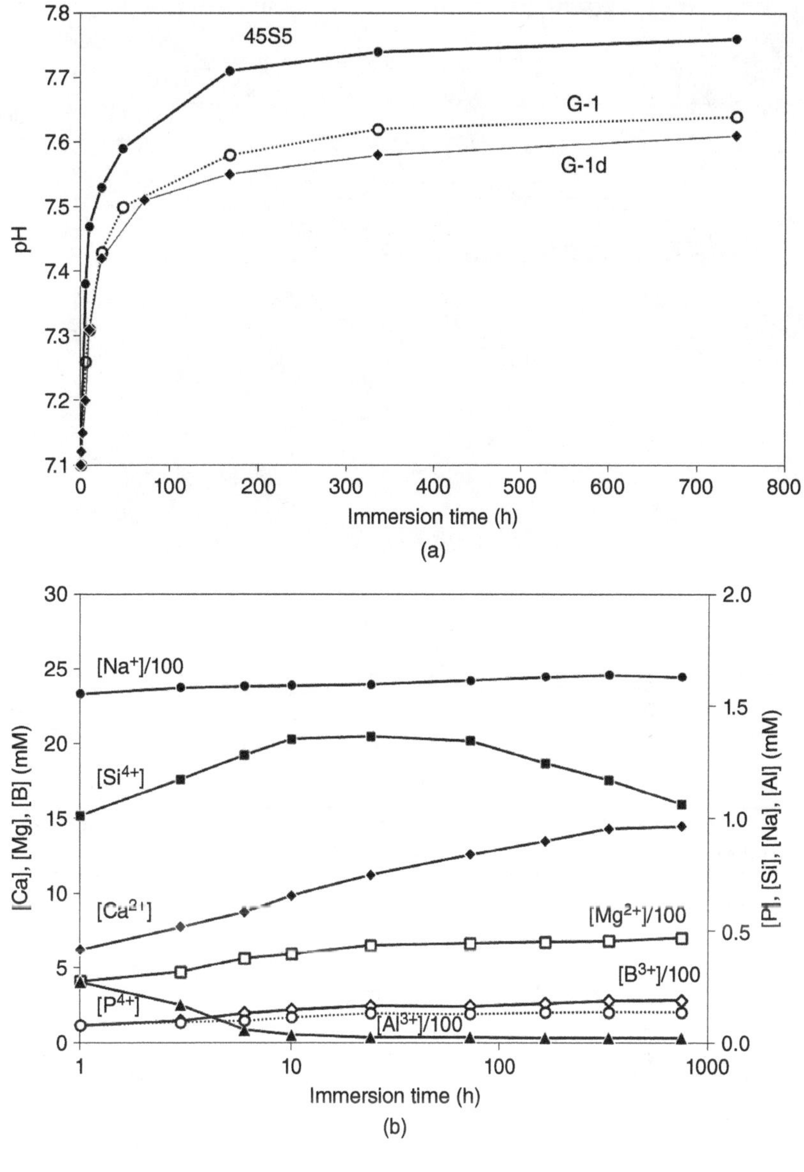

Figure 6.14 Typical evolution of (a) pH (along with the curve for the 45S5 Bioglass, for comparison purposes) (0.002 g glass powder/ml SBF) and (b) ionic concentrations in SBF over immersion time for the powder of the investigated glasses (0.2 g glass powder/ml SBF); (the dashed line corresponds to the concentration of Al in the glass G-A1); (the concentrations of Na, B, Mg, and Al were divided by 100).

glass. The increase of pH (Figure 6.14a) to approach the acidity constant of silicic acid, $pK_{Si(OH)2} = 9.6$, seemingly supports the existence of stage (ii), whereby silica is hydrolyzed to silicic acid. Silicates, which also greatly dissolve from the glasses (Figure 6.14b), may be actively involved in this process, as well.

With the aid of Raman and IR spectroscopy we shed light in the mechanism of the formation of HA in these glasses and the relationship between dissolution capability and bioactivity performance and the network connectivity of the glasses. In general, glasses comprising networks with dense cross-linking feature more rigid structures which undergo less dissolution, while flexible structures with lower network connectivity can promote dissolution and then mineralization. Beyond the influence of the structure of the initial glass, we also propose that the resulting structure of the surface of the glass, derived after the leaching of stage (i) of mineralization mechanism, should be enough flexible to favor apatite formation. Therefore, we analyzed the surfaces of glasses after short immersion times in SBF with these two spectroscopic techniques. The obtained Raman (Figure 6.16) and IR spectra (Figure 6.17) provide evidences that modifications at the glass surface have occurred from the very first day of the immersion in SBF. This early activity of glass surface is also reflected in the changes of the ion concentrations plotted in Figure 6.14.

In particular, the Raman spectra in Figure 6.16 that correspond to the glass G-1b (similar behavior was obtained in G-1, G-2, G-3, and G-1a glasses) show that there are noticeable differences between the Raman spectrum of the intact glass (i.e. stretching vibrations of Q^2 at $956\,cm^{-1}$, Q^1 $882\,cm^{-1}$, and Si–O–Si bending motions at 648 and $720\,cm^{-1}$) and that of the newly formed tiny

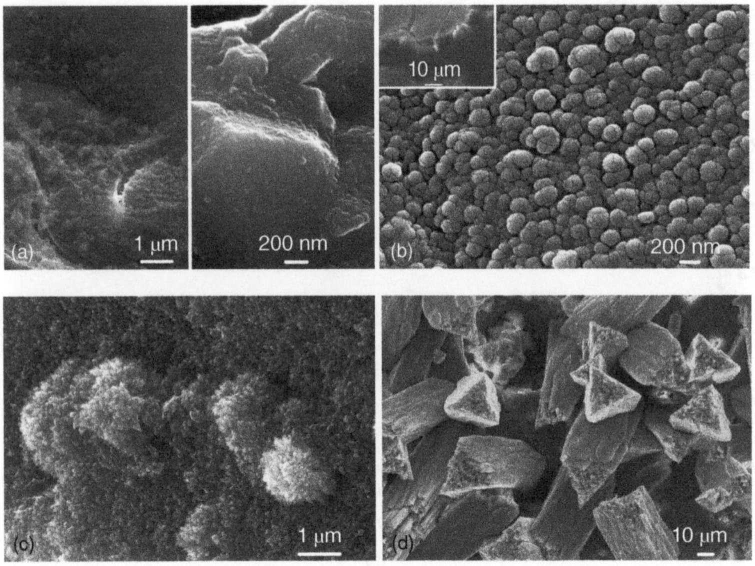

Figure 6.15 Formation of Ca-P precipitates and corrosion evidences at the surface of the investigated materials after immersion in SBF at 37 °C. (a) G-A1 glass after seven days in SBF (left-hand side) and glass-ceramic heat treated at 800 °C after 31 days in SBF. (b) Glass G-1 (b) after three weeks (and inset corresponds to glass G-1d three weeks) and (c) after one month in SBF. (d) Glass G-1e after three weeks in renewed SBF.

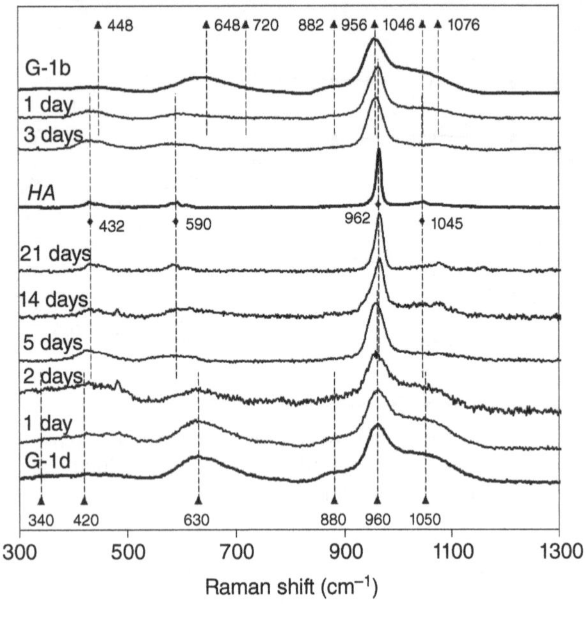

Figure 6.16 Evolution of Raman spectra obtained from the surface of the glass G-1b and G-1d over increasing immersion time in SBF. The spectrum of hydroxyapatite (HA) is also plotted. (For facilitating comparison, the spectra have been normalized.)

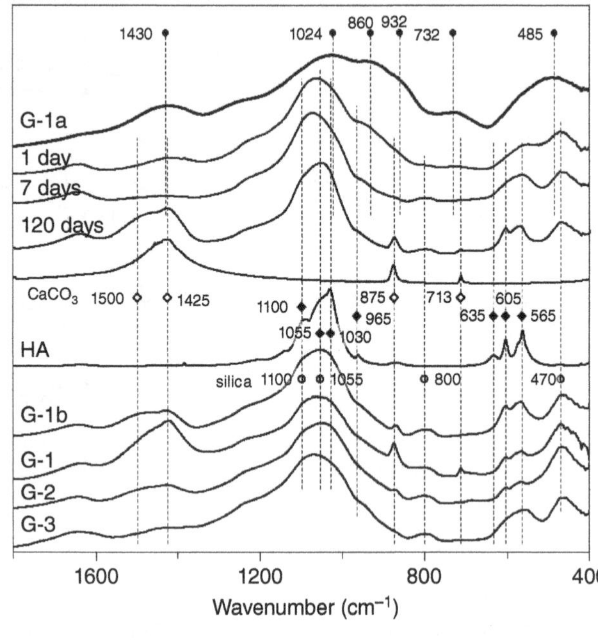

Figure 6.17 Evolution of FT-IR spectra of the glass G-1a over increasing immersion time in SBF (1 day, 7 days, and 120 days) and FT-IR spectra of the glasses G-1, G1b, G2, and G-3 after immersion in SBF for 120 days. The spectra of hydroxyapatite (HA) and $CaCO_3$ are also plotted. The frequencies which correspond to the presence of silica are also marked.

crystallites formed onto the surface of the glass after one day of immersion in SBF, whose spectra showed a shift of the peak of the principal band to 960 cm^{-1}, almost vanishing of the bands at 648 and 1045 cm^{-1}, while the overall appearance of the spectrum resembles that one of the synthetic HA. The Raman spectrum of HA exhibits a very strong peak at 960 cm^{-1} and a number of weaker ones at around 1045, 590, and 430 cm^{-1}, originated from the internal modes of PO_4^{3-} ions. The rapid decrease of phosphorous concentration showed in Figure 6.14b indicates an active role of P on the transformation of glasses' surface during immersion in SBF. These features are more evident in the spectrum obtained after three days of immersion in SBF.

In the FT-IR spectra of Figure 6.17, which correspond to the surface layer formed in glass G-1a (where the spectra of HA and $CaCO_3$ are also plotted for comparison purposes), noticeable alterations are observed even after one day of immersion in SBF, when compared to the untreated glass. The bands of the intact glasses assigned to Si–O$^-$ and B–O$^-$ vibrations (1024, 932, 860, 1430, and 732 cm^{-1}) were reduced in intensity, and the low frequency band at 485 cm^{-1} was split into two bands at 565 and 470 cm^{-1}. We can assign these changes to the formation of both silica and apatite layers on the glass surface. In particular, the peak at 1055 cm^{-1} can be attributed to the superimposition of the P–O stretch of HA phase (see spectrum of HA) and the Si–O vibration of the silica phase. The peak at 565 cm^{-1} can be assigned to the O–P–O bending mode of HA and the peak at 465 cm^{-1} to the Si–O–Si bending mode of silica. (The weak absorption peaks at 1430, 932, and 732 cm^{-1} are contributions from the original glass structure.) All these changes become more evident (i.e. development of stronger bands) after seven days of soaking in SBF. Similar changes were observed in all the investigated glasses. To shed light in the stage (ii) of the biomineralization mechanism, the characteristic absorption peaks at 1110 cm^{-1} (high frequency shoulder of the main band of the spectrum), at 800 cm^{-1}, and at 470 cm^{-1} are attributed to the vibrations of silicon-oxygen units in silica network.

With regard to the carbonate substitution of HA formed onto the surface of the investigated Al-free glasses, the FT-IR spectra after 120 days soaking in SBF (Figure 6.17) suggest that it is carbonated hydroxyapatite phase (CHA). The spectrum shows new peaks at 1425, 1500, 875, 713, and 605 cm^{-1}, which can be attributed to A- and B-type CHA. It is known that typical peaks of the A-type CHA are centered at 880, 1450, and 1540 cm^{-1}, while peaks at 1425, 870, and 713 cm^{-1} are due to the B-type carbonate-substituted apatite phase. It must be also noticed that sharp bands were found neither at 3570 cm^{-1} nor at 630 cm^{-1} due to the stretching mode of ν_{OH} of hydroxyl group in any of the treated glasses. This is in agreement with the existence of B-type CHA, in which the occupancy of CO_3^{2-} ions at the OH$^-$ positions reduces the infrared absorption at the above referred frequencies. A contribution of this effect is also possible from the presence of fluorine ions in glass structure that can cause a coupling effect OF--OH, which masks the characteristic band of hydroxyl group.

The differences among the spectra of the five investigated glasses after 120 days in SBF (Figure 6.17) reveal that the development of HA phase depends on the composition of the initial glass. The peaks attributed to carbonated species and apatite become weaker in intensity or completely vanished as the CaO and SiO_2 content increases. For instance, the peaks due to the carbonate ions vibrations at 1425, 875, and 714 cm^{-1} gradually vanish in the order G-1 > G-2 > G-3. Similar trends appear for the case of the multiple low frequency bands (605, 565 cm^{-1}), which are attributed to the vibrations of HA, where these bands gradually merge to form a broad band centered at 560 cm^{-1}. Furthermore, the spectrum of glass G-1b, which has the highest P_2O_5 content, indicates the highest amount of A-type carbonated HA, as it is evident by the peaks at 1500 and 870 cm^{-1}.

The Al content in bioactive glasses is an issue of particular interest. The results of Figure 6.14b suggest that Al has low leaching capability from the glass G-A1, comparing to other elements. We have also obtained similar evidences in our earlier study in the system fluorapatite–anorthite, where Al was not detected in the SBF solution after 108 days of immersion of glass powders in SBF. Therefore, the strong adherence of Al in the glass structure should cause intrinsic structural constraints with regards to the freedom of the glass structure for undergoing the necessary transformations anticipated in stage (ii) at the maximum extent. In the literature, it has been conjectured that alumina inhibits some of the stages of apatite formation, retarding therefore the mineralization of osteoids into bone. Kokubo experimentally determined the Al_2O_3 concentration threshold between bioactivity and bioinertness regimes in Al_2O_3-containing wollastonite glasses, which is in the range of 1.5–1.7 mol%, while glasses with 5% Al_2O_3 were entirely inert. However, the investigated glasses had lower amount of Al_2O_3 (Table 6.1). Therefore, the surface of the glass G-A1, after the stage (i) of leaching, was probably enriched in Al whose content exceeded locally this concentration threshold.

The two B-free glasses G-1d and G-1e showed similar bioactivity to the previous Al-free glasses and HA formed from the early stages of mineralization and was well developed on their surfaces after three weeks, as confirmed by SEM (inset of Figure 6.15b), EDS elemental analysis (molar ratio Ca/P = 1.67), XRD, Raman (Figure 6.16), and IR spectroscopy. Significant changes occurred at the surface of glass G-1e after only one day in SBF, whereas the modifications in the glass G-1d are seemingly slower.

However, experiments with daily renewing SBF favored the formation of monetite ($CaHPO_4$) at the surfaces of both glasses G-1d and G-1e. In particular, XRD, Raman and IR spectroscopy confirmed the formation of monetite in the glass G-1d after seven days in renewing SBF, but HA eventually forms after 21 days in daily renewing SBF. However, the experimental results from the same experimental techniques suggested that monetite forms on the surface of the glass G-1e from the very beginning (three days immersion) up to three weeks in renewing SBF. Big prismatic (with triangular aspect) well-developed crystals of monetite (according to EDS chemical analysis, where the molar ratio Ca/P ≈ 1) were observed on the surface of the glass G-1e after three weeks in daily renewing SBF (Figure 6.15d).

In general, HA layer forms faster in static systems than in slow-flowing and circulating systems, but the *in vitro* tests carried out under flowing SBF simulate better the *in vivo* conditions, making the latter tests more precise and reliable. Monetite ($CaHPO_4$) is a Ca-deficient (with respect to HA) compound which is stable under acid pH (whereas HA is stable in alkaline pH). Hence, it is suggested that the daily renewing of SBF ceases Ca2+ supersaturation (with respect to HA) in the solution and/or locally at the surface of the glass as well as did not allow the pH to be highly alkaline, favoring monetite formation. However, monetite is a precursor of HA since it serves as a substrate for the oriented reprecipitation of HA crystallites, and its bioactivity has been well-documented.

The aforementioned small differences in the mineralization behavior between the glasses G-1d and G-1e under either regular (static) or renewing SBF immersion tests can be related to the particular structural features of the two investigated glasses, which were thoroughly analyzed in Section 6.5.3, using the corresponding Raman spectra. In the case of regular (static) SBF tests, the faster bioactivity response of glass G-1e (than G-1d) might be assigned to the less covalent network and the larger number of NBOs units (Si–O$^-$) than that in glass G-1d, since both factors are of high relevance for the bioactivity mechanism of silicate glasses. With regard to the role of Ca2+, the higher concentration of phosphate units in glass G-1e might cause slowing of the mobility of Ca2+ toward glass surface because Ca2+ ions prefer to interact with NBOs of phosphate units than with silicate ones. The kinetics of Ca2+ leaching from the glass is important in the case of renewing SBF tests because monetite formation indicates lower Ca2+ supersaturation regime in comparison to the conditions favoring the formation of HA. Accordingly, the above hypothesis anticipates a faster kinetics for the local increasing of Ca2+ supersaturation onto the surface of glass G-1d in comparison to glass G-1e. This would explain the preferential formation of HA onto the surface of glass G-1d after three weeks in renewing SBF, whereas monetite remains stable on the surface of glass G-1e.

The behavior of the G-1d glass demonstrates some similar features with 45S5 Bioglass in SBF tests (e.g. the pH curve in Figure 6.14a). For instance, both glasses remain amorphous (confirmed by XRD analyses) after three days of immersion in SBF, and HA forms after three weeks, which is slightly more crystallized in G-1d than in 45S5 Bioglass. It is also worth to note that it has been postulated that the higher solubility of 45S5 Bioglass than G-1d may also favor the formation of calcite in 45S5 Bioglass (together with HA) over prolong immersion in SBF, whereas the poorer solubility of G-1d and the lower values of pH (Figure 6.14a) efficiently suppress this tendency and favors the formation exclusively of HA on the surface of the glass G-1d. The above results and the aforementioned bioactivity mechanism for the B-free glasses suggest that particulates of these glasses can be complimentary to 45S5 Bioglass in clinical applications. This assumption has to be confirmed by further experimentation; thus it is thoroughly discussed in Section 6.8 for the particular case of periodontitis, which involves progressive loss of the bone around teeth and may lead to loosening and eventual loss of teeth if untreated.

6.7 Cell Culture Testing and Tissue Response

In biomaterials which generally undergo significant surface modifications, such as the glasses investigated in the present study, the degradation products of bioactive glasses can stimulate the production of growth factors, cell proliferation, and activate the gene expression of osteoblasts. The *in vitro* experiments in the present work were carried out according to the methodology described in literature for primary culture of osteoblasts. The aim was to preliminarily examine the influence of the materials on cell biology following internationally accepted criteria.

Osteoblasts were isolated from the calvaria of one- to five-day-old neonatal Wistar rats. The cells were seeded into 25 ml tissue culture flasks, and allowed to grow in a controlled 5% CO_2, 95% humidified incubator at 37 °C. After confluence, the cells were used for next experiments. To test the stimulation of osteoblasts with a medium containing glass powder, osteoblasts were plated 1×10^5 cell density, in 24-well plates. After two hours, the medium was changed to a medium containing glass powder (grain size of powder <35 μm). The concentration used was 0.005 g powder/1 ml of culture medium. After 72 hours of incubation, osteoblasts' morphology, viability/proliferation, and secretion capability (i.e. collagen, alkaline phosphatase) were tested. The cellular proliferation and viability tests were done after 72 hours of incubation in the presence of each glass powder, evaluated by MTT assay. The osteoblast collagen production was analyzed by SIRCOL assay. The alkaline phosphatase production was evaluated by BCIP–NBT assay. The results are presented as means ± SDs (the numbers of the experiments are mentioned in the legend of the figure). The statistical significance was measured by ANOVA and Bonferroni's posttest.

Under light microscopy, osteoblasts showed no evidence of toxicity or other detrimental effects on the functionality of osteoblast cells or any morphological change after 24, 48, or 72 hours of incubation in the presence of the G-A1, G-1d, and G-1e glasses, when compared to control. The viability/proliferation of osteoblasts was not altered in the presence of these glass powders, when compared to control (Figure 6.18a). However, the powder of glass G-1d induced significant increase of proliferation when compared to control and glass G-1e, which was also higher than control. The collagen secretion of osteoblasts was not altered when the cells were incubated in the presence of the Al- and B-free glass powders G-1d and G-1e and increased about 20% in the presence of the glass G-A1, when compared to control (Figure 6.18b). The production of alkaline phosphatase was slightly higher in the presence of the glass G-A1 and decreased in the case of G-1d and G-1e glass powders, comparing to control (Figure 6.18c).

These results are in accordance with earlier studies on silicon-containing glasses, where it has been reported that the release of silicic acid enhances the production of collagen type I as well as that bioactive glasses containing wollastonite components stimulates *in vitro* biomineralization. The increased osteoblasts' proliferation and viability in the presence of the glasses G-1d and G-1e, especially in the case of the glass G-1d (Figure 6.18a), supports the important role of silicon (glass G-1d is richer in Si than G-1e). The higher abundance of glass modifier Na^+ cations in glass G-1d may also enhance the viability and proliferation of osteoblasts. On the other hand, the higher content of CaO in glass G-1e may reduce the flexibility of Ca2+ bound to phosphate units and annul the positive effect of Na^+ cations.

Osteoblasts' differentiation starts with proliferation of preosteoblasts, which are cells with lower potential to secrete alkaline phosphatase comparing to mature osteoblasts. Calvaria-derived bone cells have high proportion of preosteoblasts. The results of Figure 6.18c suggest that the glasses G-1d and G-1e may cause a delay in preosteoblast differentiation, which is not a serious concern. However, the presence of these two glass powders did not cause any difference in collagen secretion (Figure 6.18b). This is consistent with a delay in preosteoblast differentiation because collagen is an osteoblast marker of the very early stages of differentiation.

With regard to tissue engineering, these results qualify the investigated glasses for further experimentation, such as studies on cellular attachment, molecular mechanisms involved in cell behavior in the presence of these materials, and gene expression patterns.

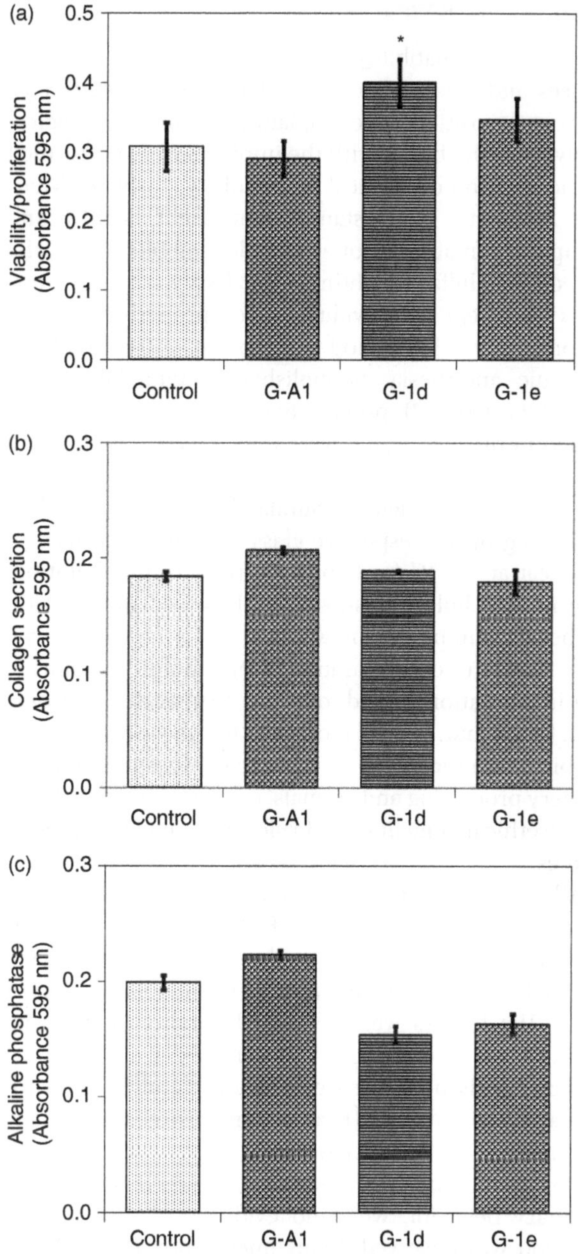

Figure 6.18 1×10^5 osteoblasts were plated in the presence of glass powders G-1A, G-1d, and G-1e. After 72 hours of incubation, viability/proliferation were evaluated by MTT assay (a), collagen production with SIRCOL assay (b), and alkaline phosphatase production by (5-bromo-4-chloro-3-indolyl-phosphate) with (nitro blue tetrazolium) for the colorimetric detection of alkaline phosphatase activity (BCIP-NBT) assay (c). Results represent mean ± SD values of duplicates from eight different experiments ($p < 0.05$).

6.8 Animal Testing and Clinical Tests

The above results suggested that the glass with composition G-1d can be qualified for further consideration and experimentation as an effective and reliable bioactive glass. In this chapter, we present the *in vivo* behavior in implantations in rabbits and the clinical trials of this glass.

6.8.1 *In vivo* Animal Tests

In vivo biocompatibility tests were conducted with bulk glasses and glass particulates of the investigated G-1d glass composition. The implantation and histological analyses of the bones with the implants were performed at the Division of Surgical Stomatology, Tashkent Medical Academy, Uzbekistan. Twenty-eight healthy and completely matured (one-year-old) rabbits from the breed "shinshilla" weighting 2.8–3.0 kg were used. Animals were kept in individuals cages, properly identified according to the period and group. After applying systemic anesthesia, nonpolished rectangular prisms (c. $2 \times 2 \times 10\,mm^3$), previously sterilized in alcohol and boiled in distilled water, were implanted in the femoral diaphysis region in a drilled hole of 2 mm diameter and about 10 mm length. Similar holes were also filled with 0.1 g of the respective glass particles, sterilized in dry heat at 180 °C for two hours prior to implantation. The incised hole was subsequently sewed up. Incision without any implantation was also performed as control. The reactions of the animals were monitored during the implantation period. one and two weeks, and one, two, three, four, and six months. After these periods, the rabbits were sacrificed by immediate decapitation. The surgery processing and animals' care were in accordance to the ethical guidelines and rules of local governmental bodies.

All femurs collected were immediately fixed in 10% phosphate-buffered formalin for 72 hours for histology or histomorphometry analysis. These femurs were decalcified in 10% formic acid formalin solution for 14 days. The femurs were sectioned parallel to the long axis of the femur through the anteromedial aspect of the defect. The tissue blocks were sectioned and stained with hematoxylin and eosin (H and E) and histopathologically observed by optical microscopy.

During the implantation period, the rabbits exhibited ordinary behavior, while no evidence of any adverse reaction was observed. Items microscopically analyzed included presence of inflammatory infiltrate, bone formation in the margins of the cavity, bone formation in the center of the cavity, and presence of giant cells (Figure 6.19). Histopathological section of the bone after one week of implantation showed low inflammatory infiltrate while an increase of blood vessel's thickness was revealed. Abundant woven bone ingrowth and ongrowth and normal fibroblast proliferation were revealed after two weeks. In particular, a newly formed bone originated from the margins of host bone toward to the center of cavities. Presence of single giant cells (macrophages) was also observed. Histological analysis in the samples after one month implantation demonstrated fragmentation of cavities by trabeculae, woven bone growth, and initial stage of blood vessels formation. Moreover, mesenchymal stem cells (MSCs) at a weak differentiation stage were observed at the periphery of cavities along with extensively developed collagen type structures of a connective tissue. The depth of bone ingrowth increased after two months and was accompanied with resorption of bone graft and formation of lamellar bone. After —three to four months, only residues of material completely embedded into bone trabeculae were observed in newly formed bone tissue, i.e. the new bone comprised osteoid type structures and remodeling occurred. The cavities were completely filled with bone structures, and matured homogeneous bone tissue was formed after six months postimplantation period.

6.8.2 Clinical Trials

According to the local arrangements, the glass samples along with the required documentation including objectives, physical-technical characteristics of the material, and the results of *in vitro* and *in vivo* tests, were submitted for evaluation to the Committee of the New Medical Techniques at the Ministry of Health of Uzbekistan in May 2007. The permission for performing clinical tests was issued by both Presidium of the Pharmacological Committee of the Ministry of Health of Uzbekistan under the reference no. 23, dated 26.11.2007, and by the National Ethical Committee of Uzbekistan under the reference no. 2, dated 05.02.2008. The protocol (program) of clinical tests was then approved by the Chief of the Department of New Medical Techniques in 13.02.2008, thereby allowing performing limited clinical trials in the following two clinics: (i) the Tashkent Medical Academy in the Clinic Hospital of the Urgent Medical Aid and (ii) the Tashkent Doctor's Qualification Upgrading Institute in the Town Clinic number 7. In both studies, the principal investigators and promoters were Professor M.E. Makhkamov (PhD and Habilitation degree from the Division of Surgical Stomatology in the Tashkent Medical Academy, Uzbekistan) and Dr. Kh. K. Karshiev (PhD surgeon from the Town Clinic No. 7), respectively. The aim of the clinical evaluation was to demonstrate the safety and efficiency of glass particulates when used for the treatment of jaw bone defects mainly after cystectomy operation. Bone grafting with bioglass will prevent the resorption of bone tissue, and thus preserve it for possible dental implantology and prosthetics restorations in the future.

Over a period of eight months, between February 2008 and October 2008, clinical tests were performed in 45 patients (21 males and 24 females), with moderate age in the range of 19–60 years old. There were patients suffering from chronic granuloma cyst (12), radicular cyst (23), follicular cyst (1), adentia (3), jaw mandible cyst (1),

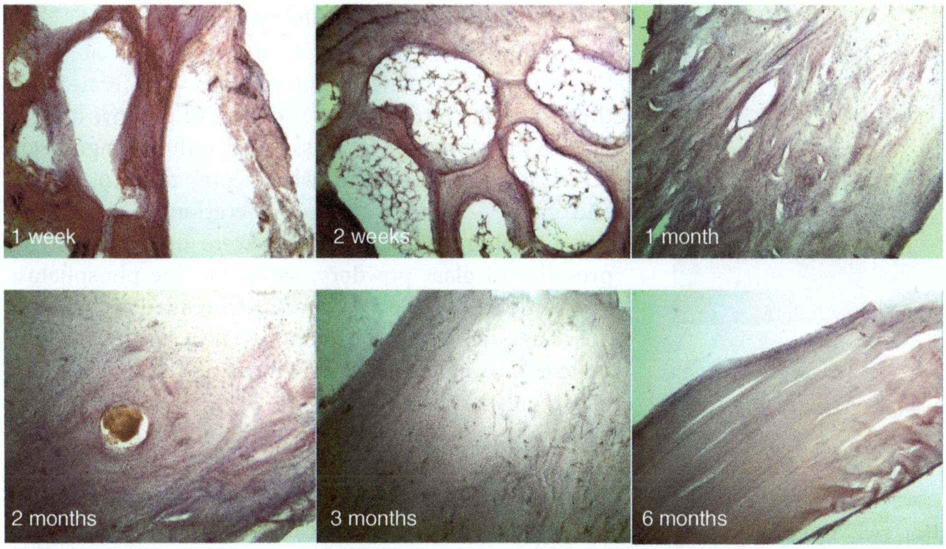

Figure 6.19 Histopathological analysis in sections of bones after different times of implantation of the glass G-1d in the femoral diaphysis of rabbits.

and periodontitis (5). The clinical trials were conducted with prior consent of all patients who agreed participating in this study on a voluntary basis. According to the protocol, all the patients were clinically examined immediately (day 0), and on 15th, 60th, and 180th day after surgery. Retroalveolar X-ray radiographs were taken at the same time periods. The clinical safety and the efficiency of bioglass particulates were assessed by both controlling the dynamics of the postoperative healing process using a standard scale ranging from 1 to 4 and by the absence of a radiolucent line between the bone graft and the osseous walls in X-rays, respectively. The bioactivity of the glass G-1d was evaluated by visual observation of the radiographic densities of the bone at the lesions sites and of the contiguous host bone.

The operation procedure and the whole treatment were as follows: on designing a surgical treatment of jaw bone cyst and periodontitis, a main objective was to follow a favorable tooth keeping tactic. Provided that this practice is successful, further application of orthopedic methods maintaining functions of neighboring teeth is feasible. Before cystectomy operation, a general clinical examination of patient, including X-ray radiography, was performed. It allowed the estimation of wound volume and the amount of bone graft to be applied. After cystectomy, the defect area and the dissected frontal wall of the jaw were carefully rinsed several times with 3% of hydrogen peroxide and 0.05% chlorhexidine solutions to wash out the cystic tissue completely. The required amount of sterilized G-1d glass particulates was mixed with the fresh blood from the defect region and then used to completely fill the bone defect. Finally, the surgical sites were closed by returning to the original position and fixed. The patients were recommended to use appropriate postoperative antibiotic and analgesic whether it was prescribed and to follow home care regime. After surgery, patients were questioned about symptoms and pain feeling using a standard scale from 1 to 5.

The glass particulates formed a cohesive mass with patient's blood, demonstrating a homeostatic effect. The graft material was easy to place and shape *in situ*. As mentioned above, the clinical safety and efficiency of bioactive glass particulates were assessed using standard scales ranging from 1 to 4. The nearest results (from the first day to the 90th day) demonstrated no high degree of pain or signs of inflammation in 95% of the cases. Only in two cases, weak inflammatory reaction adjacent to a lesion gingival region were revealed during first three postoperative days followed by normal healing process. In none of the patients was observed an occurrence of adverse clinical reactions or infectious complications in the postoperative phase. The average time of hospital stay postprocedure was one day (range: 0–33 days). Usually, patients were admitted on the day of surgery and discharged the next day. Complete clinical healing was considered when gums recuperated their natural color, jaw could open and close easily, and the teeth came together and separate easily. The patients' satisfaction was confirmed by their availability to undergo the procedures again if necessary. Furthermore, they would recommend the procedures to other patients.

X-ray radiography was performed for all 45 patients before and postoperative (Figure 6.20). A typical example of radiographic images from a patient having radicular cysts in the mandibular region is shown in the left-hand

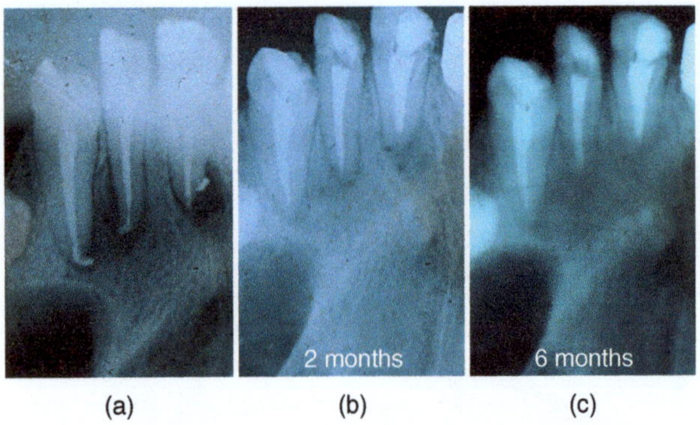

Figure 6.20 X-ray images before implantation (a) and (b) 2 and (c) 6 months after implantation of the glass G-1d in jaw bone defects after cystectomy operation.

side image in Figure 6.20. After two months postoperatively, the lesions were filled up with trabeculae of new bone, and a radioopaque line between bone graft and host bone was observed. The absence of radiolucent line suggests a good integration of biomaterial into the bone with no signs of disruption of bone, i.e. osteolysis effect. Progressive disappearance of the radioopaque line outlining the defect and the increase in radiographic density with time is observed. A significant decrease in the visible surface of the implantation sites and almost total disappearance after six months occurs. The lesions were gradually filled with new bone structures and no hypertrophy phenomenon was recorded.

6.9 Concluding Remarks

The work presents the synthesis and characterization of bioactive glasses designated in the multicomponent Na_2O–CaO–MgO–SiO_2–P_2O_5–CaF_2 system. The effect of small addition of Al_2O_3 and B_2O_3 on glass structure and glass properties was also investigated.

All the investigated glasses featured liquid–liquid glass immiscibility phenomenon while crystallization occurred from the surface. Glass compositions in the aforementioned system devitrify with the formation of diopside, wollastonite, and fluorapatite, while the presence of Al_2O_3 favors the formation of akermanite. Due to the desirable sequence of events, where sintering precedes crystallization, dense sintered glass-powder compacts with high flexural strength (up to 140 MPa) were obtained after heating at 800 °C for one hour.

The presence of Al_2O_3 suppresses formation of HA in SBF testing, while the presence of B_2O_3 causes moderate bioactivity in glasses. Glasses free of Al_2O_3 and B_2O_3 demonstrated faster formation of HA on immersion in SBF solution.

The *in vitro* biocompatibility tests of the Al- and B-free glasses G-1d and G-1e showed high viability of the osteoblasts, which continued to proliferate after three days in culture in the presence of the investigated glasses. The powder of glass G-1d induced significant increase of proliferation when compared to control and glass G-1e. The collagen secretion of osteoblasts was not altered when the cells were incubated in the presence of glass powders, while alkaline phosphatase production decreased comparing to control. In general, the results of *in vitro* tests do not show any evidence of toxicity or other detrimental effects on the functionality of osteoblast cells.

In the *in vivo* animal studies, the glass G-1d demonstrated low inflammatory infiltration and was fully compatible with the surrounding tissue without showing any significant adverse reaction. Formation of new bone occurred, which originated from the margins of host bone toward the center of cavities. In clinical trials, the particulates of the glass G-1d formed a cohesive mass with patients' blood, demonstrating a homeostatic effect. This glass was particularly interesting in conventional treatment of bone defects after the removal of a jaw bone cyst due to its ability for being gradually substituted by newly formed bone structures and completely substituted by homogeneous bone tissue.

Glass-ceramic materials in the investigated Na_2O–CaO–MgO–SiO_2–P_2O_5–CaF_2 system will be tested using standard protocols applied in bioglasses and in order to develop materials that can meet the requirements for tissue engineering needs.

Beyond the above properties and the potential applications in field of biomaterials, the results of this study indicate the investigated system as a model system for improving the technology and the properties of conventional glass-ceramics and glazes and to decrease their production cost.

Acknowledgments

The authors greatly appreciate fruitful advices and valuable help of Professor J.M.F. Ferreira, University of Aveiro, Portugal; Professor M.A. Karakassides, University of Ioannina, Greece; and Dr. O. Fabrichnaya, Max Planck Institut fuer Metallforschung, Germany, for much of the work performed and presented in this paper. Furthermore, the authors would like to thank CICECO (Portugal) and the Portuguese Foundation of Science and Technology, the Greek Secretariat of Science and Technology, and the Committee for Coordination Science and Technology Development under the Cabinet of Ministers of Uzbekistan for their financial support.

Bibliography

1 Agathopoulos, S., Tulyaganov, D.U., Marques, P.A.A.P. et al. (2003). The fluorapatite-anorthite system in biomedicine. *Biomaterials* **24** (7): 1317–1331.

2 Agathopoulos, S., Tulyaganov, D.U., Valerio, P., and Ferreira, J.M.F. (2005). A new model formulation of the SiO_2–Al_2O_3–B_2O_3–MgO–CaO–Na_2O–F glass-ceramics. *Biomaterials* **26**: 2255–2264.

3 Agathopoulos, S., Tulyaganov, D.U., Ventura, J.M.G. et al. (2006). Formation of hydroxyapatite onto glasses of the CaO–MgO–SiO_2 system with B_2O_3, Na_2O, CaF_2 and P_2O_5 additives. *Biomaterials* **27**: 1832–1840.

4 Agathopoulos, S., Tulyaganov, D.U., Ventura, J.M.G. et al. (2006). Structural analysis and devitrification of glasses based on the CaO–MgO–SiO_2 system with B_2O_3, Na_2O, CaF_2 and P_2O_5 additives. *J. Non-Cryst. Solids* **352**: 322–328.

5 Andrade, A.L., Valerio, P., Goes, A.M. et al. (2006). Influence of morphology on in vitro compatibility of bioactive glasses. *J. Non-Cryst. Solids* **352**: 3508–3511.

6 Best, S.M., Porter, J.A.E., Thian, E.S., and Huang, J. (2008). Bioceramics: past, present and for the future. *J. Eur. Ceram. Soc.* **28** ([7]): 1319–1327.

7 Brauer, D.S., Karpukhina, N., O'Donnell, M.D. et al. (2010). Fluoride-containing bioactive glasses: effect of glass design and structure on degradation, pH and apatite formation in simulated body fluid. *Acta Biomater.* **6**: 3275–3282.

8 Day, R.M. (2005). Bioactive glass stimulates the secretion of angiogenic growth factors and angiogenesis in vitro. *Tissue Eng.* **11**: 768–777.

9 Dee, K.C., Puleo, D.A., and Bizios, R. *Tissue-Biomaterials Interactions*, 2002. Hoboken, NJ: Willey.

10 Dorozhkin, S.V. (2010). *Calcium Orthophosphate-Based Biocomposites and Hybrid Biomaterials.* New York: Nova Science Publishers.

11 Eustathopoulos, N., Nicholas, M.G., and Drevet, B. *Wettability at High Temperatures*, 1999. Oxford: Elsevier.

12 Hench, L.L. (1998). Bioceramics. *J. Am. Ceram. Soc.* **81**: 1705–1728.

13 Hench, L.L. The discovery of bioactive glasses. In: *Science, Faith and Ethics*, 2001. London: Imperial College Press.

14 Hench, L.L. and Ethridge, E.C. *Biomaterials – An Interfacial Approach*, 1982. New York: Academic Press.

15 Hench, L.L. and Wilson, J. (1984). Surface-active biomaterials. *Science* **226**: 630–636.

16 Hench, L.L. and Wilson, J. *An Introduction to Bioceramics*, 1993. Singapore: World Scientific.

17 Hench, L.L., Splinter, R.J., Allen, W.C. Jr., and Greenlee, T.K. (1971). Bonding mechanisms at the interface of ceramic prosthetic materials. *J. Biomed. Mater. Res. Symp.* **2**: 117–114.

18 Hill, R. (1996). An alternative view of the degradation of bioglass. *J. Mater. Sci. Lett.* **15**: 1122–1125.

19 Höland, W. and Beall, G.H. (2012). *Glass-Ceramic Technology*. Hoboken, NJ: Wiley.

20 Jones, J.R. and Clare, A.G. (2012). *Bioglasses.* West Success, UK: Wiley.

21 Kansal, I., Tulyaganov, D.U., Goel, A. et al. (2010). Structural analysis and thermal behavior of diopside-fluorapatite-wollastonite glasses and glass-ceramics. *Acta Biomater.* **6** (11): 4380–4388.

22 Karamanov, A., Arriza, L., Matekovits, I., and Pelino, M. (2004). Properties of sintered glass-ceramics in the diopisde-albite system. *Ceram. Int.* **30**: 2119–2135.

23 Karlsson, K.H. (1998). Bioactivity of glass and its relation to glass structure. *Glass Phys. Chem.* **24**: 280–284.

24 Karlsson, K.H. (2004). Bioactivity of glass and bioactive glasses for bone repair. *Glass Technol.* **45**: 157–161.

25 Kokubo, T., Shigematsu, M., Nagashima, Y. et al. (1982). Apatite-and wollastonite-containing glass-ceramics for prosthetic application. *Bull. Inst. Chem. Res.* **60**: 260–268.

26 McMillan, P.W. (1964). *Glass-Ceramics.* London: Academic Press.

27 Ohtsuki, C., Kokubo, T., and Yamamuro, T. (1992). Compositional dependence of bioactivity of glasses in the system CaO–SiO_2–Al_2O_3: its in vitro evaluation. *J. Mater. Sci. - Mater. Med.* **3**: 119–125.

28 Rahaman, M.N. (2003). *Ceramic Processing and Sintering*. Boca Raton, FL: CRC Press.

29 Ratner, B.D., Hoffman, A.S., Schoen, F.J., and Lemons, J.E. *Biomaterials Science – Introduction to Materials in Medicine*, 2004. San Diego: Elsevier.

30 Salinas, A.J., Roman, J., Vallet-Regi, M. et al. (2000). In vitro bioactivity of glass and glass-ceramics of the $3CaO{\cdot}P_2O_5$–$CaO{\cdot}SiO_2$–$CaO{\cdot}MgO{\cdot}2SiO_2$ system. *Biomaterials* **21**: 251–257.

31 Shelby, J.E. (1997). *Introduction to Glass Science and Technology*. London: The Royal Society of Chemistry.

32 Siriphannon, P., Kameshima, Y., Yasumori, A. et al. (2000). Influence of preparation conditions on the microstructure and bioactivity of α-$CaSiO_3$ ceramics: formation of hydroxyapatite in simulated body fluid. *J. Biomed. Mater. Res.* **52**: 30–39.

33 Strnad, Z. *Glass-Ceramic Materials*, 1986. Amsterdam: Elsevier.
34 Tulyaganov, D.U. (2000). Phase equilibrium in the fluorapatite-anorthite-diopside system. *J. Am. Ceram. Soc.* **83**: 3141–3146.
35 Tulyaganov, D.U., Agathopoulos, S., Ventura, J.M. et al. (2006). Synthesis of glass-ceramics of CaO–MgO–SiO_2 system containing B_2O_3, P_2O_5, Na_2O and CaF_2. *J. Eur. Ceram. Soc.* **26**: 1463–1471.
36 Tulyaganov, D.U., Agathopoulos, S., Fernandes, H.R., and Ferreira, J.M.F. (2006). Processing of glass-ceramics in the SiO_2–Al_2O_3–B_2O_3–MgO–CaO–Na_2O–(P_2O_5)–F system via sintering and crystallization of glass powder compacts. *Ceram. Int.* **32**: 195–200.
37 Tulyaganov, D.U., Agathopoulos, S., Valerio, P. et al. (2011). Synthesis, bioactivity and preliminary biocompatibility studies of glasses in the system CaO–MgO–SiO_2–Na_2O–P_2O_5–CaF_2. *J. Mater. Sci. – Mater. Med.* **22**: 217–227.
38 Tulyaganov, D.U., Makhkamov, M.E., Urazbaev, A. et al. (2013). Synthesis, processing and characterization of a bioactive glass composition for bone regeneration. *Ceram. Int.* **39** (3): 2519–2526.
39 Valerio, P., Pereira, M.M., Goes, A.M., and Leite, M.F. (2004). The effect of ionic products from bioactive glass dissolution on osteoblast proliferation and collagen production. *Biomaterials* **25**: 2941–2948.
40 Vogel, W. and Höland, W. (1987). Development of glass-ceramics for medical application. *Angew. Chem. Int. Ed. Engl.* **26**: 527–544.
41 Zanotto, E.D. (2010). A bright future for glass-ceramics. *Am. Ceram. Soc. Bull.* **89** (8): 19.

7

Electrical Functionalization and Fabrication of Nanostructured Hydroxyapatite Coatings

Vladimir Bystrov[1], *Anna Bystrova*[2], *Yuri Dekhtyar*[2], *Igor A. Khlusov*[3,4], *Vladimir Pichugin*[4], *Konstantin Prosolov*[5,6], and *Yurii Sharkeev*[5,6]

[1] *Institute of Mathematical Problems of Biology, Keldysh Institute of Applied Mathematics, Russian Academy of Sciences, 142290, Pushchino, Russia*
[2] *Institute of Biomedical Engineering and Nanotechnologies, Riga Technical University, Riga, Latvia*
[3] *Department of Morphology and General Pathology, Siberian State Medical University, 634050, Tomsk, Russia*
[4] *National Research Tomsk Polytechnic University, Research School of Chemistry & Applied Biomedical Sciences, 634050, Tomsk, Russia*
[5] *National Research Tomsk Polytechnic University, Research School of High-Energy Physics, 634050, Tomsk, Russia*
[6] *Institute of Strength Physics and Materials Science of SB RAS, Russia*

7.1 Introduction

Hydroxyapatite (HA) is a popular material to fabricate bioimplants for bone replacement/bone tissue regeneration. Because HA mechanical properties are not similar to the bone material the implants are fabricated from the eligible material (titanium is mostly in use), it surface being coated with HA. To be in accordance with the bone tissue where HA is presented as a nanostructured net imbedded into the organic matrix, the coatings are typically nanostructured as well. After the implant is inserted into a human it starts chemically/biochemically communicate with the organism. The implant exterior surface is the gate for implant – organism signals exchanges. Both surface roughness and its electrical potential (EP) have an influence on cells to control biocompatibility of the inserted material. The surface roughness was focused by the researches for a long time. For instance, the SCOPUS data base referred 306 publications since 1990 related to the roughness (search 20 April 2016 for the keyword "HA implant surface roughness"). However, there are just a few (nine) publications directed to the EP of the HA surface, the first publication coming just six years ago (search 20 April 2016 for the keyword "HA implant surface electrical potential").

The current report considers the aspects of the electrically functionalized HA (EHA) nanostructured surface coating to control bone tissue regeneration. Section 7.2 (was written by MSc, PhD student A. Bystrova) considers necessity and prerequisites for HA electrical functionalization. The approach to computed designing of HA is presented in Section 7.3 (by Professor V. Bystrov). Possibilities to characterize EHA are considered in Section 7.4 (by Professor Yu. Dekhtyar [item 4.2.] and Prof. V. Pichugun [item 4.1.]). Fabrication of the nanostructured HA coatings are presented in Section 7.5 (by Professor V. Pichugin, MSc student K. Prosolov, and Professor Yu. Sharkeev). The biological eligibility of the EHA coatings are analyzed in Section 7.6 (by Professor I. Khlusov). The general scientific editorial job for the report was supplied by Professor Yu. Dekhtyar.

7.2 Necessity and Prerequisites of Electrical Functionalization of Hydroxyapatite to Control Bone Cell Attachment

Molecular formula of HA is $Ca_5(PO_4)_3OH$. Mostly HA is presented in ceramics, thin films, and nanoparticle (NP) forms [1, 2].

The cell must sit on the surface of the bioimplant for the start of bone tissue producing. Adhesion of the cells is the process cells interact and attach to a surface, substrate, mediated by interactions between molecules of the cell surface. Cell adhesion occurs from the action of transmembrane glycoproteins (another name is cell adhesion molecules [CAMs]). These proteins are typically transmembrane receptors and are composed of three domains: an intracellular domain that interacts with the cytoskeleton, a transmembrane domain, and an extracellular domain that interacts either with other CAMs of the same kind (homophilic binding) or with other CAMs of the extracellular matrix (ECM) (heterophilic binding). There are a lot of different type of CAMs.

Bioceramics and Biocomposites: From Research to Clinical Practice, First Edition. Edited by Iulian Antoniac.

The DLVO (Derjagin, Landau, Verwey, Overbeek) theory, named after Boris Derjagin, Lev Landau, Evert Verwey, and Theodoor Overbeek, is a dispersion stabilizing theory in which zero potential is used to explain that as two particles approach one another their ionic atmospheres begin to overlap and a repulsion force is developed [3]. The theory explains the aggregation of aqueous dispersions quantitatively and describes the force between charged surfaces interacting through a liquid medium. In this theory, two forces are considered to impact of colloidal stability: Van der Waal forces and Coulombic (Entropic) forces of the electrostatic repulsion due to the so-called double layer of counterions. The total potential energy is described as the sum of the attraction potential and the repulsion potential. When two particles approach each other, electrostatic repulsion increases and the interference between their electrical double layers increases. Meanwhile, the Van der Waals attraction increases as they get closer. At each distance, the net potential energy of the smaller value is subtracted from the larger value [4].

The electrostatic part of interaction, described at DLVO theory, is computed in the mean field approximation in the limit of low surface potentials – that is when the potential energy of an elementary charge on the surface is much smaller than the thermal energy scale, $k_B T$. For two spheres of radius each having a charge Z (in units of the elementary charge) separated by a center-to-center distance r in a fluid of dielectric constant ε_r containing a concentration n of monovalent ions. The electrostatic potential takes the form of a screened-Coulomb or Yukawa repulsion.

Any particle, cell as well, can be presented as a dipole. So, we can speak here about interaction of surface and dipole. But in real situation, it is not just surface of implant and cells. It is also the blood stream around it. Human blood consists of a liquid portion of the plasma and suspended corpuscles therein – formed elements: erythrocytes, leukocytes, and platelets [5]. The plasma fraction represents 55–60% of blood volume. It is composed of water (90–92%) and dry matter (8–10%). Dry matter consists of organic and inorganic substances. Organic substances include plasma proteins that are 7–8%. Proteins are presented by albumin (4.5%), globulins (2–3.5%), and fibrinogen (0.2–0.4%).

The proportion of formed elements make up 40–45% of the blood volume. Red blood cells, which should be at normal blood for men 4 000 000–5 000 000 erythrocytes per 1 μl, for women – 4 500 000 to 1 μl, preferably have the shape of biconcave disc with a diameter of 7.5–2.5 μm periphery in the center – 1.5 μm. They have a lot of functions, including a protective function – adsorbing on the surface toxic substances and participation in the process of blood coagulation due to the content of coagulation and anticoagulation systems of blood factors.

Leukocytes, or white blood cells, are from 8 to 20 μm. The number of leukocytes in peripheral blood of an adult ranges about 4000–9000 in 1 μl. All types of leukocytes in the body perform a protective function. However, the implementation of its depending from various types of leukocytes occurs differently:

(1) Neutrophils, which are from 46% to 70%, the first to come to the damage. Neutrophils exert the cytotoxic effect and produce interferon, which has antiviral effect.
(2) Eosinophils (1–5%) also neutralize and disrupt toxins protein origin, foreign proteins and antigen–antibody complexes. Their content in the peripheral blood is subject to daily fluctuations and it is linked to the level of glucocorticoids. At the end of the afternoon and early in the morning there are of 20% less than the average daily level, and at midnight – a 30% increase.
(3) Basophils contain and produce biologically active agents (heparin, histamine, etc.), and this is their function in the body. Heparin contrary, unlike all of the above components of the blood prevents blood clot in the inflammation. Histamine dilates capillaries that promotes resorption and healing.
(4) Monocyte – largest peripheral blood cells – phagocytose bacteria, dead white blood cells, injured cells tissue inflammation, purified place and ready it for regeneration. They produce factors that increase clotting and also factors stimulating fibrinolysis.
(5) Lymphocytes are central to the body's immune system. They carry out the formation of specific immunity, the synthesis of protective antibodies, lysis of foreign cells, and transplant rejection. All leucocytes are formed in the bone marrow from a single stem cell and differentiated at tissue.

Platelets are flat cells, which looks like irregular round shape with diameter of 2–5 μm. The number of platelets in human blood is 180 000–320 000 μl^{-1}. Also, there are daily fluctuations: platelet are longer in day than in the night. They are able to stick to foreign surfaces (adhesion) and stick together (aggregation) due to various causes. Platelets are also produced in red bone marrow from megakaryocytes. Number of them increases in inflammation, irreversible platelet aggregation.

The relative density of blood – 1.050–1.060 depends mainly on the amount of erythrocytes. Relative density of blood plasma – 1.025–1.034, determined by the concentration of proteins. Blood viscosity – 5 a.u., plasma viscosity – 1.7–2.2 a.u., if the viscosity of water taken as 1. It is caused by the presence of red blood cells and less plasma protein.

A blood, as red blood cell suspension in the protein solution – plasma, is a non-Newtonian fluid as a result of red blood cell aggregation, that is, its viscosity depends on the velocity gradient. The red blood cells aggregate to form a so-called "coin columns," consisting of six to eight erythrocytes, at nonmoving blood. While stirring they are destroyed, after termination of stirring again reversed. When blood flow through the capillaries, units of red blood cells break down and the viscosity decreases.

In almost all parts of the vascular system, a blood flow is laminar – blood moves by individual layers parallel to the axis of the vessel. The layer adjacent to the vessel wall remains essentially stationary, the second layer slips on it, and on it, in turn, the third, and so on. Blood cells comprise central, axial flow, plasma moves closer to the wall. Also into the vascular system, there is a turbulent flow with characteristic twist blood. Blood particles move not only parallel to the axis of the vessel, as in the laminar blood flow, but also perpendicular thereto. The result of such a complex movement is a significant increase in internal friction. Turbulent motion usually occurs in places of branches and narrowing of the arteries in areas of steep bends of vessels.

The zeta potential (ζ-potential) is the potential difference across phase boundaries between solids and liquids [6–9]. Even neutral particles are surrounded by ions and due to this a charged complex is obtained. Liquid with this complex is characterized by the ζ-potential.

In solution, the presence of a result charge affects the distribution of ions surrounding a particle, resulting in an increase in the concentration of counter-ions. The region over which this influence extends is called the electrical double layer. Conventionally, this layer is thought of as existing as two separate regions:

- an inner region of strongly bound ions known as the Stern layer
- an outer layer of loosely associated ions called the diffuse layer.

As the particle moves through solution, due to gravity or an applied voltage, the ions move with it. At some distance from the particle, there exists a "boundary," beyond which ions do not move with the particle. This is known as the surface of hydrodynamic shear, or the slipping plane, and exists somewhere within the diffuse layer. So that is the potential that exists at the slipping plane that is defined as the ζ-potential. The widely used technique for measuring ζ-potentials is electrophoresis. It is possible to calculate ζ-potential by Henry equation in Smoluchowski approximation [8]:

$$Z = \frac{\eta \times U}{\varepsilon} \tag{7.1}$$

where

ε – dielectric permittivity
η – dynamic viscosity of blood
U – electrophoretic mobility.

Because last parameters are flexible, so Z has also nonstable value, but it has a value in a few tens of millivolts [10, 11].

The presence of the ζ-potential on the boundaries of the slip of the dispersed particles forms on them the charges and electrostatic repulsive force, which ensures the stability of the colloidal solution and prevents aggregation. The magnitude of this potential significantly higher in plasma albumin than in other proteins. Since albumin in plasma is significantly greater, colloidal stability of plasma is predominantly determined by these proteins, providing colloidal stability not only of other proteins, but also carbohydrates and lipids.

There are two general processes during the rooting of bioimplant:

(1) overgrowing of open wound
(2) accretion of bones.

The overgrowing of open wound occurs in several stages: inflammation, proliferation, and remodeling [12]. The first stage begins immediately after injury. The wound invariably leads to damage of blood vessels with the development of bleeding of varying severity, from capillary leakage to severe blood loss with the involvement of large arteries and veins. Damage of the vascular leads to the opening of endothelium, which produces procoagulants that binding with platelets causes their activation. The platelet activation, in turn, triggers a cascade of reactions leading to the formation as a result of platelet thrombus. Together with that activated platelets serve as a platform for the coagulation factors involved in the conversion of circulating blood soluble fibrinogen into insoluble fibrin network. The resulting network consists of intersecting strands of fibrin that capturing the circulating erythrocytes and activating more of platelet, leads to the formation of a haemostatic clot. Next, leukocyte activation is stimulated, which followed by coagulation, causes the development of inflammation. Activated platelets and endothelial cells release cytokines that attract neutrophils and macrophages to the damaged area. In the presence of thrombin, endothelial cells under the influence of leukotrienes C4 and D4 synthesize platelet-activating factor (PAF) for assisting the adhesion of neutrophils. Thus, neutrophils are the predominant cells by the end of the first hour and the next two to three days after injury. The main function of neutrophils is bacteria phagocytosis and the formation of reactive oxygen species involved in the "respiratory burst." It leads to the formation of large amounts of reactive oxygen species and destroying nonviable cells and tissues. Unfortunately, this also leads to indiscriminate damage to healthy cells. Upon completion of the function, the neutrophils undergo apoptosis and macrophages removed them during the process that is not related to inflammation. Of all the cells involved in wound healing, macrophages play a crucial role. Activation of platelets, endothelial cells, and other cells in the wound leads to the formation of proinflammatory substances, including fibrinogen. These substances are characterized by many different properties, including increased capillary permeability as a result of damage of the endothelial integrity, and also the attraction of other inflammatory cells. The monocyte migration enhanced as a result of increased capillary permeability and interstitial edema, which in turn are a consequence of the action of proinflammatory substances, thus, the number of monocytes to the end of 1.5 days after the damage reaches a maximum. A wound microenvironment induced transition monocytes into macrophages, which together with tissue macrophages control the wound healing process. Macrophages are central between all cells in the process of wound healing with the main function of phagocytosis. During cleansing of wounds from bacterias, macrophages produce growth factors that enhance endothelial cell activation and are chemoattractants for different cells. Activated endothelial cells have on their surface adhesion molecules, by which new cells are involved by binding to them in the wound healing process. Activation of endothelial cells, the release of chemoattractants and growth factors together are the next stage of wound healing. At this stage of wound healing at 72 hours after the formation of wound fibroblasts migrate to a temporary matrix consisting of fibronectin and fibrin, and proliferate there. They form a wound structure by producing of collagen, the protein responsible for the strength of the wound; proteoglycans, and trace amounts of other matrix molecules. In the third stage of wound healing for two or three weeks after the formation of the wound increases the number of inflammatory cells and begins growing into the area of damage of newly formed capillaries. During this stage, "remodeling," which can last from several months to two years of age, of the collagen fibers are much more organized and connected cross-linked. Thus, in the first 24 hours in a wound dominate polymorphonuclear leukocytes.

An accretion of bones [13] has four different parts:

(1) *Clot formation*: First, the blood is collected at the ends of the broken bone, forming a viscous mass called a clot. A fibers that are the basis for new bone growth form from the clot.
(2) *Filling in a clot by healing cells*: The osteoclasts and osteoblasts, which heal a bone, fill in a clot. Osteoclasts are beginning to smooth out the jagged edges of bone, and osteoblasts fill the gap between its ends. After a few days a granular bridge connecting the bone ends forms from these cells.
(3) *Formation of callus*: Within 6–10 days after the fracture, the bridge of granular cells become bone mass, known as callus. It is fragile and can break under sudden movements. Callus later converted into solid bone.
(4) *Fusion of the bone ends*: After 3–10 weeks after fracture new blood vessels begin to supply calcium to the site of the fracture. It strengthens the new bone tissue. This process, called ossification, connects the ends of the bones. After that, the bone becomes strong and is considered to be healed. It will take about a year for the healed bone to become as strong as before the fracture.

Thus, a lot or processes are going on when an implant is placed inside a real body. However, mainly the implant is covered by protein films.

The electric field from charged surface penetrates the blood plasma on Debye wavelength (λ_D) [14]:

$$\lambda_D = \left(\sqrt{\frac{e^2}{T\varepsilon\varepsilon_0 k_B}\sum_i c_i^0 Z_i^2}\right)^{-1} \tag{7.2}$$

Z_i – the valency of ith ion sort. $T = 36\,°C$. ε (for water) – 74.5. Human blood plasma contains 143 mM Na^+, 5 mM Ca^{2+}, 1 mM Mg^{2+}, 103 mM Cl^-, 27 mM HCO_3^-, 1 mM HPO_4^{2-}, 0.5 mM SO_4^{2-}. So $\lambda_D = 0.78$ nm.

The diameter of protein is about 10 Å [15]. The corresponding thickness of the protein film provides the weakness of field inside this film. Let's compare the dielectric constant with and without this protein films: ε (for protein) = 90, ε (for pure blood) = 85.5 [16]. So, the electrical field will be less, but almost the same.

The field to polarize proteins is equal $E \sim 10^3$–10^4 V/m. However, the field that is delivered by the charged surface at the thickness of the protein is equal to $\sim 10^8$ V/m, which is still enough for proteins polarization. For example, if the proteins are located on negatively charged implants surface, then a negative charge is also on the reverse side of the protein film [17].

There are two main ways according to the technology to engineer the surface charge of HA surface could be employed:

(1) structural reconstruction of HA
(2) induction of EP.

One of the possible mechanisms for surface charge formation is the protons transfer through columnar HA structure (OH-channels) and their trapping in the "frozen" states on the HA surface [2, 18–28]. The charge is inducible on HA ceramics by the proton transport along the OH chains in columnar channels. The

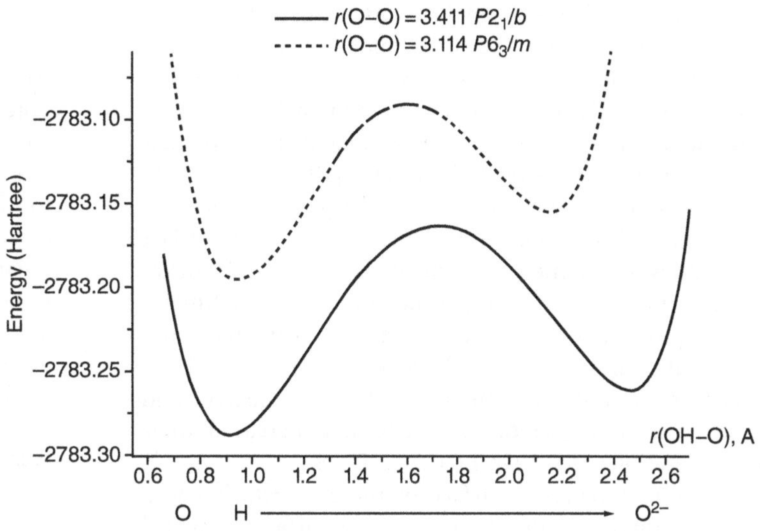

Figure 7.1 Double-wall potentials curve for monoclinic and hexagonal phases. The potential barrier between neighboring proton position in the chain of OH–OH–OH, is high >2 eV, as was shown in the experiment too [18, 22, 23, 30, 31] and calculations. To go through such potential energy barrier proton needs additional energy. It could be supplied by external electric field of the order of 109 V/m, but proton tunneling is possible at 106 V/m, as mentioned above, or by heating up to the temperature of the order of 1000 K. Both influences were used in several experimental studies [18, 22, 23, 30]. After access on HA surface, protons could be trapped and if temperature (or electric field) switches off cannot come back inside sample volume.

calculated values of barrier scan explain long storage of polarization charge, which is observed in experiments. The value of applied electric field could switch asymmetry of double-wall potential and made the proton transfer possible is ~10^9 V/m, but proton tunneling is possible at 10^6–10^7 V/m [19, 23, 29].

Figure 7.1. [19, 23, 29] shows the profile of the potential energy for the direction $z1$ (between the oxygen atoms in the OH-channel) in HA. The distance between the oxygen atoms in the chain for the hexagonal phase is equal to 3.114 Å, for the monoclinic – 3.411 Å. Similar potential energy curves in the direction $z2$ (between the oxygen atoms inside the OH-channel and oxygen of the phosphate group) give different from the first direction the energy barrier $\Delta E1$. For the hexagonal phase, distance between oxygen intrachannel OH chain and oxygen of the phosphate group is equal to 3.3 Å, for the monoclinic – 3.069 Å. As it can be seen, the value of the first barrier $\Delta E1$ approximately two times greater for direction $z2$, then for direction $z1$. This means that the proton is much more advantageous to move along the OH channel, than jump through the oxygen atom of the phosphate group.

At room temperature this leads to long proton relaxation time, so, as a result, protons going out on HA surface could be trapped and frozen in this positioning state, and therefore, change the surface charges in local site, or create local polarization.

HA can store a large charge up to 0.1 C/m^2 for a time significant for biological purposes – more than 1.5 months [2, 18, 30] at the biological temperature of 37 °C. Thus, the hydrogen atoms are embedded from the outside surface of HA, which changes its surface charges and electric properties.

In order to initiate the transfer of the proton in these conditions ("switch" position of the proton in double-wall potential and create polarization) to an external electric field of about 10^9 V/m (at room temperature), and with the possibility of proton tunneling or thermalization at elevated temperatures magnitude of the field may be the order of 10^6–10^7 V/m, which is equal to the experiment [18, 30, 32]. To initiate the transfer of the proton in these conditions or, how it is possible to say, "switch" position of the proton in double-wall potential and create polarization, it is necessary to apply an external electric field at the minimal value about ~0.15–0.22 eV [19, 23]. Such an effect is due to the quantum properties of protons and the quantum effect of proton energy splitting and tunneling, described in details in [32–34].

As a result, proton can move between these two states under energy barrier of double-wall potential. The values of these lowest proton energy levels are approximately 0.15–0.22 eV. Therefore, the energy barrier high (for usual thermal activation energy transfer) could be smaller on this value. The time of this switching between two wall position is approximately 9–12 ps, which corresponding to microwave diapason ~50–100 GHz. But this frequency (determined by energy barrier high) very depend from distance between oxygen atoms. For example, at the distance ~2.6 A, these two lowest levels is comparable with energy barrier high, and, therefore proton can be in both two wall at the same time [32, 33].

From other side, it was known that for hexagonal disordered HA the distance between two close oxygen atoms could be very small up to r = 2.7 A [23]. So, in this case, proton can move easily through barrier by tunneling effect.

Experiments of the polarization of hydroxyapatite ceramics have shown that it can be obtained by a very large surface charge Q_p (up to 14.9–15 μC/cm^2 [18, 30]). Very important point is that it was also shown that the polarization charge is to maintain sufficient time for medical use about 6.4×10^8 seconds [18, 30]. From the other side, in several works was obtained the estimated value of HA surface polarization ~$0.1\ C/m^2 = 10\ \mu C/cm$ influences movement of living cells and leads to their adhesion on the charged HA surface [19–21, 35]. It was also found that the polarization charge was large and long enough to enhance the biological reactivity of HA ceramics for biomedical implants [2, 18, 19, 30]. EP of the surface could be employed to control attachment. Such procedure enhances attachment of osteoblast and generation of tissue [35–37]. The negatively charged HA surface in contrast with the uncharged one attached 10 times more osteoblastic cells and increased their proliferation capacity in 1.6 time [35–38].

To functionalize a surface of the HA, which has a direct contact to the human cells, a surface electrical charge deposition has also been achieved by means of hydrogenation technology [24, 36, 37, 39]. The engineered charge was estimated from measurements of the photoelectron emission work function [37, 40, 41]. For example, the above increment of φ had an effect on the differentiation of mesenchymal stromal cell pool (MSCP) immobilized on the calcium phosphate (CP) coatings. *In vivo* experiments (BALB/c mice) demonstrated that hydrogenation of CP coatings could effect MSCP differentiation into fibroblasts or osteoblasts. The technique of intracellular ribonucleic acid (RNA) staining detected the actively synthesizing osteoblasts and bone marrow stromal cells [37]. We must only remark here, that CP is different from HA with variation of Ca content and changes of hydroxyl group or water molecules [17, 42].

An induction of EP can be employed by:

(a) *Temperature*: Temperature influence on the processes of proton transport, because it determined by activation energies through which must go protons. As it was shown above theoretically investigated proton transfer along a chain of OH-ions in the structure of the HA and detailed calculations of the potential energy profile, carried out in [19, 23, 24] have shown that at room temperature, the energy barrier of the order $f \sim 0.68–0.84$ eV. This is close to the experimental ~0.72–0.89 eV [18, 30] and corresponds to maintain long-term stability of the polarized state. To overcome the energy barrier it is not enough, needs also temperature ~1500 °C. The HA unit cell contains PO_4 tetrahedra and OH groups formed by covalent P—O and H—O bonds. Ca ions play a role for connecting the PO_4 tetrahedra and OH groups in an ionic character of bonding. It is found that OH^- vacancies with accompanying H^+ vacancies are dominantly formed and that their spontaneous formation takes place at temperatures above 1000 K [43]. Temperature could also influences on changes at surface charge of HA. Polarization of sintered HA ceramics by application of an external DC field at higher temperature was analyzed by thermally stimulated depolarization current (TSDC) measurements.
(b) *Pressure*: Another way to overcome the energy barriers is creation of an excessive external pressure. HA specimens were placed in the chamber filled with hydrogen at high pressure [24, 34, 36–38, 44]. The surface was charged negatively.
(c) *Microwave radiation*: The time of switching between two wall position (Figure 7.2) is approximately 9–12 ps, that corresponding to microwave diapason ~50–100 GHz [32, 33]. Therefore, because the microwave radiation with $E \sim 50–100$ GHz induces the proton transfer through double well potential, it is also possible to receive the same results as we wrote above. These estimates are approximate, because they are based on simplified models. But

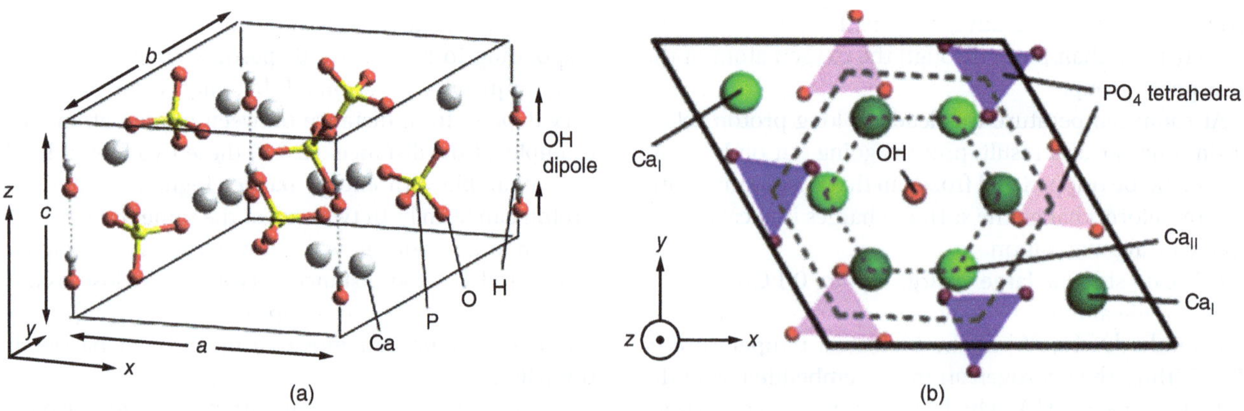

Figure 7.2 Hexagonal HA unit cell ordered structure. All OH groups are oriented in the same direction and are positioned at the four corners of this unit cell, but only one pair in one corner belongs to this unit cell, the other three pairs belonging to neighboring unit cells (i.e. one OH per unit cell): (a) 3D-view of bulk hexagonal unit cell. Source: Bystrov et al. 2015 [45]. Reproduced with permission of IOP Publishing, (b) top view of the hexagonal primitive cell. Source: Slepko and Demkov 2011 [46]. Reproduced with permission of American Physical Society.

in actual cases, it work very well. For example, if we also consider the influence of the pressure on the proton ground state are $E_0 \sim 0.15–0.22$ eV and with width ~0.0002–0.0004 eV, which correspond directly to microwave diapason ~50–100 GHz, as results – we obtain that the application of microwave irradiation with $E \sim 50–100$ GHz could be influence on protons jumping between neighboring minima in double-wall potential and protons could to propagate along OH-channels in HA, and insert most deep into HA structures. Thus, the effect of the charge on the supplied hydrogen amorphous HA structure, first of all, is dependent on the introduced admixtures and irregular structure. Because the structure is irregular (amorphous), we cannot use such an amorphous HA for formation and management of surface charges, especially under influence by protons. It is possible to reconstruct HA by changing its ionic structure: one ion is removed and another one is placed in its position. This is due primarily to the fact that the breach of the periodic structure of the crystal destroys OH^- HA channels through which proton transfer occurs that affects the change of the charge on the surface.

(d) *Electrical field*: In order to initiate the transfer of the proton in these conditions ("switch" position of the proton in double well potential and create polarization) to an external electric field of about 10^9 V/m (at room temperature), and with the possibility of proton tunneling or thermalization at elevated temperatures magnitude of the field may be the order of $10^6–10^7$ V/m, which is equal to the experiment [18, 30, 32]. But, in the case of tunneling effect this switching could be modulated by quantum effect too. The same situation could be in HA during electric field influences. As a result, protons have more opportunity for propagation through OH^- channels.

The attachment of the cell to the HA surface could be controlled both because of the cells' properties and implant surface charge. The latter is available for engineering by means of proton tunneling, electrical field. Alongside doping of HA could be employed that is considered at the following section.

7.3 Computed Designing of Nanostructured Hydroxyapatite Electrical Potential (Structurally Depended Functionalization)

7.3.1 Introduction: Nanostructured HA as Assembled from Nanoclusters

Hydroxyapatite (HA) $[Ca_{10}(PO_4)_6(OH)_2]$ has structural features that define its basic physical properties, charge distribution, and electric potential, which have especially important role at the surface, and is one of the most abundant materials in human bone [26, 27, 47]. Since, it is known that HA can exist in two main phases (hexagonal and monoclinic), which differ doubling of the unit crystalline cell along a particular axis and are energetically quite similar, and also has selected the direction of the formation of the hydroxyl OH groups (OH-channels) along which can place (occur) proton transfer [18, 19, 23–25, 48–54]. Modeling and computational study of the structure of the HA and its possible changes during the formation of the various defects to determine the electric potential of the surface charge density (polarization) and their changes is an important and necessary task for the creating of new nanostructures HA modifications for wide biomedical applications [1, 19, 23, 24, 55–57]. These results of these studies allow us to establish the further mechanisms for the effect of structural changes in the electrical properties of the HA as a whole and on the surface properties of the HA (EP, charges, and polarization). And this, in turn, will allow carrying out purposeful change the structural properties of the HA and controlling its functions. First of all, to improve the efficiency of interactions of the HA with the living bone cells (osteoblasts, osteoclasts, etc.) and thus improve the quality of the input of bone implants [1, 24, 55, 56]. Thus, we get a tool computer-aided design of nanostructured HA having the desired electrical properties given – i.e. manage its surface electric potential and charge density. And here lately it has been developed and applied to various computational methods, including the most contemporary first-principles (ab initio) and density functional theory (DFT) as well the quantum semi-empirical approaches [2, 20, 21, 39, 43, 45, 46, 57–66]. Below, we consider the most important results of these computational studies of HA structures and properties. It is important to note that the HA – in the body of all living organisms – is a biological, rather than mineral material. Therefore it differs from the more perfect crystal structure of the minerals. Its difference from the ideal mineral – primarily stoichiometry in defects, particularly, such as an O and OH groups vacancies, interstitials of H, various atomic impurities, and substitutions of several atoms (such as phosphorus for silicon, calcium by such atoms as magnesium, selenium, strontium, etc.).

It is, therefore, important in all modeling and computer researches and calculations to take into account these effects, and to bring artificially created HA coating to being most close to the biological original HA. Moreover, it is now clear that the influence of surface charge and electric potential of the HA surface on the osteo adhesion of the living cells and their growth, i.e. bone regeneration activity, is very high and important. Studies have shown that the creation of such surface charges (or HA polarization) increases the adhesion of the osteo-blasts cells and to enhance their reproduction and growth. According to [34, 35, 37, 38, 67], it is especially noticeable on the negatively charged surfaces of HA. Therefore, the second important aspect of the computer modeling and calculations of the properties of HA is to build such corresponding models and structural modifications of HA. In this chapter, we consider, first, the developed models for HA NPs, based on cluster approach. And, second, we investigate the following from this model the HA surface charges (polarization) distribution and changes of electron work function in comparision with the obtained experimental data. Third, we explore the HA crystal structure model with different vacancy (H, O, and OH), interstitials, and substitutions (e.g. of Ca) using the corresponding HA cluster models, with obtained changes of electron work function in comparision with the photoelectron emission (PEE) data. Physical properties of HA NPs, which are urgent for nanoscience and nanomedicine, were explored computationally and experimentally [19, 23, 24, 55, 64, 65, 68, 69]. Computer simulation was employed to understand the HA NPs structural, electrical (dipole momentum and polarization – surface charges) properties as by molecular mechanics as well by quantum-mechanical semi-empirical (in PM3 method) in restricted Hartree–Fock (RHF) and unrestricted Hartree–Fock (UHF) approximation, and by DFT methods using HyperChem 7.5/8.0 and AIMPRO code [70–72]. More computational details are described in [2, 39, 43, 45, 46, 61, 64–66].

7.4 HA Clusters and Nanoparticles (NPs)

7.4.1 Formation of HA Crystal from HA NPs in Various Conditions, Size, and Shape Effects

Investigations of the HA crystal growth processes in various conditions show that the main growth units of HA crystals are the initial clusters and that growth proceeds through the accumulation of these clusters, with diameter of about ~1 nm [73]. Naturally, HA is occurring in mineral form of calcium apatite with the formula $Ca_5(PO_4)_3(OH)$, but it is often written as $Ca_{10}(PO_4)_6(OH)_2$ to denote that the crystal unit cell comprises *two* molecular units. The specific feature of HA is that the OH^- ions form inner channels along the *c* axis with various random OH-dipoles orientations at different external conditions, which allows the transfer of protons along this axis under special conditions (e.g. such as increasing temperature and applied electric field with necessary critical values) [2, 20, 21, 39, 64, 65]. Usually, HA has two main distinct forms of the nano-crystalline structures (in hexagonal $P6_3/m$ and monoclinic $P2_1/b$ space group structures) and amorphous. Experimentally, the various HA structures were determined by X-ray diffraction (XRD) method and all these obtained experimental data are stored in special crystallographic databases [25]. The examples of these data are $a = b = 9.417$ Å, $c = 6.875$ Å for $P6_3/m$ and $a = b/2 = 9.48$ Å, $c = 6.83$ Å for $P2_1/b$. Corresponding HA hexagonal unit cell consisting of 44 atoms is shown in Figure 7.2, with the inner OH-channels. For monoclinic phase consisting of 88 atoms, it differs from hexagonal by doubling of the unit cell along the *b* axis and has different orientation of OH groups dipoles. It is important to note that for such ideal crystallographic structures the relation of atoms Ca and P is very strict adherence to the correct stoichiometry, with a ratio of Ca/P of 1.67 [27, 39, 48]. In real mineral, there could be many deviations from such ideal structures, including defects, such as various vacancies, interstitials, and replacements of several atoms [39, 65].

The amorphous calcium phosphate (ACP or a-HA) phase is in the form of spherical grains of diameter ~300–1000 Å, while the HA crystal forms needle-like crystal structures [27, 74]. An X-ray radial distribution study concluded that the a-HA contained definite local atomic order and microcrystallinites (or ordered domains) about ~8.0–9.5 Å in extent rather than a random network structure [74]. The main clusters revealed from HA structures was projected in [73]. Given that the size of these clusters is 0.8–1.0 nm and that their composition has a Ca/P ratio of 1–8. If it is, in this case, it is a $Ca_9(PO_4)_6$ cluster measuring 0.815 nm along the *a*-axis and 0.87 nm along the *c*-axis. This cluster forms close a hexagonal packing in the *ab*-plane. This provides a very convenient explanation for the "maturation phenomenon" in which the Ca/P ratio of apatite gradually increases toward the stoichiometric ratio of 1.67 after the crystal has been deposited. A particularly interesting aspect of this cluster accumulation model is that the stacking clusters along the *c*-axis.

Often considered Posner's cluster (PC) as it appears in crystalline HA has C_3 symmetry [74], $Ca_9(PO_4)_6$, when it is extracted without relaxation from HA (Figure 7.3b,c). It has a layered structure, with each of two parallel layers containing three PO_4 groups, and three Ca's, and each triad forming an equilateral triangle.

Bystrov et al. [2], pick out another cluster, shown in Figure 7.2a,b,d, and undertaken the study of the various sizes and shapes of HA NPs formation under different conditions, particularly with variation of protons or pH of media. The main peculiarity of this cluster is that it has inside the *OZ* axis along *c* unit cell axis, coincided with direction of OH-column and orientation of OH-dipoles. One of the main results obtained by this approach was

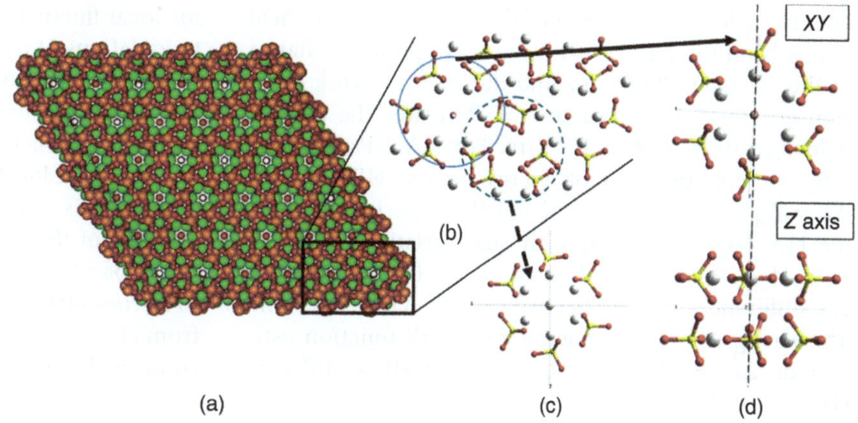

Figure 7.3 Clusters of HA extracted from the hexagonal HA crystal model with 36 OH-channels: (a) top view of big HA cluster with 36 OH-channels, (b) schematics of various minimal clusters extraction, (c) Posner cluster (PC), and (d) minimal cluster with one OH-channel, named as "HAP 3-411."

that the interaction and aggregation of HA NPs must depend on the concentration of bonded hydrogen atoms (protons). To test this point authors performed a series of various calculation of the HA NPs interaction depending on protons.

The obtained results confirm and clarify the mechanism of the earlier discovered size effect of HA NPs, which is related to the electrical properties of HA NPs (dipole moment, polarization, surface potential, and electron work function) [34, 35, 37, 67, 69]. Second, the interaction of HA NPs and the resultant shapes of their growth and aggregation directly depend on the concentration of hydrogen atoms (protons):

- when the pH is high (low protons), the HA NPs interact and formation of needle-like tubes or columnar structures oriented preferably along the OZ axis occurs;
- when the pH is low (high protons), the HA NPs interact perpendicular to the OZ-axis direction to form conglomerates in hexagonal orientation and sphere- or bundle-like shapes.

The obtained data could serve as a background for studies of the intrinsic formation of various shapes of HA following precipitation from various aqueous solutions [1, 2, 68, 75, 76] and in-body solutions.

7.4.2 Main Features of Electrical Field, Charges, and Potential Inside and Outside of HA Surface

Other important results in [2] were connected with the obtained changes of dipole moments, polarizations, and electrical field, as well as forbidden zone energy and work function changes. First, it is worth noting that the emerging dipole moment's orientation has a certain variation. Second, it is seen that the component Dy, especially in the presence of saturated dangling hydrogen bonds with additional H (protons), has expressed an orientation to the plane XOY and rise of dipole moment D with sizes [2]:

- The electron energy band structures of initial HA clusters computed by PM3 methods correspond well to reported data [28, 46, 53, 59, 63, 73, 74] and obtained values of the energy gap are $E_g \sim 3.54$ eV for fixed PC (C_3 symmetry), $E_g \sim 4.56$ eV for relaxed PC (C_1 symmetry) compared with data $E_g \sim 4.43$ eV [73, 74], $E_g \sim 5.41$ eV for HA NP (C_1 symmetry) compared with $E_g \sim 5.38$ eV for bulk HA [74].
- the computed data show the variations of the energies of the electronic band structures with the addition of hydrogen atoms and variations of E_g (4.02–5.56 eV) and having the tendency for decrease of E_g at the finally filled hydrogen bonds – these data are in line with the experimental measured $E_g < 4.0$ eV [28]. It is very urgent result for practical applications, because the recent study of the influence of electrical charge on HA specimens surface EP on the osteoblast behavior and bone tissue rise clearly shows that the deposition on the HA surface of a negative charge enhances attachment and proliferation of the osteoblasts and rise of bone tissue [34, 35, 37, 38, 67]. Moreover, it was established that the hydrogenation [24] of the HA specimens increased their surface electron work function. Let us look, how it connects with considered model. The obtained value of polarization is $P \sim 0.5\ \mu C/cm^2$. This polarization is essential for this HA NP structure, because it appears and exists as spontaneous self-induced polarization similar to the ordered dipole momentum in ferroelectrics [77]. In this model, the shift of the surface level energy under the influence of the internal electric field depends on the NP size and consequently on the corresponding change of the electron work function for NPs with size variation [2].

There is experimentally established [28] fact that the surface level with the energy $E_5 = E_v + 3.3$ eV gives a major contribution to the photoelectric effect and influences on the electron affinity χ and the electron work function φ. So, the shift of the surface level energy under the influence of the internal electric field depends on the NP size with the corresponding change of the electron affinity $\Delta\chi$ and the electron work function φ. This surface charge $\sigma = P$ creates the electric field $E_{el} \sim (0.28–0.30) \times 10^8$ V/m. For HA NPs with the size $x \sim 5$ nm the shift of energy on the NPs' surface $\Delta E = E_{el}{}^{*}x = \sim 0.14–0.15$ eV. For the experimental data for HA NPs [2, 39, 69] with size variations between NPs of ~20–60 nm and sizes of ~100 nm, the average differences in the effective radii is Δx ~10–20 nm. The change of surface energy and work function estimated: $\Delta\varphi = \Delta E = E^{*}\Delta x \sim (0.28–0.30) \times 10^8$ V/m (10–20) $\times 10^{-9}$ m ~0.28–0.60 eV. This value is close to the observed shift of the electron work function $\varphi_e = 0.3$ eV directly measured by photoelectron spectroscopy [2, 39, 69].

7.4.3 Bulk HA Crystal Structures Design (Infinite Periodical Lattice) and Electrical Potential

In this section, we describe the results of the modeling and calculations based on the initial pure bulk HA hexagonal unit cell model in the frame of the DFT in local density approximation (LDA) using AIMPRO code [70, 78, 79] in combination with HyperChem modeling [71, 80]. The computational details and all obtained data presented in our paper [39]. Using the data [25] were calculated initial hexagonal bulk HA unit cell structure (see Figure 7.2) and optimized data through AIMPRO code. The calculated equilibrium HA unit cell parameters were $a = b = 9.4732$ Å and $c = 6.9989$ Å for pure hexagonal $P6_3/m$ phase, and $a = 18.950$ Å, $b = 6.997$ Å, c = 9.474 Å for pure monoclinic $P2_1/b$ ones. These compare well with data [25, 46, 53, 61, 63].

One of the main peculiarities of the results is that the computed data clearly show that the HA monoclinic phase (with opposite oriented OH^- ions in the neighboring channels) has lower energy compared with the HA hexagonal phase, to value of ~24 meV [39], what is close to similar data [46].

All computed results are in line with the data from other authors: obtained value of $E_g = \sim 4.6$ eV [39, 65, 66] are very close to data $E_g = \sim 5.4$ eV [52], $E_g = \sim 5.23$ eV [46], $E_g = \sim 4.51$ eV [63]. The calculation of the ordered $P2_1$ form (with parallel oriented OH^- ions in channels) has a higher energy in comparison to the hexagonal $P6_3$ form, by value of ~+1.63 meV. These values are not very large, and are within the frame of the usual thermal energy at room temperature of <25 meV. This is a very important result, as it means that all these different phase structures of HA can co-exist at room temperature, and HA can easily transfer from one to another, depending on environmental conditions (and changes of the stoichiometry ratio). This leads to the opportunity for local fluctuations between the phases in space, and to variations of the HA surface profile due to occasional changes of the neighboring phase. Evidence for this fact could be confirmed by results obtained using the atomic force microscopy (AFM), shown coexisting of the double-phase local regions at the nanoscale [81–84]. This problem was analyzed in [77], where the polarization per unit cell of the order of $P \sim 0.0038$ C/m^2 was obtained, due to parallel orientation of OH dipoles, that it is similar to ferroelectric phase and this value is close to obtained from HA cluster models ($P \sim 0.005$ C/m^2) [2]. These data confirm the existence of HA surface charges. Another important remark is that the performed DFT calculation of the electronic density of states (DOS) determines the top of valence band E_v, bottom of conductive band E_c, and corresponding value of the forbidden energy gap $E_g = E_c - E_v$, as well as allowing us to study the influence of lattice charge changes on the shift and changes of the values for these E_v, E_c, and E_g [39, 65]. These results are in principal agreement with experimental data [34, 35, 37, 38, 67], and predict the shift of the HAP electron work function φ corresponding to the bulk HAP lattice charge changes, because the value of φ is directly connected with DOS parameters E_v, E_c, and E_g.

7.4.4 Imperfect Crystal with Defects

Using computed data of HA unit cell modeling by DFT LDA method, it is possible to construct and to calculate the models of several defects in HA structure: O and OH vacancies, H interstitials, etc. For each optimized HA unit cell structure, it was calculated that the corresponding DOS for wide energy spectrum range [39, 65, 70, 78, 79]. Calculation of DOS allows not only to determine the forbidden energy gap $E_g = E_c - E_v$ and its changes, but also the creation of the new additional energy levels, E_i, which are inside the forbidden zone and correspond to modeled defects of the unperfected HA unit cell.

Let us consider the main schematic of the computed DOS structure (Figure 7.4), which presents connections with PEE experimental data. The upper right DOS image in Figure 7.4a presents the DOS structure for the initial hexagonal HA, and consists of several peaks (A, B, C, and D), as well as several deep levels [66], which is in good agreement with the data from other authors [46, 53, 60–63] and by synchrotron technique [45, 66]. On Figure 7.4, represent the computed results from work [45], and all the states, which are occupied by electrons, are marked by "green" color and all the states, which are unoccupied by electrons, are marked by "red" color. When photoelectron excitation is applied for samples with sufficient energy (equal to or larger than the forbidden energy gap, $E_g = E_c - E_v$), electrons can be excited to

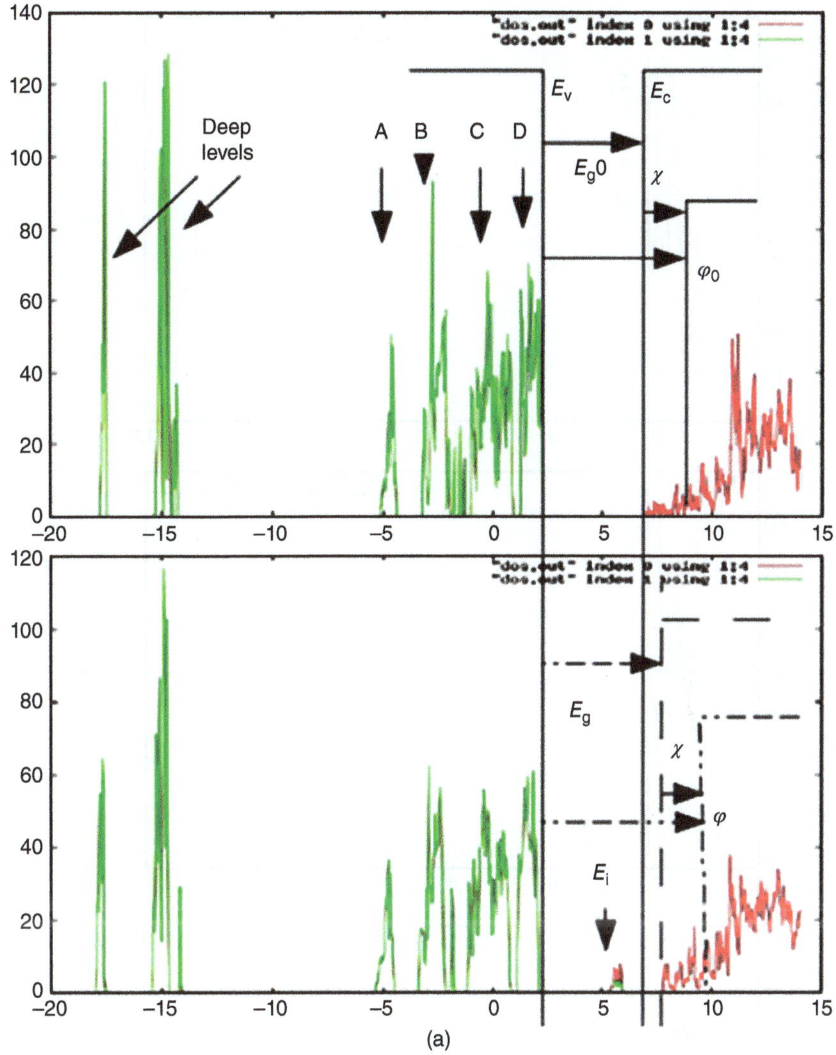

Figure 7.4 Density of states (DOS) for pure HA hexagonal structure: (a) (upper right image) and with OH vacancies (bottom right image = OH vacancy energy levels in the one lattice model); (b) DOS of H and O vacancies (upper and middle), and H interstitial (bottom). Energy scale is shown for the main part only. Green shows energy levels occupied by electrons, red shows unoccupied.

the conductive band. If additional energy is then applied, larger than the electron affinity χ, then electrons with a total energy $\varphi = \chi + E_g$ can escape from the HA sample. This border energy level is the electron work function φ, measured by the photoelectron emission (PE) technique [45, 66]. For further analysis, here introduced E_{g0} and φ_0 as the energy gap and work function for initial pure HA, while for all the cases with defects, the new values are E_g and φ. In the case, if $\chi < \sim 1$ eV [28], the changes can written as $\Delta\varphi = \varphi - \varphi_0 = \sim E_g - E_{g0} = \Delta E_g$. So, the calculated change ΔE_g corresponds to measured $\Delta\varphi$ corresponding to various defects.

However, this is correct only for the case when any additional energy levels (E_i) are absent inside the forbidden zone E_g. If additional energy levels, or thin band, arise inside the E_g, electrons can be excited from these levels too, by photo-excitation, contributing to total electron flow and influencing $\Delta\varphi$ changes. Such a situation is shown in the middle DOS image in Figure 7.4b, where a thin energy band E_i arises inside E_g. This energy level (or band) can also be occupied or unoccupied. The case under consideration is half-occupied (OH vacancy case). It must be stated that an important factor for the experimental observation of such levels (bands) is that the sensitivity of the experimental system be sufficient to detect ones. Because the usual sensitivity of the intensity of PEE is ~5% (ratio of ~0.05), if the ratio of intensity of the E_i peak inside E_g is less than this value, this PEE technique cannot accurately be used to observe such energy levels. Therefore, these results were really on the borderline of what could be experimentally observed, and may not be reliable.

7.4.5 DOS for O, H, and OH Vacancies and H and OH Interstitials

In [45], the calculations of such important defects as H, O, and OH vacancies, as well as H interstitials, by making

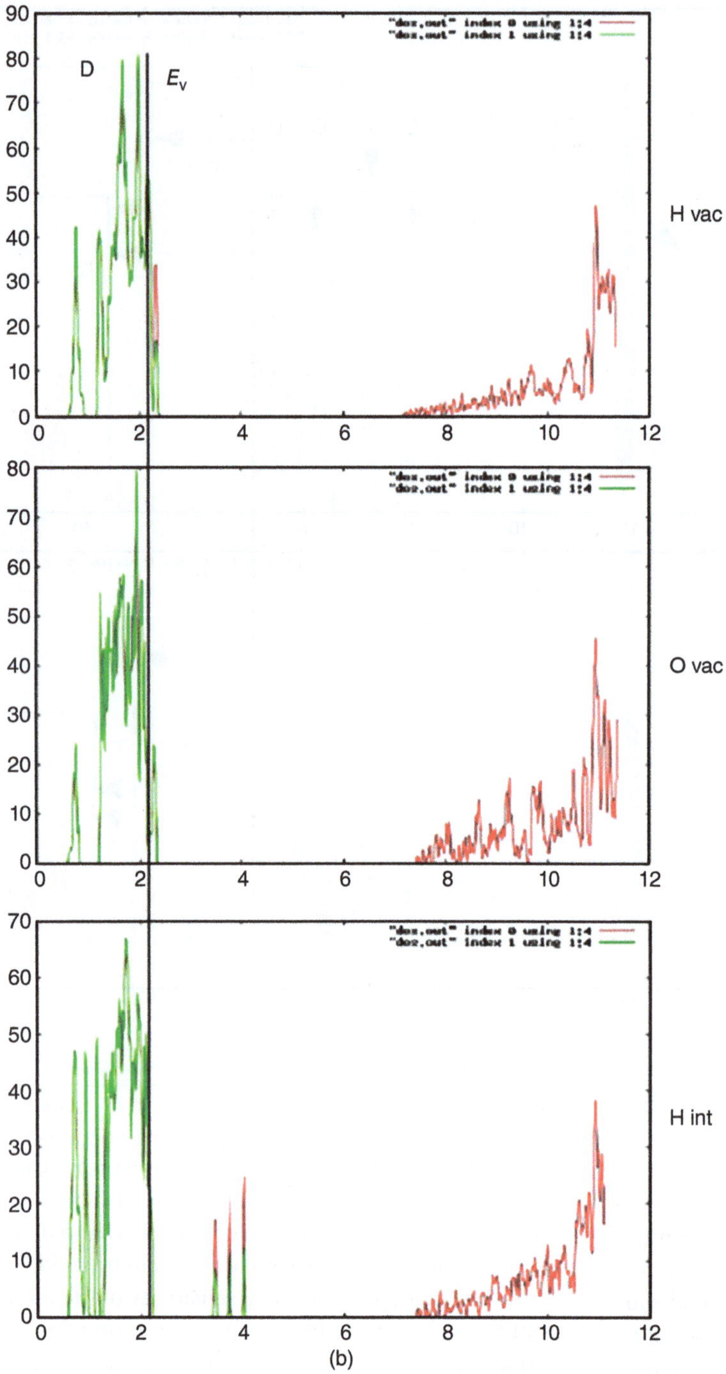

Figure 7.4 (Continued)

the changes of the corresponding atoms were considered. The energies obtained at the level of ~0.1 eV obtained for O and H vacancies are very close to data from [43]. These energy levels created in the forbidden zone are very close to the top of the valence band, while OH vacancies form a wider trapped band (with several peak levels), placed in the middle of the E_g: $E_i = {\sim}E_v + (3.11–3.82)$ eV. Such regularity has been recently observed experimentally by using the synchrotron spectroscopy technique [45, 66]. These data are confirmed in [28], which leads to a rise in the energy level $E_i = {\sim}E_v + 3.5$ eV connected with the rise of OH vacancies. Therefore, ***OH vacancy influence is very important***, because it leads to:

(1) A high increase of E_g of $\Delta E_g \sim 0.86$ eV; from $E_g \sim 4.6$ eV for pure bulk HA to $E_g \sim 5.49$ eV;

(2) The creation of trapping levels in the middle of the forbidden band with $E_i = {\sim}E_v + (3.11–3.82)$ eV having several peaks at ~3.40, 3.53, and 3.66 eV, which serve as traps for electrons and recombination with holes. As a result, photo-luminescence could be observed in this case, after preliminary excitation of electrons from the valence band to the conductive band (see experiments with the synchrotron technique [45, 66]).

Another important result of these computational studies is that the H interstitials create three close, half-occupied energy levels with $E_i = E_v + 1.20$, 1.45, and 1.75 eV (Figure 7.4b, lower DOS image), and all with rather high intensity – approximately half of the *D* peak intensity. It means that existence of these energy levels due to H interstitials lead to the opportunity of the high concentration of electrons trapped on these levels. These levels can arise in HA samples after hydrogenation procedures under high pressure or microwave irradiation, and can serve as traps for electrons as mentioned in [45, 66]. So, it could be serving for negative charges accumulation after insertion of hydrogen atoms (protons).

7.4.6 Exploration of Influences of Various Atoms Substitutions in HA Structure and Properties

Based on the previous investigations of HA structures studies, we performed the investigation of the influence on the HA properties the substitutions of the various atoms in the HA unit cell lattice structure in this section. Experimental preparation of HA samples was made as it is described in detail in [39, 45, 65, 66].

7.4.7 Studies of the Substitution Influences of Mg, Sr, and Si Atoms

As was established during this work, based on the performing of the calculations of DOS in the hexagonal HA unit cell (using described above LDA DFT methods), the main peculiarity of the Mg, Sr, or Si atoms as the substitutions in HA structure with these atoms does not create any new electron energy levels inside the forbidden zone E_g. They only resulted in a shift of E_g width value, and therefore a change in the electron work function φ [45]. Because the total energy is increased for the Sr/Ca and Si/P substitutions in HA, it could be suppose that the resulted HA structure could be less stable, and therefore the possible effects could rise the reactivity/solubility, especially with temperature rise. The variations of E_g for the new optimized structures are very small. Thus, these substitutions in the pure initial HA do not have much influence on surface electrical charges.

7.4.8 Studies and Calculations of Mn and Se Substitutions

For the same atomic positions in the HA hexagonal unit cell, substituting Ca atoms with Mn and Se (which are often used in biological HA) were observed that the new energy levels, E_i, which led to a rise inside forbidden zone E_g, in comparison with the initial pure HA [39]. In this case, additional energy levels (E_i), occupied by electrons, arise inside the forbidden zone E_g, with very high intensities (I), which can serve as additional excitation centers during photoelectron emission experiments, making a contribution to the emitted electrons. The resulting electron work function can be shifted to the positions of the E_i energy levels inside E_g: $\Delta\varphi = \varphi - \varphi_0 = {\sim}(E_g - E_{g0}) = \Delta E_g = {\sim}(E_c - E_i) - E_g = E_v - E_i$. Therefore, we can consider from which initial position of E_{g0} will calculate this shift – in comparison to the initial pure HA having E_{g0}, or in comparison with this new HA structure, which now has another shifted value of E_g. In this case, this additional E_g shift is larger, being approximately $\Delta E_g \sim +0.2$ eV.

7.4.9 Combined DOS from Substituted Atoms and OH Vacancy

The most interesting results that were obtained when atom substitutions in a HA unit cell with an existing OH vacancy are considered. The results obtained are presented in [39] (for substitution with Mn and Se atoms). Calculated data shows that the E_g shift is larger for all atomic substitutions (Mg or Sr for Ca, and Si for P), when combined with OH vacancies. The DOS data for atomic substitution of Ca by Mn or Se, with OH vacancies, have more complicated structure with several peaks and band from OH vacancy [39].

Further detailed studies of the atomic substitutions in HA [24, 28, 34, 35, 37, 38, 67, 69] show the following:

(1) simple substitutions changed only E_g, without arising of any new energy levels inside;
(2) substitutions with changes in E_g and with arising of additional energy levels inside it;
(3) complex substitutions in combination with OH vacancy leads to arising of half-occupied energy band.

Finally, all these computed data compared with experimentally measured shifts of the electron work function by PE for several substitutions in HA samples. In this case the computed E_g shift of Mg, Sr, and Si atoms is very close to the experimental data: computed data (with OH vacancy) for Mg and Sr substitutions of Ca atom lies close within the main observed trend with changes of atomic radius [45].

It means that proposed model with OH vacancy influence on such substitutions is probably in good agreement with experimental data for these samples. It is known that in HA samples OH vacancy is presented in high concentration [64, 69, 85]. The data is similar for Mn and Se atoms, the E_g shift (in this case both without and with OH vacancy) being due to the electron excitation from occupied energy levels E_i [45], and corresponding more to the experimentally observed shift of the electron work function.

The values for substitution of Ca by Sr and Mg atoms close correspond to calculations with combinations of the OH vacancy in the unit cell [45]. For Se substitutions electron excitation is going from additional energy level inside forbidden zone and the computed work function shift is equal $\sim\Delta\varphi \sim(E_c - E_i) - E_g \sim 1.0$ eV. All these studies are devoted to the modeling of several imperfections in the initially perfect bulk HA. But for investigation of the HA interactions with living cells, etc., here are urgently needed some studies of initially perfect HA surface models. And further, on the next stage, the studies of the various defects models, which can be arisen in the HA surfaces.

7.4.10 First Principle to Design HA Nanostructured Surface Properties

Using obtained data for optimized HA unit cell lattice atomic positions in first principle AIMPRO calculations, we can constructed the HA crystal structures consisting from several unit cells and cluster models of various sizes for hexagonal and monoclinic phase. The initial lattice unit cell for hexagonal HA structure consists of 44 atoms (Figure 7.2). Several axes and planes of HAP structures must be presented to compare all models with the basic theory [45, 65, 66, 86, 87] must be presented several axes and planes for HA structures.

In recent experiments by AFM using functionalized tips, it has been found that pure HA mineral surfaces are close to isoelectric at pH = 6 with negative surface charge average of $-0.02\,C/m^2$ and varying between -0.0037 and $-0.072\,C/m^2$ [85, 87, 88]. This result is correlated with the considered data for monoclinic ordered HA [43], where it was obtained that the polarization values are on the same order $0.0038\,C/m^2$. Note, that the estimation of polarization is in the order of $\sim$0.005 C/m^2 for HA NPs too [2], and maximal data *0.072* C/m^2 (in absolute value) is close to estimated value for HA crystal structure $\sim$0.1 C/m^2 [2, 19–21, 23, 24] and $\sim$0.149 C/m^2 [18]. Note that in work [89] registered surface charge (0.000 033 C/m^2), which is two orders lower of [2, 66, 85] and four orders smaller than in [18], is very strange, have a doubt of its validity, because is in contradiction with known data [2, 19–21, 23, 24].

Finally, it is worth noting that obtained value of the polarization and the surface charge density ($P \sim 0.0038\,C/m^2$) through the general law of the electromechanical coupling (i.e. the connection between polarization and piezoelectric coefficients, inherent of all ferroelectrics) [90, 91] leads to the value of the piezoelectric coefficient at the order of $d \sim 15.7$ pm/V, which is only twice larger than values $\sim$7.62–8.48 pC/N (pm/V) measured by Halperin et al. [91, 92]. Such a deviation may occur when the magnitudes of registered piezoelectric signals from the different grains with various values of local polarity are averaged [83]. The most important conclusion is that it could be due to negative surface charges distribution with average value in the range of $\sim -(0.0038-0.1)\,C/m^2$. Therefore, we must emphasize here that on the different open HA surfaces arise a various breaking chemical bonds (OH, PO_4, Ca atomic groups), and having different charged states.

7.4.10.1 Super-Cell and Slabs Approaches for HA "Surface-Vacuum" Nanostructure Modeling – Various Versions of the Contemporary Developed Models and Calculations, Based on Different ab Initio/DFT Approaches

To study HA surface properties in more details it is necessary to clearly determinate, which of the surfaces of HA structure is in the focus of the research. As we can see above from modeling of HA clusters, several different surfaces could be presented the HA sample in border with surrounded open space (vacuum).

First, for correct modeling usually consider the several most often used HA surfaces. Various authors use different approaches, but mainly were studied surfaces with Miller indexes (001), (101), and (010), which representing the plane perpendicular to the corresponding direction [001], [101], or [010] [46]. For hexagonal structures often used indexes, including three coordinate axes [*uxy*] in the plane (0001) perpendicular the *OZ*-axis. For example, in Figures 7.4 and 7.5 HA structures with such direction and planes are shown from [60, 61, 63].

Second, various surfaces, corresponding to some layers in HA structure, it can be with various stoichiometric contents and value of ratio of Ca/P can differ from value = 1.67. For example, such situation is shown in Figure 7.4 from [61]. Such structure is very similar and comparative with the formation of HA cluster detailed in [73] and close to the rise of cluster shown in [2].

Third, important feature of HA surface properties modeling and HAP surface electrical field and charges properties calculations by using first principle DFT method is the special presentation of the modeled HA structures as layered *slab supercells* units, where a *vacuum is located* between the layers of forming surface slabs. One of the examples of such approach was considered in [63]. Similar super-cell construction are used by various authors with different DFT methods

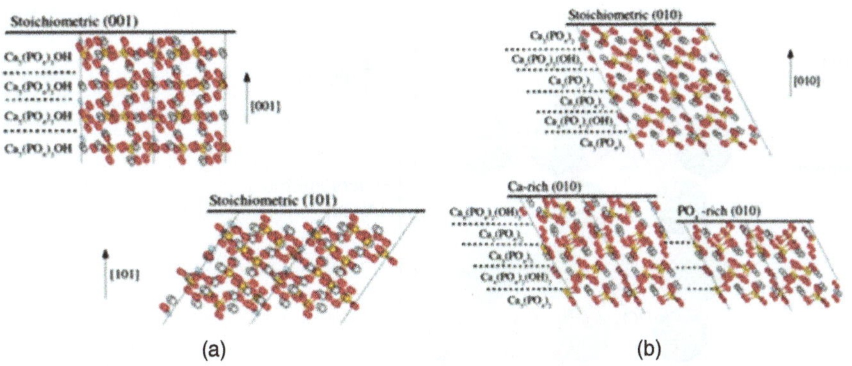

Figure 7.5 (a) a side view of the stoichiometric (001) and (101) slabs. Multiple unit cells of the periodic structure are shown. The tetrahedral groups are PO_4 ions, the large spheres are Ca atoms, and the small spheres are H atoms. For the (001) surface, the $Ca_5(PO_4)_3OH$ layers have been highlighted. Note the orientation of OH ions in the channel, which breaks the symmetries between the tops and the bottoms of the slabs. (b) A side view of the (010) surface slabs. Multiple unit cells of the periodic structure are shown. The layered structure has been highlighted.

of local basis (LDA) [66, 70, 77, 78] and plane-wave (or general gradient approximation: GGA) in VASP codes [46, 60, 72, 93, 94].

It is noted that the only case of hexagonal phase as the simplest case is used to investigated surface properties, because hexagonal and monoclinic phases are energetically close to each other (as it was pointed out in several works [39, 45, 46, 61, 65, 77, 93]). The similar presentation of modeled HA slab structures with the vacuum spaces on surface plane was used in (Figure 7.6) [46, 60, 93].

For most deep understanding of computational approaches and its principal features let us consider first the model from [72]. The used bulk HA has a hexagonal structure consists of layers of PO_4 groups and Ca ions and of OH ions that occupy channels running along the *c* direction (see Figure 7.4a). *Supercells periodic* in three dimensions were used in this models. Three different surface facets were considered: (010), (001), and (101). The surfaces were modeled using slabs cut from bulk HA so that the crystalline periodicity in the in-plane directions was retained. In the normal direction, the slabs were separated from their periodic images by *vacuum layers* of *17 Å thick*, which is enough to make the interaction between the slabs negligible. The *slabs were charge neutral*. Since the breaking of P—O or O—H bonds is likely to be energetically costly, the surface cuts were chosen so that PO_4 and OH ions were left intact. In the (001) and (010) directions, the structure consists of layers providing natural cuts that maintain charge neutrality (Figure 7.4a,b). In the (001) direction, all these layers have the same stoichiometric composition of $Ca_5(PO_4)_3OH$. Note that because the OH ions are aligned in the (001) direction, there are two slightly different (001) surfaces, depending on the OH orientation. In considered slab model, the top and the bottom of the slab have different OH orientations. Here, we must to emphasize that the full similar situation are considered in [63]. The finally optimized super-cell slabs structure for this case have one common and principal peculiarity of the HA – the OH groups formed the OH-channels structure – and each OH dipole orientation on the different sides of slabs OH has different direction.

Let us consider more carefully the model from [61]. For the (010) direction, there are two different types of layers. First, there are A-type layers composed of $Ca_3(PO_4)_2$ that have a Ca/P ratio of 1.5 and are therefore *PO_4 rich* compared to stoichiometric HA with a Ca/P ratio of 1.67. Second, there are B-type layers of $Ca_4(PO_4)_2(OH)_2$ that have Ca/P ratio of 1.75, and are *Ca rich*. These form the AABAAB stacked HA structure so that cutting between the layers yields three chemically distinct terminations (Figure 7.4b). The ABA termination is stoichiometric. Removing the outmost A-type layer gives BAA termination, which leaves the slab Ca rich because the PO_4-rich layer has been removed. Finally, removing the Ca-rich B-type layer gives AAB termination and a PO_4-rich slab. These lead to three different (010) surface facets that are denoted stoichiometric, Ca rich, and PO_4 rich, respectively. These are important features of HA slabs layered structures, revealed various surfaces and such peculiarities were used by other authors too.

Note here that in [61] the construction of surface slabs began by taking single unit cells of HA that had both the lattice parameter and atomic coordinates relaxed and then stacking these cells in the surface normal direction. The stoichiometric slabs had two HA unit cells stacked in the surface normal direction. The nonstoichiometric (010) surfaces were constructed by starting from the stoichiometric two-cell slab and cleaving off layers from the top of the slab. It is noteworthy that the thicknesses of slabs (10–16 Å) are close to that of natural bone platelets (15–40 Å). On the Ca-rich (010) surface, the topmost Ca

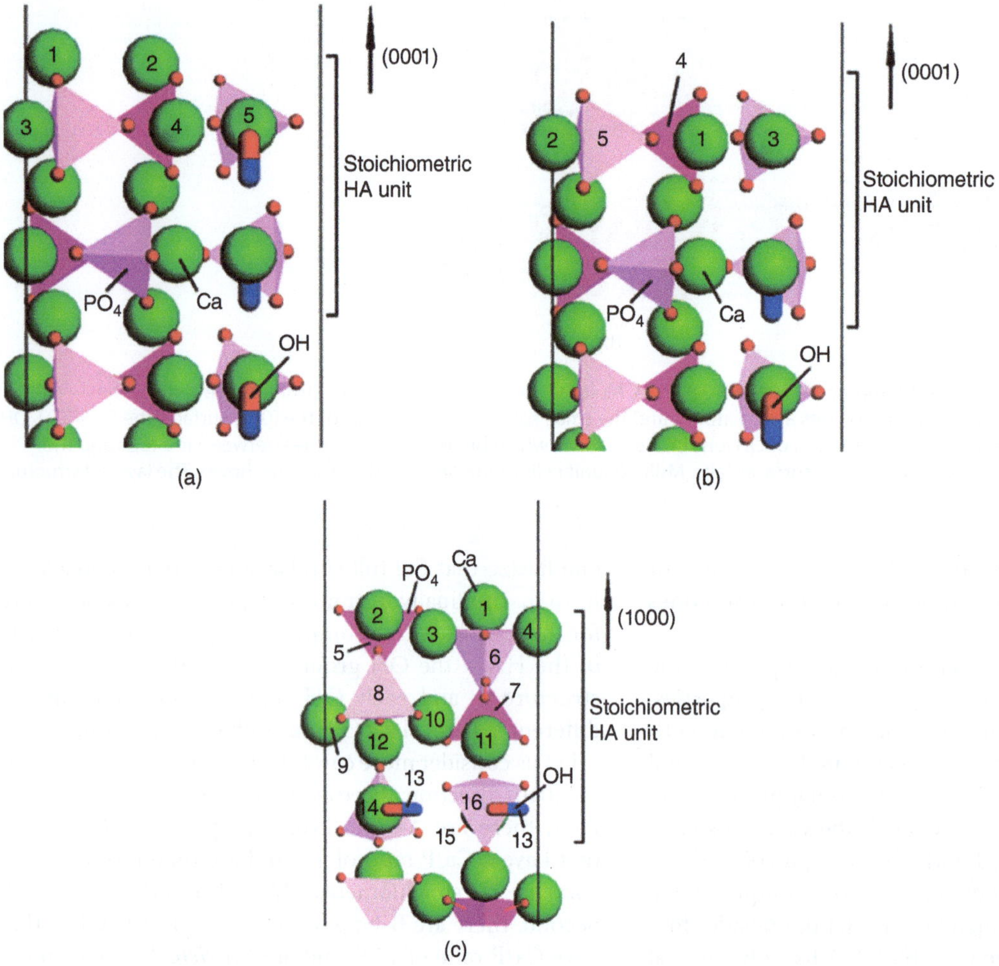

Figure 7.6 (a)–(c) Three prototype HA surface structures. From these three models, we derive all other model surfaces by continuously removing the numbered particles. In total, here are constructed 29 surface models. The classifications of surface models are in Table 7.1 in work. Source: Slepko and Demkov 2013 [60]. Reproduced with permission of AIP Publishing.

atoms can have two different positions. The (101) surface was constructed in a similar way to the other surfaces by cutting a stack of HA unit cells; only one surface cut was found that yielded a stoichiometric charge neutral slab without broken P—O or O—H bonds. With (101), there are again two slightly different surfaces due to two possible OH orientations. Important features are that in all modeling cases authors were used the DFT techniques for the total energies and forces were calculations. For the optimized surface studies they used optimization methods, where the positions of all atoms in the slabs were relaxed using a conjugate gradients algorithm or similar [58, 60, 62, 66], while the lattice parameters in the surface plane were held fixed. In some cases, the lattice optimized too [45]. The similar construction and distinctions between slabs in super-cell models were used by various authors. For example, in [63] the fully relaxed (001) surface models for HA are considered and after relaxation, the cell dimensions for HA (001) are $a = b = 9.4320$ Å and $c = 22.1992$ Å. For the HA (001) model, the symmetry obtained of the two surfaces (upper and lower) is broken due to the orientation of the OH group on the c axis. As a result, the upper and lower surfaces in HA (001) are slightly different. Rulis et al. [63] analyzed here also the shifting and rotation of all atomic positions after relaxation.

But, the key features of the relaxed structure of HA (001) are due to the effects of the different-axis ions in a system. Further, the differences between the upper and lower surfaces in HA (001) are related to the fact that the OH group is a polar bond and thus has a distinct orientation.

Finally, the surface charges distribution was obtained in [63]. It is interesting that from first principles point of view, that HA surface could have various charges, because HA surface has both positive as well as negative charges due to the charged Ca^+ ions and PO_4^{3-} groups. But, it was [63] directly shown that HA surface must be most positively charged in the region of Ca ions close to surface. From other side, the possible surface charges distribution depend also from which crystallographic surface occur at the real HA surface, which may be arranged with negative oxygen ions too. Moreover, in real situation, we have no crystallographic homogeneous samples, but ceramics, consisting from many small micro-crystals with different surface orientations close composed one with another with a stochastic regime. Therefore, this leads to irregularities on the common HA sample surfaces and their surface charge signs.

A similar as in [63] but more detailed analysis were made in [46, 60, 61, 93], using DFT method in generalized gradient approximation (GGA) by VASP code [110]. They were made again similar simulation super-cells with on average of the size 10 Å × 10 Å × 40 Å. These models consist of 15–20 Å thick slabs separated by a 20 Å thick vacuum region in the *c*-direction to suppress interactions between neighboring cells when applying periodic boundary conditions. The surface models are built in a quasi-symmetric fashion to prevent the macroscopic electric fields across the slab. By quasi-symmetric authors mean that the atomic compositions of the top and bottom surfaces are the same. However, as a consequence of the low crystal symmetry, the PO_4 molecules and Ca atoms in the surface planes may be rotated and translated with respect to each other. The deviation from this rule is allowed only in the (001) models, because the OH groups have hydrogen pointing towards the bottom surface and oxygen pointing towards the top surface (Figure 7.5a). In these models, the top and bottom surfaces of each model differ in the orientation of OH groups. Further, Slepko and Demkov [60] studied the surfaces (0001) and (1000) (which are similar to (001) and (100) in another known notation), allowing for both stoichiometric and non-stoichiometric models. By stoichiometric model, here it means that the model slab contains an integer number of HA formula units. The considered surface terminations must keep the OH and PO_4 groups intact. In total, they constructed *29* distinct atomic level surface models. Three prototypes are shown in Figure 7.6a–c. The numbers in Figure 7.6 indicate how they cleaved these models.

For example, removing particle "1" in Figure 7.6a yields a new model, removing particles "1" and "2" yields another one, and so on. From the model depicted in Figure 7.6a, authors deduced a total of 6 atomistic surface models, from Figure 7.6b a total of 6 surface cleavages, and from Figure 7.6c they deduced a total of 17 models. The deviation in stoichiometry from HA bulk is denoted in [60, 93] by a sub-index, where a positive sub-index denotes a Ca-rich model, and a negative sub-index denotes a P-rich model – similar as in [61]. To indicate by how many OH, Ca, and PO_4 formula units used models deviate from the HA bulk stoichiometry and the bulk ionic charge per cell for each model [93]. The bulk ionic charge is calculated by assigning formal charges −3e, −1e, and + 2e to the PO_4, OH, and Ca chemical units, respectively. Overall, the models are charge neutral. To differentiate between models with same stoichiometry here authors used an upper index.

Authors considered a wide range of Ca-rich and Ca-poor models to account for the large Ca/P range of 1.3–1.9 found in natural bone [95]. Authors obtained [60, 93] two stoichiometric models, one with the (0001) and one with (1000) orientation, and have three more surfaces with zero bulk ionic charge. Finally, all models consist of 15–20 Å thick slabs separated by a 20 Å thick vacuum region in the *c*-direction to suppress interactions between neighboring cells. Due to quasi-symmetric it means that on average, the atomic compositions of the top and bottom surfaces are the same. The PO_4 groups and Ca atoms at the two surfaces can be rotated and translated in the surface planes with respect to each other as a consequence of crystal symmetry. The deviation from the (0001) model rule is present, because the OH group have hydrogen pointing towards the bottom surface and oxygen pointing towards the top surface (Figure 7.6a). In these models, the top and the bottom surfaces of each model differ in the orientation of OH groups.

7.4.10.2 Surface Charges and Surface Energy for Different HA Surfaces with Different Stoichoimetry in Various Models

For calculation of the surface energy, various authors used some small different approaches.

In [61] authors, first write most simple equation. The surface energy E_{surf} for a slab of stoichiometric composition can be defined as the energy difference between the slab E_S and the equivalent number of bulk formula units E_B, divided by the surface area *A*:

$$E_{surf} = \frac{E_s - E_B}{A} \quad (7.3)$$

For the (001) and (101) surfaces, which have two different OH orientations, this formula yields an average. In order to define the surface energy in non-stoichiometric cases, Astala and Stott [61] assumed equilibrium conditions so that the chemical potential of each species of ion is equal to its value in some external reservoir. Thus, the energy to create a surface is the energy difference between the surface slab and the bulk, plus the energy to add or remove ions to reach the correct chemical composition. This chemical potential dependent surface energy can be written as

$$E_{surf}(\mu[X_1], \ldots, \mu[X_n]) = \left(E_S - \sum_{i=1}^{n} \mu[X_i] \right) /A \quad (7.4)$$

where $\mu[X_i]$ is the chemical potential of ion species X_i, which can be estimated by using chemical potentials of appropriate bulk phases as references. Using bulk HA, this yields

$$\mu[\mathrm{HA}] = 10\mu(\mathrm{Ca}) + 6\mu(\mathrm{PO_4}) + 2\mu(\mathrm{OH}) \qquad (7.5)$$

At $T = 0\,\mathrm{K}$ and $p = 0\,\mathrm{Pa}$, the $\mu[\mathrm{HA}]$ equals $E_{\mathrm{HA}} = E_{\mathrm{B}}$: the energy of a bulk HA unit cell. Authors considered here several different cases and denote the surface energies of stoichiometric, Ca-rich, and PO_4-rich (010) surfaces, respectively. After analysis of each surface using Eq. (7.4), they concluded that it is possible to write the surface energies as a function of a single chemical potential variable $3\mu[\mathrm{Ca}] - 2\mu[\mathrm{PO_4}] = \mu[\mathrm{Ca_3(PO_4)_2}]$ for an external reservoir that is in equilibrium with the surface. Because the prefactors of $\mu[\mathrm{Ca_3(PO_4)_2}]$ differ: −1 for Ca-rich (010), +1 for PO_4-rich (010), and 0 for stoichiometric surfaces, the relative values of surface energies will depend on this variable. By producing a plot of the surface energies and tracing the lowest-energy envelope, the most stable surfaces can be found. When the surface energies are plotted as a function of $\mu[\mathrm{Ca_3(PO_4)_2}]$ (Figure 7.7), the stoichiometric (001) is found to have the lowest surface energy over a wide range of chemical potential. At high values of $\mu[\mathrm{Ca_3(PO_4)_2}]$, the Ca-rich (010) becomes favorable, while at low values, the PO_4-rich (010) is favored. The stoichiometric (010) and (101) surfaces always have higher energies than stoichiometric (001). The lower energy of the (001) may be related to the coordination of O atoms in the top layer, as shown in [61].

As for atomic relaxation in this model: the (001) surface showed only minor relaxation with the dominant effect being a collective motion of ions in the normal direction, probably to reduce the surface electric dipole. The relaxed stoichiometric (010) and (101) surfaces exhibited a larger spread of P—O bond lengths than the bulk HA. The top OH groups on the (101) surface underwent about 90° rotation to become oriented perpendicular to the c channel direction so that the outermost surface layers are close to symmetry equivalent. Similar detailed studies based on this approach were performed in [61] for water molecules adsorption and Ca atom loss. Important that in vacuum, the (001) surface is the most stable. Another important result is that, it is possible to obtain the connection between surface charges, determined by changes of main charged groups (Ca^+ and PO_4^-), and surface energy for different surfaces and corresponding models of perfect HA surfaces. It is very important for following experimental investigations. The identification of stable surface structures and the role of H_2O adsorption give a promising starting point for future investigations, such as the studies of impurities and adsorption of different molecules. It will be as basic platform for studies of surface defects and irregularities, important for applications and form electric field and electrostatic potential in surrounded media.

Some simplest ways were used in [63], where authors attempted a total of four (001) surface models for HA with different surface cuts. The relaxed total energies of the models with different cuts vary quite significantly, with differences ranging from 0.35 to 2.09 eV in HA (001). However, the one with the lowest energy in HA the same surface cut. Accordingly, they were adopted as the HA (001) surface models. Omitting gross details of other surface models and construction techniques, note that authors adopted the strategy of approximating Gibb's free energy by the total energy from the DFT

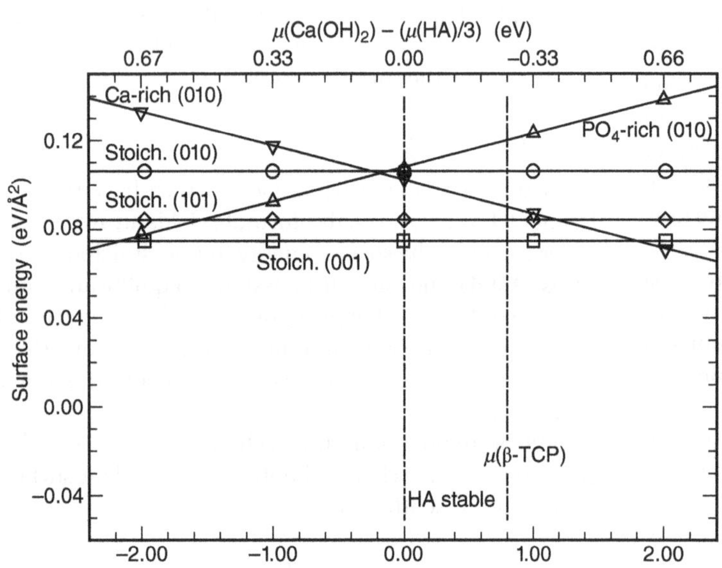

Figure 7.7 The surface energies as a function of $Ca_3(PO_4)_2$ chemical potential in vacuum: squares, stoichiometric (001); circles, stoichiometric (010); diamonds, stoichiometric (101); up triangles, PO_4-rich (010); and down triangles, Ca-rich (010). For the (001) and (101) surfaces, the energy is the average over two OH polarizations. The top *x*-axis shows the corresponding $Ca(OH)_2$ chemical potential, calculated using Eq. (7.5).

calculation [63] and finally have calculated the average formation energies of the two surfaces in reaction. The resulted calculated surface energy for HA (001) according to [63] is in average 0.871 J/m^2 = 0.0544 eV/Å^2, that is somewhat lower than in [61] and more lower than in the similar oxides, e.g. such as in [96] for the measured surface energy of the HA nuclei growing on oxadiazole homopolymer to be 0.158 J/m^2.

In [46, 60, 93] some another way were used. For OH and PO_4 molecules, the energy per corresponding isolated molecule as a reference were used. The calculated formation energy in these works [60, 93] is of −111.7 eV per $Ca_{10}(PO_4)_6(OH)_2$ molecular unit and it is in line with the heat of formation of −138.9 eV [93, 97]. The surface energy is then estimated as:

$$\sigma = [E_{\text{slab}} - N_{\text{Ca}}(E_{\text{Ca}} + \widetilde{\mu}_{\text{Ca}}) - N_{\text{OH}}(E_{\text{OH}} + \widetilde{\mu}_{\text{OH}}) - N_{\text{PO}_4}(E_{\text{PO}_4} + \widetilde{\mu}_{\text{PO}_4})]/2A \quad (7.6)$$

The range of chemical potentials is determined by relation $10\widetilde{\mu}_{\text{Ca}} + 2\widetilde{\mu}_{\text{OH}} + 6\widetilde{\mu}_{\text{PO}_4} = -E_f, -E_f < \widetilde{\mu}_i < 0$, similar to (7.5). With these boundary conditions, authors calculated the surface energy (Figure 7.8a) [60, 93].

With increasing ionic charge and the deviation from bulk stoichiometry the surface energy increases. The large ionic charge [60], indicates that the stoichiometry of HA surface layers strongly deviates from HA volume stoichiometry. This leads to under-coordinated functional groups Ca, OH, and PO_4 that while overall considered these models have charge neutral, however, under-coordinated functional groups on the surface creates additional surface dipoles that in turn increase the slab energy.

The obtained surface energy ranges between −0.23 and +0.62 eV/Å^2. To interpret the data authors [60, 93] assumed that this is the relative energy rather than its absolute value. Alternatively, the negative energy may be interpreted in this case as the surface being more stable than the bulk, which would suggest etching under the certain choices of chemical reference potentials and therefore unstable under given conditions. The obtained here stoichiometric $(0001)_0$ and $(1000)_0^2$ surfaces have energy 0.055 and 0.076 eV/Å^2, respectively, in good agreement with the 0.075 and 0.105 eV/Å^2 reported in [61], and the 0.054 eV/Å^2 reported in [63] for the $(0001)_0$ (or (001)) orientation. Furthermore, the stoichiometric $(1000)_0^1$ and $(1000)_0^3$ models correspond to [61] PO_4-rich and Ca-rich surfaces, respectively, and resulted surface energies are 0.11 and 0.10 eV/Å^2 for the PO_4-rich and Ca-rich surfaces, respectively. In works [60, 93] were found the average values 0.05 and 0.06 eV/Å^2 for these two surfaces with respect to $Ca_3(PO_4)_2$ and $Ca(OH)_2$. Such deviation between [60, 61] works could be interpreted to difference in used their method of constructing the HA surface.

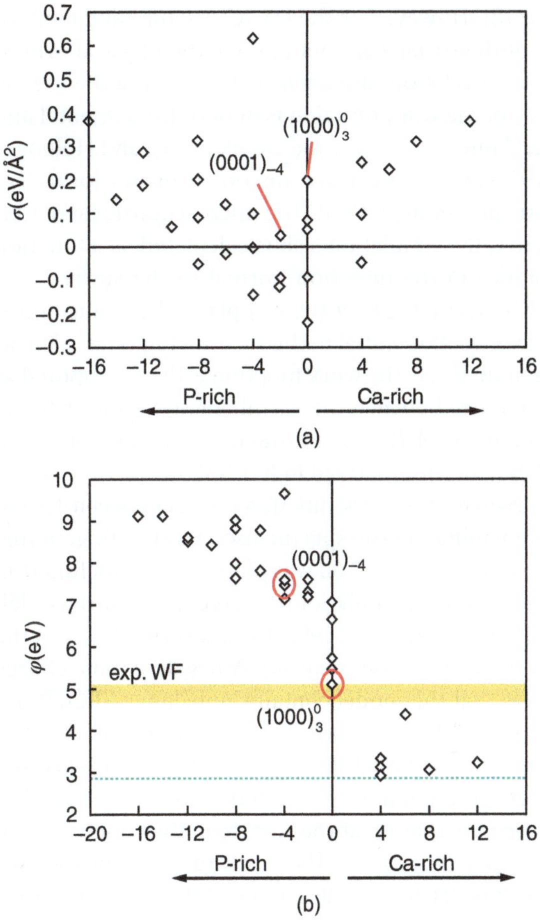

Figure 7.8 (a) Surface energy averaged over the entire chemical range plotted as function of the stoichiometry of the models. Negative stoichiometry indicates P-rich conditions, while positive stoichiometry indicates Ca-rich models. The models $(0001)_{-4}$ and $(1000)_0{}^3$ are most stable under OH-rich conditions. (b) Work function as function of the stoichiometry of the models. Negative stoichiometry indicates P-rich conditions, while positive stoichiometry indicates Ca-rich models. Bystrov et al. [23] point out the models $(0001)_{-4}$ and $(1000)_0{}^3$ which are most stable under OH-rich conditions. The work function strongly depends on the stoichiometry, ranging from 3 to 9.5 eV. The range of experimental work function is indicated by the shaded bar.

7.4.11 The Electron Work Function (from Data of the HA DFT Modeling) to Characterize HA Surface Electrical Charge

The very important question is how the surface structure and charges influence the work function of HA. The work function is one of the key parameter determining charge transfer at the material's interface. In photoelectron emission measurements, the work function is found to range between 4.7 and 5.1 eV [2, 69] and to correlate with the size of the HA particles used for the measurement and with concentration of hydrogen atoms at the surface [2]. However, as the exact structure and composition of the surface are not known, the physical origins of these correlations are unclear. Therefore, a theoretical analysis of the work function is of both fundamental and practical interest. Slepko and Demkov [60] and Hollinger et al. [93] calculate the work function using the local electrostatic potential method. The microscopic local potential across the simulation slab is calculated as a function of distance in the direction normal to the surface (the z-axis) by averaging over the x–y plane. The value of this plane averaged potential in the vacuum region is taken as the vacuum level. The work function is then computed as the difference between the Fermi energy of the slab and the vacuum level. Results for the work function obtained in [60, 93] are summarized in [60, 93].

Surprisingly, the work function ranges between 10 and 3 eV, depending on the specific used model. To gain further insight, in Figure 7.6b was plotted the work function as a function of the bulk ionic charge in the surface slab (note, that as before, this reflects the stoichiometry of the model which is overall neutral). A negative ionic charge indicates that the model contains unbalanced $PO_4^{3-}$and OH^- groups. Positive net ionic charge means that the surface contains unbalanced Ca^{2+}. The plot reveals that the large variation in the work function can be traced to a significant variation at the surface in the concentration of Ca and PO_4 groups. The work function of the two surface models most stable under OH-rich conditions (model $(0001)_{-4}$ and $(1000)_0{}^3$) is pointed out by the large circles in Figure 7.8b. For model $(0001)_{-4}$ was found value of 7.5 eV. Interestingly, for model $(1000)_0{}^3$ were found value of 5.1 eV in the closest agreement with the value [25, 30]. This suggests that it may be a good model for the OH-terminated HA surface described by Sato et al. [60, 93, 96].

Obtained results allow us to make further targeted study for design of nanostructures HA surface with desired electrical properties – charges, electric field and potential, and could control the electron work function. This result is the most important, because, it show direct connection between construction and charges of the surface for initially HA structures and corresponding work function and open the way how it is necessary to change the HA surface, if we want to reach some specific desirable value of work function and how we can to reach this value of work function by targeted reconstruction of HA surfaces.

Finally, we must remember that in this last approach the thermoelectronic work function was considered , but not the photoelectron emission work function. This values differ by shift from Fermi level F on to the valence band top E_v, for excited by photons and emitted electrons. But, it is possible to take into account for experimental conditions and will make the necessary shift of energy. So:

1) Stoichiometry is the main origin to increase in the vacuum-cleaved surface energy. For the biologically relevant OH-rich environment two dominant surface structures, one with the (0001) orientation and one with the (1000) orientation were identified. The (1000) surface has OH groups directly facing vacuum. The surface undergoes major reconstruction to stabilize the OH groups. The estimated work function of HA is found to range from 3.0 eV for the Ca-rich termination to 9.7 eV for Ca-poor surfaces. The work function of the OH-terminated surface is 5.1 eV, in very good agreement with the reported values that range from 4.7 to 5.1 eV [2, 24, 69].
2) The developed models allow the description of properties of HA and design/predict its surface EP.

7.4.12 Characterization of Electrical Functionalization

To characterize the electrical charge/potential both contact and contact less technique could be in use. Both of these approaches are considered in this section. The advanced Eguchi originated and prethreshold photo electron spectroscopy instruments are described in respect to HA.

7.4.13 Eguchi Originated Technique

The method of the lifting electrode (the Eguchi method) [97] was used to measure the surface charge density and EP of the surface. For this the homemade device described in [98] was used for measuring the EP of the surface at the macroscale. This device measures the electric field potential of weakly charged bodies in the condition of high environmental electrostatic field. The measurements carry out at ambient conditions. The longitudinal resolution of the device is 5 mm and the measured potentials ranged from tens of millivolts to hundreds of volts [99]. The resistance of device input insulation is not less than 10^{16} Ω and input capacitance C_{in} is no more than 5 pF.

A block diagram of measurement is shown in Figure 7.9a and the equivalent circuit of the sample with electrode is presented in Figure 7.9b,c.

A charge q is induced at the measuring electrode of device when it installed on the coating with thickness L at the distance $l = 0.5$ from surface. This charge q is compensated by the influx of free charge carriers through a normally closed switch S. The charge equal to q and with opposite sign will be distributed on the capacitors C_{in} and C_l when placing the measuring electrode of the

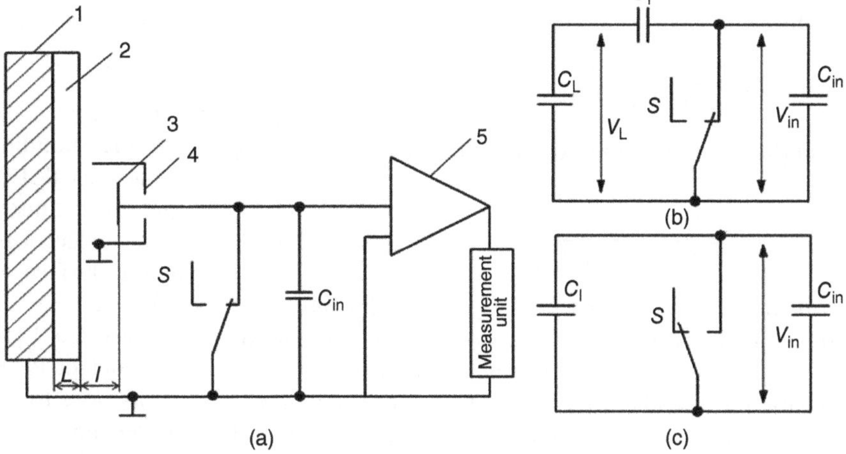

Figure 7.9 (a) Block diagram of surface charge density measurement: 1, substrate; 2,coating; 3,measuring electrode; 4, screen; 5, an amplifier; (b, c) the equivalent circuit of the sample with the electrode placed on coating (b); placed on metallic plate (c).

device at a grounded metallic surface at the open switch S (Figure 7.9c). This charge is

$$q = V_{in}(C_{in} + C_l) \tag{7.7}$$

The measuring electrode of the device is screened from environmental electrostatic field. The surface density of electric charge induced at the measuring electrode equals

$$\sigma_{in} = \frac{|q|}{S} = \frac{V_{in}(C_{in} - C_l)}{S} \tag{7.8}$$

where S is the electrode area; C_l is the measuring capacitance relative surface of coating or metallic surface. Considering the coating as thin plane electret creating the field in the gap between shorted electrodes we can get an equation for density of induced charge σ_{in} [100]

$$\sigma_{in} = \frac{\sigma_{eff}}{(\varepsilon l/L) + 1} \tag{7.9}$$

where σ_{eff} is effective charge density on the coating; ε is the coating permittivity. From Eqs. (7.4) and (7.5), we get the expression for σ_{eff}

$$\sigma_{eff} = \frac{V_{in}(C_{in} - C_l)((\varepsilon l/L) + 1)}{S} \tag{7.10}$$

Electric potential of the coating surface can be calculated by formula

$$V_L = \frac{\sigma_{eff} L}{\varepsilon \varepsilon_0} \tag{7.11}$$

where ε_0 is electric constant.

The potential induced at the measuring electrode V_{in} is connected to the potential of the surface V_L by the expression:

$$V_L = \frac{C_{in} + C_l}{C_l} V_{in} \tag{7.12}$$

where C_{in} is input capacitance of the measuring instrument and C_l is the measuring capacitance.

Table 7.1 EP and surface charge density of calcium phosphate coatings prepared by rf-magnetron sputtering on SS L316.

Substrate	Thickness of coating (nm)	Surface electric potential (EP) (V)	Surface charge density ($\sigma_{eff} \times 10^{-8}$ C/cm^2)
L316	500	0.45	0.79
	600	0.68	1.00
	700	0.85	1.10

EP and surface charge density of substrate SS L316 are zero.

An installation Cathode 1M (Russia) with a radio frequency (rf)-magnetron source (working gas is Ar), with operation frequency 13.56 MHz was used to deposit the calcium phosphate coatings [101]. Plates (10 mm × 10 mm × 0.5 mm) of stainless steel L316 were used as substrates. Before sputtering, all samples were mechanically polished to the roughness with $R_a < 0.1$ μm.

The results of measurement of surface EP are presented at Table 7.1.

The data of Table 7.1 show positive sign of surface charge. So, calcium phosphate coating prepared by rf-magnetron sputtering is insulator and electret. There are different ways to create an electret state of insulator and in this case deal with electric charge acquire by coating during grows in plasma of magnetron discharge. Spectral analysis shows that in rf-magnetron plasma there are the cations Ca^+, O^+, and positively charged molecular ions CaO^+, HPO^+ [102]. The content of calcium and phosphorus within the coating depends on the presence of molecular ions CaO^+ and PO_4^{3-} in the plasma [101].

The problem of estimation of electric field strength in calcium phosphate (with HA structure) coating have been discussed in [103] where external electric field and those inside coating were estimated on the base model of two metallic plates with insulator between. In this case, the strength of the field inside insulator determines by expression

$$E_{in} = \frac{\sigma_{eff}}{(L/l)((\varepsilon l/L) + 1)\varepsilon_0} \quad (7.13)$$

and the strength of the external field close to the surface is

$$E_{ex} = \frac{\sigma_{eff}}{((\varepsilon l/L) + 1)\varepsilon_0} \quad (7.14)$$

In the case of contact of the coating with biological tissue when the distance "surface of coating – cell monolayer" is in order of intercellular spacing $l = 10\,\mu m$ and separation boundary surface coating – cell medium is considered as a capacitor filled by intercellular liquid with a dielectric permeability $\varepsilon' = 80$. The electric field strength inside such capacitor is [103]

$$E'_{in} = \frac{\sigma_{eff}}{((\varepsilon l/L) + 1)\varepsilon'\varepsilon_0} \quad (7.15)$$

Calculated strength of electric field of the coating with thickness $L = 0.5\,\mu m$ and charge surface density $\sigma = 7.64 \times 10^{-9}\,C/cm^2$ at the boundary with cell medium is $E = 5.4\,V/cm$ and potential $V_0 = E^*L$ induced at the cell monolayer is $V_0 = 0.27\,mV$. This value with considering of cellular polarization is in the limit of cell potential. Thus, CP coatings deposited by rf-magnetron spattering are electrically biocompatible with biological medium.

7.4.14 Prethreshold Photoelectron Spectroscopy

To characterize gentle nano-objects/nanostructured materials and to avoid their possible influence on measurements the contact less measurements are preferable, the prethreshold photoelectron emission (PE) being among them. PE delivers low energy (a couple of eV or less) electrons that have a mean free path in a solid that is in order of nanoscale [104–106]. To reach this an energy of the emitting electron should be slightly higher that an electron work function (an energy threshold to escape the electron). In this case, an energy of the energized electron is just several eV [100] and its mean free path (L) in the solid corresponds to the nanodimension [101].

A current (I) of the PE is described by the classical formula

$$I = K(h\nu - \varphi)^m \quad (7.16)$$

where

K – coefficient
$h\nu$ – energy of exciting photon
φ – electron work function
m – power index

For the materials having an energy gap (HA belonging to them) the value of φ is defined as:

$$\varphi = E_g + \psi_s + \chi \quad (7.17)$$

E_g, ψ_s, χ – energy gap, surface potential, electron affinity, correspondingly.

Formula (7.17) demonstrates that the value of φ is directly connected with ψ_s, that is provided by the surface electrical charge. In this connection, alteration of the surface charge density influences the electron emission current I. Moreover, I works as amplifier of φ because $m > 1$ [107].

To detect PE the photon energy should be as possible as close to the electron work function: $h\nu \approx\geq \varphi$. To supply the single photon electron emission mode and to avoid multiphoton effects as well as heating of a tested object, the flux of the photons should be rather weak. This stipulates small values of I. Because of this very sensitive electron detectors must be in use. Typically the secondary electron multipliers that have a noise 0.1–1 electron/second are applied.

On the other hand, the value of I should excess its uncertainty (to reach reliable measurements) that is minimally equal to $I^{1/2}$ as the current obeys the Poisson statistics. For the reasonable <10% uncertainty, if the current measurement unit is electron/second:

$$I^{1/2}/I < 0.1 \quad \text{or} \quad I > 10^2 \text{ electron/second}$$

The value of ψ_s could be effected by ions/dipoles sorption/desorption on/from an emitter surface. This asks for stable and "passive" environment (preferably vacuum; 10^{-2} to 10^{-7} Pa [105, 106]) for electron emission measurements.

Typically the surface of the emitter is not uniform in sense of φ. As a result, a contact potential difference is induced between the surface areas. This decreases/increases I from the places with lower/higher φ, correspondingly [104]. In fact, when characterization of φ distribution is the aim of measurements, their results could become false. To avoid this, an external compensating electrical field $\sim 10^{2-3}$ V/cm directed from the surface to the detector should be provided [107].

To select the photon energy, the eligible monochromator should be provided, too.

To characterize nano-objects PE technique has some limitations:

Geometrical limitation: As a priori condition, a mean free path of the emitting electrons must not exceed a size of the nano-objects. In this case, the energy $h\nu$ supplied to the electron to escape, it should fit L that is placed in a range from 10 to 100 nm. Typically the value of $h\nu$ is around several eV or less.

Charge limitation: Because the electrons leave the surface, it is able to acquire the induced electrical charge.

In this case, the values of ψ_s and χ could be affected. Therefore the emitting charge cannot be very large. Typically the emitting charge is around $\sim 10^{-16}$ to 10^{-15} Q/cm^2 [108] that is just 10^{-15}% to 10^{-13}% of the emitter electron concentration ($\sim 10^{23}$ cm^{-3}). This is below the measurement accuracy and therefore one could assume that emission of electrons does not influence the properties of the measured nano-object.

Quantum mechanical limitation: When the electron leaves the atom, the latter acquires location uncertainty Δx because of the Heisenberg principle:

$$\Delta x \geq \frac{h}{4\pi \Delta p}$$

where

H – Planck constant, $h = 4.14 \times 10^{-15}$ eV s
Δp – uncertainty of the atom's momentum p.

To ensure that the emitted electron escapes from the nano-object, the size of the latter should be larger than Δx.

Assuming that the atom had the zero momentum before interaction with the photon, the "bumping" of the atom by the photon increases p until the photon momentum value ($h\nu/c$, c – speed of the light). Therefore,

$$\Delta p = \frac{h\nu}{c}$$

Because the magnitudes of the photon energy should be in accordance with the condition $h\nu \geq \varphi$, and typically $\varphi \approx 5$ eV and one could estimate that $\Delta x \approx 0.2$ nm. However, in some cases, φ could be rather small and therefore corresponding Δx increases.

To identify the value of φ experimentally the following condition must be achieved (in connection with (7.12)):

$$I = 0, \text{ i.e. } h\nu = \varphi \quad (7.18)$$

However, the electronic technique that is in use to detect electrons delivers a noise. This means that never (7.18) could be reached. In this case, the above should be transformed as

$$I \to 0, \text{ i.e. } h\nu \to \varphi \quad (7.19)$$

To get φ the current I (7.16) should be extrapolated to zero from the applied range of $h\nu$. Such procedure could be complicated, if the tested specimen has a disordered/amorphous structure. The latter induces both localized electron states and a tail of the states in the energy gap, the tail connecting the ceiling of the valance band.

In a case of the localized states, the value of φ is recognized as a distance from the highest localized state to the vacuum level (E_{vac}). To detect the localized states, the (7.16) is differentiated as [108]:

$$\frac{dI}{d(h\nu)} \sim N_i(W)N_f(W, h\nu) \quad (7.20)$$

N_i (W), N_f (W, $h\nu$) – density of the states that electron emits from and the density of the states that electron emits to, correspondingly,

$$W = h\nu + E_i - E_{vac}$$

E_i – energy of the states that electron emits from.

The derivation (7.20) plotted at the diagram in dependence on $h\nu$ identifies position of the local states.

When tail is extended from the valance band ceiling to the energy gap the emission current is could supplied both from the tail and the edge of the valance band. However, just the range of $h\nu$ exciting electrons from the tail should be in use to identify φ. To separate the current that is delivered from the tail the (7.16) is transformed as:

$$\ln I = \ln K + m \ln(h\nu - \varphi) \quad (7.21)$$

Because $h\nu - \varphi < 1$ eV (i.e. easy supplied by the experiment) the ln ($h\nu - \varphi$) is transformed as

$$\ln(h\nu - \varphi) \approx (h\nu - \varphi - 1) - \frac{(h\nu - \varphi - 1)^2}{2} + \frac{(h\nu - \varphi - 1)^3}{3} - \cdots \approx h\nu - \varphi - 1$$

and therefore

$$\ln I = \ln K + m(h\nu - \varphi - 1) = \ln K - m(\varphi + 1) + mh\nu \quad (7.22)$$

Equation (7.18) describes the straight line ln $I - h\nu$ at the area of φ. Therefore, the range of $h\nu$ ($h\nu > \varphi$; $I > 0$) should be in use to identify φ, the value of φ being identified from the spectrum $I - f(h\nu)$ within the $h\nu$ range obeying the condition (7.22).

To get the value of φ(4.15) could be written after the differentiating as

$$\frac{I}{dI/d(h\nu)} = \frac{1}{m}(h\nu - \varphi) \quad (7.23)$$

Because $h\nu$ is close to $\varphi dI/d(h\nu) \approx$ const. (linear approximation). In this case, the value of φ is available from the linear function

$$I \sim h\nu - \varphi \quad (7.24)$$

Searching for the condition $I(h\nu) = 0$.

The uncertainty of the identified value of φ is connected to the accuracy to measure both I and $h\nu$. The uncertainty ($\Delta\varphi$) of φ could be calculated from (7.16):

$$\Delta\phi = \Delta\left(h\nu - \left(\frac{I}{K}\right)^{\frac{1}{m}}\right) = \Delta h\nu + K^{-\frac{1}{m}} m^{-1} I^{\frac{1-m}{m}} \Delta I$$

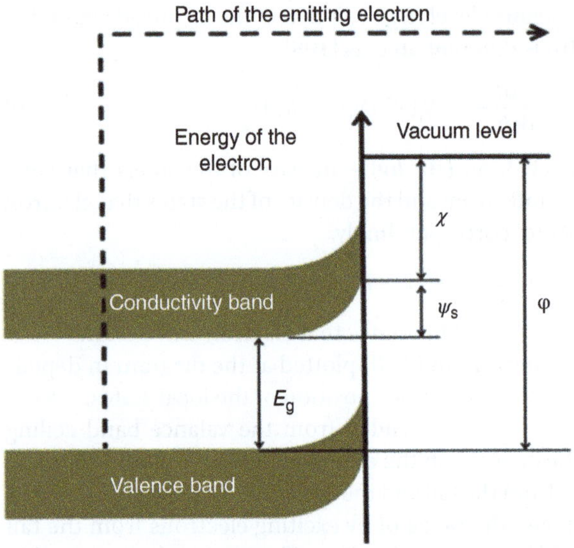

Figure 7.10 Energy diagram for the emitting photoelectron.

Because a number of radiated particles detected at some time interval obeys Poisson statistics the $I^{1/2}$ is the minimal value of ΔI. Therefore

$$\Delta\varphi = \Delta h\nu + K^{-\frac{1}{m}} m^{-1} I^{\frac{2-m}{2m}} \quad (7.25)$$

For example, if $m \approx 2$, the range $h\nu - \varphi \approx 1$ eV, $K \approx 250$ ($I \approx 1000$ electrons/second), [109], $\Delta h\nu = 0.02$ eV (at $\varphi = 5$ eV and the monochromator wave length dispersion is 0.001 μm), $\Delta\varphi \approx 0.03$ eV. Such the value is reasonable because it is close to the room conditions that supplies energy uncertainty ~0.03 eV.

Figure 7.10 demonstrates the example to apply PE measurements to identify φ influenced by the HA NPs size (X).

Both Eguchi originated and prethreshold photoelectron emission techniques deliver information about the HA surface EP. The Eguchi originated instrumentation provides the contact measurements, however the photoelectron emission detection provides contact less identification [109, 110].

7.5 Fabrication of Nanostructured Hydroxyapatite Coatings

7.5.1 rf-Magnetron Technique

Thin films are material layers with thickness ranging from a few nanometers (few atomic layers) to a few micrometers. Today, thin films can be produced by virtually any material for a wide range of applications and in some forms are today used in practically any high-tech product, e.g. semiconductors, medicals, etc. Combining different elements opens for an opportunity to tailor fit the film for the specific application. Development of biocomposites for replacement of damaged sites of tissues is the most intensive field of modern medical material science. In this connection, it is necessary to obtain biocompatible coatings on the medical implants.

A lot of methods are known to produce biocompatible coatings on implants: plasma-spraying [111], crystallization techniques [112], electrophoretic deposition [113], deposition by ablation [114], and micro-arc techniques [115] and there are a number of reviews [116, 117] summarizing carried out by researchers. Every technique has its own restrictions due to insufficient physico-mechanical characteristics or difficulties to control their phase composition. Radio-frequency magnetron (rf-magnetron) sputtering technique to deposit calcium phosphate (CP) coatings have been developed the last decade [101, 102, 118, 119] and can be regarded as very promising because it allows preparing coatings with required quality.

Magnetron sputtering is a technique where an external magnetic field is applied to an object to confine plasma. Ions from the plasma are used to bombard the target and evaporate material. Usually the plasma is sustained by applying a negative voltage to the object and current is drawn through the plasma. There are a number of ways to apply the voltage to the cathode depending on the nature of the discharge: DC, pulsed DC, rf (usually 13.56 MHz), bipolar pulses of various frequencies, and high power pulses.

rf-Magnetron spattering technique is the most suitable for spattering of dielectric target (e.g. made from HA) since the plasma discharge has mostly capacitive characteristics [120, 121]. Practical rfs range from 5 to 30 MHz, and 13.56 MHz has been reserved for plasma processing. This technology uses powerful magnets to confine the "glow discharge" plasma to the region closest to the target. That vastly improves the deposition rate by maintaining a higher density of ions, which makes the electron/gas molecule collision process much more efficient.

The current situation on the rf-magnetrons was described perfectly in the review of Kelly and Arnell [121]. In the basic sputtering process, a target (or cathode) plate is bombarded by energetic ions generated in glow discharge plasma, placed in front of the target. The bombardment process causes the removal, i.e. sputtering, of target atoms, which may then condense on a substrate as a thin coating. Secondary electrons are also emitted from the target surface as a result of the ion bombardment, and these electrons maintain the plasma. The magnets are arranged in such a way that one pole is positioned at the central axis of the target and the second pole is formed by a ring of magnets around the outer edge of the target. Trapping the electrons in this way substantially increases the probability

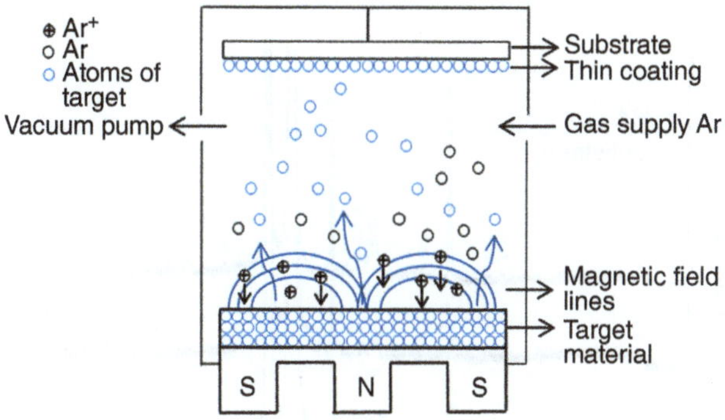

Figure 7.11 Schematic diagram of the typical rf-magnetron sputtering process.

of an ionizing electron-atom collision occurring. The increased ionization efficiency of a magnetron results in a dense plasma in the target region. Sketch of the typical rf-magnetron sputtering process illustrated in Figure 7.11.

The fulfilled works showed that the rf-magnetron CP coating had chemical composition similar to that of HP, high adhesion, and cohesion properties, high biocompatibility. However, process of osseointegration depends on the surface roughness. If roughness parameter R_a is less than 1 μm osseointegration is not observed and the behavior of CP coating is similar to those of bioinert coating. rf-magnetron sputtering deposition is extremely versatile technique that provides the ability to control phase composition, crystallinity, surface topography, and bioactivity of the coatings firstly, by variation of the sputtering conditions (viz, operation frequency, discharge power, working gas composition, substrate bias a temperature) and mainly by changing the sputter target material [122–126].

7.5.2 Engineering of CP Coatings Having Different Morphology and Structures

The following are the results of thorough researches of the properties of calcium phosphate coatings deposited by means of rf-magnetron sputtering versus target and plasma composition as well as different operating modes of magnetron discharge. These materials are based on the results obtained by authors jointly with Maria Surmeneva and Roman Surmenev.

An installation type Cathode 1M (Russia) was used to prepare the CP coating. The following parameters were applied in the sputtering process: operation frequency was 13.56 MHz, working gas argon (0.5 Pa), and incident power of the rf-generator 2 kW. A target was sintered from microcrystalline synthetic hydroxyapatite prepared from a powder with a particle size of 80 nm by pressing at 70 MPa and subsequent sintering at 1000 °C in air for one hour. A coating growth rate was 8 nm/s [101, 118].

Scanning electron microscopy showed that the calcium phosphate coating was dense and free of pores. The elemental distribution (Figure 7.12) and calcium to phosphorus (Ca/P) ratio of deposited coatings were computed from Rutherford backscattering (RBS) data. The Ca/P ratio was about 1.8, which is a little greater than for stoichiometric hydroxyapatite (1.67).

This deviation from the stoichiometric ratio finds the explanation whereas rf-magnetron growth conditions: implantation of Ca ions into the growing coating; phosphorus escaping from the chamber during spattering; phosphorus re-sputtering from the growing coating by impinging particles [101, 102]. The data concerning phase composition obtained by XRD demonstrate the presence only slightly broadened hydroxyapatite peaks, indicating a good crystallinity of the coatings (Figure 7.13).

Figure 7.12 The elemental composition of the calcium phosphate coating of 1.1 μm thickness on a titanium substrate as a function of depth computed from RBS data.

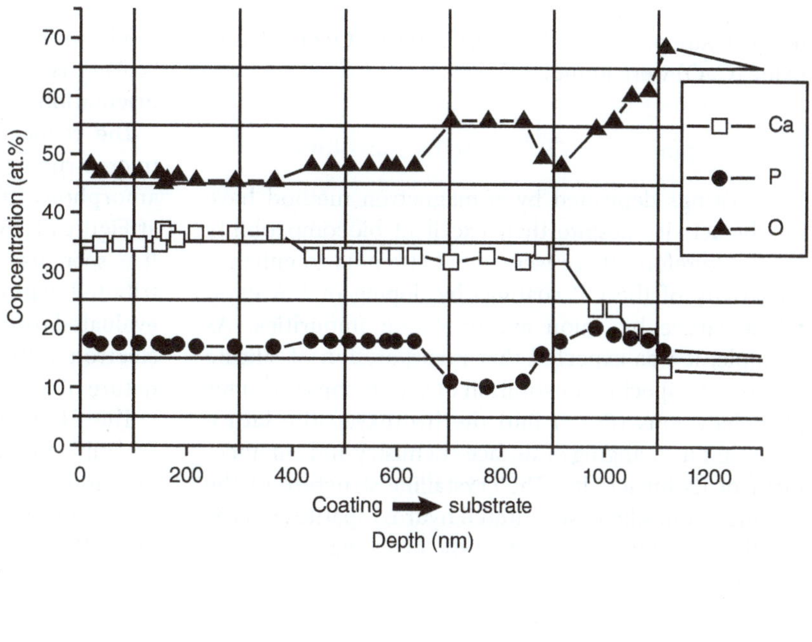

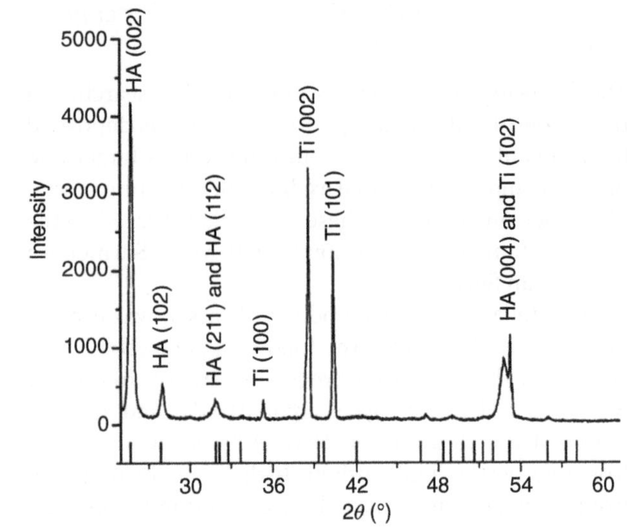

Figure 7.13 X-ray diffraction pattern of an as-deposited calcium phosphate coating on titanium (thickness: 1.5 μm). Besides the substrate (Ti), only HA was found. The peak positions of HA are indicated at the bottom of the spectrum.

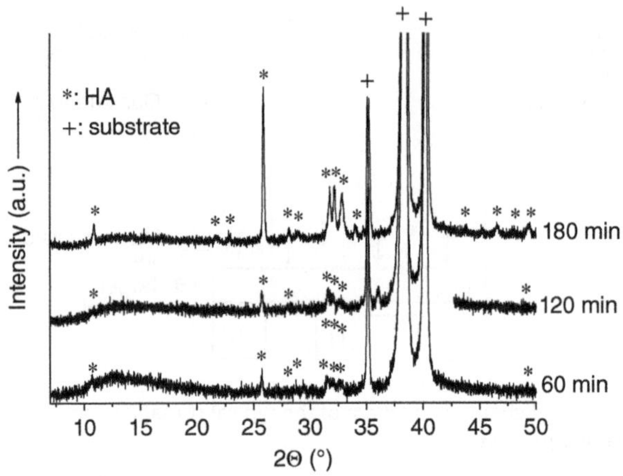

Figure 7.14 The typical XRD-patterns of as-deposited Si-HA coating.

The crystalline structure of the CP coating depends on the power of magnetron discharge [102]. This is confirmed by data [102] with rf-magnetron source 5.28 MHz and different average power density of 30 W (W/cm^2) and 290 W (W/cm^2). The coating deposited at 30 W was fully amorphous in the first hour of deposition and the peaks typical for crystalline hydroxyapatite appeared only after one hour. An rf-power level of 290 W resulted in an amorphous coating until 30 minutes of the deposition and crystallization of the coating to the hydroxyapatite with a preferred crystallographic (002) orientation occurs with increasing of deposition time from 30 to 180 minutes.

Besides the peaks assigned to crystalline HA no other phases like β-tricalcium phosphate (β-TCP; $Ca_3(PO_4)_2$), tetracalcium phosphate (TTCP; $Ca_4(PO_4)_2O$) or calcium oxide (CaO) were found.

7.5.3 Doping of the CP Coating by Substitutions

HA coatings deposited by rf-magnetron method have low bioactivity despite their excellent biocompatibility [127]. Therefore, there were some attempts to enhance bioactivity of the CP coatings by doping of HA crystalline lattice by anion and/or cation impurities. As example, it was expected that incorporation of silicate ions by site-specific substitution of silicate ions (Si_4^{4-}) for phosphate ions (PO_4^{3-}) into the hydroxyapatite lattice will result in changing of surface chemistry and enhancement of its bioactivity. The crystalline structure of the coatings from silicon substituted hydroxyapatite (Si-HA) was the aim of investigations at the first stage.

The rf-magnetron source (5.28 MHz) was used to deposit Si-HA coatings. The target for sputtering was prepared from powder of Si-HA ($Ca_{10}(PO_4)_{6-x}(SiO_4)_x(OH)_{2-x}$, $x = 0.5$) by ceramic technology. The target had a three-phase composition: 12% of HA, 50% of β-TCP, and 38% α-TCP. The EDS analysis has shown Ca/P and Ca/(P + Si) ratios of 1.74 and 1.56, respectively whereas the theoretical molar Ca/P ratio for Si-HA ($x = 0.5$) and stoichiometric HA are 1.82 and 1.67, respectively. XRD-patterns of Si-HA coating are shown in Figure 7.14. In opposition of target which is three-phase the coating is monophase and consists of crystalline HA with crystallites of 33 nm average size according to Rietveld analysis. Similar structure was observed and for pure rf-magnetron HA coatings [102, 128]. The preferred orientation of grains growth is (002) and that is typically for rf-magnetron deposited HA coatings [101, 119, 129]. Observed crystallographic texture is due to the growth of the grains along *c*-axis of HA, which is more thermodynamically preferable. So, the overall energy of the coating is thus minimized by the development of this orientation.

The rf-magnetron coatings are uniform with dense microstructure and composed of crystalline and amorphous phases. TEM-images of Si-HA coating at Figures 7.15 and 7.16 illustrate this affirmation [128]. It is seen also that nanocrystals are non-uniformly distributed within the coating. The average crystal size evaluated from the TEM image is 30 ± 20 nm. The spotty electron diffraction rings revealed the polycrystalline nature of Si-HA coating with amorphous inclusions.

The ED-patterns and determined *d*-spacings closely resemble the structure of HA phase (ICDD No. 24-0033, hexagonal, $P6_3/m$, $a = 9.432$ Å, $c = 6.881$ Å) without any impurity phases. Analysis with a highly magnified HRTEM images (Figure 7.16) revealed that the

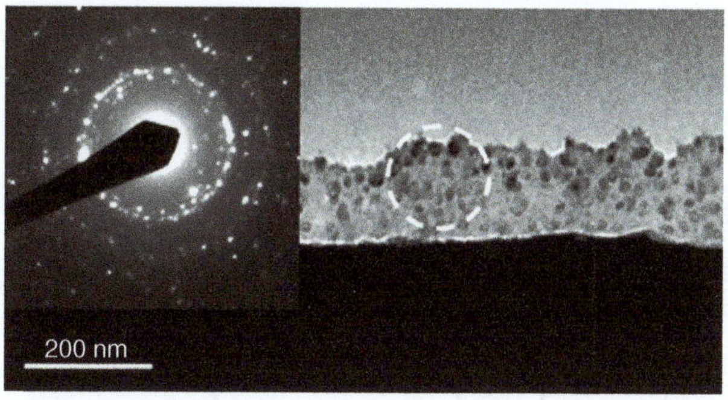

Figure 7.15 TEM-image of Si-HA coating. Inset: ED-pattern.

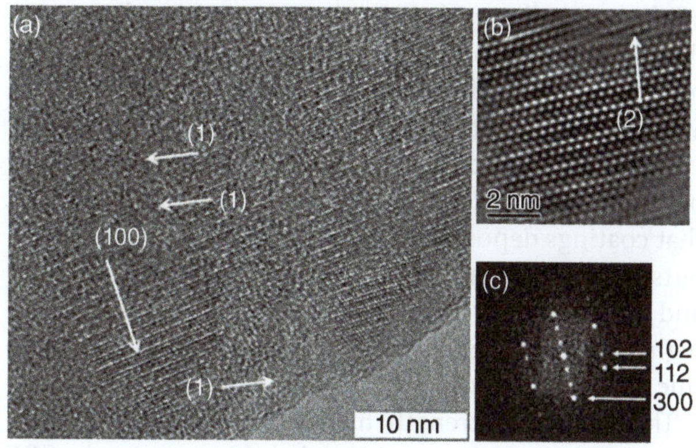

Figure 7.16 A typical HRTEM-pattern (a) of the crystallites in Si-HA coating (the crystallographic orientation [100] is shown as arrows). Insets: a fragment of HRTEM-image after filtering (b) and a corresponding Fourier picture with Miller indices (c). Amorphous regions are marked by arrows as (1), and dislocation is also shown (2).

grain clusters are composed of several nanocrystals which in Si-HA coatings preferentially grow in the same crystallographic direction ([100] is shown).

In Figure 7.16b,c HRTEM images (after filtering) of the layered structure of Si-HA and a corresponding Fourier picture with the Miller indices are shown. Slight misorientations of crystallites relative to each other are visible in the images. Misfit edge dislocations are presented Figure 7.16b. The corresponding Fourier transform (FT) picture of the nanocrystal is shown in Figure 7.16c. This pattern was indexed according to the HA structure.

The effect of cation substitution takes place also. Nowadays, in dental practice there exists important and not yet solved problem – peri-implantitis. That problem is connected with unwanted bacteria colonization in the near to implant site which eventually cause bone marrow loss. Therefore, many of scientific groups are trying to enhance CP coatings with regard to its antimicrobial activity. One of the approaches would be to introduce doping agents, metals that have antimicrobial activity. Subsequently, when coating will slowly dissolve in the body fluids, ions of the metals will be released and become active against unwanted bacteria, e.g. *Escherichia coli*. In Figure 7.17, the most used ions of metals in terms of their antimicrobial activity are shown.

7.5.4 Characterization of Coatings: Physical and Chemical Properties of rf-Magnetron CP Coatings

It was known that implant coatings for orthopedic should have low porosity (≤1 μm), high adhesive property, high crystallinity, and high chemical and phase stability [116, 117]. HA chemical purity should be 95% or higher. Ca/P ratio should correspond to stoichiometric HA and equals to 1.67. There is no predefined parameter

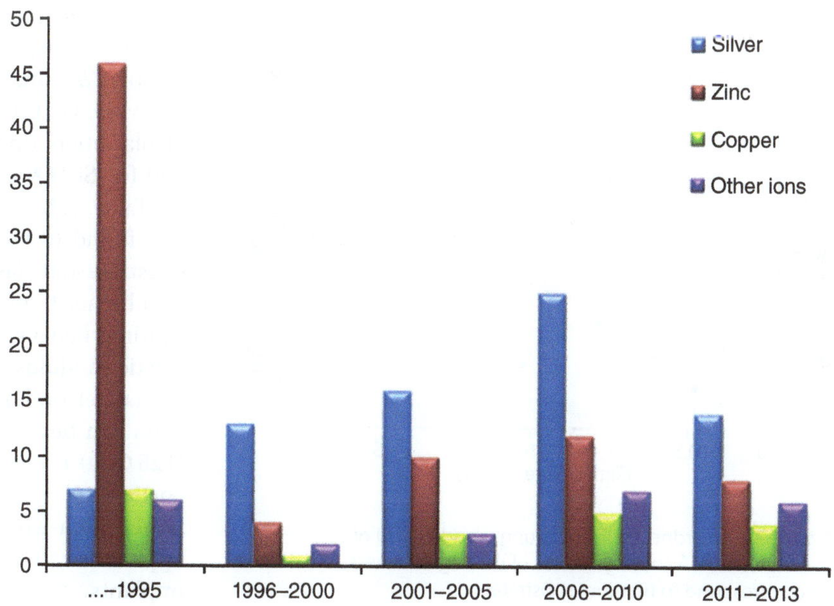

Figure 7.17 Flow chart of the number of publications for the most studied metal ions (silver, zinc, and copper) versus year of publication. The literature search was conducted using web-of-science, with "metal ions," "silver," "zinc," "copper," "periodontitis," "gingivitis," and "peri-implantitis" as keywords. Source: Mostafa et al. 2007 [59]. Reproduced with permission of Elsevier.

of the crystallinity, but in the most research papers, this parameter is on the level of 70%. Variation of the mechano-chemical parameters could be possible with applying different techniques for the coating deposition.

The HA coating thickness and crystallinity increased in proportion with discharge power [117]. It is well known that coatings deposited by rf-magnetron sputtering have outstanding properties with regard to adhesion strength and homogeneity. Due to the nature of the deposition, high level of homogeneity is shown in nearly every scientific report that addressing rf-magnetron sputtering.

The adhesion strength higher than 60 MPa did not change much even after 14 weeks of immersion in SBF [130]. The multi-layered composite coatings had the advantages of high and non-declining adhesion strength and high resistance to SBF attack.

Mechanical properties are very important for long-term performance of implants with HA coating. Hardness (H) and Young's modulus (E) of rf-magnetron coatings determined by dynamic nanoindentation method as a function of the coating thickness are presented at Figure 7.18 [101, 118].

It is seen from Figure 7.18 that nanohardness of a titanium substrate is about 4 GPa and its Young's modulus is 110 GPa in good agreement with known data (http://www.swissprofile.com/data/documents/fiches-techniques/EN/TitaneGrade5.pdf). The nanohardness of the HA coating is at the range of (5–13) GPa (average value is 10 GPa) depending on the coating thickness, and Young's modulus is (100–130) GPa (average value is 110 GPa) (Figure 7.19). Nanohardness (H) and reduced modulus (E) of the Si-HA coatings are calculated from loading–unloading curves which typical patterns Si-HA coating deposited for three hours and Ti substrate are shown in Figure 7.20.

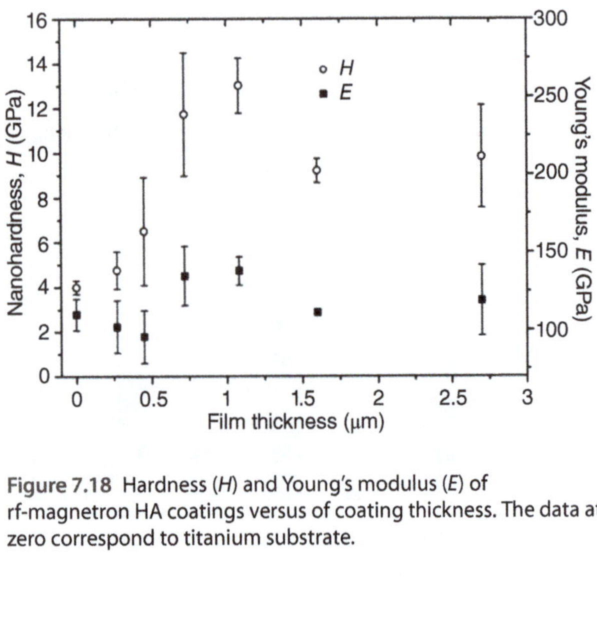

Figure 7.18 Hardness (H) and Young's modulus (E) of rf-magnetron HA coatings versus of coating thickness. The data at zero correspond to titanium substrate.

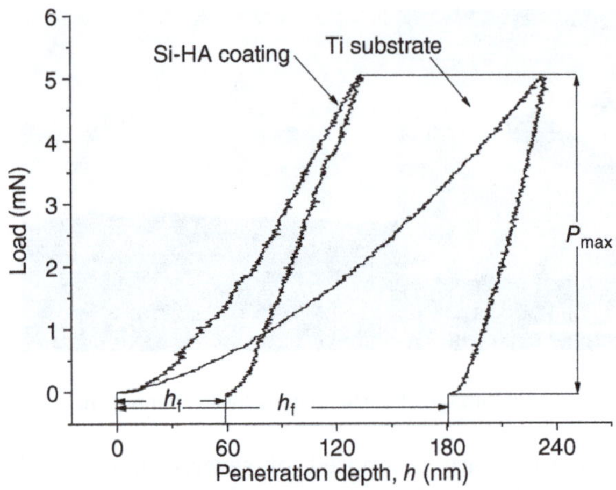

Figure 7.19 The loading–unloading (P–h) curves for Si-HA coating and Ti substrate.

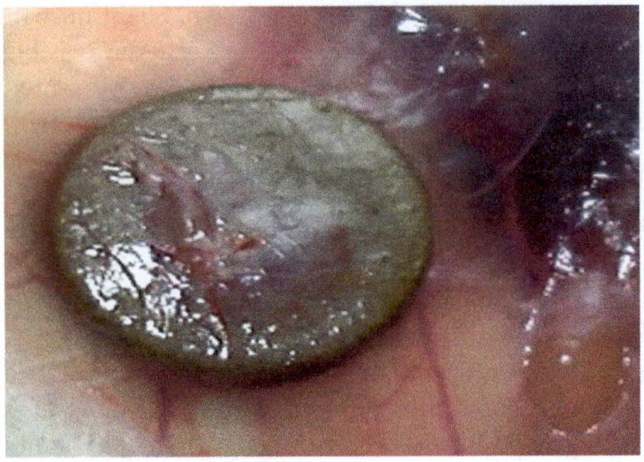

Figure 7.20 Subcutaneous tissue state around the specimen with electrically functionalized (hydrogenated) hydroxyapatite coating.

The values of H and E, elastic strain to failure ratio (H/E), the displacements of a Vickers indenter into the sample "h_f," maximal penetration depth "h_{max}," elastic recovery, i.e. the ratio of h_f/h_{max} and elastic recovery of displacement on unloading $W_e(\%) = [(h_{max} - h_f)/h_{max}] \times 100$ for Si-HA coatings and Ti substrate are presented in Table 7.2. The elastic recovery of Si-HA coatings was found to be 2.67, which is higher than that of the substrate and elastic recovery of Si-HA coatings (62%) is also higher than that of the substrate (43%). The Si-HA coatings had a values of hardness H (11.6 ± 1.7) GPa and elastic modulus E (125 ± 20) GPa closed to that of pure rf-magnetron HA coatings.

As can be seen, that elastic modulus of Si-HA films (125 GPa) is significantly greater than that of a human cortical (E = 7–30 GPa) and trabecular (15–19.4 GPa) bone. Such great difference substantially reduces the opportunity to apply this type of coatings for bone implants.

Table 7.2 The experimental parameters for Si-HA coating and Ti substrate.

Sample	h_{max} (nm)	h_f (nm)	h_{max}/h_f	H (GPa)	E (GPa)	H/E	W_e
Uncoated Ti	240 ± 20	135 ± 20	1.77	4.0 ± 0.3	115 ± 10	0.04	0.43
Si-HA coating	120 ± 15	45 ± 15	2.67	11.6 ± 1.7	125 ± 20	0.09	0.62

The adhesion parameters of rf-magnetron HA coatings were determined by the scratch test method with measurement of acoustic emission, friction coefficient, and visual inspection of the damaged area [101, 118]. The data show that the mechanical parameters of the coatings with a thickness of less than 1.6 μm possess both a sufficient adhesion strength and cohesive resistance. The destruction of the coatings with a thickness of less than 1.6 μm occurred only after its perforation. Vice versa, the mode of damaging of a HA coating with a thickness greater than 1.6 μm differed from that of the thinner HA coatings. The coatings with a thickness greater than 1.6 μm collapsed by exfoliation, splits, and chips along the scratching direction. Cracking and detachment of the thick (>1.6 μm) coating starts at a loading force that is four times less than for thin (<1.6 μm) coating. The effect of the substrate is noticeable if the film is thinner than 1 μm.

7.5.5 The Biomedical Properties of rf-Magnetron CP Coatings

The outcome of implantation (engraftment and rejection of the implant) is mediated through the direct interaction of cells with an artificial surface and secretory activity of the resident and immuno competent cells. The bone resorption around implant occurs in the case of negative development of events and that leads to its slacking, accession infection, and finally the removal of implant.

The problem of bioactivity, i.e. ability to be osteoinductive or osteoconductive is not defined sufficiently for rf-magnetron HA coatings. The numbers of factors determine these properties of the HA coatings: (i) the surface roughness (relief), availability of "cell niches"; (ii) the phase composition and crystalline structure of the coating; (iii) the chemical composition of the coatings, the presence of doping elements. These questions have been the subject of studies [131, 132].

In [131], CP coatings were deposited by rf-magnetron sputtering (5.28 MHz, generator power of 250 W) of targets prepared of pure HA and Si-HA (synthesized by the mechanochemical method) with a silicon content in the target of 4.9 wt%, which corresponds to the formula $Ca_{10}(PO_4)4.28(SiO_4)1.72(OH)_{0.28}$. The latter target was phase containing silicon-stabilized crystalline HA (the Si-HA phase) and tricalcium phosphate. The effect of the artificial surface relief, phase, and chemical composition of the coatings on the response of cell culture and osteogenic potential of coatings in a comparative respect (HA versus Si-HA) was studied with a culture of fibroblast-like stem cells of a light man.

XRD analysis of coating showed the absence of crystalline phases corresponding to calcium phosphates. So, the coatings grown in this mode have amorphous structure. It was shown that "smooth" rf-magnetron CP coatings (HA, $R_a < 1$ μm) have no osteoinductive ability despite the ratio Ca/P is higher than 1.67. The probability of bone growth from a bone marrow column on such coatings is negligible despite their excellent biocompatibility. The presence of silicon in the CP magnetron coating (Si-HA, $R_a < 1$ μm) leads to their transfers from the class of bioinert to the class of osteoinductive materials. One of the mechanisms of the detected effect can be associated with an increased solubility of the Si–CP layer because of its amorphous structure.

In [132], the reaction of *T*-cells of Jurkat line on the direct contact *in vitro* with rf-magnetron CP coatings of two types: pure HA and Si-HA was investigated. Data of XRD-analysis demonstrate crystalline structure of the coatings with a crystallite size about (10–50) nm. Culture human cells line Jurkat tat standardized to 2.0×10^6 viable mononuclear cells per 1 ml of culture medium was used to assess the cellular–molecular reaction on model implants with coating. The viability of cells in the test with 0.4% trypan blue was 90%. The data show that HA and Si-HA coatings have no effect on the secretory capacity of Jurkat cell line culture. Immunomodulatory effect of cultured cells with rf-magnetron CP HA and Si-HA coatings is negligible. Cytokines are the most studied group of bioactive substances whose epigenetic effect on processes and mechanisms of death, differentiation, and maturation of normal and leukemic cells is proved and used in various protocols of immune biotherapy. In this segment of immunochemical reactions rf-magnetron HA and Si-HA coatings are practically bioinert. So, bioactivity of rf-magnetron HA coatings related directly to the level of their crystallinity: increase in crystallinity reduces the bioactivity.

rf-Magnetron deposition method has been realized in a set of installations. The method is able to engineer of HA coatings with different structure, grain morphology, element, and phase composition that provides a wide range of their structural, physical, mechanical, and biological properties. The electrical functionalization of HA coatings could be achieved at coatings formation due to control of the process parameters and application of magnetron HA doped target.

7.6 Biological Properties of the Electrically Functionalized Hydroxyapatite Coatings

7.6.1 Introduction

Biomaterials are rapidly being developed to display and deliver stem-cell-regulatory signals in a precise and near-physiological manner, and serve as powerful artificial microenvironments in which to study and instruct stem-cell fate both in culture and *in vivo*. The ability to better engineer cellular microenvironment as ECM that controls cell behavior, through physical as well as molecular interactions, may further extend our capabilities in engineering tissue substitutes from stem cells [133, 134].

The biophysical properties of the ECM are important to understand the role of blood flow, matrix mechanical properties, geometry, topography, and the transmission of mechanical or other biophysical factors to the cell [135, 136]. The ECM of different tissues (bone, marrow, brain, muscle, etc.) is physically–chemically diverse. To control the stem cells, biomaterial science mimics the properties of ECM.

Besides, the materials applying for the bone implants should satisfy a number of requirements, namely: do not corrode, have the mechanical characteristics close to the ones of bone tissue, not to cause reactions of the immune system, to be integrated with bone tissue, and to stimulate osteogenesis. Various researchers and clinicians consider a biocompatibility and functional activity of implants for osteosynthesis depending to a large extent on processes which take place at the bone/implant interface [137]. Nevertheless, the unified mechanisms of cell and biomolecule adhesion lack up to now.

Fine physicochemical properties of artificial surface (relief, polarization, surface energy, chemical composition) regulate behavior of various cell types (fibroblasts, osteoblasts, osteoclasts) *in vitro* and *in vivo* [126, 138–140]. Van der Vaals forces, hydrogen, electrostatic, hydrophobic – hydrophilic and receptor interactions, adhesion factors (lectin, fibronectin, collagen, arginine–glycine–aspartic acid [RGD] motives, and so on) are considered as possible applications [141–143].

As a result, electrical, optical, electrochemical, and other methods, which common feature is modification of initial surface energy and substrate properties connected with it (wettability, adsorption, adhesion, and so on) have been developed to adapt biological substrates. Electrical polarization of hydroxyapatite (HA) ceramics improves essentially its biological properties [18, 144], which can be important for adherence of osteogenic cells and realization of their potential for differentiation and maturation. Dekhtyar et al. discovered the positive effect of calcium phosphate (CP) surface hydrogenation on osteoblasts attachment *in vitro* [145].

In the present study, an ability of bone marrow stromal stem cells to form the bone tissue on nanostructured and electrically functionalized CP surface was investigated *in vivo* with the help of well-known test of ectopic osteogenesis. Its features are presented below.

To achieve the purpose, nanosized powders of synthetic $Ca_{10}(PO_4)_6(OH)_2$ for manufacturing of surfaces have been obtained by mechanochemical method, which has been described us previously [146]. Electron microscopy (JEM-200CX, Japan) of HA powder showed particles with diameters of 10–40 nm and their aggregates with sizes up to 100 nm. The phase composition and crystallinity of HA nanopowders were confirmed by data of XRD (Bruker D8 Advance).

Commercially pure titanium (99.58 Ti, 0.12 O, 0.18 Fe, 0.07 C, 0.04 N, 0.01 H wt%) plates (10 mm × 10 mm × 1 mm) were used as substrates for the deposition of calcium phosphate (CP) coatings. The specimens were cleaned ultrasonically by Elmasonic S10 (Elma Schmidbauer GmbH, Sigen, Germany) for 10 minutes in distilled water immediately before deposition. The micro-arc CP bilateral coating was prepared in the anodal regime as described previously in [147, 148] using the apparatus Micro-Arc 3.0 (ISPMS, Tomsk, Russia). An aqueous solution prepared from 20 mass% phosphoric acid, 6 mass% dissolved synthetic HA NPs, and 9 mass% dissolved calcium carbonate was used to obtain CP. The specimens were dried in the dry-heat manner with Binder FD53 (Binder GmbH, Tuttlingen, Germany) at 453 K for one hour.

The substrate surface roughness was assessed with a Talysurf 5–120 profilometer (Taylor Hobson Ltd, Leicester, UK). Ten randomly selected traces were recorded for each specimen. The average roughness (R_a) and peak-to-valley roughness (R_z) were estimated.

The part of specimens was processed by application of hydrogen gas at 6 MPa at room temperature for one hour. An alteration of the surface charge was estimated by measurement of the photoelectron emission electron work function (φ). Detection of I was provided in vacuum applying a hand-made spectrometer [149]. The specimens were tested before (untreated samples) and after hydrogenation.

To testify biologically, the untreated (eight plates) and hydrogenated (six plates) specimens were sterilized by dry-heart manner (Binder FD 53, Germany) during 60 minutes at 160 °C. Adequate experimental approach to defining of CP material osteogenic properties is a variant of ectopic bone formation (bioreactor *in vivo*), when artificial scaffold with applied bone marrow is implanted under mouse skin without injection of additional growth factors [150].

The animal experiments were carried out with the approval of Local Ethics Committee of Siberian State Medical University (Permission No. 948 from 9 February 2009). Twenty-eight male CBA mice were used for bioreactor *in vivo*. The specimens tested were subcutaneously implanted into 14 mice under ether anesthesia. Each animal get one specimen with column of singenious bone marrow taken from femur [150].

For stromal cells adhesion the mouse bone marrow was preliminary cultured on the sample surface for 45 minutes in culture medium containing 95% DMEM (Gibco Life Technologies; Grand Island, NY, USA) medium and 5% fetal bovine serum (Sigma-Aldrich, St. Louis, MO, USA). Donor syngeneic bone marrow served as a source of multipotent mesenchymal stromal cells (MMSCs) and growth factors. Tissue platelet growth from bone marrow column is a result of donor MMSCs adhesion, migration, proliferation, and differentiation. In turn, the bone marrow lacunes formation by recipient's macrophages and osteoclasts, and their following colonization by recipient's hematopoietic stem cells (HSCs) migrated from blood occurs in case of bone formation in tissue lamina [151].

Implants were explanted from mice in 45 days, and were photographed. Tissue peri-implant reaction was investigated in mice (Figure 7.21, Table 7.3). Tissue growth was evaluated on the specimens, and it was quantified by histomorphometry. Quantitative morphometry of digital images (8 megapixels resolution) was carried out according to gray levels statistics as it is described early [152] by means of ImageJ 1.43 software. The areas (μm^2) of the bone marrow columns before implantation (see Figure 7.21a) and tissue laminae (see Figure 7.21b) after one were determined.

Specimens with tissue laminae were fixed in neutral formalin for 24 hours. Tissue platelets were subsequently decalcified and dehydrated and embedded in wax, then thin (5–8 μm) perpendicular sections were prepared and stained using with hematoxylin–eosin by usual technique. Besides, intracellular RNA expression was studied on the tissue sections using pyronin Y staining by Unna-Brashe method [153]. Sections from the middle part of the tissue laminae were analyzed histologically by light microscopy at different magnifications and the tissues formed ectopically were evaluated (see Figure 7.23). Standard method of light microscopy (Axioskop 40, Carl Zeiss, Germany) was implied for histological analysis. Digital images (14 megapixels resolution) of tissue sections were done by Canon PowerShot A 630 camera.

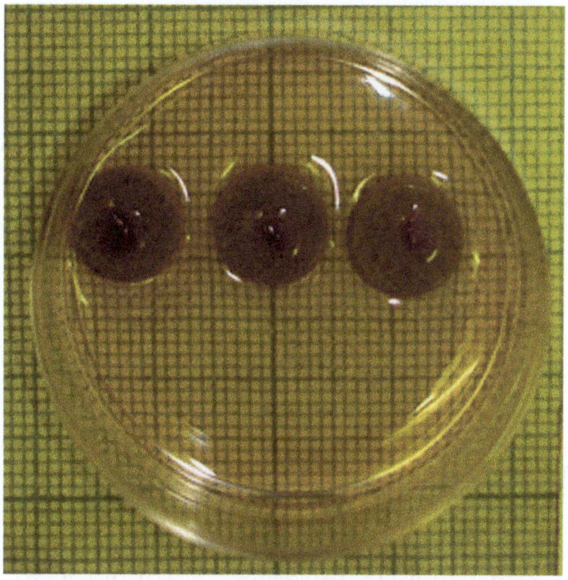

(a)

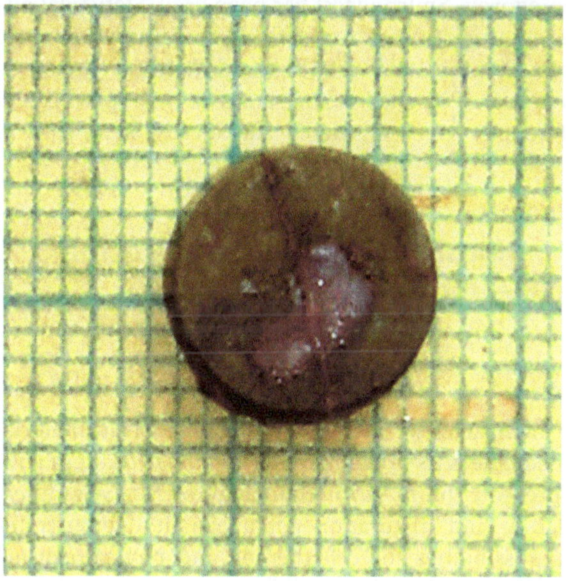

(b)

Figure 7.21 Digital images of donor syngeneic bone marrow *in vitro* and tissue platelets growth *in vivo* for investigation of their areas before and after specimens are subcutaneously implanted in mice, respectively.

Bone marrow, connective, adipose, muscle, and bone tissues were revealed to be potential histological compounds of tissue laminae on CP materials implanted subcutaneously [150]. Bone and marrow formation was considered as positive result of ectopic osteogenesis test. No formation of tissue laminae was observed when or CP substrates or bone marrow fragments were implanted singly.

Data were shown as mean $(X) \pm$ standard deviation (SD) and standard error of mean (SEM). To

Table 7.3 Subcutaneous biocompatibility of nanostructured electrically functionalized hydroxyapatite coatings.

Samples studied	Tissue peri-implant reaction		
	Inflammation	Capsule thickness	Implants cohesion with surrounding tissue
1	No	±	+
2	No	+	++
3	No	+	+
4	No	+	+
5	No	+	++
6	No	+	+

Note: (+) corresponds to grade 1 according to semiquantitative 1 (weak), 2 (middle), and 3 (high-grade) scoring of tissue reaction.

analyze the available data sets a normal distribution Kolmogorov–Smirnov test has been used. Statistical differences were estimated with the help of non-parametric Mann–Whitney's *U*-test (P_U) and Wilcoxon matched pairs test (P_T). Regression analysis was performed. Differences were considered statistically significant at $p < 0.05$.

7.7 Biocompatibility of Nanostructured and Electrically Functionalized Hydroxyapatite Coatings: Subcutaneous Model

The main factor for successful application of any material in medicine is its preliminary testing *in vitro* and *in vivo*. At present, the *in vitro* technology of MMSCs differentiation and maturation got ahead. It demonstrates vast possibilities for cell therapy and bioengineering. MMSCs are capable to differentiate in osteoblasts, chondroblasts, fibroblasts, adipocytes, muscle cells, and hematopoiesis-supportive stromal cells [154]. Nevertheless, a selection of differentiation outcome is unclear in conditions of multicellular system.

It is well known that the *in vitro* results require their obligate *in vivo* verification [155]. The test of ectopic (heterotopic) osteogenesis [150, 156–158] is one of the manners to validate soft tissue biocompatibility and osteogenic features of implants. To study the biocompatibility of the hydrogenated HA coatings *in vivo*, experiments were carried out in CBA mice as described above. Results demonstrated that subcutaneous implantation of samples treated had no side effects of inflammatory and allergic origin (see Figure 7.20, Table 7.3). No blood vessels sensation, edema, and cell infiltration have been shown in peri-implant tissues.

Thin encapsulation and slight/middle cohesion of implants with surrounding tissue were revealed (see Table 7.3). The results obtained confirm good biocompatibility of hydrogenated hydroxyapatite surfaces with subcutaneous tissue.

7.7.1 Tissue and Bone *in Vivo* Growth on Electrically Functionalized Hydroxyapatite Coatings on the Titanium Substrate

The test of ectopic osteogenesis to study osteogenic properties of native and artificial materials is developing since 1950s of the twentieth century. Urist and McLean [156] have investigated this phenomenon one of the first in 1952. They demonstrated a capability of bone organic matrix to form the bone *de novo*.

Osteogenetic features of HA and tribasic calcium phosphate, which are the main components of mineral bone matrix, proved obviously an ectopic osteogenesis phenomenon, when bone tissue was generated on the surface of CP materials. M.R. Urist was one of the first scientists, who described this phenomenon in 1965 [159].

Different specimens of CP materials have diverse ability for osteogenesis depending on their physical–chemical properties (crystallinity, solubility, wettability, porosity, surface roughness, surface charge, etc.). A key combination of biomaterials structure, thickness, and dissolution rate for realization of MMSCs osteogenous potential is not found till now.

Thus, Yang et al. [160] observed ectopic osteogenesis in porous CP implanted in dogs, pigs, but not in rats, and rabbits. Similar data in dogs were presented by Klein et al. [161]. Vice versa, other scientists revealed osteoconduction in conditions of mouse and rabbit subcutaneous introduction of CP materials [162].

Immature bone tissue is forming in one to two months following the subcutaneous implantation of CP materials [161] without bone morphogenetic proteins superinduction [27].

CP roughness effect on its ectopic osteogenic potential was described in [163].

Transplanted bone marrow-derived MMSCs are capable of generating donor's ectopic bone with stem cell niches and of organizing hematopoietic progenitors of recipient origin [164]. Ectopic bone formation through a stage of cartilage endochondral ossification is required for HSCs niche formation in bone tissue [165].

We showed an essential effect of physical–chemical properties of CP surfaces on realization of osteogenous potential of MMSCs *in vivo*. Thick micro-arc CP coatings with $R_a = 1.5–6\,\mu m$ have a three-dimensional (3D) scaffold bone-like topography with a multilevel structure consisting of spherulites, valleys, sockets, and pores [150]. Interestingly, an attachment and differentiation

Table 7.4 An effect of hydrogenated micro-arc calcium phosphate (CP) nanostructured coatings on ectopic osteogenic activity of mouse bone marrow *in vivo*.

	Electron work function (φ)			Before implantation	Tissue plates composition (after implantation)		
Samples studied	Untreated surface (eV)	Hydrogenated surface (eV)	$\Delta\varphi$	Bonemarrow area (A1) (mm^2)	Area of tissue plate (A2) (mm^2)	A2/A1 (%)	Histological composition
Untreated calcium phosphate coatings (n = 8)							
X ± SD (SEM)	–	–	–	4.82 ± 2.17 (1.26)	8.25 ± 2.87 (1.66) $P_T = 0.04$	179 ± 32 (18)	Connective tissue in five cases; connective tissue with muscular fibers in two cases; bone with marrow in one case
Electrically functionalized calcium phosphate coatings (n = 6)							
1	5.200	5.287	0.087	4.91	19.62	400	Connective tissue, muscular fibers
2	5.199	5.160	−0.039	6.07	17.54	289	Bone tissue, bone marrow; actively RNA synthesized osteoblasts and osteoclasts
3	5.209	5.335	0.126	8.65	12.12	140	Bone tissue, connective tissue; actively RNA synthesized osteoblasts and osteoclasts
4	5.225	5.308	0.083	5.72	27.11	474	Connective tissue, muscular fibers, adipose tissue
5	5.220	5.324	0.104	6.70	19.83	296	Connective tissue, muscular fibers, adipose
6	5.215	5.300	0.086	4.51	12.41	275	Connective tissue, muscular fibers
X ± SD (SEM)	5.211 ± 0.011 (0.004)	5.286 ± 0.064 (0.036) $P_T = 0.046$	0.075 ± 0.058 (0.024)	6.09 ± 1.48 (0.60)	18.11 ± 5.57 (2.27) $P_T = 0.03$	312 ± 115 (47) $P_U = 0.02$	—

Note: Each data shown are the average of three measurements; n = the number of samples tested; statistical differences in each group and between groups are shown according to Wilcoxon's T-test ($P_T < 0.05$) and Mann–Whitney's U-test, respectively.

of osteoblasts versus osteoclasts have been recently established *in vitro* to be greater on more complex, micro-rough HA surfaces (roughness index R_a = 2 μm) than on smoother topographies (R_a = 1 μm) [166]. Ectopic bone and marrow growth overshoot has been *in vivo* determined earlier on rough (R_a = 2–3 μm) CP micro-arc coatings by us [167]. Thus, artificial CP surface is a scaffold for *de novo* bioengineering of cell microenvironment that is necessary for regeneration of bone/bone marrow system.

Correlation interrelations of physical (porosity and roughness) and biological properties of micro-arc CP coatings have been established earlier. The probability of tissue lamina formation on CP microstructured surfaces has to be 80–100% [150].

Virtual output of tissue laminae on eight samples of untreated CP nanostructured coatings reached 100% in current experiment (see Table 7.3). The area of tissue laminae (see Figure 7.21b) increased up to 179% of initial value (bone marrow before implantation; see Figure 7.21a) that testified an adhesion and advancement (conduction) of bone marrow cells on artificial surfaces.

Only one case from eight specimens (12.5%) was estimated by thin histological sections of tissue laminae on CP nanostructured coatings as the bone and marrow growth *de novo* (see Table 7.3). Therefore, the bone tissue growth on untreated CP surface seems to be extremely low. Vascularized loose connective tissue mixed sometimes with muscular and adipose cells was mainly formed from donor bone marrow. Vice versa, rough micro-arc CP coatings applied from micrometer HA particles

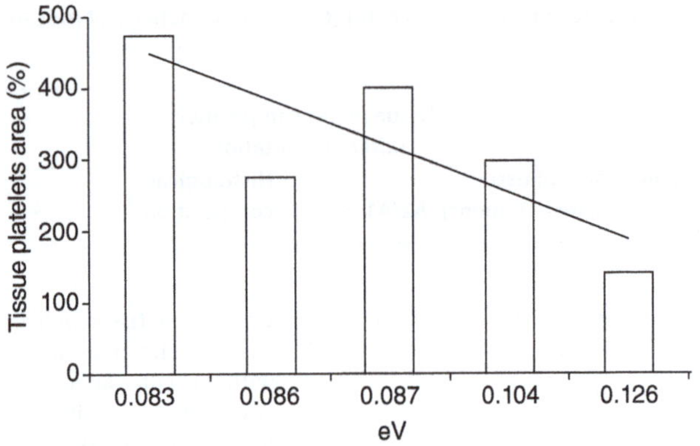

Figure 7.22 Correlation of the tissue platelets (laminae) growth with φ increment of the electrically functionalized CP nanostructured coatings.

promoted 67–100% bone formation. Roughness of micro-arc CP nanostructured coatings corresponded to that for usual micro-arc CP surfaces deposed from HA microparticles (R_a = 5–6.5 μm; R_z = 18–24 μm). Expected bone growth on micro-arc CP microstructured coating has to be 63–83% by R_a and 45–60% by R_z [20]. Thus, CP coating applied from HA nanopowder seems to diminish dramatically the ectopic bone tissue engineering.

Detailed study of photoelectron emission in CP nanostructured coatings showed the average amplitude of electron work function (φ) 5 eV (see Figure 7.22). It is similar to data of Rosenman et al. that HA ceramics is semi-conductor of p-type with large-band-gap semiconductor being about 4 eV [168].

We found φ augmentation followed by electrical functionalization (hydrogenation) of CP nanostructured coatings, and $\Delta\varphi$ achieved +0.075 eV (P_T = 0.046 in comparison with respective initial level), in average. As a result, an area of tissue laminae increased sharply from 179% to 312% (P_U = 0.02) as compared with untreated surfaces (see Table 7.3). Results were estimated as enhanced histoconduction on CP surface caused by hydrogenation.

Surprisingly, reverse linear regression of φ (excluded one point with negative $\Delta\varphi = -0.039$ eV) and relative area of tissue laminae was revealed with approximation value R^2 = 0.64 (see Figure 7.22). Perhaps, $\Delta\varphi$ addition more than 0.1 eV is crucial for subcutaneous tissue growth on electrically functionalized rough CP nanostructured coatings.

Bone and marrow tissues bioengineering *de novo* on hydrogenated CP nanostructured surface was shown histologically in 2/6 (33%) cases rather than 12.5% in untreated CP coatings (see Table 7.3, Figure 7.23a). Connective, adipose and muscular cells and tissues was noted in other cases (see Table 7.3, Figure 7.23b).

Actively RNA synthesized bone marrow cells, osteoblasts (see Figure 7.24a), and osteoclasts (see Figure 7.24b) were estimated in histological sections by Unna-Brashe staining. It argues for bone and marrow development and remodeling on electrically functionalized CP coatings.

Thus, electrically functionalized micro-arc CP coatings deposed with HA nanopowder have good subcutaneous biocompatibility, strongly promote the histoconduction, and stimulate the bone (osteoinduction) and marrow growth in ectopic test (bioreactor *in vivo*). Surface hydrogenation is prospective method to improve biological features of implants for osteosynthesis.

7.8 General Conclusions

1) Electrical functionalization of nanostructured HA coating surface enhances biocompatibility of the corresponding implants. This is based on the cell

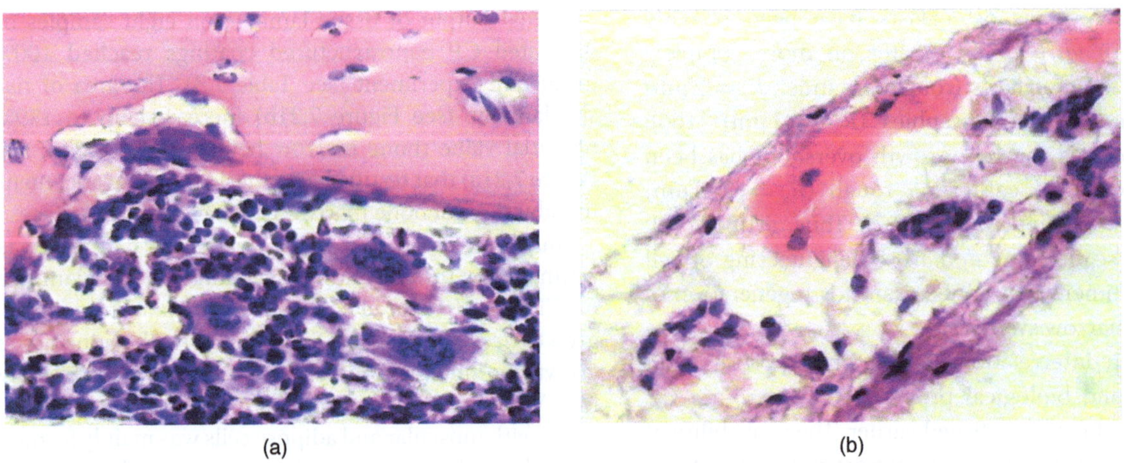

(a) (b)

Figure 7.23 Histological sections of tissue laminae on the hydrogenated nanostructured calcium phosphate surface. Bone tissue with bone marrow cells (a), and connective tissue with muscular fibers (b) are shown. Hematoxylin – eosin staining. Magnification, 700x.

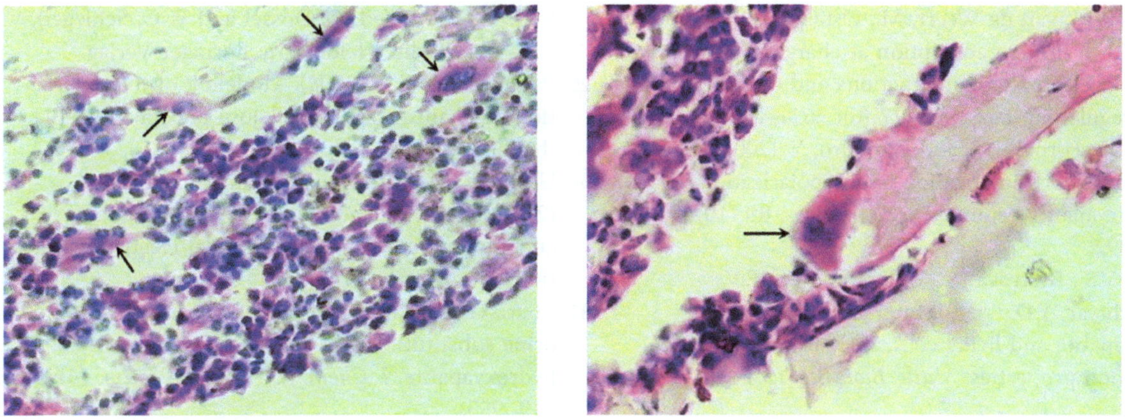

(a) (b)

Figure 7.24 Histological sections of tissue platelets on the hydrogenated nanostructured calcium phosphate surface. Unna-Brashe staining of RNA is shown as pink color in cytoplasm of osteoblasts and marrow cells (a), and osteoclast (b). Some of target cells are marked by black arrows. Magnification, 700×.

attachment control due to HA surface electrical charge.

2) The HA surface charge could be engineered because of HA lattice stoichiometry, doping, and reconstruction.
3) The Eguchi originated and prethreshold photoelectron emission techniques are offered to reach the simple procedures aimed to the HA coating surface EP measurement.
4) rf-magnetron deposition is the powerful technique to fabricate the HA nanostructured coatings to deliver them on demand properties.

References

1 Dorozhkin, S.V. (2010). Nanosized and nanocrystalline calcium orthophosphates. *Acta Biomater.* **6**: 715–734.

2 Bystrov, V.S., Paramonova, E., Dekhtyar, Y. et al. (2011). Computational and experimental studies of size and shape related physical properties of hydroxyapatite nanoparticles. *J. Phys. Condens. Matter* **23**: 065302.

3 LCSC (2014). Overview of DLVO Theory Gregor Trefalt and Michal Borkovec. September 29, 2014 Direct link www.colloid.ch/dlvo.

4 NPTEL – Chemical Engineering – Interfacial Engineering. Module 3: Lecture 5. DLVO Theory and Non-DLVO Forces. Dr. Pallab Ghosh, Guwahati–781039 India.

5 Chiras, D.D. (2011). *Human Biology*, 494. Jones & Bartlett Publishers.

6 Das, S.K., Choi, S.U., Yu, W., and Pradeep, T. (2007). *Nanofluids: Science and Technology*, 485. Wiley.

7 IUPAC (1997). *Compendium of Chemical Terminology*, 2e, Compiled by A.D. McNaught and A. Wilkinson. Oxford: Blackwell Scientific Publications.

8 Zetasizer Nano Series User Manual (2004). Malvern Instruments Ltd., Man0317, Issue 1.1 February 2004.

9 Colloidal Dynamics (1999). The Zeta Potential, Electroacoustics Tutorials.

10 Greenwood, R. and Kendall, K. (1999). Electroacoustic studies of moderately concentrated colloidal suspensions. *J. Eur. Ceram. Soc.* **19** (4): 479–488.

11 Hanaor, D.A.H., Michelazzi, M., Leonelli, C., and Sorrell, C.C. (2012). The effects of carboxylic acids on the aqueous dispersion and electrophoretic deposition of ZrO_2. *J. Eur. Ceram. Soc.* **32** (1): 235–244.

12 Kuzin, M.I. and Kostyuchenok, B.M. (1990). *Wounds and Wound Infection*. Moscow: Medicine (in Russian).

13 Leonkin, V. , Sitkalieva, E., Sokolova, M. et al. (2008). Handbook of Rehabilitation After Diseases, EKSMO (in Russian).

14 Butt, H.-J., Graf, K., and Kappl, M. (2006). *Physics and Chemistry of Interfaces*, 373. Wiley.

15 Erickson, H.P. (2009). Size and shape of protein molecules at the nanometer level determined by sedimentation, gel filtration, and electron microscopy. *Biol. Proced. Online* **11**: 32–51. https://doi.org/10.1007/s12575-009-9008-x.

16 http://tehtab.ru/Guide/Engineers/HumanBeing/HumanBeingPhysics/ (accessed 13 January 2019).

17 Hartvig, R.A., van de Weert, M., Østergaard, J. et al. (2011). Protein adsorption at charged surfaces: the role of electrostatic interactions and interfacial charge regulation. *Langmuir* **27** (6): 2634–2643.

18 Satoshi, N., Hiroaki, T., and Kimihiro, Y. (2001). Proton transport polarization and depolarization of hydroxyapatite ceramics. *J. Appl. Phys.* **89** (10): 5386–5392.

19 Bystrov, V.S., Bystrova, N.K., Paramonova, E.V., and Dekhtyar, Y.D. (2009). Interaction of charged hydroxyapatite and living cells. I. Hydroxyapatite polarization properties. *Math. Biol. Bioinf.* **4** (2): 7–11.

20 Bystrov, V., Paramonova, E., Bystrova, N. et al. (2005). Computational molecular nanostructures and mechanical/adhesion properties of hydroxyapatite. In: *Micro- and Nanostructures of Biological Systems* (ed. G. Bischoff and M. Luther), 77–93. Aachen: University Halle-Wittenberg, Germany, Shaker Verlag.

21 Bystrov, V., Bystrova, N., Paramonova, E. et al. (2006). Modeling and computation of hydroxyapatite nanostructures and properties, advanced materials forum III. *Mater. Sci. Forum* **514–516** (1–2): 1434–1437.

22 Kobayashi, T., Nakamura, S., and Yamashita, K. (2001). Enhanced osteobonding by negative surface charges of electrically polarized hydroxyapatite. *J. Biomed. Mater. Res.* **57** (4): 477–484.

23 Bystrov, V.S., Paramonova, E.V., Bystrova, N.K., and Sapronova, A.V. (2008). Hydroxyapatite polarization properties, Scientific Proceedings of Riga Technical University. *Mater. Sci. Appl. Chem.* **17** (1): 30–37.

24 Cordis (2007). PERCERAMICS: Multifunctional percolated nanostructured ceramics fabricated from hydroxyapatite, NMP3-CT-2003-504937 FP6 project. Riga Technical University. http://cordis.europa.eu/publication/rcn/12743_en.html; Permalink: http://cordis.europa.eu/result/rcn/51676_en.html © European Union, 2015 (Retrieved 11 March 2015).

25 Hughes, J.M., Cameron, M., and Crowley, K.D. (1989). Structural variations in natural F, OH, and Cl apatites. *Am. Mineral.* **74**: 870–876.

26 Elliot, J.C. (1994). *Structure and Chemistry of the Apatites and Other Calcium Orthophosphates.* Amsterdam: Elsevier.

27 Kay, M.I., Young, R.A., and Posner, A.S. (1964). Crystal structure of hydroxyapatite. *Nature* **204**: 1050.

28 Bystrov, V., Bystrova, N., Dekhtyar, Y. et al. (2009). Size depended electrical properties of hydroxyapatite nanoparticles. In: *World Congress on Medical Physics and Biomedical Engineering*, IFMBE Proceedings 25/VIII, WC 2009 (ed. O. Dossel and W.C. Schlegel), 230–232. Berlin, Heidelberg: Springer-Verlag.

29 Paramonova, E.V. (2008). Modeling of the polarization mechanisms of the calcium phosphates. PhD thesis, 20 p. Moscow: MSU.

30 Ueshima, M., Nakamura, S., and Yamashita, K. (2002). Huge, millicoulomb charge storage in ceramic hydroxyapatite by bimodal electric polarization. *Adv. Mater.* **14** (8): 591–595.

31 Maiti, G.C. and Freund, F. (1981). Influence of fluorine substitution on the proton conductivity of hydroxyapatite. *J. Chem. Soc., Dalton Trans.* (4): 949–955.

32 Janoschek, R., Weidemann, E.G., Pfeiffer, H., and Zundel, G. (1972). Extremely high polarizability of hydrogen bonds. *J. Am. Chem. Soc.* **94** (7): 2378–2396. https://doi.org/10.1021/ja00762a032.

33 Zundel, G. (2000). Hydrogen bonds with large proton polarizability and proton transfer processes in electrochemistry and biology. In: *Advances in Chemical Physics*, vol. **111** (ed. I. Prigogine and A. Rice). Wiley. ISBN: 0-471-34990-9.

34 Dekhtyar, Yu., Bystrov, V., Khlusov, I. et al. (2011). Hydroxyapatite surface nanoscaled characterization and electrical potential functionalization to engineer osteoblasts attachment and generate bone tissue. In: Society For Biomaterials Annual Meeting, Orlando, FL, USA (11–16 April 2011), Abstract # 519.

35 Dekhtyar, Y., Bystrov, V., Bystrova, A. et al. (2013). Engineering of the hydroxyapatite cell adhesion capacity. In: *International Symposium on Biomedical Engineering and Medical Physics*, IFMBE Proceedings, , vol. **38** (10–12 October 2012), 182–185. Riga, Latvia.

36 Dehtjars, J., Līvdane, A., Poļaka, N., and Timofeeva, A. (2006). Methods to process surface layer of the bioprostheses. Latvian Patent LV13522.

37 Dehtjars, J., Dvornichenko, M., Karlov, A. et al. (2010). Electrically functionalized hydroxyapatite and calcium phosphate surfaces to enhance immobilization and proliferation of osateoblasts in vitro and modulate osteogenesis in vivo. In: *World Congress on Medical Physics and Biomedical Engineering*, IFMBE Proceedings. vol. 25/10, Vācija, Munich (7–12 Septembris 2009), 245–248. Berlin, Heidelberg: Springer-Verlag. ISBN: 978-3-642-03899-0. e-ISBN: 978-3-642-03900-3. ISSN: 1680–0737. https://doi.org/10.1007/978-3-642-03900-3_70.

38 Dekhtyar, Y., Polyaka, N., Sammons, R. et al. (2008). Electrically charged hydroxyapatite enhances immobilization and proliferation of osteoblasts. In: *14th Nordic-Baltic Conference on Biomedical Engineering and Medical Physics*, IFMBE Proceedings, vol. **20**

(ed. A. Katashev, Y. Dekhtyar and J. Spigulis), 23–25. Berlin, Heidelberg: Springer-Verlag.

39 Dekhtyar, Y., Khlusov, I., Polyaka, N. et al. Influence of bioimplant surface electrical potential on osteoblast behaviour and bone tissue formation. In: *Proceedings of the 12th Mediterranean Conference on Medical and Biological Engineering and Computing*, IFMBE Proceedings, vol. **29** (Munich: MEDICON), Greece, May 2010 (ed. P.D. Bamidis and N. Polikarakis), 800–803. Berlin, Heidelberg: Springer-Verlag.

40 Hertz, H. (1887). Ueber einen Einfluss des ultravioletten Lichtes auf die electrische Entladung. *Ann. Phys. Chem.* **267** (8): 983–1000.

41 Soboleva, N.A. and Melamid, A.E. (1974). *Photoelectronic Devices*. Moscow: Vysshaya Shkola (in Russian).

42 Barinov, S.M. and Komlev, V.S. (2005). *Calcium Phosphate Based Bioceramics*, 204. Moscow: Nauka (in Russian).

43 Matsunaga, K. and Kuwabara, A. (2007). First-principles study of vacancy formation in hydroxyapatite. *Phys. Rev. B* **75**: 014102.

44 Kronik, L. and Shapira, Y. (1999). Surface photovoltage phenomena: theory, experiment, and applications. *Surf. Sci. Rep.* **37**: 1–206.

45 Bystrov, V.S., Coutinho, J., Bystrova, A.V. et al. (2015). Computational study of the hydroxyapatite structures, properties and defects. *J. Phys. D: Appl. Phys.* **48**: 195302.

46 Slepko, A. and Demkov, A.A. (2011). First-principles study of the biomineral hydroxyapatite. *Phys. Rev. B* **84**: 134108.

47 Rather, B.D., Hoffman, A.S., Schoen, F.J., and Lemons, J.E. (1996). *Biomaterial Science*. London: Academic Press.

48 Elliot, J.C., Mackie, P.E., and Young, R.A. (1973). Monoclinic hydroxyapatite. *Science* **180** (4090): 1055–1057.

49 Young, R.A. (1967). Dependence of apatite properties on crystal structural details. *Trans. N.Y. Acad. Sci.* **29** (7): 949–959.

50 Ikoma, T. and Yamazaki, A. (1999). Preparation and structure of refinement of monoclinic hydroxyapatite. *J. Solid State Chem.* **144**: 272–276.

51 Ma, G. and Liu, X.Y. (2009). Hydroxyapatite: hexagonal or monoclinic? *Cryst. Growth Des.* **9** (7): 2991–2994.

52 Calderin, L., Stott, M.J., and Rubio, A. (2003). Electronic and crystallographic structure of apatites. *Phys. Rev. B* **67**: 134106.

53 Tofail, S.A.M., Haverty, D., Stanton, K.T., and McMonagle, J.B. (2005). Structural order and dielectric behaviour of hydroxyapatite. *Ferroelectrics* **319**: 117–123.

54 Hitmi, N., LaCabanne, C., and Young, R.A. (1986). OH^- dipole reorientability in hydroxyapatites: effect of tunnel size. *J. Phys. Chem. Solids* **47** (6): 533–546.

55 Epple, M., Ganesan, K., Heumann, R. et al. (2010). Application of calcium phosphate nanoparticles in biomedicine. *J. Mater. Chem.* **20** (1): 18–23.

56 Leon, B. and Janson, J.A. (2009). *Thin Calcium Phosphate Coatings for Medical Implants*. Springer.

57 de Leeuw, N.H. (2010). Computer simulations of structures and properties of the biomaterial hydroxyapatite. *J. Mater. Chem.* **20**: 5376–5389. https://doi.org/10.1039/B921400C.

58 Haverty, D., Tofail, S.A.M., Stanton, K.T., and McMonagle, J.B. (2005). Structure and stability of hydroxyapatite: density functional calculation and rietveld analysis. *Phys. Rev. B* **71**: 094103.

59 Mostafa, N.Y. and Brown, P.W. (2007). Computer simulation of stoichiometric hydroxyapatite: structure and substitutions. *J. Phys. Chem. Solids* **68** (3): 431–437.

60 Slepko, A. and Demkov, A.A. (2013). First-principles study of hydroxyapatite surface. *J. Chem. Phys.* **139**: 044714.

61 Astala, R. and Stott, M.J. (2008). First-principles study of hydroxyapatite surfaces and water adsorption. *Physiol. Rev. B* **78**: 075427.

62 Rulis, P., Ouyang, L., and Ching, W.Y. (2004). Electronic structure and bonding in calcium apatite crystals: hydroxyapatite, fluorapatite, chlorapatite and bromapatite. *Phys. Rev. B* **70**: 155104, 8 p.

63 Rulis, P., Yao, H., Ouyang, L., and Ching, W.Y. (2007). Electronic structure, bonding, charge distribution, and x-ray absorption spectra of the (001) surfaces of fluorapatite and hydroxyapatite from first principles. *Phys. Rev. B.* **76**: 245410.

64 Bystrov, V., Costa, E., Santos, S. et al. (2012). Computational study of hydroxyapatite properties and surface interactions. In: *Proceedings of ISAF-ECAPD-PFM 2012*, 1–3. IEEE Conference Publications https://doi.org/10.1109/ISAF.2012.6297766.

65 Bystrov, V.S., Paramonova, E.V., Costa, M.E.V. et al. (2013). Computational study of the properties and surface interactions of hydroxyapatite. *Ferroelectrics* **449** (1): 94–101. https://doi.org/10.1080/00150193.2013.822774.

66 Bystrova, A.V., Dekhtyar, Y.D., Popov, A.I., and Bystrov, V.S. (2014). Modeling and synchrotron data analysis of modified hydroxyapatite structure. *Math. Biol. Bioinf.* **9** (1): 171–182.

67 Onuma, K. (2006). Recent research on pseudobiological hydroxyapatite crystal growth and phase transition mechanisms. *Prog. Cryst. Growth Charact. Mater.* **52**: 223–245.
68 Ye, F., Guo, H., and Zhang, H. (2008). Biomimetic synthesis of oriented hydroxyapatite mediated by nonionic surfactants. *Nanotechnology* **19** (24): 245605.
69 Bystrov, V.S., Dekhtyar, Y., Paramonova, E. et al. (2012). Polarization of PVDF and P(VDF- TrFE) thin films revealed by emission spectroscopy with computational simulation during phase transition. *J. Appl. Phys.* **111**: 104113, 8 p. https://doi.org/10.1063/1.4721373.
70 Britney, P.R. and Jones, R. (2000). LDA calculations using a basis of Gaussian orbitals. *Phys. Status Solidi B* **217**: 131–171.
71 Terpstra, R.A., Bennema, P., Hartman, P. et al. (1986). F faces of apatite and its morphology: theory and observation. *J. Cryst. Growth* **78**: 468–478.
72 Yamashita, K., Oikawa, N., and Umegaki, T. (1996). Acceleration and deceleration of bone-like crystal growth on ceramic hydroxyapatite by electric poling. *Chem. Mater.* **8**: 2697.
73 Yin, X. and Scott, M.J. (2003). Biological calcium phosphates and Posner's cluster. *J. Chem. Phys.* **118** (8): 3717–3723.
74 Bystrov, V.S. (2015). Piezoelectricity in the ordered monoclinic hydroxyapatite. *Ferroelectrics* **475** (1): 148–153. https://doi.org/10.1080/00150193.2015.995581.
75 Aronov, D., Chaikina, M., Haddad, J. et al. (2007). Electronic states spectroscopy of hydroxyapatite ceramics. *J. Mater. Sci. - Mater. Med.* **18**: 865–870.
76 Martins, M., Santos, C., Almeida, M., and Costa, E. (2008). Hydroxyapatite micro- and nanoparticles: nucleation and growth mechanisms in the presence of citrate species. *J. Colloid Interface Sci.* **318** (2): 210–216.
77 Menendez-Proupin, E., Cervantes-Rodríguez, S., Osorio-Pulgar, R. et al. (2011). Computer simulation of the elastic constants of hydroxyapatite and fluorapatite. *J. Mech. Behav. Biomed. Mater.* **4** (7): 1011–1020.
78 Briddon, P.R. and Rayson, M.J. (2011). Accurate Kohn-Sham DFT with the speed of tight binding: current techniques and future directions in materials modeling. *Phys. Status Solidi B* **248** (6): 1309–1318.
79 HyperChem (2002). *Tools for Molecular Modeling* (release 7, 8) Professional edition. Gainesville, FL: Hypercube, Inc. http://www.hyper.com/?tabid=360.
80 Stewart, J.J.P. (1989). Optimization of parameters for semi-empirical methods I. Method. *J. Comput. Chem.* **10** (2): 209–220; I. Applications. *J. Comput. Chem.* **10** (2): 221–264.
81 Lang, S.B., Tofail, S.A.M., Kholkin, A.L. et al. (2013). Ferroelectric polarization in nanocrystalline hydroxyapatite thin films on silicon. *Sci. Rep.* **3**: 2215.
82 AIMPRO. http://aimpro.ncl.ac.uk (accessed 12 May 2014 and now in 2015).
83 Lang, S.B., Tofail, S.A.M., Gandhi, A.A. et al. (2011). Pyroelectric, piezoelectric, and photoeffects in hydroxyapatite thin films on silicon. *Appl. Phys. Lett.* **98**: 123703.
84 Bystrov, V.S., Seyedhosseini, E., Kopyl, S. et al. (2014). Piezoelectricity and ferroelectricity in biomaterials: molecular modeling and piezoresponse force microscopy measurements. *J. Appl. Phys.* **116** (6): 066803.
85 Horiuchi, N., Nakaguki, S., Wada, N. et al. (2014). Polarization-induced surface charges in hydroxyapatite ceramics. *J. Appl. Phys.* **116**: 014902.
86 Jiang, W., Pan, H., Cai, Y. et al. (2008). Atomic force microscopy reveals hydroxyapatite-citrate interfacial structure at the atomic level. *Langmuir* **24**: 12446–12451.
87 Hu, Y.-Y., Rawal, A., and Schmidt-Rohr, K. (2010). Strongly bound citrate stabilizes the apatite nanocrystals in bone. *Proc. Natl. Acad. Sci. U.S.A.* **107** (52): 22425–22429.
88 Vandiver, J., Dean, D., Patel, N. et al. (2005). Nanoscale variation in surface charge of synthetic hydroxyapatite detected by chemically and spatially specific high-resolution force spectroscopy. *Biomaterials* **26**: 271–283.
89 Johann, F. and Soergel, E. (2009). Quantitative measurement of the surface charge density. *Appl. Phys. Lett.* **95**: 232906.
90 Bystrov, V.S., Bdikin, I., Heredia, A. et al. (2012). Piezoelectricity and ferroelectricity in biomaterials: from proteins to self-assembled peptide nanotubes. In: *Piezoelectric Nanomaterials for Biomedical Applications*, Chapter 7 (ed. G. Ciofani and A. Menciassi), 187–211. Berlin, Heidelberg: Springer-Verlag. ISBN: 978-3-642-28043-6.
91 Halperin, C., Mutchnik, S., Argonin, A. et al. (2004). Piezoelectric effect in human bones studied in nanometer scale. *Nano Lett.* **4** (7): 1253–1256.
92 (a) Kittel, C. (1978). *Introduction to Solid State Physics*. New York: Wiley. (b) Slepko, A. (2013). Theory of biomineral hydroxyapatite. Dissertation on PhD, 160 p. University of Texas at Austin.
93 Hollinger, J.O., Einhorn, T.A., Doll, B., and Sfeir, C. (2004). *Bone Tissue Engineering*, 91. Washington, DC: CRC Press.
94 VASP (Vienna ab initio Simulation Package). https://www.vasp.at/ (accessed 13 January 2019).

95 Kanakis, J., Chrissanthopoulos, A., Tnaetos, N.P. et al. (2006). Crystallization of hydroxyapatite on oxadiazole-based homopolymers. *Cryst. Growth Des.* **6**: 1547.

96 Sato, K., Kogure, T., Iwai, H., and Tanaka, J. (2002). Atomic-scale {101¯0} interfacial structure in hydroxyapatite determined by high-resolution transmission electron microscopy. *J. Am. Ceram. Soc.* **85**: 3054.

97 Eguchi, M. (1925). On the permanent electret. *Philos. Mag.* **49**: 178.

98 Gostischev, E.A. (2004). A noncontacting manner to determine the potentials of charged surface of objects and the device for its realization: Russian Federation. Patent 2,223,511, 10. February 2004.

99 Electrets, G.M. and Sessler, G.M. (eds.) (1987). *Topics in Applied Physics*, 2e, vol. **33**. Berlin: Springer-Verlag.

100 Chang, J.-S., Kelly, A.J., and Crowley, J.M. (eds.) (1995). *Handbook of Electrostatic Processes*, 756. New York, Basel, Hong Kong: Marcel Dekker, Inc.

101 Pichugin, V.F., Surmenev, R.A., Shesterikov, E.V. et al. (2008). The preparation of calciumphosphate coatings on titanium and nickel–titanium by rf-magnetron-sputtered deposition: composition, structure and micromechanical properties. *Surf. Coat. Technol.* **202**: 3913–3920.

102 Surmenev, R.A., Surmeneva, M.A., Evdokimov, K.E. et al. (2011). The influence of the deposition parameters on the properties of an rf-magnetron-deposited nanostructured calcium phosphate coating and a possible growth mechanism. *Surf. Coat. Technol.* **205**: 3600–3606.

103 Gostischev, E.A., Surmenev, R.A., Khlusov, I.A., and Pichugin, V.F. (2011). *The Research of Bioelectrical Compatibility of Thin Calcium–Phosphate Coatings, Formed by Rf-Magnetron Spattering Method*, vol. **319**, no. 2, 108–113. Izvestia of Tomsk Polytechnic University.

104 Dekhtyar, Y. (2008). Photo-, dual- and exoelectron spectroscopy to characterize nanostructures. In: *Functionalized Nanoscale Materials, Devices, and Systems for Chem.-Bio Sensors, Photonics, and Energy Generation and Storage*, 169–183. Springer.

105 Dekhtyar, Y.D. and Sagalovich, G.L. (1988). Exoelectron emission of monocrystalline silicon and its practical application. *Proc. USSR Acad. Sci., Phys. Ser.* **52**: 1611–1613. (in Russian).

106 Kortov, V.S., Shifrin, V.P., and Gaprindashvili, A.I. (1975). Exoelectron spectroscopy of semiconductors and insulators. *Microelectronics* **8**: 28–49. (in Russian).

107 Dobrecov, L.N. and Gomoyunova, M.V. (1966). *Emission Electronics*. Moscow: Nauka (in Russian).

108 Dekhtyar, Y. (2012). Emission of weak electrons towards sensing nanoobjects. In: *Technological Innovations in Sensing and Detection of Chemical, Biological, Radiological, Nuclear Threats and Ecological Terrorism* (ed. A. Vaseashta), 171–178. Springer.

109 Dekhtyar, Y. (1993). *Exoelectron Spectroscopy of the Single Defects in Semiconductors*, 59 p. . Riga: Riga Polytechnic Institute (in Russian).

110 Bystrov, V., Bystrova, N., Dekhtyar, Y. et al. (2006). Size depended electrical properties of hydroxyapatite nanoparticles. *IFMBE Proceedings* **14**: 3149–3150.

111 Topić, M., Ntsoane, T., and Heimann, R.B. (2006). Microstructural characterisation and stress determination in as-plasma sprayed and incubated bioconductive hydroxyapatite coatings. *Surf. Coat. Technol.* **201** (6): 3633–3641.

112 Choi, J., Bogdanski, D., Koller, M. et al. (2003). Calcium phosphate coating of nickel–titanium shape-memory alloys. Coating procedure and adherence of leukocytes and platelets. *Biomaterials* **24** (21): 3689–3696.

113 Urch, H., Franzka, S., Dahlhaus, D. et al. (2006). Preparation of two-dimensionally patterned layers of functionalised calcium phosphate nanoparticles by laser direct writing. *J. Mater. Chem.* **16**: 1798–1802.

114 Struts, V.K., Petrov, A.V., Matvienko, V.M. et al. (2011). Properties of calcium phosphate coatings deposited by high-power ion beam ablation plasma. *J. Surf. Invest.* **5** (3): 497–499.

115 Sharkeev, Y.P. and Kulyashova, K.S. (2014). Regularities of forming calcium phosphate coatings on zirconium from electrolytes based on synthesized and biological hydroxyapatite. *Russ. Phys. J.* **56**: 1170–1175.

116 Sergey, V. (2015). Dorozhkin Calcium orthophosphate deposits: Preparation, properties and biomedical applications. *Mater. Sci. Eng., C* **55**: 272–326.

117 Surmenev, R., Surmeneva, M., Pichugin, V. et al. (2012). Nanostructured hydroxyapatite coatings for medical implants deposited by rf-magnetron sputtering: properties and biomedical application. In: *Calcium Phosphate: Structure, Synthesis, Properties, and Applications* (ed. R.B. Heimann), 498. Nova Science Publishers, Inc.

118 Pichugin, V.F., Eshenko, E.V., Surmenev, R.A. et al. (2007). Application of high-frequency magnetron sputtering to deposit thin calcium-phosphate biocompatible coatings on a titanium surface. *J. Surf. Invest.* **1** (6): 679–682.

119 Surmenev, R.A., Ryabtseva (Surmeneva), M.A., Shesterikov, E.V. et al. (2010). The release of nickel from nickel-titanium (NiTi) is strongly reduced by

a sub-micrometer thin layer of calcium phosphate deposited by rf-magnetron sputtering. *J. Mater. Sci. – Mater. Med.* **21**: 1233–1239.

120 Surmenev, R.A. (2012). A review of plasma-assisted methods for calcium phosphate-based coatings fabrication. *Surf. Coat. Technol.* **206**: 2035–2056.

121 Kelly, P.J. and Arnell, R.D. (2000). Magnetron sputtering: a review of recent developments and applications. *Vacuum* **56**: 159–172.

122 Lin, D.-Y. and Zhao, Y.-T. (2011). Preparation of novel hydroxyapatite/yttria-stabilized-zirconia gradient coatings by magnetron sputtering. *Adv. Eng. Mater.* **13** (1–2): B18–B24.

123 Ivanova, A.A., Surmeneva, M.A., Surmenev, R.A., and Depla, D. (2015). Influence of deposition conditions on the composition, texture and microstructure of RF-magnetron sputter-deposited hydroxyapatite thin films. *Thin Solid Films* **591**: 368–374.

124 Grubova, I.Y., Surmeneva, M.A., Ivanova, A.A. et al. (2015). The effect of patterned titanium substrates on the properties of silver-doped hydroxyapatite coatings. *Surf. Coat. Technol.* **276**: 595–601.

125 Surmeneva, M.A., Mukhametkaliyev, T.M., Tyurin, A.I. et al. (2015). Effect of silicate doping on the structure and mechanical properties of thin nanostructured RF magnetron sputter-deposited hydroxyapatite films. *Surf. Coat. Technol.* **275**: 176–184.

126 Surmenev, R.A., Surmeneva, M.A., and Ivanova, A.A. (2014). Significance of calcium phosphate coatings for the enhancement of new bone osteogenesis – a review. *Acta Biomater.* **10**: 557–579.

127 Nelea, V., Morosanu, C., Iliescu, M., and Mihailescu, I.N. (2004). *Appl. Surf. Sci.* **228**: 346.

128 Surmeneva, M.A., Chaikina, M.V., Zaikovskiy, V.I. et al. (2013). The structure of an RF-magnetron sputter-deposited silicate-containing hydroxyapatite-based coating investigated by high-resolution techniques. *Surf. Coat. Technol.* **218**: 39–46.

129 Surmeneva, M.A., Surmenev, R.A., Pichugin, V.F. et al. (2011). In-vitro investigation of magnetron-sputtered coatings based on silicon-substituted hydroxyapatite. *J. **Surf. Invest.*** **5**: 1202–1207.

130 Ding, S.J. (2003). Properties and immersion behavior of magnetron-sputtered multi-layered hydroxyapatite/titanium composite coatings. *Biomaterials* **24** (23): 4233–4238.

131 Pichugin, V.F., Surmeneva, M.A., Surmenev, R.A. et al. (2011). Study of physicochemical and biological properties of calcium phosphate coatings prepared by RF magnetron sputtering of silicon-substituted hydroxyapatite. *J. Surf. Invest* **5** (5): 863–869.

132 Khlusov, I.A., Surmeneva, M.A., Surmenev, R.A. et al. (2012). Cellular and molecular aspects of immunologic compatibility of implants with nanostructured calcium phosphate coating. *Bull. Siberian Med.* (4): 78–85.

133 Ratner, B.D., Hoffman, A.S., Schoen, F.J., and Lemons, J.E. (eds.) (2004). *Biomaterials Science: An Introduction to Materials in Medicine*, 2e. San Diego, CA, London: Elsevier Inc.

134 Metallo, C.M., Mohr, J.C., Detzel, C.J. et al. (2007). Engineering the stem cell microenvironment. *Biotechnol. Progr.* **23**: 18–23.

135 Discher, D.E., Mooney, D.J., and Zandstra, P.W. (2009). Growth factors, matrices, and forces combine and control stem cells. *Science* **324** (5935): 1673–1677.

136 Guilak, F., Cohen, D.M., Estes, B.T. et al. (2009). Control of stem cell fate by physical interactions with the extracellular matrix. *Cell Stem Cell* **5** (1): 17–26.

137 Nepola, J.V. (1996). External fixation. In: *Rockwood and Green's Fractures in Adults*, 4e, vol. **1** (ed. C.A. Rockwood Jr., D.P. Green, R.W. Bucholz and J.D. Heckman), 229–304. Philadelphia, PA: Lippincot-Raven.

138 Kovacs, P. and Davidson, G.A. (1996). Chemical and electrochemical aspects of the biocompatibility of titanium and its alloys. In: *Medical Applications of Titanium and Its Alloys: The Material and Biological Issues*, ASTM STP 1272 (ed. S.A. Brown and J.E. Lemons), 163–178. American Society for Testing and Materials.

139 Ponsonnet, L., Reybier, K., Jaffrezic, N. et al. (2003). Relationship between surface properties (roughness, wettability) of titanium and titanium alloys and cell behaviour. *Mater. Sci. Eng., C* **23**: 551–560.

140 Thian, E.S., Ahmad, Z., Huang, J. et al. (2010). The role of surface wettability and surface charge of electrosprayed nanoapatites on the behaviour of osteoblasts. *Acta Biomater.* **6** (3): 750–755.

141 McCaig, D. and Zhao, M. (1997). Physiological electrical fields modify cell behaviour. *BioEssays* **19**: 819–826.

142 Lahann, J. and Langer, R. (2005). Smart materials with dynamically controllable surfaces. *MRS Bull.* **30**: 185–188.

143 Zhou, H., Chen, W., Weir, M.D. et al. (2012). Biofunctionalized calcium phosphate cement to enhance the attachment and osteodifferentiation of stem cells released from fast-degradable alginate-fibrin microbeads. *Tissue Eng. Part A* **18** (15–16): 1583–1595. https://doi.org/10.1089/ten.TEA.2011.0604.

144 Yamashita, K., Kitagaki, K., and Umegaki, T. (1995). Thermal instability and proton conductivity of ceramic hydroxyapatite at high temperatures. *J. Am. Ceram. Soc.* **78**: 1191–1197.

145 Dekhtyar, Y., Bystrov, V., Khlusov, I. et al. (2011). Hydroxyapatite surface nanoscaled characterization and electrical potential functionalization to engineer osteoblasts attachment and generate bone tissue. In: *35th Annual Meeting and Exposition* (13–16 April 2011). Orlando, FL: Society for Biomaterials.

146 Chaikina, M.V., Uvarov, N.F., Ulihin, A.S., and Khlusov, I.A. (2008). Mechanochemical synthesis of nanosized functional materials with the apatite-type structure. *Prob. Mater. Sci.* **54** (2): 219–232.

147 Sharkeev, Y.P., Legostaeva, E.V., Eroshenko, A.Y. et al. (2009). The structure and physical and mechanical properties of a novel biocomposite material, nanostructured titanium-calcium-phosphate coating. *Compos. Interfac* **16**: 535–546.

148 Legostaeva, E.V., Kulyashova, K.S., Komarova, E.G. et al. (2013). Physical, chemical and biological properties of micro-arc deposited calcium phosphate coatings on titanium and zirconium-niobium alloy. *Materialwiss. Werkstofftech.* **44**: 188–197. https://doi.org/10.1002/mawe.201300107.

149 Akmene, R.J., Balodis, A.J., Dekhtyar, Y.D. et al. (2013). Exoelectron emission specrometre complete set of surface local investigation. *Surf.: Chem. Phys. Mech. (Russian Journal)* **8**: 125–128.

150 Khlusov, I.A., Karlov, A.V., Sharkeev, Y.P. et al. (2005). Osteogenic potential of mesenchymal stem cells from bone marrow in situ: role of physicochemical properties of artificial surfaces. *Bull. Exp. Biol. Med.* **140** (1): 144–152.

151 Friedenstein, A.J., Chailakhyan, R.K., Latsinik, N.V. et al. (1974). Stromal cells responsible for transferring the microenvironment of the hemopoietic tissues. Cloning in vitro and retransplantation in vivo. *Transplantation* **17**: 331–340.

152 Karlov, A.V., Usikov, V.D., Khlusov, I.A., and Khohlov, A.V. (2000). Dynamometrische einschatzung der fixationsfestigkeit von bioimplantaten in kaninchenwirbeln. *Biomed. Tech.* **45** (1): 125–126.

153 Potvin, C. (1979). A simple, modified methyl green – pyronin Y stain for DNA and RNA in formalin-fixed tissues. *Lab. Med.* **10**: 772–774.

154 Aerts, F. and Wagemaker, G. (2006). Mesenchymal stem cell engineering and transplantation. In: *Genetic Engineering of Mesenchymal Stem Cells* (ed. J.A. Nolta), 1–44. The Netherlands: Springer.

155 Lutolf, M.P., Doyonnas, R., Havenstrite, K. et al. (2009). Perturbation of single hematopoietic stem cell fates in artificial niches. *Integr. Biol. (Camb.)* **1**: 59–69.

156 Urist, M.R. and McLean, F. (1952). Ostegenetic potency and new bone formation by induction in transplants to anterior chamber of eye. *J. Bone Joint Surg.* **34**: 443.

157 Yamasaki, H. and Sakai, H. (1992). Osteogenic response to porous hydroxyapatite ceramics under the skin of dogs. *Biomaterials* **5**: 308–312.

158 Claase, M.B., de Bruijn, J.D., Grijpma, D.W., and Feijen, J. (2007). Ectopic bone formation in cell-seeded poly(ethylene oxide)/poly(butylene terephthalate) copolymer scaffolds of varying porosity. *J. Mater. Sci. – Mater. Med.* **18** (7): 1299–1307. https://doi.org/10.1007/s10856-006-0077-y.

159 Urist, M.R. (1965). Bone: formation by autoinduction. *Science* **150**: 893–899.

160 Yang, Z., Yuan, H., Tong, W. et al. (1996). Osteogenesis in extraskeletal implanted porous calcium phosphate ceramics: variability among different kinds of animals. *Biomaterials* **17**: 2131–2137.

161 Klein, C., de Groot, K., Chen, W. et al. (1994). Osseous substance formation induced in porous calcium phosphate ceramics in soft tissues. *Biomaterials* **15**: 31–34.

162 Kurashina, K., Kurita, H., Kotani, A. et al. (1998). Experimental cranioplasty and skeletal augmentation using an alpha-tricalcium phosphate/dicalcium phosphate dibasic/tetracalcium phosphate monoxide cement: a preliminary short-term experiment in rabbits. *Biomaterials* **19**: 701–706.

163 Yuan, H., Kurashina, K., de Bruijn, J.D. et al. (1999). A preliminary study on osteoinduction of two kinds of calcium phosphate ceramics Zhang Xingdong. *Biomaterials* **20**: 1799–1706.

164 Miura, Y., Gao, Z., Miura, M. et al. (2006). Mesenchymal stem cell-organized bone marrow elements: an alternative hematopoietic progenitor resource. *Stem Cells* **24** (11): 2428–2436.

165 Chan, C.K.F., Chen, C.C., Luppen, C.A. et al. (2009). Endochondral ossification is required for hematopoietic stem cell niche formation. *Nature* **457** (7228): 490–494.

166 Costa, D.O., Prowse, P.D.H., Chrones, T. et al. (2013). The differential regulation of osteoblast and osteoclast activity by surface topography of hydroxyapatite coatings. *Biomaterials* **34**: 7215–7226.

167 Gnedenkov, S.V., Sharkeev, Y.P., Sinebryukhov, S.L. et al. (2011). Formation and properties of bioactive surface layers on titanium. *Inorg. Mater. Appl. Res.* **2** (5): 474–481.

168 Rosenman, G., Aronov, D., Oster, L. et al. (2006). Photoluminescence and surface photo-voltage spectroscopy studies of hydroxyapatite nano-bio-ceramics. *J. Lumin.* **122–123**: 936–938.

8

Bioactive Micro-arc Calcium Phosphate Coatings on Nanostructured and Ultrafine-Grained Bioinert Metals and Alloys

Yurii Sharkeev[1,2], Ekaterina Komarova[2], Maria Sedelnikova[2], Igor A. Khlusov[3,4], Anna Eroshenko[2], Larisa Litvinova[5], and Valeria Shupletsova[5]

[1] National Research Tomsk Polytechnic University, Research School of High-Energy Physics, 634050, Tomsk, Russia
[2] Institute of Strength Physics and Materials Science of SB RAS, Russia
[3] Department of Morphology and General Pathology, Siberian State Medical University, 634050, Tomsk, Russia
[4] National Research Tomsk Polytechnic University, Research School of Chemistry & Applied Biomedical Sciences, 634050, Tomsk, Russia
[5] Laboratory of Immunology and Cellular Biotechnology, Immanuel Kant Baltic Federal University, 14 A. Nevskogo Street, 236041 Kaliningrad, Russia

8.1 Bioinert Alloys in Nanostructured and Ultrafine-Grained States and Bioactive Calcium Phosphate Coatings for Medical Applications

During the last few decades, there has been a research development boom in the area of biocompatible material production. More and more advanced medical technologies, materials, and items are being developed, including metal-based implants and biocompatible coatings, which, in its turn, could replace injured and disable areas of the bone tissue. The functional reliability of such materials depends on such factors as biochemical, cellular, tissue, and biomechanical compatibility.

It should be noted that there are two highly important and progressive research prospects. The first is the development of metal-based materials for biomechanical compatible implants which would exclude possible degenerating processes in the bone tissue itself and even reoperation, if it is necessary. The second is the development of newly compositional, structural, and morphological gradient calcium phosphate (CaP) coatings enhancing osteogenetic potential of the organism itself during osseointegration.

The implant function is defined by complex biological media factors, embracing physical, chemical, and mechanical effects. It is these factors that impose high requirements to the biological and mechanical compatibility of implant materials. However, most biocompatible metal materials lack required biological and mechanical properties. This fact could be explained that there is a significant number of noneffective implantation results, including implant failure [1–4].

The material for implants should be not only endurable and highly plastic but also harmless and biocompatible with the living body. European Society for Biomaterials (1986) defined the term "biocompatibility" as "the ability of a material to perform with an appropriate host response in a specific application" [1]. According to the existing concept of host response to biological organism structure [1, 4], it is possible to define the basic properties of biocompatible products as following. Material should not provoke local inflammatory reactions, should not have toxic and allergic effect, have no cancer effect, and should preserve effective functional properties during its lifetime. Although above-stated properties are essential for this specific item, they are still inadequate. Depending on the implantation site and purpose, new requirements are applied to the item. Implantation material should possess significant mechanical strength and effective bone tissue-implant healing [4]. Additionally, finished implants after processing and sterilization should preserve their properties including mechanical properties, excluding fading or changing. This fact in itself furthers the research and the development of newer and newer applicable medical materials.

Nowadays, approximately 70–80% of all implants are produced from metals and alloys. Metal implant structures for osteosynthesis in orthopedics and traumatology are made of noncorrosive alloys (for example vitallium–cobalt–chrome alloy, stainless steel, titanium nickelide alloys with shape memory effect, titanium alloys). These alloys are used in the production of pins, nails, plates, and bolts for anchoring fractured joints and bones, as well as developing artificial joints. Titanium has been widely used in surgery since 1952 and is the basic production material for different implants [5].

Bioceramics and Biocomposites: From Research to Clinical Practice, First Edition. Edited by Iulian Antoniac.

The most abundantly used alloys in medicine are commercially pure titanium Grade 4, titanium alloys Ti–6Al–4V, Ti–6Al–4V ELi and vanadium-free alloys as Ti–6Al–7Nb and Ti–6Al–2.5Fe. However, preferred alloys are those without any toxic alloying elements, such as A1, V, Mo, and others [6–8] that could affect the organism. In this case, the most perspective ones are valve bioinert metals, such as titanium, zirconium, niobium, hafnium, tantalum, and their alloys. The main advantages of these materials are high corrosion resistance and good biocompatibility, hypotoxicity, low thermal linear expansion and thermal conductivity, nonmagnetization, and insignificant specific gravity. Examining applied metal materials, such as stainless steel, cobalt–chrome alloy, commercially pure titanium, Ti–6Al–4V titanium alloy, and titanium nickelide in produced implants from the point of view escaping ions in the human body and their toxicity, it has been noted that the formation of an oxide coating on the metal material surface is an antioxidant for effusing ions. Dense oxide film on titanium and its alloy surfaces protects the metal from corrosion in most media, including biological ones. Besides, titanium ions, effusing into the tissue, don't show a toxic effect on the human organism [9].

Commercially pure titanium Grade 2 and Grade 4 have been approved for dental implant production. Some dentistry, such as "Konmet" (Moscow, Russia) and "Calcitek" (France) use Grade 4 and Grade 5 as implant material. The latter (Grade 5) contains 7% aluminum and 4% vanadium, which under specific conditions could have some negative effects during implantation and implant service life.

Low strength properties, especially low ultimate strength, restrict the further application of pure titanium as implant material. The solution for this problem is using commercially pure titanium in nanostructured and ultrafine-grained state lacking toxic alloying elements, whereas the mechanical property values are corresponded to the mechanical properties of titanium alloys.

Currently, the main problem of forming ultrafine-grained and nanostructured state in commercially pure titanium is being successfully solved by different research teams [10–17]. Nanostructured and ultrafine-grained state in bulk titanium billets is attained by applying equal channel angular pressing (ECAP) and its combinations as ECAP–conform; uniaxial pressing to deformation axis pressing (*abc*-pressing); extrusion and severe plastic deformation (SPD) methods and rolling; combined methods, for example, severe deformation rolling methods; different tribological processes, for example, friction stir and others [10–20].

Application fields of nanostructured and ultrafine-grained titanium with significantly high mechanical properties after SPD are primarily orthopedics, traumatology, and dental surgery. Application examples of ultrafine-grained titanium are described by Valiev et al. [14] and include the following: metal plates for osseosynthesis, conical bolts for fixation of spinal discs. Nowadays, nanostructured titanium Grade 4 with high mechanical properties is being applied as dental implants [10, 13–15].

The mechanical characteristics of ultrafine-grained titanium produced by SPD methods are presented in Table 8.1. It can be stated that refining titanium structure up to ultrafine-grained state resulted in a significant increase of the mechanical properties.

Materials used for implants should have not only high strength properties (yield strength, ultimate strength, fatigue strength, cycle life, wear resistance, etc.) but also low elastic properties, such as elastic modulus. Elastic modulus is an important biofunctional characteristic of implant materials. Rather low elastic modulus furthers the uniform distribution of deformation strain and stress where bone–implant interfaces and excludes possible breakdown at rigid fixation of the implant to the bone and bone resorption in area of no mechanical stress [6, 7]. Elastic modulus of titanium and its alloys ranges from 100 to 120 GPa, which is significantly higher than the elastic modulus of bone tissue which ranges from 15 to 55 GPa. Accordingly, the most promising research area in medical materials science is the application of β-titanium alloys with low elastic modulus, for example Ti–Nb or Ti–Nb–Zr systems. Thus, niobium alloyed titanium (~40 mass% of niobium) could decrease the elastic modulus to 55–60 GPa [6, 21]; however, in this case, mechanical properties as material tensile yield and ultimate strength decrease.

Traditional methods used in producing the titanium–niobium alloys are extraction metallurgical methods. Nevertheless, the application of traditional methods in producing titanium–niobium alloys with homogeneous microstructures is not always effective. Formation of nanosized and ultrafine-grained structures in titanium alloys by SPD methods increases the structural strength without additional alloying and the composition of which lacks toxic alloying elements; while mechanical properties are close to the mechanical properties of the coarse-grained medium strength titanium alloys applied in implantology. Formation of nanostructured and ultrafine-grained state in alloys does not deteriorate its biocompatibility and other biological properties.

Thus, titanium and niobium-based alloys in nanostructured and ultrafine-grained states are perspective in the production of orthopedic and dental implants improving implant mechanical properties. Applying CaP coatings provides appropriate biological properties.

Table 8.1 Mechanical properties of ultrafine-grained titanium produced after variable severe plastic deformation methods [11–17].

Severe plastic deformation method	Mean grain size (μm)	$\sigma_{0.2}$ (MPa)	σ_B (MPa)	δ (%)
Initial coarse-grained titanium	15–20	400–580	270–380	23–43
Pressing torsion	0.1	790	950	14
ECAP	0.1	915	1100	9
ECAP–conform	0.3	880	1020	13
abc-pressing	0.15	635	710	14
ECAP (eight passes) with cold extrusion (73%) and annealing at 300 °C for one hour	—	942	1037	12.5
ECAP (eight passes) with cold extrusion (75%)	—	970	1050	8
Helica extrusion (three passes) with cold rolling	—	760	795	27
abc-pressing in a press mold at 700–390 °C and rolling at 250 °C for one hour	0.06	1100	1010	6
abc-pressing in a press mold at 700–390 °C and rolling (90%) and annealing at 300 °C for one hour	0.11	1000	940	7
Multi-pressing in a press mold at 700–390 °C and rolling (90%) and annealing at 350 °C for one hour	0.17	780	860	9
abc-pressing with rolling (75%) and annealing at 250 °C for one hour	0.16	1240	1000	6
abc-pressing with rolling (75%) and annealing at 350 °C for one hour	0.27	1070	870	6–7
Multi-pass cold rolling with annealing at 300 °C for one hour	0.2–0.4	1000	840	7

σ_B, ultimate strength; $\sigma_{0.2}$, yield strength; δ, plasticity value.

To provide reliable osteointegration of bone tissue–implant interface integration, the implant surface should possess specific morphology and porosity. To solve this task, as well as to impart bioactive properties, metal surfaces are covered with bioactive coatings. Hydroxyapatite (HA), tricalcium phosphate (TCP), and fluoro-hydroxyapatite (F-HA) possess the optimal bioactive properties. The latest trend is to use such materials that would further similar natural processes when implanted into the organism. For example, simultaneous dissolution (bioresorption) and precipitation (osteogenesis) of acid calcium phosphate resulting in the intensive osteointegration of the coated implant itself. To define the correlation between material biogradation rate and osteogenesis behavior and intensity, it is necessary to study the influence of phase and structural compositions on the triggering resorption process [22].

Conditionally, all orthocalcium phosphates (OCPs) are divided into two categories: low-temperature OCPs that are synthesized at relatively low temperatures without additional thermal treatment for crystallization of synthesis product, and high-temperature OCPs that are subjected to thermal treatment. Low-temperature OCPs include monocalcium phosphate monohydrate, $Ca(H_2PO_4)_2{\cdot}H_2O$ (MCPM); dicalcium phosphate dihydrate, $CaHPO_4{\cdot}2H_2O$ (DCPD); anhydrous dicalcium phosphate, $CaHPO_4$ (DCPA); octacalcium phosphate $Ca_8H_2(PO_4)_6{\cdot}5H_2O$; precipitated apatite calcium, $Ca_{10-x}(HPO_4)_x(PO_4)_{6-x}(OH)_{2-x}$; and amorphous calcium phosphate, $Ca_3(PO_4)_2{\cdot}nH_2O$ (ACP) (n = 3.0–4.5) [23–26]. The specific feature of these systems is that the solid phase is in equilibrium with a rather acid solution in comparison to the solid phase composition. This could explain the fact that calcium phosphate partially dissolves forming subsalts and phosphate acid [25].

MCPM is highly acidic and is a water-soluble calcium phosphate. At temperatures more than 100 °C, it reacts to form anhydrous monocalcium phosphate (MCPA). MCPM and MCPA have the lowest ratio of Ca/P = 0.5 and they cannot be biocompatible due to its acid reaction [23].

DCPD and DCPA have limited solubility region, while precipitated hydroxyapatite (calcium-deficient hydroxyapatite [CDHA]) is practically insoluble in water. DCPD has Ca/P ratio of 1.0, while CDHA has Ca/P ratio ranging within 1.5–1.67. Variable composition structure of precipitated hydroxyapatite could be explained by the existing solid solutions in it and low transformation rate of metastable indissolvable calcium phosphate into HA [25]. OCPs (Ca/P = 1.33) precede bone tissue crystallization and are the intermediate phase in CDHA synthesis. ACP (Ca/P = 1.0) is unstable, having high solution reaction and converts into calcium in aqueous media, i.e. deficient CDHA.

Among the low-temperature OCPs, the most similar to natural tissue and having promising practical application are DCPD, OCP, precipitated hydroxyapatite, and ACP. Another important factor is that all these phosphates can be found in the bone tissue [23].

The basic high-temperature OCPs are MCPA, $Ca(H_2PO_4)_2$; α-TCP, α-$Ca_3(PO_4)_2$; β-TCP, β-$Ca_3(PO_4)_2$; hydroxyapatite, $Ca_{10}(PO_4)_6(OH)_2$; and tetracalcium phosphate (TTCP), $Ca_4(PO_4)_2O$.

β-TCP (Ca/P = 1.5) is "apparent orthocalcium phosphate" as it does not precipitate from aqueous solutions and is produced only at high temperature annealing, i.e. more than 800 °C. If the temperature increases to 1125 °C, it converts into α-TCP [27]. β-TCP is biocompatible and is applicable for bone tissue replacement, not only in a pure state but also in combination with CDHA. As α-TCP cannot be found in biologically calcium phosphate, it is applied only in bone cement.

TTCP (Ca/P = 2.0) is produced at 1300 °C and it is unstable in water (hydrolysis occurs forming HA and hydroxide calcium). TTCP cannot be found in biological calcium phosphates and it is applied as bone cement in medicine [23].

Hydroxyapatite (HA or HAP, Ca/P = 1.67) is the most stable and insoluble calcium phosphate. HA is associated with biological active materials, having structure similar to bone tissue and is extensively applied as material in traumatology and orthopedics [28]. HA is related to apatite group with $M_{10}(ZO_4)_6X_2$ composition. Crystalline apatite lattice including 42 ions has a wide spectrum of substitution – two cation positions and two anion sublattice positions. This could be explained by the various natural calcium phosphate apatites, wherein the M position could be occupied by cations Ca^{2+}, Sr^{2+}, Ba^{2+}, Pb^{2+}, etc.; the ZO_4 position in anion sublattice is occupied by groups PO_4^{3-}, CO_3^{2-}, SiO_4^{4-}, etc.; the X position is occupied by anions F^-, Cl^-, OH^-, CO_3^{2-}, etc. [29]. Fluor-hydroxyapatite (F–HA) $Ca_{10}(PO_4)_6F_x(OH)_{2-x}$ is a rather new and understudied bioactive material. However, the latest research has proved that this material possesses excellent osseostimulative properties, and, in some cases, it is preferred to HA [30].

Calcium phosphate solubility depends on pH and under normal physiologic conditions (pH = 7), solubility decreases as follows MCPM > α–TCP > TTCP > DCPD > DCPA > OCP > β–TCP > HA [25].

Advanced tendencies in fields of bioactive coating application involve the optimal selection of coating parameters ensuring significant bioactivity and effective osseointegration. The foremost method in today's regenerative medicine is based on applying resorbed materials triggering bone tissue generation and newly forming replacement [22]. Various calcium phosphate (CaP) materials, in terms of their physicochemical properties (crystallinity and porosity, solubility, surface roughness, and morphology) exhibit different effective bone formation. It is presupposed that osseoinductive and osseoconductive properties could occur if CaP surface imitates the structure of bone tissue. In this case, HA and TCP have the most significant bioactivity and potential osseointegration. TCP is applied in combination with HA as a composite, thus increasing resorption rate and replacement of newly formed bone tissue [26].

HA of different nature is used to produce CaP coatings. Until recently, biological powdered HA was produced from cattle bones [30]. Currently, it has been noted that biological HA has some disadvantages, including the risk of infection transmission and potential immunological potency due to the foreign material, as well as the content of heavy metals which accumulate in the animal bones throughout its life [3]. This problem could be solved by using chemically pure synthesized HA, which, in its turn, has several advantages. They are ethical and medical ones.

There are several well-known method classifications of HA synthesis, whereas the prevailing classification was suggested by Barinov [23, 26]. According to this classification, all the methods could be divided into three groups: solution deposition ("aqueous" method), solid-phase synthesis ("dry" method), and hydrothermal synthesis. One of the perspective methods is the mechanochemical method in producing HA [31]. This method uses different calcium- and phosphorus-containing materials, as well as other elements to synthesize HA with different crystalline structures which embrace a wide spectrum of isomorphous replacement.

There are various deposition methods for producing CaP biocoatings on the metal implant surface. One should consider the application area of the implant itself when selecting the coating method. The CaP coatings improving the implant osseointegration with bone tissue are more attractive as in the case of plastic (reconstruction) surgery. In dentistry, maxillofacial surgery, and traumatology, more attention is paid to the biocoatings, namely improving rigid fixation of the implant to the bone. At the same time such coatings should be stable in a biological media and possess high adhesion strength to the substrate. The increasing demand for biocompatible coatings in practical medicine could be satisfied by different types of biocoatings with various thicknesses, porosity, adhesion strength, and other properties. This problem could be resolved by applying different coating formation methods, such as plasma spraying [32, 33], electrophoresis [34], sol-gel method [35, 36], biomimetic method [37, 38], high-frequency magnetron sputtering [39, 40], detonation-gas spraying (DGS) [41, 42], and micro-arc oxidation (MAO) [43–45].

Plasma spraying method is the most commonly used process in biocoating formation, including HA [32]. In plasma spraying, the material to be deposited, typically as a powder, is introduced into the plasma jet, emanating from a plasma torch. The material is melted and propelled toward a substrate. When contacting with the substrate surface, the particles deform, flatten, crystallize, and form agglomerates. Precipitating and crystallizing the particles form the coating layer by layer. Coating properties are defined by thermal-physical, chemical, and mechanical properties of material particles, spraying distance, arc current, particle velocity, atmosphere composition and plasma forming, and carrier gas type [33]. This method allows to produce coatings with thickness of up to 100 µm.

Another CaP coating process is electrophoresis, which produces coatings with thickness to 2 mm. Electrophoresis is based on the deposition of electrically charged HA particles dipped in a solution or other media and is used to form coatings on complex-shaped units. However, low-energy particles at room temperature result in the formation of HA coatings with asymmetrical porosity and heterogeneity. Such coatings often have different defects and cracks. Sintering is the final stage in this process involving a prolonged interval and high temperatures. This, in its turn, could change the structure and properties of the titanium substrate, as well as the coating phase composition. Such coatings generally have low adhesion strength to titanium substrate [34].

CaP coatings produced through slip process and sol-gel process are also applicable. These methods are relatively cheap and do not require expensive equipment and devices for filtration, rinsing, and drying. These methods are based on the preparation of a suspension as a coating base material, then processing the metal surface in the ready-made suspension without applying electrical or magnetic fields, and further annealing at the temperature corresponding to crystallization of dispersed substance phase. CaP coatings with thickness of 200–300 µm can be produced by applying the HA dispersion phase and water-dispersed media [35, 36].

The biomimetic method in producing CaP coatings are commonly used for biomedical applications due to similar natural coating formation. Precipitation and growth of biologically compatible coatings on titanium-based substrate is immersed in a simulating human intertissue liquid as simulated body fluid (SBF) solution wherein HA particles are dissolved. The titanium-based substrate is preliminarily alkalized (NaOH) forming sodium titanate on the surface, which, in its turn, subsequently promotes complete apatite precipitation from SBF solution [37, 38].

Magnetron sputtering methods are also used for producing biocompatible coatings [39, 40]. This methods involves ejecting material from a "target" that is a source onto a substrate by ion and atom bombardment forming a highly dense film. Current density and ion sputtering rate increase significantly. This method produces thin film homogeneous coatings. However, there are difficulties at deposition of coatings on complex-shaped items. Another type of magnetron sputtering method is radio frequency (RF) magnetron sputtering used to produce ultrafine dense biocompatible CaP coatings of up to 5 µm in thickness and with high adhesion strength to substrates. RF magnetron sputtering method produces coatings from dielectrics including HA without destructing the stoichiometric composition and the initial ratio of the sputtering target components.

Nowadays, impulse energy source is used in heating and precipitation of deposited powdered materials, particularly, combustion gas mixture blast energy with oxidizing agents. This method is termed as DGS [41, 42]. It involves CaP material powder spraying on the substrate surface by direct gas mixture blasting. This method has serious advantages in practical medicine, mainly, identical phase composition in sprayed-on material and produced coating.

During the last few decades, MAO method is being widely used as electrical and chemical surface treatment for forming oxide and CaP coatings on metals. It employs high potentials as the discharges occur and the resulting plasma modifies the structure of the oxide layer [43–45]. The coating formation is the result of substrate material oxidization and transport of ultrafine-dispersed phase from electrolyte. Such coatings have a wide spectrum of physical and chemical properties, including high corrosion resistance, wear resistance, hardness, chemical stability in aggressive media, and so on.

8.2 Production, Structure, and Mechanical Properties of Bioinert Alloys Based on Titanium and Niobium in Nanostructured and Ultrafine-grained States

Today's current issue of the production of nanostructured and ultrafine-grained titanium billets from pure titanium is being solved. In this case SPD is applied, particularly ECAP and its different types as uniaxial pressing to deformation axis pressing (*abc*-pressing) and others [11, 12, 14–17]. Combined SPD methods are also considered. In spite of the rather advanced development of above-mentioned SPD methods, their further application is hindered due to processing complexity associated with designing required tools, improving work piece sizes, and forming dimensional nanosized homogeneous structures. Development of SPD methods in producing nanostructured Ti–Nb alloys and conducting further research is currently important [46–48]. This is due to the diversity of forming structures and phase transformation mechanisms of alloying β-alloys as a result of SPD. Depending on the alloying element concentration and thermal deformation impact, both equilibrium phase transformations could proceed and metastable states (α′,α″, ω phases) could form in the Ti–Nb alloys [49, 50]. This, in itself requires newly developed methods, for example, SPD in constrained conditions providing high mechanical strain and megaplastic deformation (strain).

The investigation results of mechanical properties of commercially pure titanium Grade VT1-0 (Ti) and Ti–40mass%Nb (Ti–40Nb) alloy in nanostructured and ultrafine-grained states formed by SPD methods are described in this chapter.

Microstructure and phase composition of the samples were investigated by optical microscopy (Carl Zeiss Axio Observer, Germany), transmission electronic microscopy (TEM; JEOL JEM 2100, Japan), and X-ray diffractometry (XRD) in CoK_{α} radiation (Dron-7, Burevestnik, Russia). Average size of structural elements (grains, subgrains, fragments) was calculated by "secant" method according to ASTM E1382–97(2010). Microhardness was measured according to Vickers on microhardness tester Duramin-500 (Struers, Denmark). Tensile deformation mechanical testing was carried out on Instron-1185 (Instron, USA). Experimental research was conducted on the equipments of Common Use Center "Nanotech" at Institute of Strength Physics and Materials Science SB RAS (ISPMS SB RAS, Tomsk, Russia).

Investigation materials were commercially pure titanium Grade VT1-0 (Ti) and Ti–40mass%Nb alloy (Ti–40Nb). In the initial state, the titanium VT1-0 microstructure included rather equiaxed α-phase grains (HCP lattice) of average grain size of 25 μm (see Figure 8.1a,b). Ti–40Nb is produced after multi-remelting by arc-melting method [51], which involves annealing at 1100 °C for one hour in argon atmosphere. Samples were cut out from the remelted billet and then exposed to deformation effect.

Figure 8.1a,c illustrate the optical images of Ti and Ti–40Nb microstructure after annealing. In the Ti–40Nb structure, polyhedral grain boundaries of primary β-phase with body-centered cubic (bcc) lattice, pitted by dendritic segregation are observed (see Figure 8.1c). The sizes of polyhedral β-grains are within the range of 120–650 μm. The β-grain volume includes acicular inclusions, characteristic of metastable martensite α″ phase (see Figure 8.1d). The analysis of phase composition, based on the results of selected area microdiffraction

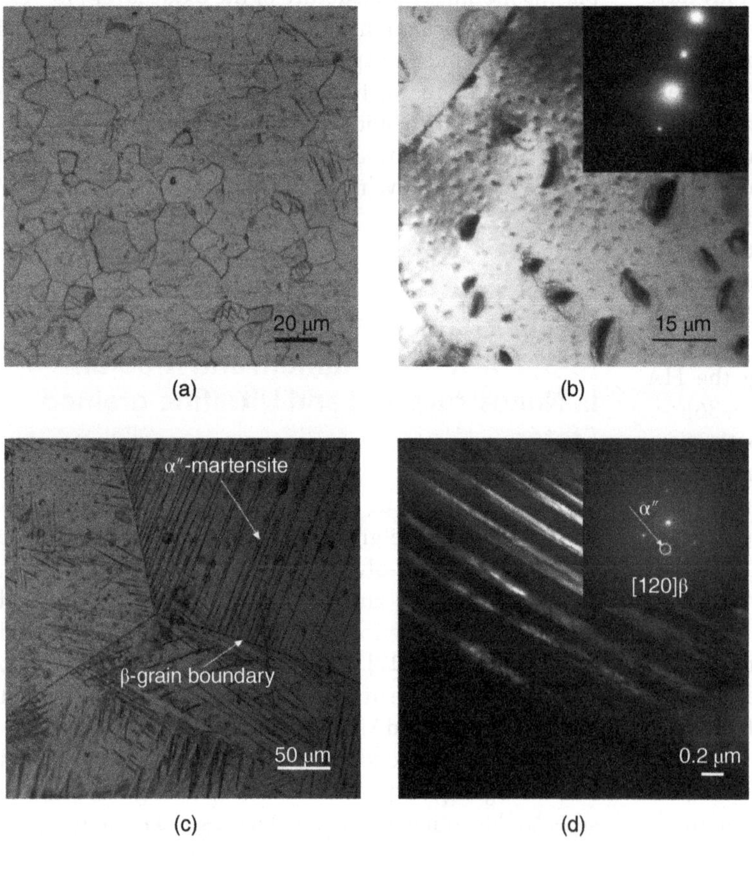

Figure 8.1 Optical images (a,c) and bright-field TEM images of microstructure with microdiffraction patterns (b,d) for Ti VT1-0 (a,b) and Ti–40Nb (c,d) in coarse-grained states.

pattern, indicated existing reflections of β-phase solid Ti and Nb solution and α″ phase. The formation of such a structure after annealing is characteristic of Ti-based alloys containing from 30 to 40 mass%Nb [52].

To produce ultrafine-grained state, two-step combined SPD method was used, i.e. *abc* pressing and multiple rolling [12]. During the first stage, the samples were deformed by *abc* pressing locomotion, consisting of three cycles (see Figure 8.2). Each cycle included three pressing phases at a constant temperature. When passing from one pressing cycle to the next one, the temperature of the samples decreased gradually by 50 °C in the interval of 500–400 °C. After every pressing cycle, the sample was rotated at 90° about the roll axis perpendicular to the previous pressing direction. The relative deformation size of a sample in each pressing cycle was not more than 40–45%. To produce the nanostructured state in Ti, the *abc* pressing in press molds was applied instead of only *abc* pressing [9, 11]. In this case, the sample shrinkage was performed in the press mold itself via three gradual compression axis changes. This is comparable to combined multi-stage *abc*-pressing and rolling. The application of press molds is to enhance constrained deformation conditions furthering more effective grain refinement at smaller number of pressing cycles. During the second stage, the samples after multi-pass rolling are deformed at indoor temperature in grooved rolls to deformation degree of 80%. Multi-stage rolling was conducted to finite deformation at shrinkage in increments of not more than 3%. For the purpose of a more effective grain refinement and homogeneous structure, the samples were placed in a press mold during the first two pressing cycles. After rolling, the billets with 6 × 6 mm^2 in section and 1000 mm in length for Ti VT1-0 and 200 mm in length for Ti–40Nb were produced. To reduce internal strain and elasticity, produced billets were annealed at 350 °C for 1 hour in argon atmosphere. As a result of two-step deformation processing (see Figure 8.2), nanostructured and ultrafine-grained state was formed throughout all billets of Ti VT1-0 and Ti–40Nb.

Figure 8.3 illustrates typical TEM images of titanium microstructures in nanostructured and ultrafine-grained states. Applying press molds in titanium *abc*-pressing effectively improves grain refinement and produces the nanostructure with specifically sized structural elements (grain, subgrain, fragment) of 0.1 μm (see Figure 8.3a) [12]. In case of no existing significant mechanical characteristics of Ti VT1-0, pressing is performed in free conditions without press molds during the first stage [12]. The average structure element size for titanium is 0.1 μm, which corresponds to ultrafine-grained state [53]. Figure 8.3b shows image of titanium microstructure in ultrafine-grained state formed as a result of applying free *abc*-pressing without press molds and further rolling

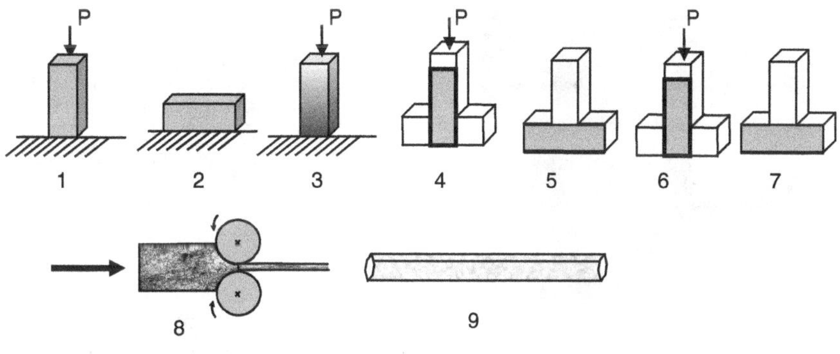

Figure 8.2 Scheme of *abc*-pressing and further rolling: 1, initial sample (arrow shows the direction of the imposed load during pressing); 2, 3, repressing cycle of samples without press mold; 4, initial sample (arrow shows the direction of the imposed load during pressing in a press mold); 5, sample after first pressing cycle in a press mold; 6, 7, repressing cycle with changing deformation axis in a press mold; 8, rolling in grooved rolls; 9, rod after rolling.

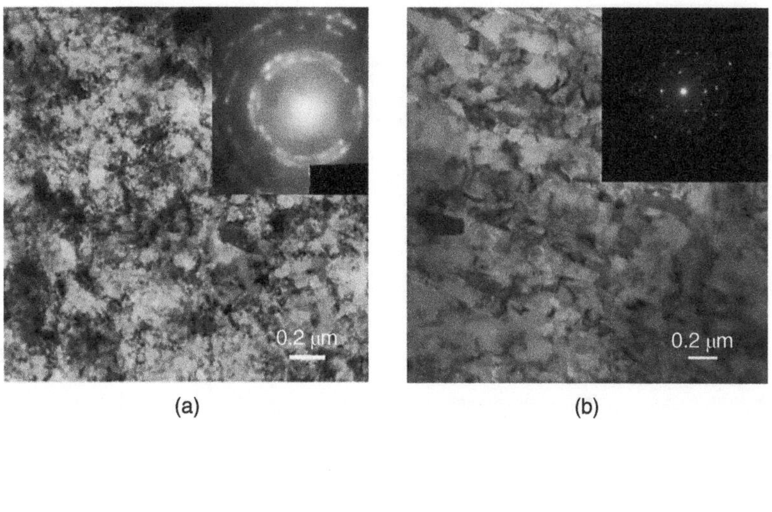

Figure 8.3 Bright-field TEM images of microstructure with microdiffraction patterns of nanostructured Ti (a) and ultrafine-grained Ti (b).

with average-sized structure elements of 0.2 μm. TEM images (see Figure 8.3) show that grain structures are barely discernible. A fragment (subgrain) is observed inside the grain itself. Existing extinction contours show the evidence of high residual stress level in the material after deformation. Cellular-dislocated subgrain with high dislocation density is located in the subgrains and fragments. Significant number of intensive reflections were observed on the microdiffraction patterns (see Figure 8.3), located peripherally, which indicates the increasing grain-boundary angle and the formation of dominating subgrains with large-angle misorientation. No reflections were observed on the microdiffraction patterns extrinsic of α-titanium. Microhardness level of Ti after combined SPD increases significantly within the interval of 3000–3300 MPa comparable to initial coarse-grained state (1800 MPa).

Figure 8.4a–c illustrates TEM images of Ti–40Nb ultrafine-grained microstructure. Bright-field TEM image (see Figure 8.4a) shows subgrains and fragments similar to equiaxial shapes. To identify β- and α-phases, the energy-dispersive X-ray spectrometry (EDX) was applied. Based on this analysis, β-phase subgrains with high niobium concentration relative to initial condition (up to 39 mass%) and α-Ti subgrains with low niobium concentration (4 mass%) were identified in the structure. The subgrain is shown by an arrow in Figure 8.4a. The average size of structure elements, including grains, subgrains, and fragments is 0.28 μm.

Identified microdiffraction patterns (see Figure 8.4b) showed reflections of intensity from β-solid Ti–Nb solution to low intensity from α-phase, supported by electron microprobe analysis. Reflections related to a thermal nanodispersed ω-phase were also observed. On the dark-field image of ω-phase reflection (see Figure 8.4), ellipsoid isolations with maximum and minimum size of 5–10 nm were observed in β-grain. Figure 8.4d shows the diagram of microdiffraction identification, where two β-phase reflection locations are presented for axis zone $[11\bar{2}0]_\omega$ and for axis zone $[1\bar{1}0]_\beta$ in the β-phase lattice. The analysis showed that ω-phase is connected with matrix bcc lattice of β-phase with oriented ratio of $[1\bar{1}0]_\beta \parallel [11\bar{2}0]_\omega$, $(\bar{1}11)_\beta \parallel (0001)_\omega$, and $(1\bar{1}2)_\beta \parallel (1\bar{1}00)_\omega$. It corresponds to the orientation relation of coherent ω-phase to the matrix in titanium alloys [54, 55]. Martensite phase of solid α″-Ti solution could not be identified. It is obvious that metastable α″-Ti phase transforms during deformation processing into stable β-phase of solid Ti–Nb solution according to $\alpha'' \rightarrow \beta + \alpha$ [52]. Under deformation effect, microhardness value comparable to

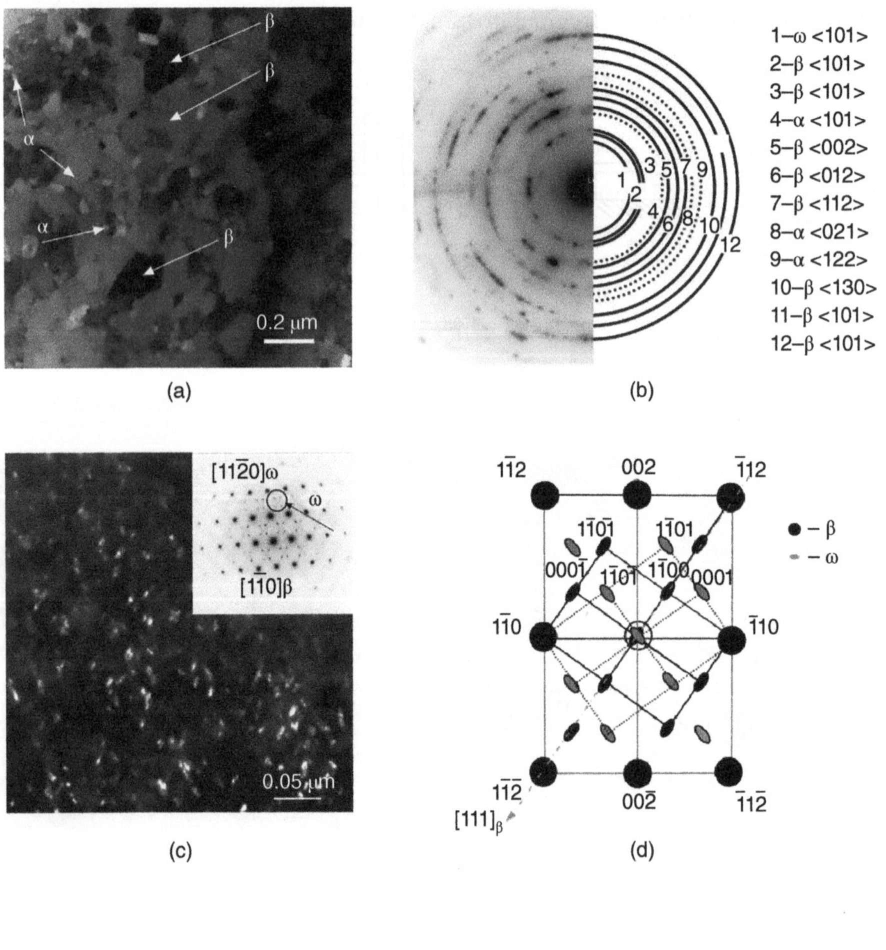

Figure 8.4 Bright-field TEM image (a) with microdiffraction pattern (b); dark-field TEM image in ω-phase reflections (c), and phase identification diagram (d) for Ti–40Nb in ultrafine-grained state.

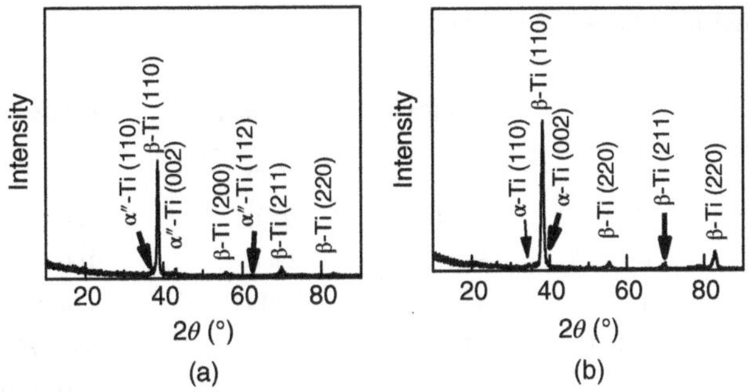

Figure 8.5 XRD patterns of Ti–40Nb after annealing (a) and after *abc*-pressing with rolling (b).

initial annealing state (1700 MPa) increases significantly up to 3300 MPa.

XRD patterns of alloy after annealing with *abc* pressing and further rolling are illustrated in Figure 8.5. Martensite α″-phase and β-phase reflections are observed in the XRD spectrum showing ultrafine-grained phase after annealing (see Figure 8.5a). Transformation of metastable α″-phase into β-phase of solid Ti and Nb solution (see Figure 8.5b) after pressing and further rolling was proved by TEM results. The ω-phase reflections were not observed on the XRD patterns, probably due to the nanodispersed size of this phase.

Flow curves for titanium in ultrafine-grained and coarse-grained states are shown in Figure 8.6a. Ultrafine-grained state in titanium provides plasticity value of up to 8%, and tensile yield $\sigma_{0.2}$ and ultimate stress σ_B are 960 and 1160 MPa, respectively (Figure 8.6a, curve 1), while $\sigma_{0.2}$ and σ_B for titanium in coarse-grained state are 270 and 400 MPa, respectively (Figure 8.6a, curve 2). Mechanical characteristics of Ti–40Nb in ultrafine-grained state are as follows: relative tensile yield $\sigma_{0.2}$ is 920 MPa (see Figure 8.6b, curve 1), which is twice more than that of Ti–40Nb in coarse-grained state – 480 MPa (see Figure 8.6b, curve 2). Ultimate stress σ_B is 1040 MPa, being 1.5 times more in comparison to the initial state – 700 MPa where plasticity value decreases to 4%. To produce increased plasticity, it is necessary to significantly increase subrecrystallization annealing after deformation processing.

Mechanical property data of investigated materials in ultrafine-grained and coarse-grained states including Ti–6Al–4V alloy are listed in Table 8.2. The latter is widely used as a base for different medical implants. Based on the comparative analysis of the mechanical characteristics of investigated alloys, it is obvious that SPD combined with *abc*-pressing and further rolling and subrecrystallization annealing makes it possible to produce nanostructured and ultrafine-grained alloys with high mechanical properties. This is comparable to the mechanical properties of medium titanium alloys such as Ti–6Al–4V and Ti–6Al–7Nb being used in medicine now. It should be noted that investigated titanium alloys contain only bioinert metal elements and no alloying elements, which are toxic for the human organism.

Thus, combined two-step SPD method, including free *abc*-pressing and *abc*-pressing in press mold with further multi-pass rolling and recrystallization annealing allows forming Ti VT1-0 and Ti–40Nb in nanostructured and ultrafine-grained states. Ultrafine-grained structure provides improved mechanical properties (yield strength, ultimate strength, microhardness) comparable to initial coarse-grained state. Bioinert ultrafine-grained Ti–40Nb alloy with low elastic modulus (55–75 GPa) is the most perspective material in the production of medical implants.

8.3 Micro-Arc Oxidation Method for the Production of Bioactive Calcium Phosphate Coatings on the Surface of Bioinert Metals and Alloys

MAO, also called plasma electrolytic oxidation (PEO) or anodic spark deposition or micro-arc discharge oxidation, is a plasma-chemical and electrochemical process.

Figure 8.6 Tensile diagrams of Ti VT1-0 (a) and Ti–40Nb (b) in ultrafine-grained (1) and coarse-grained states (2).

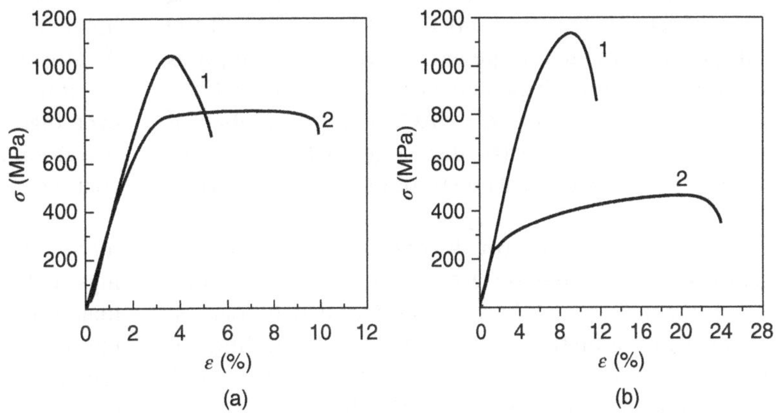

Table 8.2 Mechanical characteristics of titanium alloys in ultrafine-grained and coarse-grained states.

Titanium alloys	$\sigma_{0.2}$ (MPa)	σ_B (MPa)	δ (%)	σ_0 MPa	H_μ (MPa)	E (MPa)
VT1-0, coarse-grained state	240	400	23	280	1800	100–105
VT1-0, ultrafine--grained state	700	1000	7	>300	3000	100
VT1-0, nanostructured state	1100	1160	6	580	3300	100
Titanium, Grade 4	≥480	≥550	15	470	2200	114
Ti–6Al–4V	1010	1100	≥8	570	3500	88–116
Ti–6Al–7Nb	820	940	7	—	2000	110–120
Ti–40Nb, coarse-grained state	200	400	15	—	2300	55–70
Ti–40Nb, ultrafine-grained state	920	480	4	—	3300	55–80

$\sigma_{0.2}$, yield strength; σ_B, ultimate stress; δ, plasticity value; σ_0, fatigue strength for 10^6 cycles; H_μ, microhardness; E, elastic modulus.

The process combines electrochemical oxidation with a high-voltage spark treatment in an aqueous electrolytic bath, which also contains modifying elements in the form of dissolved salts (e.g. silicates) to be incorporated into the resulting coatings [56].

During the MAO process, the specimen is immersed in an aqueous electrolyte bath and connected to a high-voltage power supply. A water-cooled stainless steel or titanium electrolyte bath as well as is the counter-electrode. When the applied voltage exceeds a certain critical value, micro-plasma discharge occurs on the surface of the component, thereby resulting in a modified surface [57]. During the process, microdischarges promptly arise and extinguish during 10^{-4}–10^{-5} seconds near the anode and heat the metal substrate to 373–423 K. Simultaneously, the local temperature and pressure in the discharge channels formed by electric sparks reach 10^3–10^4 K [58] and 10^2–10^3 MPa, respectively [59]. Such temperature and pressure are sufficient to induce plasma thermochemical interaction between the substrate and electrolyte. These internal interactions lead to the formation on the surface of melted-cooled high-temperature oxides and complex compounds consisting of oxides of the substrate material and modified electrolyte elements. Due to the strong electric field (10^6–10^8 V/m) between the anode and the cathode, electrolyte ions penetrate into structural pores where they can participate in electrochemical reactions [58–62]. In the course of MAO, a great number of short-living sparks (electric discharges) arise as a result of localized electric breakdowns of the growing coating. These discharges, certainly, play an important role in the mechanism of coating growth. They leave characteristic "craters" on the free surface of the growing coating. Dunleavy et al. [63, 64] have shown that such discharges, as a rule, have lifetimes of several tens or hundreds of microseconds; moreover, they often arise in "cascades" in the same place and lasted several milliseconds.

The MAO process having a sufficiently complex mechanism can be tentatively subdivided into several stages proceeding in series or simultaneously [65]:

1. chemical interaction of the material basis and coating being formed with the electrolyte;
2. electrochemical processes occurring before and after the ignition of an electric discharge in sections of the surface being treated in places, where no electric discharge is present at the moment (anodizing in water solutions of electrolytes and electrolysis);
3. MAO itself including short initial stages of luminescence and arching; the main stage of micro-arc discharge burning;
4. transition of the micro-arc discharge into an arc after formation of the coating of definite thickness.

The heart of the MAO process is anode oxidation of metals. Nowadays it is unambiguously established that anode oxide films on aluminum and other valve metals formed in electrolytes moderately dissolving oxide consist of two layers: barrier, a thin dense porous layer adjoining the metal, and an external porous layer. However, the MAO process has an advantage in comparison with conventional anodizing, allowing coatings with a more developed and complex structure to be formed, including coatings with higher degree of crystallinity. As already reported, during MAO treatment, specimens are immersed into acidic or alkaline electrolyte; however, higher voltages are applied than during anodizing; therefore, electric local plasma discharges allow thicker coatings to be obtained and thus the microstructure of the coatings being formed to be controlled. The MAO method is often used to deposit various functional coatings with porous structure on the titanium, aluminum, magnesium, zirconium, and their alloy surfaces, providing an effective chemical barrier against the escape of the substrate metal ions and increasing the corrosion resistance of metal materials [66, 67]. Since the MAO can be performed at room temperature for specimens with complex geometry, this method of coating deposition on the surface of metals and alloys is considered simple, economic, and nonpolluting to obtain oxide ceramic coatings.

It is well known that the MAO is a complex process whose characteristics depend on both *external factors* (elemental composition, concentration, pH, and electrolyte temperature; MAO mode: polarity, frequency, porosity, amplitude and waveform of voltage, and current pulses and their parity; treatment time, etc.) and *internal factors* (alloy structure, its heat treatment and roughness and porosity of the material, etc.). These factors determine the coating thickness, composition, structure, density, porosity, microhardness, and strength of coupling with the substrate, wear and corrosion resistance, electrical and thermal conductivity, breakdown voltage, and other properties. An analysis of the influence of external and internal factors on the formation of coatings during MAO and its properties allows us to conclude that the decisive influence have the *electrolyte composition, electric* and *time parameters* of the MAO mode, and the *composition of the substrate material* [68].

To obtain biocoatings by the MAO method, electrolytes comprising calcium and phosphorus compounds are employed. Moreover, all electrolytes can be subdivided into three groups: by the acid indicator (*acid, alkaline*, and *neutral*), by the number of components (*single component* and *multicomponent*), and whether the electrolyte is a *solution* or a *suspension*. In the first group, *acid electrolytes*, as a rule, are based on sulfuric, phosphoric, fluoric, and acetic acids or their mixtures [69, 70]; *alkaline electrolytes*, for example, are based on potassium and sodium hydroxides, and hydrolyzed salts ($NaSiO_3$, $NaAlO_2$, etc.) [71]; *neutral electrolytes*, for example, are based on salts (NaCl, etc.) [72]. The second group comprises *single-component* electrolytes, for example, silicate ones based on silicates of alkaline metals ($NaSiO_3{\cdot}9H_2O$, etc.) or solutions of liquid glass ($mNa_2O{\cdot}nSiO_2$, $M = n/m = 2–4$, etc.) [73]; *two-component* electrolytes, for example, silicate-alkaline ($KOH + NaSiO_3{\cdot}9H_2O$, etc.) [70, 72]; *three-component* electrolytes, for example, comprising soluble aluminate, hexaphosphate, and alkaline ($KOH + Na_6P_6O_{18} + NaAlO_2$) [74]; and *multicomponent* electrolytes, for example, comprising soluble hexaphosphates, aluminates, and alkali and complex salt [71]. *Electrolytes* belonging to the third group – the *suspensions* comprising various insoluble compounds to assign special characteristics to coatings, for example, apatites ($Ca_{10}PO_4(OH)_6$), oxides (TiO_2, $A1_2O_3$, SiO_2, and MgO), nitrides (TiN and BN), and carbides (SiC) [75]; *electrolytes – true solutions*, for example, based on solutions of calcium acetate, calcium glycerophosphates, and ethers of phosphoric acid [72].

The composition of the substrate material also has an important effect on the structure, composition, and properties of the coatings formed in the course of MAO. As already indicated above, micro-arc treatment can be performed only for metals and alloys of the valve group. In particular, titanium and its alloys are widely used for biomedical applications as implant materials due to their biological compatibility (technically pure Ti, Ti–6Al–4V, etc.) as well as alloys based on Ti–Nb–Zr due to their biomechanical compatibility (Ti–6Al–7Nb, Ti–13Nb–13Zr, Ti–35Nb, Ti35Nb15Zr, etc.). Alloys based on Cr–Ni and Co–Cr (18Cr–8Ni, 18Cr–14Ni–2.5Mo, Co–Cr–Mo (F75), Co–Cr–Mo (F799), Co–Cr–W–Ni (F90), Co–Ni–Cr–Mo–Ti (F562), etc.) are also widely used [76–78]. Increasing interest has recently been focused on biodegradable Mg-based alloys (Mg–Al (AZ31, AZ61, AZ91D), Mg–Zn–Cu (ZC71, ZE41, WE43), etc.) [79, 80].

Numerous works (for example see [72, 81]) demonstrated that the applied voltage and the process duration are two important parameters of the MAO process having the greatest impact on the structure and property of coatings being formed. Thus, for example, in [82] by means of anodizing of titanium in a direct current at low voltages ($\leq$20 V), a nanotube surface structure was obtained. However, in [72] it was shown that to form HA as a part of coatings in the course of MAO, a pulsed current with a high voltage ($\sim$350 V) creating sufficient electric field between the anode and the cathode is required in order that dissolved ions of the electrolyte can take part in chemical and electrochemical reactions.

Over the last 10 years, a group of scientists from the Laboratory of Nanostructured Biocomposite Physics at the Institute of Strength Physics and Materials Science of the Siberian Branch of the Russian Academy of Sciences (ISPMS SB RAS, Tomsk, Russia) has been engaged in the development and investigation of the structure and properties of biocomposites based on bioinert (titanium, zirconium, and niobium) alloys and bioactive CaP coatings formed by the MAO method. The technological process of micro-arc deposition of CaP coatings has several subsequent stages: preparation of the substrate surface, electrolyte preparation, deposition of coatings by the MAO method, washing and drying of specimens with coatings, and quality control.

8.3.1 Stage 1: Specimen Preparation

The specimens were cut from billets of technically pure titanium (Ti) and Ti–40Nb alloy in nanostructured and ultrafine-grained conditions and their sizes were $10 \times 10 \times 1\ mm^3$. Specimens were prepared with silicon carbide papers of 120, 480, 600, 1200 grit, respectively, using the grinding and polishing machine "TegraSystem" (Struers, Denmark) at two speeds of 150 and 300 rpm. Then specimens were ultrasonically cleaned (Elmasonic, Germany) in distilled water and ethanol for 10 minutes and further dried in air.

8.3.2 Stage 2: Preparation of Electrolyte

Previously, the structure of electrolyte based on aqueous solution of orthophosphoric acid (30 mass%) and calcium carbonate (9 mass%) with addition of biological HA (6 mass%) was suggested and patented [83]. It was shown that the use of this electrolyte allows CaP coatings on titanium having quasi-amorphous structure, roughness in the range of 2–5 μm, strength of the coating adhesion to the substrate 20–25 MPa, and Ca/P ratio up to 0.7 to be formed [68, 84]. At present, the given composition of the electrolyte is modified. Thus, to form the hydrophilic CaP coatings with new functional and biological properties, it was suggested to use HA with stoichiometric composition synthesized by the mechanochemical method. Also to provide the antibacterial properties of CaP coatings, it was suggested to use the Zn- or Cu-substituted HA. HA substituted in cation sublattice by Zn^{2+} or Cu^{2+} ions with concentration of substitutes ($Ca_{10-x}Zn_x(PO_4)_6(OH)_2$ or $Ca_{10-x}Cu_x(PO_4)_6(OH)_2$, $x = 0.1$) was prepared by mechanochemical synthesis in an AGO-3 planetary mill at the Institute of Solid State Chemistry and Mechanochemistry of the Siberian Branch of the Russian Academy of Sciences (ISSCM SB RAS, Novosibirsk, Russia) [31, 85]. The above-indicated modifying additives will balance the concentrations of microelements in biocoatings and bone structures and will improve conditions for implant adaptation to organism environments. It is well known that long-term treatment with Zn and Cu in microquantities produces antimicrobial effect and minimizes the danger of growth of pathogenic microorganisms.

In addition to HA, bioceramics and $CaO–SiO_2$ type compounds to which wollastonite $CaSiO_3$ belongs have high bioactivities [86, 87]. These compounds are partially dissolved in body liquids, releasing Ca^{2+} ions. Silicon stimulates intercellular reactions, promoting the formation of the bone tissue [88]. In addition, as has been established recently, silicon plays an important role in the process of collagen mineralization [89]. To increase the biological activity and strength characteristics of the coating, wollastonite $CaSiO_3$ was added to the electrolyte structure [45, 90]. Natural wollastonite possesses clearly expressed needle-like crystal habit that allows reinforced structure to be formed by incorporation of wollastonite into the material [91].

To prepare the given electrolytes, calcium carbonate was added to orthophosphoric acid and partly reacted with it forming calcium phosphates (MCPM and DCPD), carbon dioxides, and water in the following reactions [68]:

$$\begin{aligned} &H_3PO_4 + CaCO_3 \rightarrow Ca(H_2PO_4)_2 \cdot H_2O + CO_2 \\ &H_3PO_4 + CaCO_3 \rightarrow CaHPO_4 \cdot 2H_2O + CO_2 \end{aligned} \tag{8.1}$$

Phosphoric acid, similar to other multibase acids, dissociated in steps with formation mainly of dihydrophosphate ions [68]:

$$\begin{aligned} &H_3PO_4 \Leftrightarrow H^+ + H_2PO_4^- \\ &H_2PO_4^- \Leftrightarrow H^+ + HPO_4^{2-} \\ &HPO_4^{2-} \Leftrightarrow H^+ + PO_4^{3-} \end{aligned} \tag{8.2}$$

MCPM and DCPD are thermally unstable, and already at temperatures above 80–100 °C are transformed into the waterless form [68]:

$$\begin{aligned} &Ca(H_2PO_4)_2 \cdot H_2O \xrightarrow{\geq 80^\circ C} Ca(H_2PO_4)_2 + H_2O \\ &CaHPO_4 \cdot 2H_2O \xrightarrow{\geq 80^\circ C} CaHPO_4 + 2H_2O_2 \end{aligned} \tag{8.3}$$

In the acid electrolyte ($1 < pH < 2$), waterless dicalcium phosphate and monocalcium phosphate are dissolved with the formation of calcium and phosphate ions [68]:

$$\begin{aligned} &Ca(H_2PO_4)_2 \xrightarrow{1 \leq pH \leq 2} CaH_2PO_4^+ + H_2PO_4^- + H_2O \\ &CaH_2PO_4^+ \xrightarrow{1 \leq pH \leq 2} Ca^{2+} + PO_4^{3-} + 2H^+ \\ &CaHPO \xrightarrow{1 \leq pH \leq 2} Ca^{2+} + PO_4^{3-} + H^+ \end{aligned} \tag{8.4}$$

Then after the termination of gas liberation into the electrolyte, HA was added with constant stirring. Despite the lowest HA resorbability among calcium phosphates, it was partly dissolved in the acidic environment.

The electrolyte was held for several days to complete chemical reactions, interaction, and dissolution of the solution components. As a result, the homogeneous electrolyte with insignificant amount of a disperse phase was formed. Application of HA and calcium carbonate as a disperse phase stabilized the process of forming of micro-arc CaP coatings on the metal matrix; as a result, uniform coatings with satisfactory adhesion to the substrate were formed [68].

To form CaP and oxide coatings by the MAO method, a Micro-arc-3.0 technological complex was developed at the Laboratory of Physics of Nanostructured Biocomposites at the ISPMS SB RAS. The setup comprised a pulse power supply, a cooled galvanic bath, a complete set of electrodes, an oscilloscope, and software for control over the electrophysical parameters. The key parameters of the pulse source varied in wide limits: output voltage 10–1000 V, pulse duration 10–500 μs, and pulse repetition frequency 10–200 Hz. Previous investigations demonstrated that for two constant parameters – pulse repetition frequency and pulse duration – the voltage applied to the specimen and the duration of the deposition process had the greatest influence on the characteristics of coatings. Therefore, in the process of forming CaP coatings, the voltage of the MAO process varied from 150 to 350 V, the process duration varied from 5 to 15 minutes, and the pulse duration varied from 100 to 500 μs. The process frequency of 50 Hz was constant.

The process of coating formation in electrolyte suspension during MAO had several successive stages: dissociation of salts into ions, diffusion of electrolyte ions toward the specimen surface, microplasma processes and electrochemical reactions, formation of the oxide or CaP coating, and then the processes were repeated [68].

On the cathode hydrogen was liberated [68]:

$$2H^+ + 2e = H_2 \tag{8.5}$$

On the *anode* surface (specimen), the high-pressure and high-temperature gas cavity, consisting of oxygen ions diffusing deep into the metal was formed on sharp edges under the action of micro-arc discharge. When the electric field strength in the gas cavity became higher than beyond it, the bubble burst and a part of metal ions, reacting with electrolyte, was hydrolyzed by the following mechanism (an example for Ti specimens) [68]:

$$\begin{aligned} &Ti^+ - 2e = Ti^{2+} \\ &Ti^{2+} + 3H_2O - e = Ti(OH)_3 + 3H^+ \end{aligned} \tag{8.6}$$

Other part was in the solution in the form of ions. Since titanium hydroxide had lower conductivity, the following microcategory arises nearby under the same scheme. Further under the influence of temperature there are the following reactions [68]:

$$\begin{aligned} &Ti^{3+} + H_2O - e = TiO_2 + 2H^+ \\ &Ti^{4+} + 2OH^- = TiO_2 + 2H^+ \end{aligned} \tag{8.7}$$

Since titanium oxides possessed good electrical conductivity, a thin anode film was formed thereby leading to the formation of the intermediate titanium oxide layer. In the process of forming the subsequent CaP layer, HA powder particles or reaction products (dicalcium phosphate and monocalcium phosphate or their waterless forms) arrived on the anode surface. Many electrochemical reactions run during coating formation in the micro-arc discharge; only some of them are given below [68]:

$$\begin{aligned} &Ti^{4+} + Ca_{10-x}(PO_4)_6^{2(1-x)} \xrightarrow{T} CaTi_4(PO_4)_6 + n \cdot Ca^{2+} \\ &Ca^{2+} + 4Ti^{4+} + 6(PO_4)^{3-} \xrightarrow{T} CaTi_4(PO_4)_6 \\ &3Ca^{2+} + 2(PO_4)^{3-} \xrightarrow{T} Ca_2P_2O_7 + CaO \\ &2CaHPO_4 \xrightarrow{T} Ca_2P_2O_7 + H_2O \\ &Ti^{4+} + 2CaHPO_4 \xrightarrow{T} TiP_2O_7 + H_2O + 2Ca^{2+} \\ &2Ti^{4+} + 2(PO_4)^{3-} \xrightarrow{T} TiP_2O_7 + TiO \\ &Ti^{4+} + Ca_2P_2O_7 \xrightarrow{T} TiP_2O_7 + Ca^{2+} \end{aligned} \tag{8.8}$$

Similar reactions will run when Ti–40Nb alloy is used for the anode.

8.3.3 Experimental Methods and Procedures for Investigations of CaP Coatings

The surface morphology and cross-sectional structure of the CaP coatings were observed by scanning electron microscopy (SEM; LEO EVO 50, Zeiss, Germany, "Nanotech" center at ISPMS SB RAS, and JEOL JSM–7001F SEM, Japan) and transmission electron microscopy (TEM; JEOL JEM–2010, Japan). In addition, the elemental compositions and distributions of the coatings were also analyzed using EDX (INCA, Oxford Instruments) in conjunction with the SEM system. The size of structural elements of the coating is measured by the secant method according to ASTM E1382–9 and DD ENV 1071–5. The porosity is calculated by the formula $P\,(\%) = \Sigma l/\Sigma L \times 100$, where L is the length of a randomly secant drawn in SEM images and l is the length of a secant part that falls on pores.

The chemical composition was determined by XRD (Dron 7, Burevestnik, Russia, "Nanotech" center at ISPMS SB RAS) in the angular range $2\theta = 10–90°$ with a scan step 0.03 with Co K_α radiation ($\lambda = 0.17902$ nm). The average roughness (R_a) was estimated as with a Homel–Etamic T1000 profilometer. Fourier transform infrared (FT-IR) spectroscopy was performed in transmission mode using an FT-IR spectrometers (Alpha FT-IR Spectrometer, Bruker, Germany) in the infrared wave region of 4000–500 cm^{-1} for the functional group analysis. For FT-IR analysis, the coating particles were mixed well with potassium bromide (KBr) and pressed into pellets.

The apparent density was calculated according to the formula: $\rho = m/(S{\cdot}D)$, where m is the mass of the coating, calculated as a difference between the mass of the sample before and after deposition of the coating; S is the area of the coating calculated for two sides of the sample; D is the coating thickness determined using SEM cross-section micrographs. To measure the adhesion strength of the coatings to the substrate, two cylinders were glued to both sides of the samples with coating by Loctite Hysol 9514. They were fixed in grips in order to be tested under tension (Instron–1185, Great Britain). The adhesion strength is the maximum stress required to tear the cylinder off the calcium phosphate coating. It was measured as $\delta_A = F/S$, where F is the breakout force of coating from substrate and S is the area of separation.

Wettability tests were carried out using an Easy Drop goniometer with the drop shape analysis software DSA1 (Kruss, Germany). We used two test liquids, i.e. distilled water as polar liquid and glycerol as dispersive one. To measure static contact angles of the liquids on the solid surface, we used a sessile drop method and the Young equation

$$\sigma_{SG} = \sigma_{SL} + \sigma_{LG}\cos\theta \tag{8.9}$$

where θ is the contact angle value; σ_{SG}, σ_{SL}, and σ_{LG} are the surface tension coefficients at the solid–gas, solid–liquid, and liquid–gas boundaries.

Furthermore, the free surface energy of the coating was calculated in accordance with the Owens–Wendt equation [92]:

$$\sigma_L(\cos\theta + 1) = 2\sqrt{\sigma_S^P\sigma_L^P} + 2\sqrt{\sigma_S^D\sigma_L^D} \tag{8.10}$$

where $\sigma_L^D, \sigma_S^D, \sigma_L^P, \sigma_S^P$ are the dispersive and polar components of the free surface energy of the liquid and solid phases, respectively, and σ_L is the free surface energy of the test liquid.

8.4 Hydrophilic Calcium Phosphate Coatings with Developed Surface Relief, Porous Morphology, and High Rate of Bioresorption

To prevent postoperative complications caused by rejection of the active metal, it is expedient to deposit coatings possessing biologically active and biocompatible properties on the implant surface to accelerate osseogenesis and osseointegration of the bone tissue as well as to improve the anticorrosive protective properties allowing an effective chemical barrier to be created against ion escape from the metal of the substrate. For these purposes it is most promising to use bioactive CaP coatings with porous morphology and developed surface relief comprising compounds "native" for the bone tissue [93].

In this chapter, it will be represented the comparative investigations of structure, composition, physical and chemical, and biological properties of Ca coatings on Ti and Ti–40Nb in nanostructured and ultrafine-grained states deposited by MAO method in electrolyte based on phosphoric acid, calcium carbonate, and synthesized HA under different oxidation voltages in the range of 200–300 V. Other electrophysical parameters have been previously defined [68]: the pulse duration of 100 μs, the frequency of 50 Hz, and process duration of 10 minutes. Addition of HA particles in the electrolyte–suspension composition is used to produce the CaP coatings by MAO method with new good biological properties. Wei et al. [71] investigated the influence of nano-HA powder concentration in electrolyte on structure and bioactivity *in vitro* micro-arc coatings. Alternative method composed of MAO and electrophoretic deposition was developed to prepare HA/TiO_2 coatings in an HA-containing electrolyte [75, 94, 95].

Figure 8.7 shows SEM images of the CaP coatings on Ti and Ti–40Nb deposited under different MAO voltages. Investigation of the CaP coatings morphology showed that the coatings are formed by layers (see Figure 8.7f–h). The structure of the CaP coatings consisted of thin porous oxide sublayer and the basic porous CaP layer. The main components of surface structure are spheroidal elements with pores. The same surface morphology with spheres and pores were obtained for CaP coatings on Ti deposited in electrolyte based on biological HA in the previous works [43, 68, 96]. The process of spheres and pores formation is similar to the process of formation and collapse of electrolyte–suspension "bubble" in the area microplasma discharges.

The size of the structural elements depends substantially on the parameters of MAO method, in particular, on the oxidation voltage. It was established that the initial oxidation voltage was 200 V. At this voltage the porous CaP layer with spheres and pores on the surface is formed. An increase of the process voltage in the range of 200–300 V leads to the increase of micro-arc discharge magnitudes and, as consequently, to the growth of structural element (spheres and pores) sizes and local destruction of spheres. In this case, plate-like crystals of the new substance form on the surface of fragments and hemispheres into the CaP coatings on Ti–40Nb (see Figure 8.7e). It was found that the thickness, roughness, and the average size of the structural elements grow linearly with increasing of the MAO voltage (see Figure 8.8). For the CaP coatings on Ti, the thickness and roughness increase from 35 to 80 μm and from 2 to 4.5 μm, respectively (see Figure 8.8a, curves 1 and 3). And for the CaP coatings on the Ti–40Nb, the thickness and roughness increase from 60 to 105 μm and from 3 to 5 μm, respectively (see Figure 8.8a, curves 2 and 4). The average sizes of spheres and pores for the CaP coatings on both substrates grow linearly from 10 to 22 μm and from 3 to 8 μm, respectively, with increasing of the process voltage (see Figure 8.8b).

In the previous work [97], it was reported about novel concepts of "niche-relief" and "niche-voltage" for stem cells and supposed that the average roughness in the

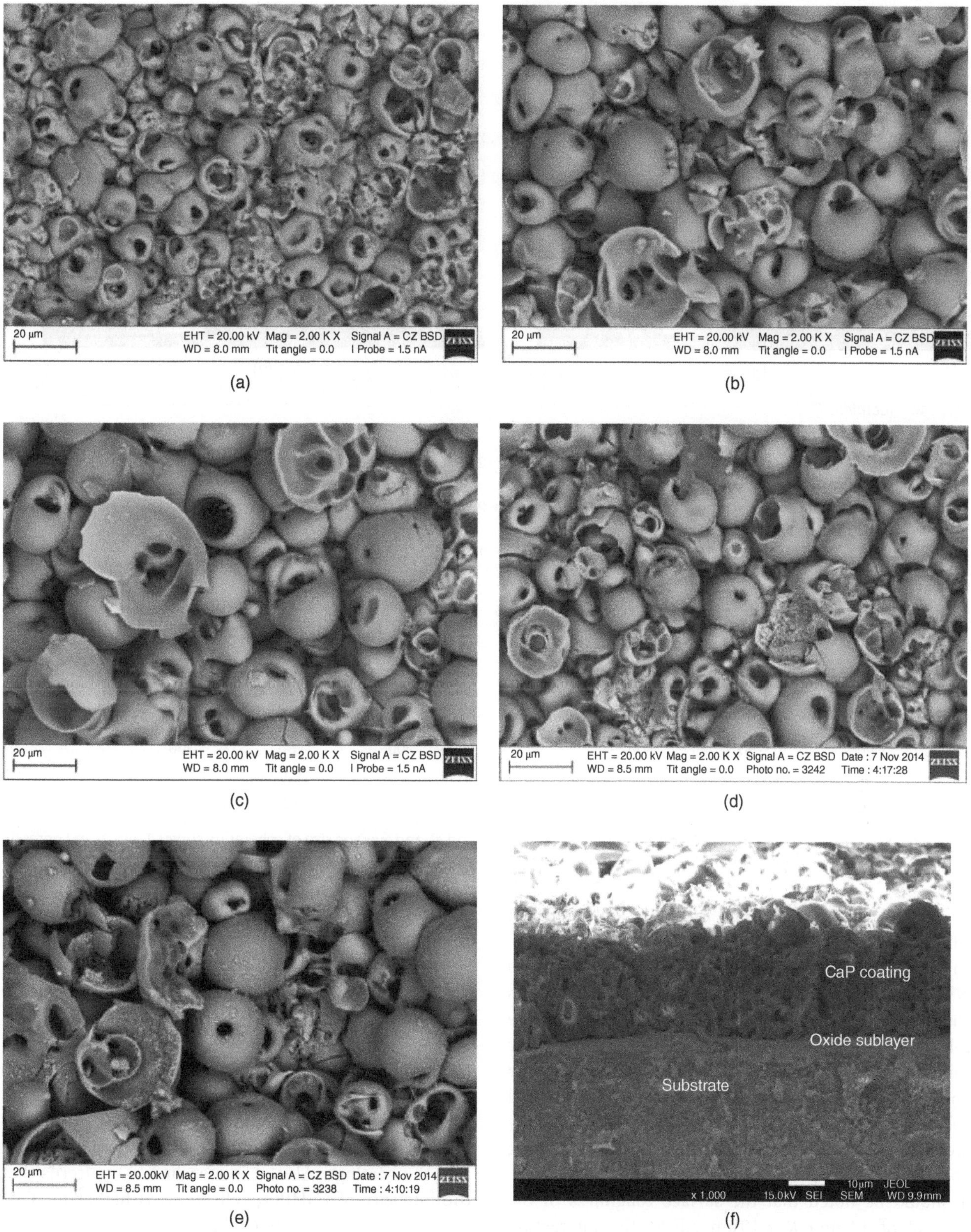

Figure 8.7 SEM images of the top (a–e) and cross-sectional (f–h) CaP coatings on Ti (a–c, f–h) and Ti–40Nb (d–e) deposited under different oxidation voltages (V): (a,f) 200, (b,c,g) 250, (d,e,h) 300.

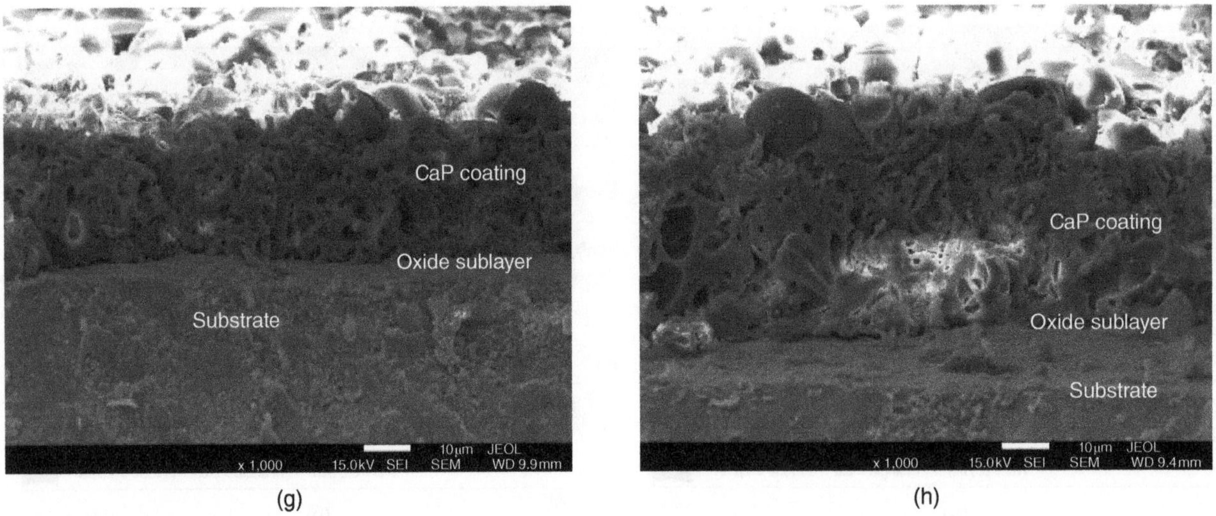

Figure 8.7 (*Continued*)

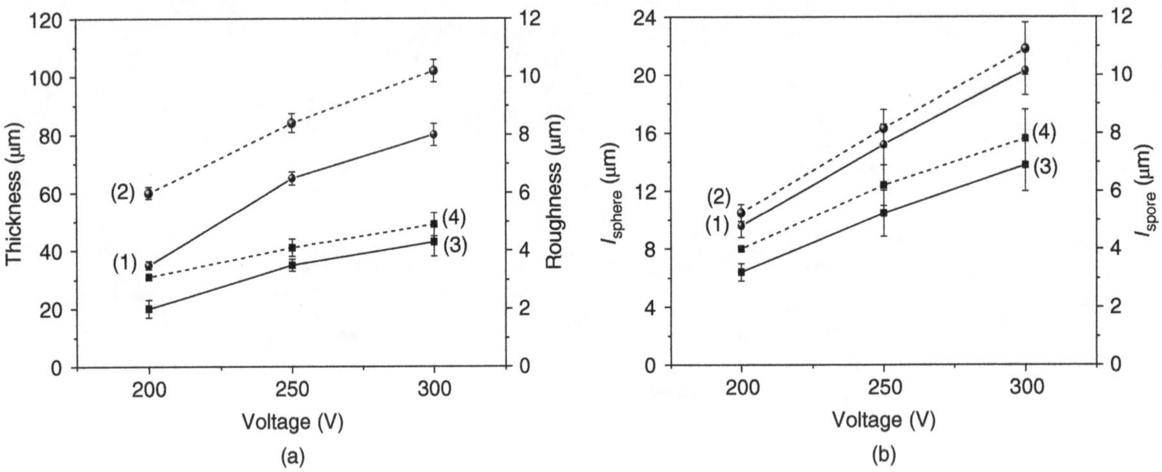

Figure 8.8 Plots of thickness (a, curves 1 and 2), roughness (a, curves 3 and 4), and average size of spheres (b, curves 1 and 2) and pores (b, curves 3 and 4) for CaP coatings on the Ti (curves 1 and 3) and Ti–40Nb (curves 2 and 4) against the MAO voltage.

range of 2.5–5 μm is optimal for successful stem cell adhesion to the coating surface and their further differentiation into the bone tissue. However, some authors [98–100] supposed that the surface of titanium implants with nanoroughness strengthens the adhesion of definite cells – osteoblasts (bone-forming cells) – and other cellular functions (for example synthesis of alkaline phosphatase (ALP) and precipitation of calcium and collagen secretion) and simultaneously suppresses the growth of the competing cells – fibroblasts (cells creating fibrous tissue and preventing normal bone integration). It should be noted that the surface roughness in the interval of $10\,\text{nm} < R_a < 10\,\mu\text{m}$ affects the interaction of the biological implants with the bone tissue because it has the same order of magnitude as cells and large biomolecules. At the same time, Giavaresy et al. [101] and Sammons et al. [102] reported that microporous rough surfaces improved osseointegration of the implants.

XRD patterns (see Figure 8.9) demonstrated that the CaP coatings on both substrates produced under process voltages of 200–250 V are mainly in X-ray amorphous state, as indicated by well-pronounced halo on the XRD patterns. There are only small reflections corresponding to β-calcium pyrophosphate (β-$Ca_2P_2O_7$). With increasing of the oxidation voltage to 300 V, the new crystalline phase of monetite ($CaHPO_4$) starts to form into the coatings. Also, it is seen in XRD patterns that the intensity of $CaHPO_4$ reflections is higher for CaP coatings on Ti–40Nb than that for the coatings on Ti. Such XRD result is in agreement with the SEM results for CaP coatings on Ti–40Nb (see Figure 8.7f), which demonstrated the platelet-shaped crystals typical for

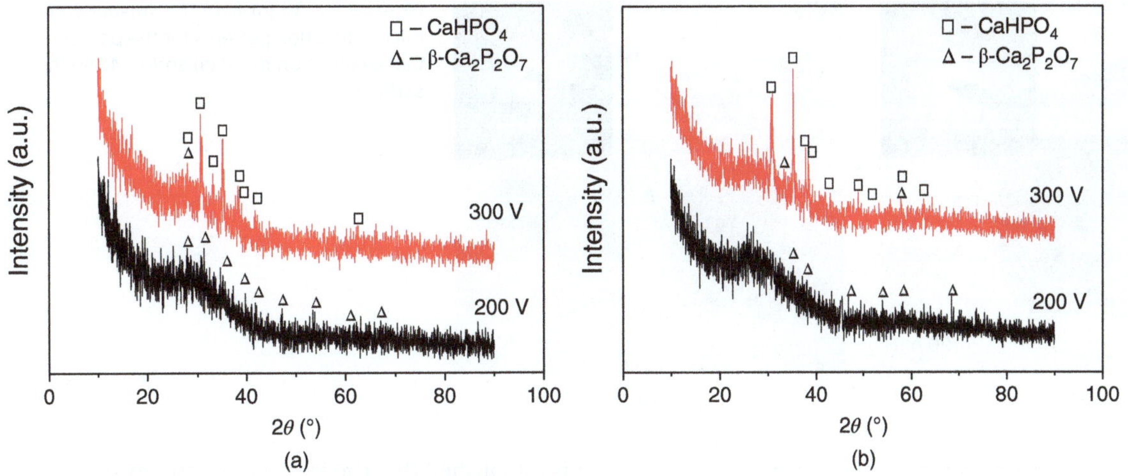

Figure 8.9 XRD patterns of CaP coatings on Ti (a) and Ti–40Nb (b) deposited under different MAO voltages.

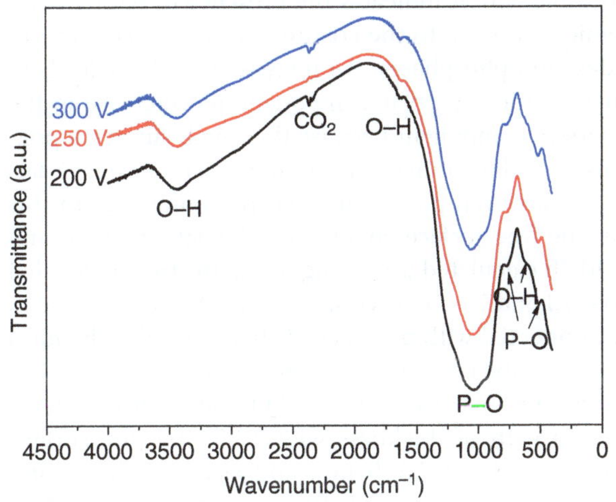

Figure 8.10 IR spectra of CaP coatings on Ti deposited under different voltages.

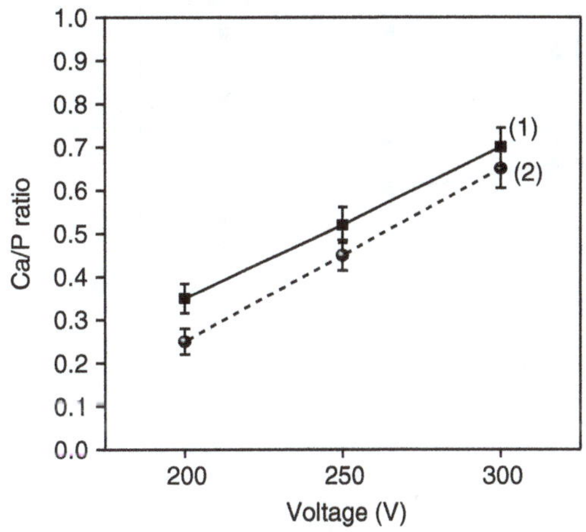

Figure 8.11 Plots of Ca/P ratio for the CaP coatings on Ti (1) and Ti–40Nb (2) against the process voltage.

monetite. The presence of X-ray amorphous structure and content of freely soluble monetite into the coating indicate a high rate of coating bioresorption, which is confirmed by previous biological tests [68].

Figure 8.10 shows the typical IR spectra of the CaP coatings on Ti deposited under different process voltages. All spectra are characterized by the presence of intense absorption bands corresponding to asymmetric and symmetric oscillations of P—O phosphate bond with maximum absorption in the region of 1130–930 cm^{-1} and the absorption bands of OH^- groups of adsorbed water at 1650–1620 cm^{-1} and 3550–3200 cm^{-1}. The shoulder in the area of 800–730 cm^{-1} also indicates the presence of oscillations of O—H bonds of acid phosphate such as HPO_4^- groups and P—O—P pyrophosphate bridge bonds. The presence of absorption band at 2400–2300 cm^{-1} can be due to absorption of atmospheric CO_2 during sample preparation for IRS analysis [103].

The EDX analysis demonstrated that the composition of the CaP coatings on the titanium surface is represented by the following elements: Ca (6.6–11.4 at.%), P (17.4–21.1 at.%), O (52.0–62.2 at.%), and Ti (12.3–17.8 at.%). The elemental composition of the CaP coatings on the Ti–40Nb was analogous to that of coatings on Ti with Nb content of 5.4–7.8 at.%. With increasing of the process voltage and, as consequently, the growth of temperature in the microplasma discharge area, the deposition of Ca^{2+} ions from the electrolyte intensify and the $CaHPO_4$ crystalline phase forms. As a result, the Ca content into the coating and the Ca/P ratio increase. The maximum value of Ca/P ratio equaled to 0.7 (for the bone tissue, Ca/P = 1.67) was found for the coatings deposited under the process voltage of 300 V (see Figure 8.11).

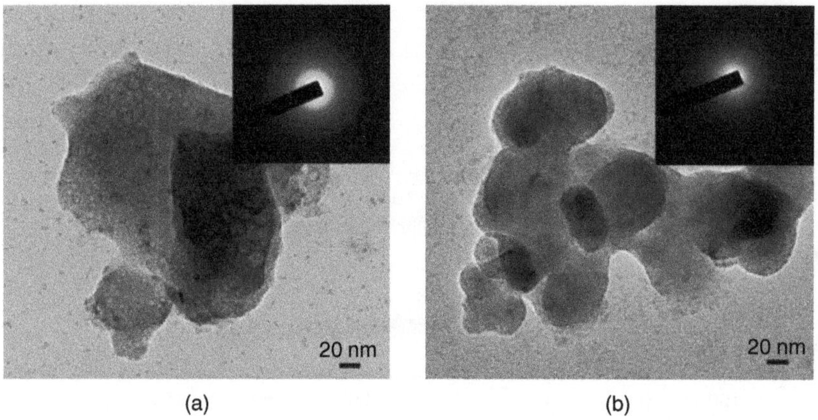

Figure 8.12 Bright-field TEM images with microdiffraction patterns for the particles of CaP coatings on the Ti (a) and Ti–40Nb (b) surfaces.

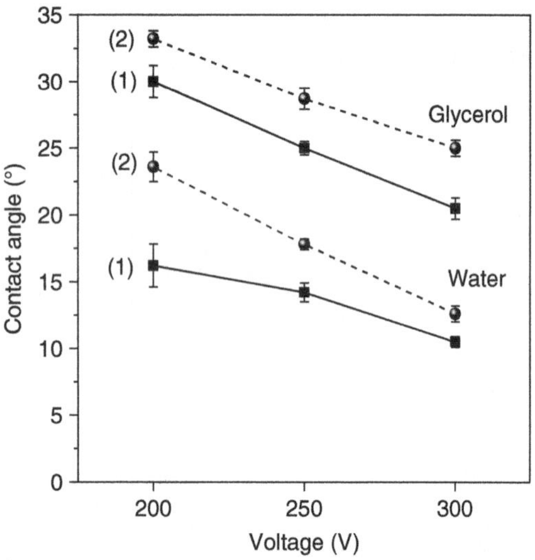

Figure 8.13 Plots of the glycerol and water contact angles with CaP coatings on Ti (1) and Ti-40Nb (2) against the process voltage.

Figure 8.12 shows the bright-field (BF) TEM images of CaP coating particles with microdiffraction patterns for the coatings on both substrates. The TEM images demonstrated that the CaP coatings on the both substrates have amorphous structured, as indicted by two diffusion halos on the microdiffraction patterns.

Wettability is an important property of biomaterials because cell adhesion, proliferation, and further differentiation occur more actively on hydrophilic surfaces [104]. The wettability studies of CaP coatings on both substrates show that maximum contact angles with water and glycerol do not exceed 35° (see Figure 8.13). This indicates a high hydrophilicity of the coatings. With increasing of the MAO voltage, the contact angles decrease linearly to 10° with water and to 20° with glycerol. This is related to the surface roughness growth. The formation of monetite plate-like crystals promotes an increase in the coating surface area and in the coating wettability.

It is established that the free surface energy of the CaP coating consists of two components, namely, dispersive and polar ones, with the predominance of the second one (see Table 8.3). It indicates the presence of strong polar chemical bonds into the coatings, such as OH^- groups, oxides, and phosphates. An increase in voltage leads to a decrease in the polar component and increase in the dispersive component because the rough surface topography of CaP coatings triggers nonpolar van der Waals forces. However, polar bonds keep dominating. In this case, the free surface energy of CaP coatings on Ti and Ti–40Nb calculated according to Eq. (8.10) and equaled to 69–73 and 74–76 mN/m, respectively (see Table 8.3). It is connected with presence of stronger polar chemical bonds into the coatings on Ti–40Nb than on Ti.

Thus, the increase of the MAO voltage leads to the linear growth of thickness within 35–105 μm, surface roughness within 2.5–5 μm, and size of spheres and pores within 10–25 and 3–10 μm, respectively, for CaP coatings on Ti and Ti–40Nb. With increasing of the process voltage, the contact angles with water and glycerol decrease linearly from 25° to 10° and from 35° to 20°, consequently, that indicate the high hydrophilicity of

Table 8.3 The free surface energy of CaP coatings on Ti and Ti–40Nb.

U (V)	σ_s^P (mN/m)	σ_s^D (mN/m)	σ (mN/m)
CaP coatings on Ti			
200	57.9 ± 0.5	10.9 ± 0.3	68.8 ± 0.8
250	60.1 ± 1.0	11.3 ± 0.6	71.4 ± 1.6
300	60.2 ± 0.4	12.5 ± 0.3	72.7 ± 0.6
CaP coatings on Ti–40Nb			
200	69.5 ± 0.4	6.5 ± 0.1	76.0 ± 0.5
250	66.1 ± 0.4	8.5 ± 0.2	74.6 ± 0.6
300	64.2 ± 0.3	10.0 ± 0.1	74.2 ± 0.5

the coatings. Also, the low contact angles of CaP coatings on both substrates indicate the high free surface energy (68–76 mN/m) due to the porous morphology, rough topography, and the presence of strong polar chemical bonds.

CaP coatings on both substrates produced under process voltages of 200–250 V are mainly in X-ray amorphous state. It indicates a high rate of coating dissolution and its ability to synthesize a new intercellular matrix around an implant [68]. With increasing of the oxidation voltage to 300 V, the new crystalline phase of monetite ($CaHPO_4$) starts to form into coatings. The maximum Ca/P ratio of 0.7 was found for CaP coatings formed under process voltage of 300 V.

8.5 Wollastonite–Calcium Phosphate Coatings with Enhanced Strength Characteristic and High Biological Activity

A CaP coating is known to improve the biocompatibility of metallic implants and to increase bone growth at the site of implantation [105]. First, apatite is the main component in bones and teeth. Second, calcium phosphate has the property of bioactivity, the ability to form bone apatite-like material such as carbonated HA [106, 107]. Bioceramics and bioactive glasses including $CaO–SiO_2$ compounds also reveal high bioactivity [86, 87]. At the present time, the nature of glass bioactivity is not clearly understood. However, it is well known that hydrolysis and repolymerization of the glass-forming base material (silicon oxide) leads to the Si—OH silane bond formation on the glass surface. These bonds are a basis for sequential changes such as calcium phosphate base – octacalcium phosphate – ACP – carbonate-substituted crystalline HA [87].

The bioceramic material based on HA and natural mineral wollastonite $CaSiO_3$ was synthesized at National Research Tomsk Polytechnic University (Tomsk, Russia) [91]. To improve the bioactivity of Ti–15Mo, the surface was modified using the PEO process [44, 108]. TCP (Ca_3PO_4), wollastonite ($CaSiO_3$), and silica (SiO_2) were selected as additives in the anodizing bath to enhance the bioactivity of the coatings formed during the PEO process. Wollastonite–calcium phosphate (W–CaP) coatings were obtained on titanium by MAO at ISPMS SB RAS (Tomsk, Russia) [45, 90].

The comparative investigation of the morphology, structure, physical, chemical, and biological properties of W–CaP coatings deposited by MAO method on Ti and Ti–40Nb is performed in this chapter. Coatings on metal substrates are synthesized by the MAO method at different pulse voltage depending on the substrate material. For Ti, the process voltage ranges from 150 to 300 V, and for Ti–40Nb, the process voltage ranges from 200 to 300 V.

How the substrate material is related to MAO parameters and coating properties was shown earlier [43]. Electrophysical, thermal, and thermodynamic characteristics of Ti and Nb metals, and TiO_2, Nb_2O_5 oxides are presented. Nb has a higher thermal conductivity (54.5 W/m K at 300 K) and lower resistivity (0.15 μΩ m) than Ti. These differences in the electrical properties lead to the formation of coatings on the Ti and Ti–40Nb in different ranges of MAO voltage.

Figures 8.14 and 8.15 demonstrate top and cross-sectional views of W–CaP coatings deposited at different MAO parameters. Coatings with a thin CaP layer (20–23 μm) are formed on the Ti substrate at the low oxidation voltage of 150 V. Wollastonite crystals with sizes of 70–150 μm incorporated into the structure of this coatings (see Figures 8.14a and 8.15a). With increasing of the oxidation voltage from 200 to 300 V, the coating thickness on Ti as well as on Ti–40Nb grows from 40 to 120 μm (see Figures 8.15 and 8.16a,d). In this case, spherical structural elements with pores are formed on the coating surface. CaP coatings with a similar surface morphology on the pure Ti and Zr–1.1Nb [43, 109, 110] and on Ti–40Nb [96] deposited at the oxidation voltages of 150–400 V in electrolyte based on biological HA are received in the previous works. Wollastonite particles are undetected in the coatings (see Figures 8.14b–f and 8.15b,c) since they were destructed at the oxidation voltage from 200 to 300 V. The change in the surface morphology of coatings with increasing of the MAO voltage is connected with an increase of microplasma discharge intensity.

The EDX results for thin W–CaP coatings on Ti deposited at voltage of 150 V for five minutes showed the presence of Si and Ca elements into elongated crystals typical for wollastonite (see Figure 8.17). Incorporation of Si and Ca elements is also observed for thick W–CaP coatings on both substrates deposited under voltages of 200–300 V but in the "diffused" state (see Table 8.4).

How the process parameters affect the coating properties was shown elsewhere [111, 112]. As a result of previous investigations it is established that the oxidation voltage and process duration are main MAO parameters influenced on physical and mechanical properties of W–CaP coatings on the Ti and Ti–40Nb [45, 90]. The W–CaP coating thickness increases linearly with increasing of the oxidation voltage from 150 to 300 V (see Figures 8.15 and 8.16a,d). This can be related to a current density growth and, as a consequence, to an increase in coating deposition rate [45]. The apparent

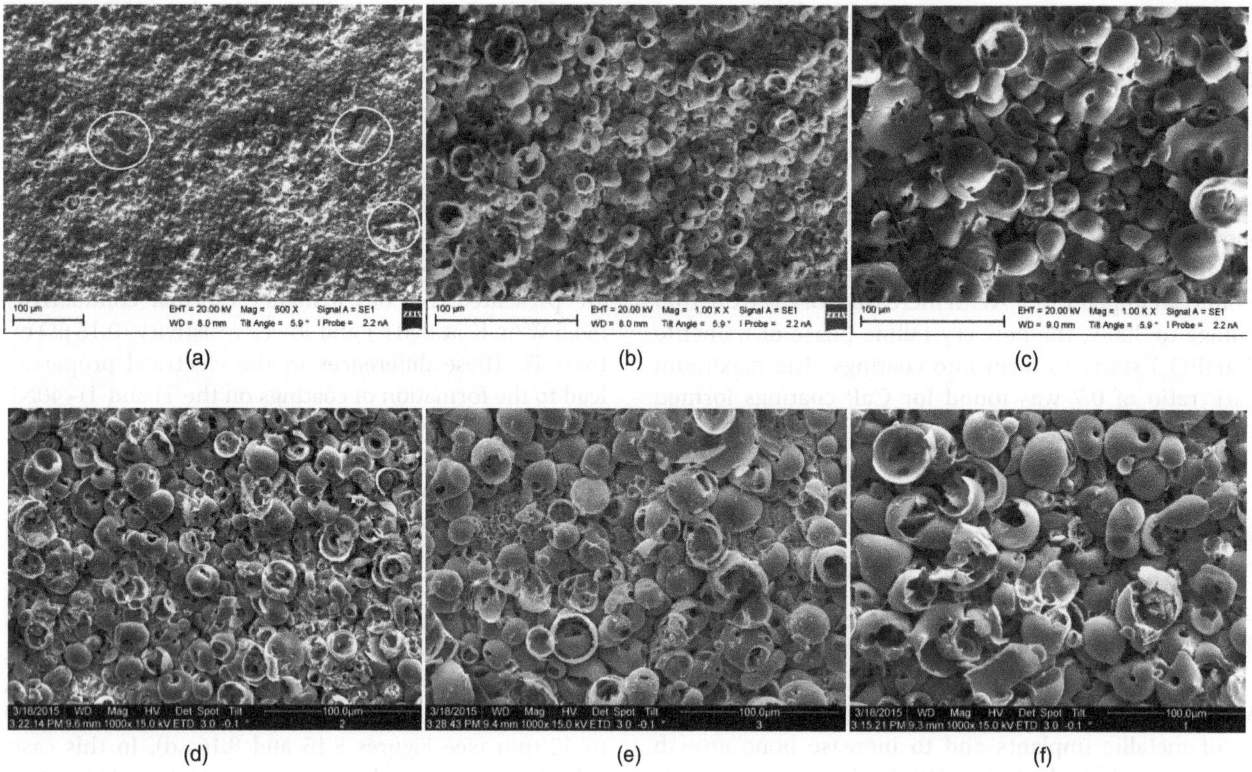

Figure 8.14 SEM micrographs of W-CaP coating on Ti (a–c) and Ti–40Nb (d–f) produced for five minutes under different oxidation voltages (V): 150 (a), 200 (b,d), 250 (e), and 300 (c,f).

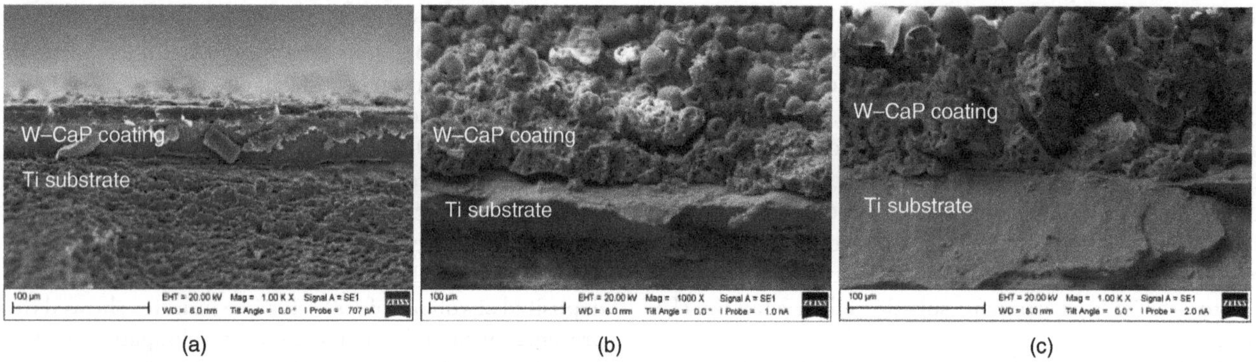

Figure 8.15 SEM images of cross-sectional W-CaP coating on Ti produced for five minutes under different oxidation voltages: (a) 150 V, (b) 200 V, and (c) 300 V.

density of coatings changes irregularly with the oxidation voltage increase. In the voltage range of 150–200 V and at the process duration of 5–10 minutes, the coating density on Ti increases slightly from 1.05 to 1.16 g/cm^3 (see Figure 8.16b,e). The apparent density decrease to 0.9 g/cm^3 is observed in the voltage range of 200–250 V for coatings on the Ti and Ti–40Nb. As the oxidation voltage increases from 250 to 300 V, the apparent density of coatings remains constant. The dependence testifies that the structure and phase composition of the coatings is mainly formed in the MAO voltage range of 150–250 V. The graph of the roughness for the coating on Ti has an inflection point corresponding to an oxidation voltage of 250 V (see Figure 8.16c,f). This is connected with the rough relief formed by spherical elements on the surface. The size of such elements grows irregularly with increasing of the oxidation voltage from 150 to 300 V. The roughness parameter R_a of coatings on the Ti and Ti–40Nb increases from 2.5 to 7.8 μm with of the increasing oxidation voltage and process duration. According to [97], the optimum values of the coating

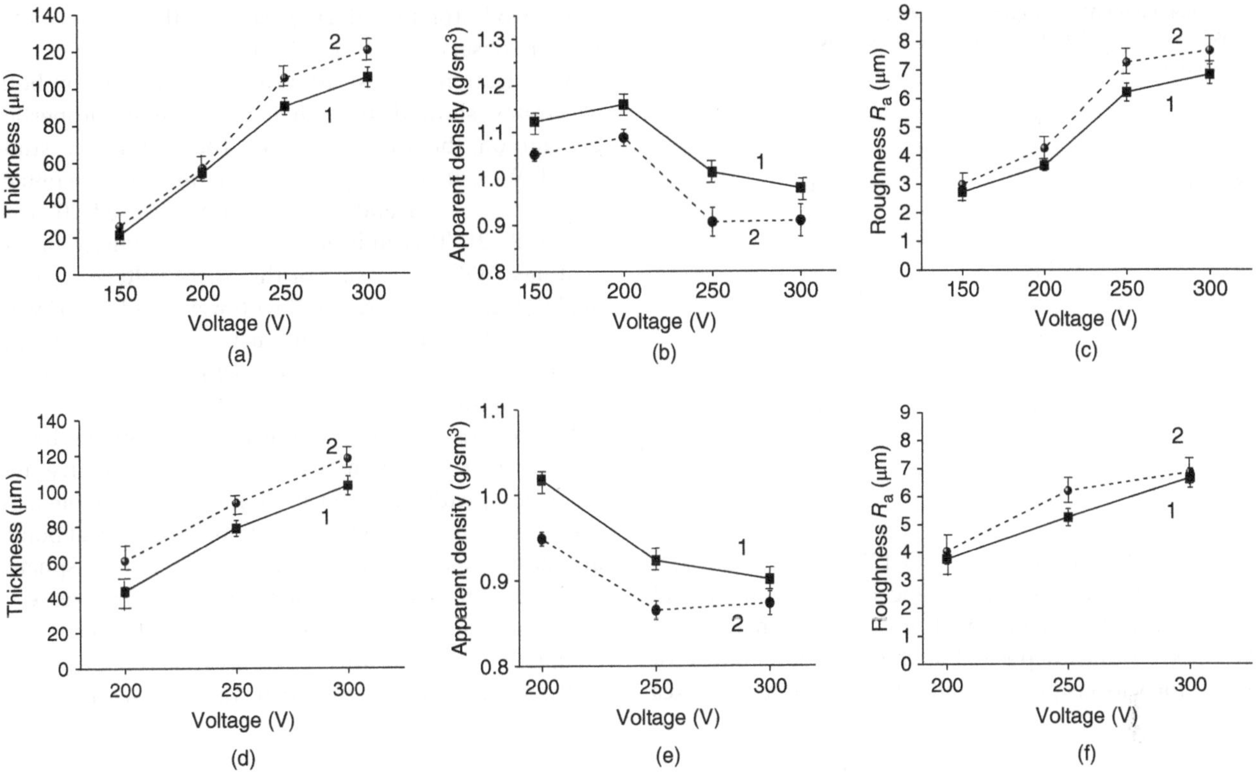

Figure 8.16 Plots of thickness (a,d), apparent density (b,e), and roughness (C,f) of W–CaP coatings on the Ti (a,c) and Ti–40Nb (b,d) deposited for 5 (1) and 10 (2) minutes against the MAO voltage.

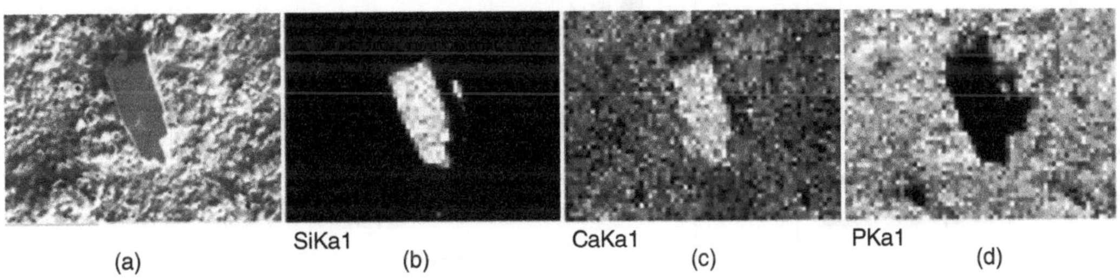

Figure 8.17 SEM micrograph (a) and distribution of elements (b–d) into the W–CaP coating on Ti produced under the process voltage of 150 V for five minutes.

roughness for the implant osseointegration with bone tissue are from 2.5 to 5.0 µm.

The XRD analysis demonstrates that the coating structure is in the X-ray amorphous state. Figure 8.18 illustrates the presence of a halo in XRD patterns. It indicates a high rate of coating dissolution and an ability to synthesize a new intercellular matrix around the implant [68]. Reflexes related to titanium, wollastonite, titanium, and niobium oxides are observed in XRD spectra.

It is found that an increase in the process duration from 5 to 10 minutes or in the pulse duration from 100 to 500 µs at the low oxidation voltage of 150 V leads to the formation of coating surface structure with circular-shaped plates, pores, and wollastonite crystals (see Figure 8.19a,b). SEM micrographs of the cross-sectional coating on the Ti also show the presence of wollastonite into the coating (see Figure 8.19c).

The graphs of the W–CaP coating characteristics depending on the pulse duration illustrate that the variation of pulse duration from 100 to 500 µs affects inconsiderably the thickness, apparent density, and roughness parameter of coatings (see Figure 8.20a). The plot of adhesion strength of W–CaP coatings has the maximum point corresponding to the pulse duration of 300 µs. The adhesion strength increases from 28 to 57 MPa with increasing of the pulse duration from 100 to 300 µs. However, a further increase in pulse duration to 500 µs leads to the adhesion strength reduction to 24 MPa. Thus, the pulse duration of 300 µs is optimum for the production of W–CaP coatings with the highest adhesion strength (see

Table 8.4 Elemental composition of W-CaP coatings produced under the voltage of 200 V for five minutes.

Element	Elemental content (at.%)	
	Ti	Ti-40Nb
C	8.3	12.9
Ti	15.8	14.9
O	53.9	50.1
Si	0.3	0.3
P	18.3	15.6
Ca	3.5	3.1
Nb	—	3.1

Figure 8.20b). According to ISO 13779-4, the adhesion strength of biocoatings for medical applications should be at least 15 MPa. Figure 8.21 presents XRD patterns of W–CaP coatings deposited at the oxidation voltage of 150 V for various process and pulse durations. Reflexes of the wollastonite and Ti phases and the presence of a halo are observed in XRD spectra.

Investigation of W–CaP coatings wettability on both substrates showed that their hydrophilic properties depend on the MAO voltage. The wettability studies of W–CaP coatings show that maximum contact angles with water and glycerol do not exceed 30° (see Figure 8.22). This indicates high hydrophilicity of the coatings. With increasing of the MAO voltage, contact angles decrease linearly to 8° with water and to 15° with glycerol. This is related to the surface roughness growth as well as to an increase in the coating surface area and coating wettability.

The free surface energy of the W–CaP coating is found to consist of two components, namely, dispersive and polar ones, with the latter predominant (see Table 8.5). It points to the presence of strong polar chemical bonds in coatings, such as OH–groups, oxides, and phosphates [68, 110]. An increase in voltage leads to a decrease in the polar component and to an increase in the dispersive component because the rough surface topography of CaP coatings triggers nonpolar van der Waals forces.

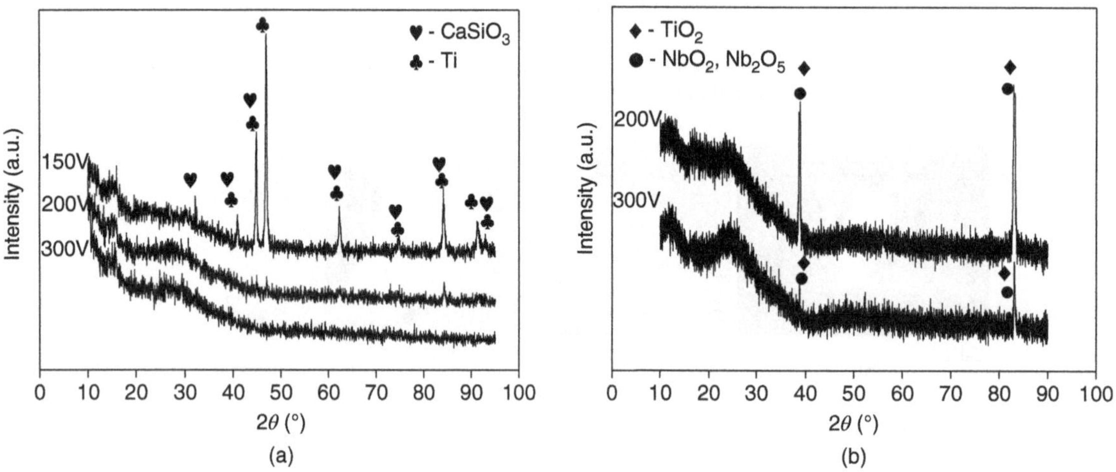

Figure 8.18 XRD patterns of W–CaP coatings on Ti (a) and Ti–40Nb (b) deposited for five minutes under different MAO voltages (150, 200, and 300 V).

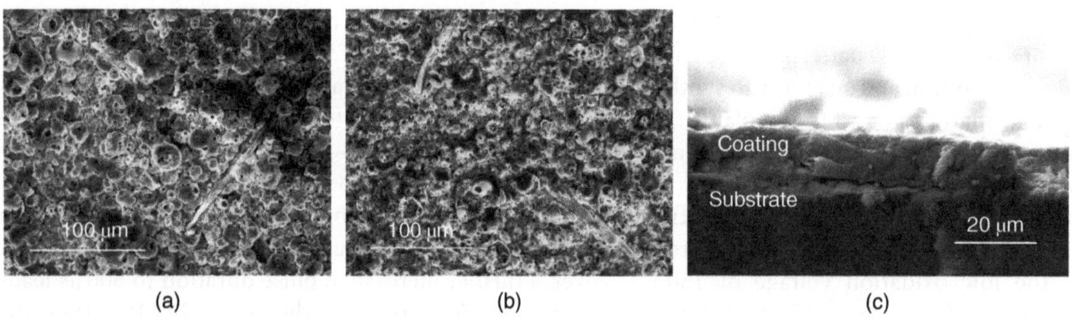

Figure 8.19 SEM micrographs of cross-sectional W–CaP coatings on Ti produced at the voltage of 150 V and various process and pulse durations: (a) 10 minutes, 100 μs; (b,C) 5 minutes, 300 μs.

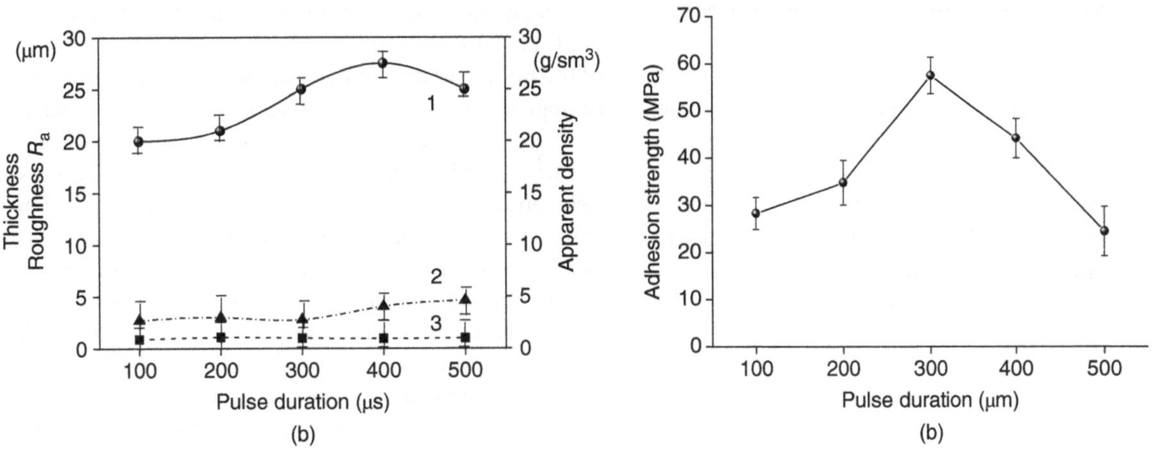

Figure 8.20 Plots of thickness (a, curve 1), apparent density (a, curve 2), roughness (a, curve 3), and adhesion strength (b) of W–CaP coatings on Ti deposited under the voltage of 150 V for five minutes against the pulse duration.

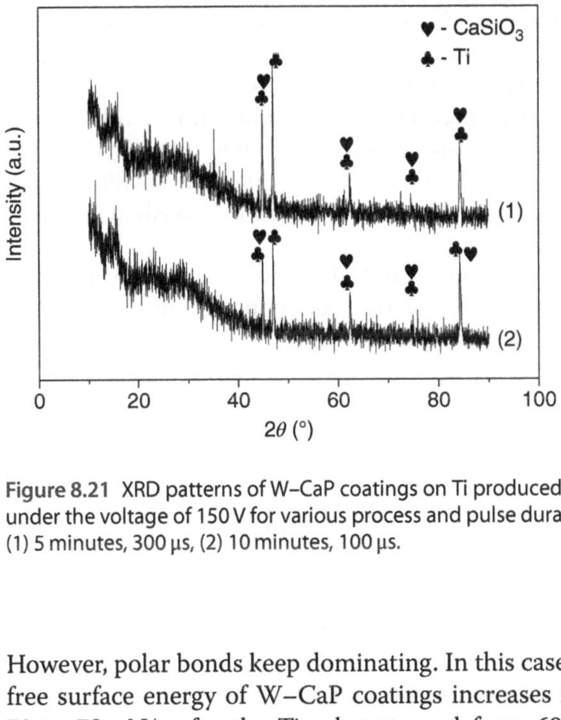

Figure 8.21 XRD patterns of W–CaP coatings on Ti produced under the voltage of 150 V for various process and pulse durations: (1) 5 minutes, 300 μs, (2) 10 minutes, 100 μs.

However, polar bonds keep dominating. In this case, the free surface energy of W–CaP coatings increases from 70 to 73 mN/m for the Ti substrate and from 69.4 to 72.7 mN/m for Ti–40Nb substrate with the increasing of the process voltage.

In conclusion, considerable differences in electrical properties of Ti and Nb lead to the formation of coatings on the Ti and Ti–40Nb in different ranges of MAO voltage. For Ti, the oxidation voltage ranges from 150 to 300 V, and for Ti–40Nb, oxidation voltage ranges from 200 to 300 V. Such MAO parameters as electrical voltage and process duration influence essentially on the W–CaP coating properties. The optimum MAO parameters are revealed: the electrical voltage of 150 V, process duration of 5–10 minutes, and pulse duration of 100–500 μs. Such MAO parameters yield W–CaP coatings with a plate-like structure, the thickness of 25–30 μm, roughness of 2.5–5.0 μm, adhesion strength of 27–57 MPa, and an enhanced ability to osseointegration. With increasing of the oxidation voltage from 200 to 300 V, thick porous Si-containing coatings are formed on Ti as well as on the Ti–40Nb. Wollastonite particles are undetected in these coatings since they were destructed at the oxidation voltage of 200–300 V.

The coating structure is in the X-ray amorphous state. Reflexes related to titanium, wollastonite, titanium, and

Figure 8.22 Plots of the glycerol (1, 2) and water (3, 4) contact angles with W–CaP coatings on Ti (a) and Ti–40Nb (b) deposited for 5 (1, 3) and 10 (2, 4) minutes against the process voltage.

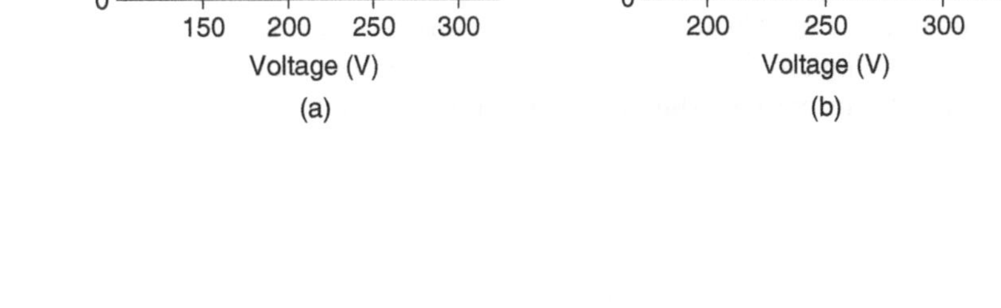

Table 8.5 The free surface energy of W–CaP coatings on Ti and Ti–40Nb.

U (V)	σ_S^D (mN/m)	σ_S^P (mN/m)	σ (mN/m)
W–CaP coatings on Ti			
150	10.3 ± 0.9	59.8 ± 1.4	70.1 ± 2.2
200	12.7 ± 0.4	57.6 ± 0.9	70.3 ± 1.3
250	14.1 ± 0.7	57.2 ± 1.5	71.3 ± 2.2
300	14.3 ± 0.6	58.8 ± 0.8	73.1 ± 1.2
W–CaP coatings on Ti–40Nb			
200	14.2 ± 0.4	55.2 ± 0.8	69.4 ± 1.2
250	14.3 ± 0.3	56.5 ± 0.5	70.8 ± 0.8
300	14.1 ± 0.3	58.6 ± 0.5	72.7 ± 0.8

niobium oxides are observed in XRD spectra of coatings deposited at the oxidation voltage of 150 V. The wettability studies of W–CaP coatings show that maximum contact angles with water and glycerol do not exceed 30°. The free surface energy of W–CaP coatings increases from 70 to 73 mN/m for the Ti and from 69.4 to 72.7 mN/m for Ti–40Nb with increasing of the process voltage. This indicates a high hydrophilicity of the coatings.

8.6 Zn- or Cu-incorporated Calcium Phosphate Coatings with Promising Antibacterial Properties

A serious problem in biomedicine is bacterial infection of medical implants. Bacterial infections result from adhesion of bacteria to the implant surface and formation of a biofilm that sometimes cannot be destroyed by antibacterial drugs coming from outside [113]. Therefore, of great interest at present are investigations aimed at the synthesis of biomaterials with antibacterial properties and at the study of bactericidal properties of implanted materials and patterns of interaction of antibacterial agents with surrounding tissues of the organism. The development of inorganic antibacterial preparations with high antibacterial activity, biosafety, and osseoconductivity is extremely necessary. Bactericidal and anti-inflammatory actions of implanted materials are mainly caused by the presence in their structure of certain chemical elements possessing natural antiseptic properties and contained in them in small amounts. It is well known that zinc and copper (Zn and Cu), in particular, in the form of free ions possess strong slowing down activity and strong antimicrobial activity against various bacteria. Zn and Cu are necessary cofactors for enzymes participating in the synthesis of various components of the bone matrix. They are especially important for the regulation of bone sedimentation and resorption [114, 115]. In addition, Zn is an important microelement of the human body and plays an important role in various biological functions, including DNA synthesis, activity of enzymes, metabolism of nucleic acids, biomineralization, and hormonal activity [116, 117]. Large Cu deficiency, as is well known, causes heavy skeleton disorders. Addition of Zn and Cu in microdosages to biocoatings will allow the directed antimicrobial activity to be obtained for a long time and the danger of growth of pathogenic microorganisms to be minimized. In addition, incorporation of the above-indicated modifying additives will promote balancing between microelement concentrations of biocoatings and bone structures as well as improving conditions for implant adaptation to organism environments.

In this chapter, it will be represented the comparative investigations of structure, composition, physical and chemical, and biological properties of Zn-contained CaP (Zn–CaP) and Cu-contained CaP (Cu–CaP) coatings on Ti and Ti–40Nb in nanostructured and ultrafine-grained states deposited by MAO method in electrolyte based on Zn- or Cu-substituted HA under different oxidation voltages in the range of 200–300 V, and with constant other MAO parameters defined previously (Chapters 3 and 4).

Zn–CaP and Cu–CaP coatings start to form on both substrates at the oxidation voltage of 200 V (see Figures 8.25a,d and 8.26a,d). The surface morphology of such coatings is presented by spheroidal formations with pores, and largely similar to the morphology of CaP coatings deposited in electrolyte based on biological HA [68] and synthesized HA (Chapter 4). An increase in the process voltage to 250 V causes structural element to grow. However, a further increase in the MAO voltage to 300 V leads to the destruction of structural elements. In this case, plate-like crystals of the new substance form on the surface of fragments and hemispheres (see Figures 8.25b,e and 8.26b,e). In this case, with increasing of the process voltage, the thickness and roughness of the Zn–CaP and Cu–CaP coatings on both substrates increase linearly from 50 to 110 μm and from 3 to 6 μm, respectively (see Figure 8.27). The change in the surface morphology, topography, and thickness of these coatings under increase of the process voltage is connected with increasing of microplasma discharge intensity.

Results of XRD analysis showed that the Zn–CaP and Cu–CaP coatings on both substrates deposited under the process voltages of 200–250 V are in the X-ray amorphous state. Low-intensive reflexes corresponding to the β-calcium pyrophosphate (β-$Ca_2P_2O_7$) phase are present in XRD patterns (see Figures 8.23c,f and 8.24c,f). With increasing oxidation voltage to 300 V, the new crystalline monetite ($CaHPO_4$) phase forms in the

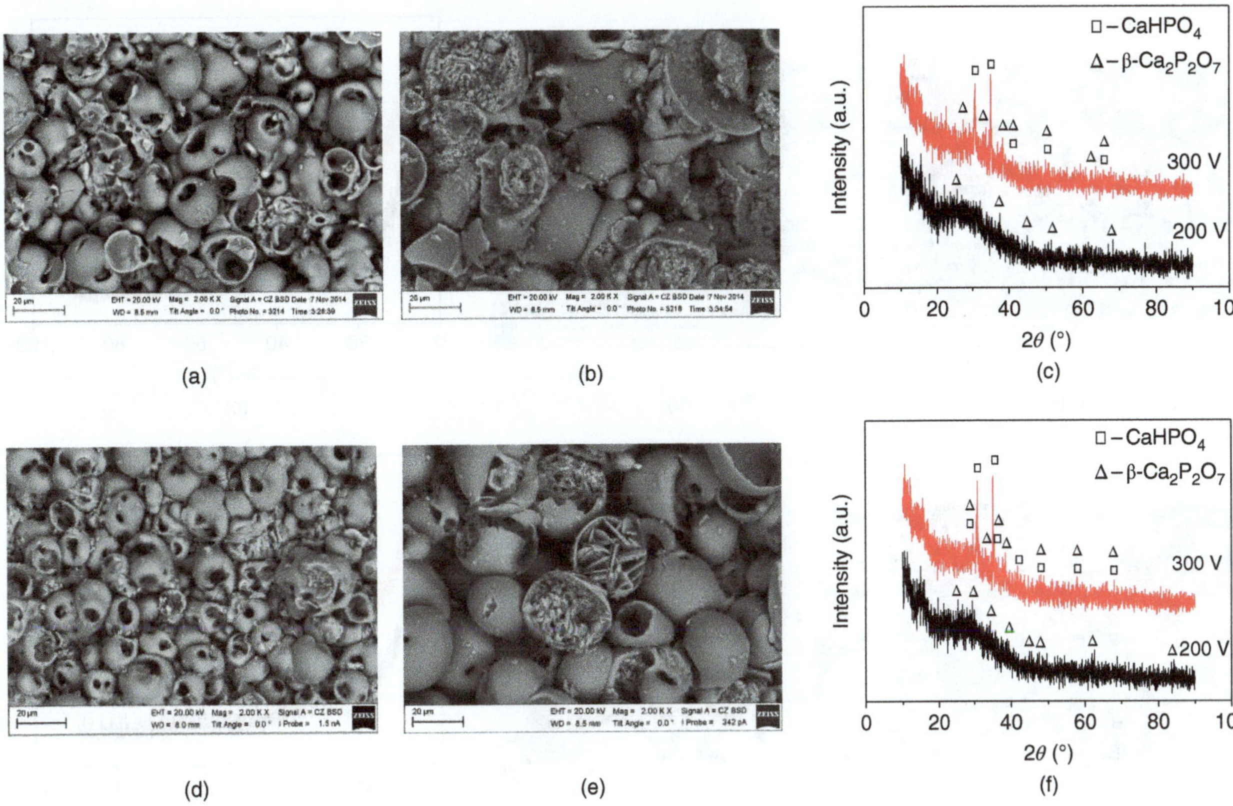

Figure 8.23 SEM images (a,b,d,e) and XRD patterns (c,f) of Zn–CaP (a–c) and Cu–CaP (d–f) coatings on Ti deposited under the oxidation voltages of 200 V (a,d) and 300 V (b,e).

coatings. Like other acid calcium phosphates, monetite exhibits osteoinductive properties. This is connected with high acid pH at the interface with the bone, which "etches" bone apatite and induces desorption of specific osteoinductive bone morphogenetic protein (BMP)-type proteins [22]. In addition, β-calcium pyrophosphate and monetite dissolve easily in the body fluids and transform into HA at subsequent mineralization [105]. The XRD results are in agreement with the SEM results (see Figures 8.23b,e and 8.24b,e), which demonstrated that the plate-like crystals are typical for monetite crystals.

The EDX results showed that the maximum Zn and Cu incorporation of 0.4 and 0.2 at.% corresponds to the coatings on Ti deposited under oxidation voltage of 250 and 200 V, respectively (see Table 8.6). With increasing of the process voltage and consequently the temperature in the microplasma discharge region, the process of Ca^{2+} ion deposition from the electrolyte intensifies and the Ca/P ratio increases [43, 68]. The maximum Ca/P ratios of 0.7 and 0.4 are obtained for the Zn–CaP and Cu–CaP coatings, respectively, deposited under the process voltage of 300 V.

All IR spectra represented in Figure 8.26 for Zn–CaP and Cu–CaP coatings on both substrates are similar and characterized by the presence of intense absorption bands corresponding to asymmetric and symmetric oscillations of P—O phosphate bond with maximum absorption in the region of 1130–930 cm^{-1} and the absorption bands of OH^- groups of adsorbed water at 1650–1620 and 3550–3200 cm^{-1}. The shoulder in the area of 800–730 cm^{-1} also indicates the presence of oscillations of O—H bonds of acid phosphate such as HPO_4 groups and P—O—P pyrophosphate bridge bonds.

The contact angle studies give information about wetting properties of the biomaterials. Figure 8.27 demonstrates the dependencies of contact angles between surface of Zn–CaP and Cu–CaP coatings on both substrates and liquid drops of water and glycerol on the MAO voltage. The coatings have low values of contact angles due to the porous morphology and rough topography (see Figures 8.23–8.25). It is seen from Figure 8.27 that with increasing of the process voltage the values of contact angle reduces linearly from 25° to 12° with water and from 42° to 22° with glycerol that indicates a high hydrophilicity of these coatings.

The free surface energy of the coatings has two components: dispersive and polar, with predominance of polar. It indicates the presence of strong polar chemical bonds in the coatings (OH–groups, oxides, and phosphates). This conclusion corresponds to XRD

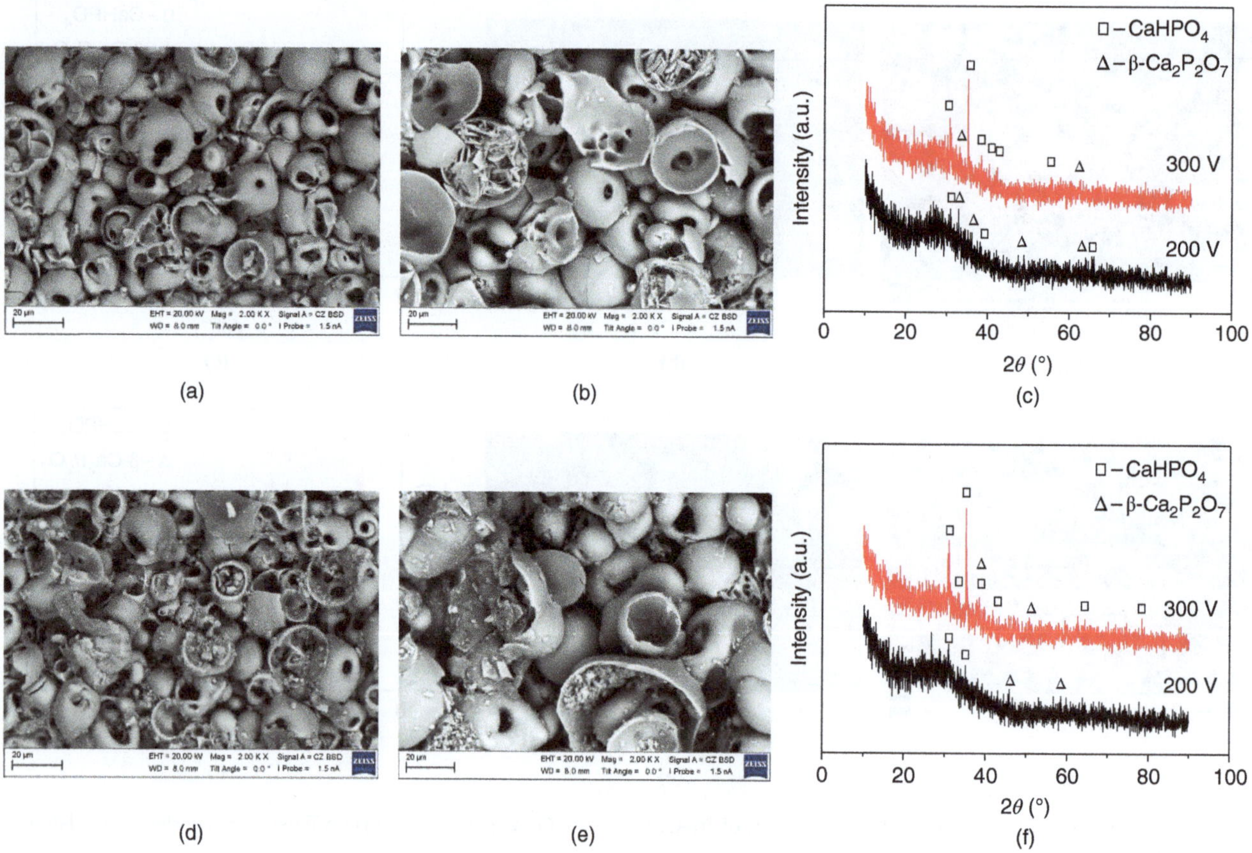

Figure 8.24 SEM images (a,b,d,e) and XRD patterns (c,f) of Zn–CaP (a–c) and Cu–CaP (d–f) coatings on Ti–40Nb deposited under the voltages of 200 V (a,d) and 300 V (b,e).

Table 8.6 Elemental composition in atomic percentage of Zn–CaP and Cu–CaP coatings on both substrates deposited under different MAO voltages.

Element	Elemental composition of Zn–CaP coatings (at.%)			Elemental composition of Cu–CaP coatings (at.%)		
	200 V	250 V	300 V	200 V	250 V	300 V
Ti substrate						
O	51.2 ± 1.7	59.5 ± 2.2	65.9 ± 2.9	61.7 ± 2.7	69.1 ± 3.3	73.4 ± 4.0
Ti	21.2 ± 1.1	12.6 ± 0.8	6.3 ± 0.3	13.6 ± 0.5	11.5 ± 0.7	7.0 ± 0.8
Zn, Cu	0.2 ± 0.1	0.4 ± 0.1	0.1 ± 0.08	0.1 ± 0.06	0.2 ± 0.1	0.1 ± 0.04
P	19.3 ± 0.9	18.5 ± 0.9	16.3 ± 0.8	19.7 ± 1.0	14.4 ± 0.8	14.3 ± 0.8
Ca	8.1 ± 0.3	9.1 ± 0.2	11.4 ± 0.5	4.6 ± 0.3	5.0 ± 0.6	5.3 ± 0.6
Ca/P	0.4	0.5	0.7	0.2	0.3	0.4
Ti–40Nb substrate						
O	51.2 ± 2.5	57.5 ± 3.5	57.8 ± 3.2	57.1 ± 3.1	63.3 ± 3.3	70.5 ± 4.1
Ti	11.5 ± 0.6	9.8 ± 0.5	8.6 ± 0.6	8.5 ± 0.3	9.0 ± 0.6	5.8 ± 0.6
Nb	4.2 ± 0.8	4.0 ± 0.4	2.6 ± 0.4	4.2 ± 0.6	3.5 ± 0.4	2.2 ± 0.4
Zn, Cu	0.2 ± 0.1	0.4 ± 0.1	0.1 ± 0.06	0.1 ± 0.05	0.2 ± 0.1	0.1 ± 0.04
P	25.2 ± 1.6	21.9 ± 1.4	21.6 ± 1.3	23.0 ± 1.3	18.1 ± 1.1	15.8 ± 1.2
Ca	7.6 ± 0.8	6.6 ± 0.6	9.6 ± 0.8	7.2 ± 0.6	5.9 ± 0.8	5.7 ± 0.8
Ca/P	0.3	0.3	0.4	0.3	0.3	0.4

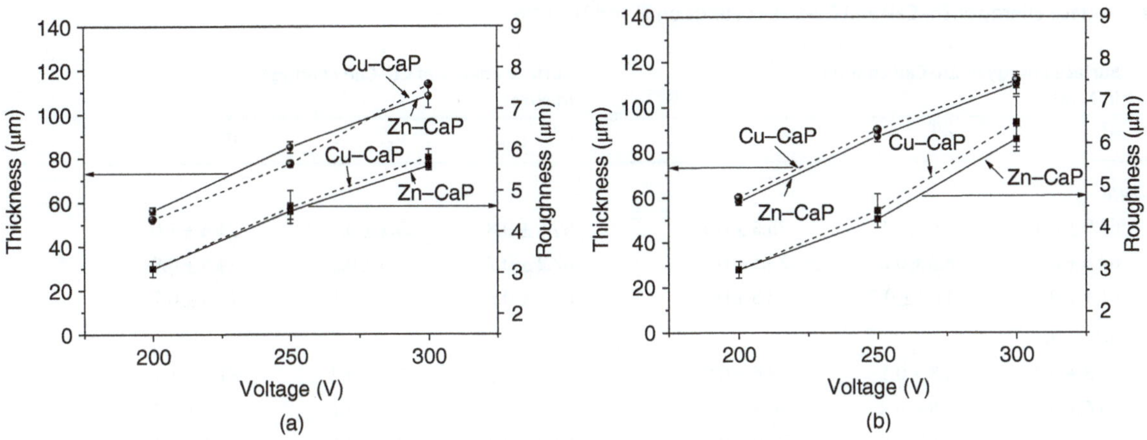

Figure 8.25 Plots of thickness and roughness of Zn–CaP and Cu–CaP coatings on both Ti (a) and Ti–40Nb (b) against the MAO voltage.

results that demonstrated the presence of crystalline monetite phases and amorphous CaP substance (see Figures 8.23c,f and 8.24c,f) and IRS results illustrated intensive P—O and O—H bonds (see Figure 8.26). Increase in process voltage leads to the decrease of polar component and increase of dispersive component, because rough surface topography of CaP coatings triggers nonpolar van der Waals forces. However, polar bonds remain dominant. It is seen from Table 8.7 that with the increasing of the voltage and process duration, the free surface energy of Zn–CaP and Cu–CaP coatings decrease from 76 to 72 mN/m for Ti substrate and from 81 to 74 mN/m for Ti–40Nb. Surface roughness growth leads to the decrease of the surface energy of CaP coatings of both substrates. Rough surface profile leads to the reduction of the attractive forces of liquid molecules inside the material, which create surface energy (Figure 8.27).

In conclusion, investigation of structure and properties of Zn–CaP and Cu–CaP coatings on both Ti and Ti–40Nb formed by MAO method in electrolyte based on substituted HA under different applied voltage in range of 200–300 V was performed. It was established that the coatings deposited under voltages of 200–250 V have X-ray amorphous structure and consequently high rate of bioresorption. Increase of the voltage to 300 V leads to the formation in the coatings of crystalline phases, such as monetite ($CaHPO_4$) and β–calcium pyrophosphate (β-$Ca_2P_2O_7$). EDX spectroscopy showed that maximum contents of 0.3 at.% zinc and 0.2 at.% copper were found into the coatings deposited under oxidation voltage of 200–250 V. Maximum Ca/P ratios of 0.7 and 0.4 were obtained for the Zn–CaP and Cu–CaP coatings, consequently, deposited under applied oxidation voltage of 300 V. It was shown that the biocoatings have high free-surface energy of 72–76 mN/m and consequently high hydrophilicity. It is supposed that

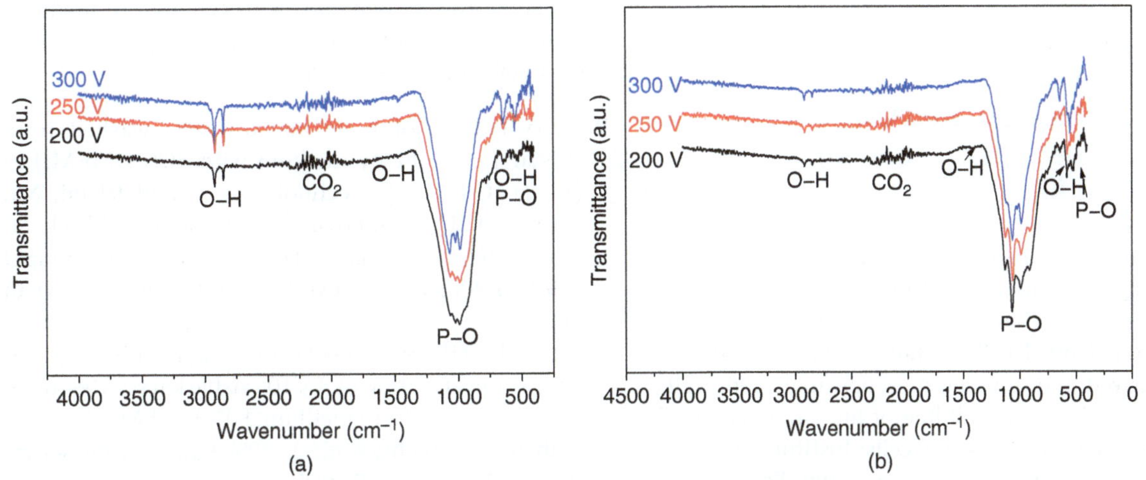

Figure 8.26 IR spectra of CaP coatings on Ti (a) and Ti–40Nb (b) deposited under different voltages.

Table 8.7 Free surface energy of Zn–CaP and Cu–CaP coatings on Ti and Ti–40Nb.

	Surface energy of Zn–CaP coatings (mN/m)			Surface energy of Cu–CaP coatings (mN/m)		
U (V)	σ_S^P	σ_S^D	σ	σ_S^P	σ_S^D	σ
For Ti substrate						
200	69.9 ± 0.4	5.6 ± 0.1	75.5 ± 0.5	69.6 ± 0.8	5.2 ± 0.2	74.4 ± 1.0
250	64.6 ± 0.5	8.5 ± 0.2	73.1 ± 0.7	67.2 ± 0.7	7.3 ± 0.2	74.5 ± 0.9
300	61.1 ± 0.4	11.3 ± 0.3	72.3 ± 0.7	60.6 ± 0.5	12.3 ± 0.3	72.9 ± 0.7
For Ti–40Nb substrate						
200	75.3 ± 0.7	3.3 ± 0.1	78.6 ± 0.9	79.0 ± 1.0	2.4 ± 0.2	81.4 ± 1.2
250	70.6 ± 0.5	5.8 ± 0.2	76.4 ± 0.7	75.0 ± 0.4	3.9 ± 0.1	78.9 ± 0.5
300	63.1 ± 0.3	10.1 ± 0.2	74.0 ± 0.4	64.2 ± 0.3	9.9 ± 0.1	74.1 ± 0.5

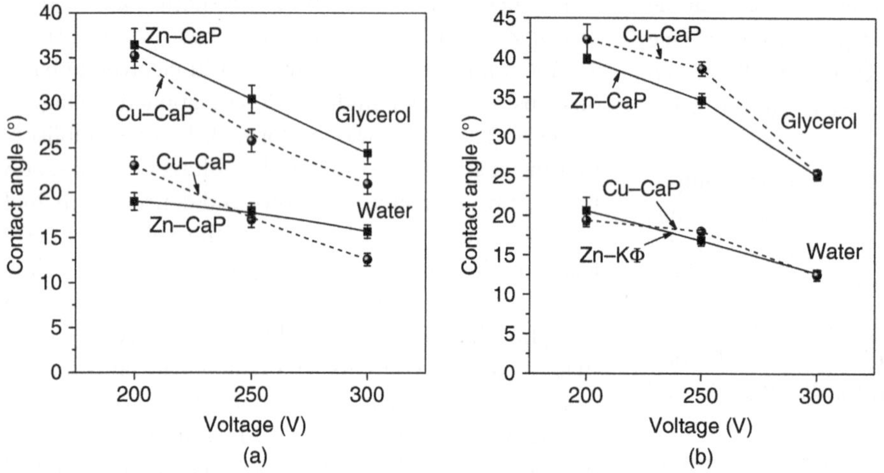

Figure 8.27 Plots of glycerol and water contact angles with Zn–CaP and Cu–CaP coatings on both Ti (a) and Ti–40Nb (b) against the MAO voltage.

antibacterial Zn and Cu elements contained in the coating may have directed antimicrobial action during the coating dissolution.

8.7 Biological Studies *In Vitro* of Wollastonite-, Zinc-, and Copper-incorporated Calcium Phosphate Coatings on Titanium and Niobium Alloys

Biological tests *in vitro* of CaP-coated samples were carried out with four cell cultures: Wistar rat femur bone marrow cells (Bank of Stem Cells, Tomsk, Russia); prenatal stromal cells of human lungs (HLPSCs); adipose-derived multipotent mesenchymal stem cells (AMMSCs); Jurkat 5332 cell line of human leukemic T lymphoblast-like cells (Jurkat T cells; Institute of Cytology, Russian Academy of Sciences, Saint Petersburg). Before the biological testing, all CaP-coated samples ($10 \times 10 \times 1\,mm^3$ in size) were dry-heat sterilized with Binder FD53 (Binder GmbH, Tuttlingen, Germany) at 453 K for one hour. One CaP-coated specimen was placed in each plastic well of a 24-well or 12-well plates (Orange Scientific, Belgium) with cell culture medium. Control wells did not have tested specimens.

Four cell culture media were used:

Primary culture of bone marrow cells washed from Wistar rat femur by medium with 80% DMEM/F12 (1 : 1) (Gibco Life Technologies; Grand Island, NY, USA) and 20% fetal bovine serum (Sigma-Aldrich, St. Louis, MO, USA) was used extempore to perform ISO 10993-5-2009 *in vitro* cytotoxic test with 0.4% trypan blue.

Second, the HLPSCs' suspension was freshly prepared with a concentration of 3×10^4 viable karyocytes/ml of the following culture medium: 80% DMEM/F12 (1 : 1) (Gibco Life Technologies), 20% fetal bovine serum (Sigma-Aldrich), 50 mg/l gentamicin (Invitrogen, UK), and freshly added L–glutamine sterile solution in a final concentration of 280 mg/l (Sigma-Aldrich). This cellular culture is useful to testify osteogenic activity of human mesenchymal stem cells *in vitro* [118].

To determine the osteogenic potency of a rough CP surface, the culture medium was not saturated by osteogenic supplements such as β-glycerophosphate, dexamethasone, and ascorbic acid. The HLPSCs suspension was added in a volume of 1 ml *per* well. The cell culture was incubated for three days in a humidified atmosphere of 95% air and 5% CO_2 at 37° C.

Third, the AMMSCs were prepared from human fat tissue after processing of lipoaspirates (Permission No. 4 from 23.10.2013 of Local Ethics Committee of Innovation Park of Immanuel Kant Baltic Federal University) as particularly described by [119]. The cell suspension was freshly prepared with a concentration of 5×10^4 viable karyocytes/ml of the following culture medium: 90% DMEM/F12 (1 : 1) (Gibco Life Technologies), 10% fetal bovine serum (Sigma-Aldrich), 50 mg/l gentamicin (Invitrogen, UK), and freshly added L–glutamine sterile solution in a final concentration of 280 mg/l (Sigma-Aldrich). The cell culture was incubated for seven days in a humidified atmosphere of 95% air and 5% CO_2 at 37 °C. The morphology of adherent cells, their motility and ability to form a monolayer in contact (in the interface) with the test specimens was studied using integrated platforms for continuous visualization of living cells Cell–IQ® v2 MLF (CM Technologies, Finland). Digital images were obtained in 20 minutes during seven-day culturing.

Minimal morphological criteria for multipotent mesenchymal stem cells (MMSCs) defining required by the International Society for Cellular Therapy (ISCT) is the ability to differentiate *in vitro* into the osteogenic, chondrogenic, and adipogenic lineages reviewed in [120]. Human AMMSCs in differentiation media StemPro® Differentiation Kit (Thermo Fisher Scientific, USA) showed positive staining on alizarin red S., alcian blue, and oil red ("Sigma-Aldrich", USA), which confirms their belonging to MMSCs pool.

Finally, the immortalized Jurkat T cells was employed at a concentration of 1×10^6 living mononuclear cells per 1 ml of nutrient medium to assess *in vitro* cell death (apoptosis and necrosis). The cell culture was incubated for 24 hours in a humidified atmosphere of 95% air and 5% CO_2 at 37 °C. The ratio between the living and dead (apoptotic and necrotic) Jurkat T cells was measured via flow cytofluorometry. To this end, the cells to be tested were transferred in a volume of 12.5 μl to an immunological plate, and 112.5 μl of the Guava ViaCount reagent (Millipore, USA) was added. The cells were then resuspended and incubated in the dark for five minutes, and the samples were analyzed with a Guava EasyCyte Plus device (Millipore, USA) using Guava ViaCount software (Millipore, USA).

Intercellular liquids (supernatants, conditioned media) of cell cultures were collected from the wells into tubes, centrifuged for 10 minutes at 500 g. Potassium (K) and sodium (Na) concentrations, and the activities of ALP were measured by a standard colorimetrical method [121] according to protocols of manufacturer (Thermo Fisher Scientific Inc., USA). Automatic biochemical Konelab60i device (USA) was used. ALP is a marker of functional activity (osteogenic differentiation and maturation) of osteoblasts. Potassium is a predominantly intracellular cation, and sodium is an extracellular cation. A significant variance of their concentrations in the intercellular fluid is connected with the disturbance of physiological mechanisms of cell membrane permeability due to the potential cytotoxicity of the tested materials in relation to transmembrane ion transport.

Osteogenic state of cells was evaluated *in vitro* by osteocalcin (OC) measurement in the supernatants. OC concentration was estimated using Osteometer BioTech A/S N–MID Osteocalcin One Step ELISA test system (Nordic Bioscience diagnostics). The analysis was performed by the standard scheme for ELISA. ALP and OC are real molecular markers of osteoblasts [122].

The results were analyzed using STATISTICA software. Data were shown as mean (X), standard deviation (SD), and standard error of mean (SEM), as well as the median (Me), 25% quartile (Q1), and 75% quartile (Q3). To analyze the available data sets, a normal distribution Kolmogorov–Smirnov test has been used. Nonparametric Mann–Whitney's U-test (P_U) was performed, and differences were considered significant at $p < 0.05$.

In the previous work [123], the absence of cytotoxicity of HA nanoparticles with cations substituted by calcium used to form CaP coatings was demonstrated.

Results of biological tests of synthesized CaP coatings showed (see Table 8.8) that cultivation of specimens with the bone marrow cells (myelocariocytes) does not lead to an increase in potassium concentration in the intercellular liquid. This demonstrates that the coatings being tested, irrespective of the metal substrate and the microelement incorporated into HA, do not cause massive destruction of cells accompanied by the escape of the intracellular content into the environment. As is well known, massive disintegration of cells leads to inflammation of tissues due to the effect of lysosomal enzymes on surrounding cells and extracellular matrix.

Hence, this suggests that the examined specimens do not possess potential to initiate peri-implant inflammations. In addition, after one hour of incubation (the period recommended by ISO 10993-5-2009 for definition of cytotoxicity), the percent of viable cells in the

Table 8.8 Potassium ion concentration in intercellular fluids and percentage of viable bone marrow cells (according to ISO 10993-5 test with 0.4% trypan blue) after one-hour cultivation with CaP-coated Ti or Ti–40Nb specimens, Me (Q1–Q3).

Groups, (n = 3)	Potassium (mM)	Viable cells (%)
Culture medium without cells; group 0, $n = 5$	5.1	—
Cells without specimens; group 1, $n = 4$	5.1 (5.1–5.1)	94.9 (94.7–95)
Zn–CaP coatings on Ti and Ti–40Nb		
Ti substrate	5.1 (5.05–5.1)	88.5* (84.6–92.3)
group 2, $n = 4$		<0.02
Ti–40Nb substrate	5.1 (5.1–5.1)	93.5 (91.7–97)
group 3		
Cu–CaP coatings on Ti and Ti–40Nb		
Ti substrate	5.1 (5.1–5.1)	94.1 (95.2–97.6)
group 4		
Ti–40Nb substrate	5.1 (5.1–5.1)	93.8 (89.7–97.1)
group 5		
CaP coatings on Ti and Ti–40Nb		
Ti substrate	5.05 (3.8–5.1)	96.4 (95.8–97.0)
group 6		
Ti–40Nb substrate	5.1 (3.2–5.1)	94.1 (91.3–97.0)
group 7		

*Statistically significant differences with values of group 1; n, the number of tested specimens.

majority of tests did not differ statistically from that for the background (myelocariocytes without addition of specimens).

The exception is group 2. Reduction of the number of survived cells by 6% in comparison with the background level was observed (see Table 8.8). Dyeing of cells by trypan blue testifies to an increase in the permeability of cellular membranes with preservation of the cell integrity since the potassium ion concentration did not change.

In other words, for direct (since the CaP surface dissolution is still insignificant for one-hour cultivation) *in vitro* contact of bone marrow cells with the majority of CP coatings being tested, the specimens did not show cytotoxic properties. The tested specimens are promising for manufacturing of a new class of products and coatings for orthopedics and traumatology possessing adjustable bioactivity that calls for their further study *in vitro* and *in vivo*. For Zn–CaP coatings, the possible antimicrobial effect can be assumed, since zinc ions are not selective in inducing destruction of prokaryotic and eukaryotic cells.

From the functional viewpoint, prenatal stromal cells extracted from human lungs (HLPSCs) secreted into the intercellular liquid enzyme ALP (see Table 8.9), which testified to their osteogenic potential. Potassium levels in supernatants did not differ statistically for all observation groups that testified to the absence of toxic influence of specimens being tested. Reduction (to 96% from the level of the reference cell culture, group 1) of sodium ion concentration in intercellular liquid of HLPSC cultures contacting with specimens on the Ti substrate (groups 2, 6, and 8) could be a manifestation of sodium delivered to cells and formation of the action potential that testifies to the activation of cells.

Thus, the developed coatings independent of the metal substrate type not only had no toxic effect on the functional status *in vitro* of HLPSC culture, but also, apparently, promoted to the osteogenic (by ALP) activation of mesenchymal stromal cells.

Various scientists consider a biocompatibility and functional activity of implants for osteosynthesis depending to a large extent on processes which take place at the bone/implant interface [124]. Results of phase-contrast microscopy Cell–IQ *in situ* showed that morphology of cell culture on plastic wells of cultured plates show absence of significant differences in behavior of human AMMSCs for various tested coated specimens. The fibroblast-like cells adhered, increased cell mass, and actively migrated to the monolayer formation (see Figure 8.28). It indicates the high life activity of

Table 8.9 Ion concentrations and ALP activity in intercellular fluids of HLPSCs after three-day cultivation with CaP-coated Ti or Ti–40Nb specimens, Me (Q1–Q3).

Groups ($n = 3$)	K (mM)	Na (mM)	ALP activity (U/l)
Culture media without cells,	7.9 (7.8–7.9)	138.5 (138.0–140.0)	388.0 (380.0–389.0)
background group 0, $n = 6$			
Cells without specimens,	7.8 (7.8–7.9)	141.5 (141.0–143.0)	400.5 (400.0–403.0)
control group 1, $n = 6$		P0 < 0.05	P1 < 0.001
CaP coatings on Ti and Ti–40Nb			
Cells with CaP-coated Ti;	7.6 (7.4–7.6)	138.0* (137.0–139.0)	407.0 (407.0–417.0)
group 2		P1 < 0.05	
Cells with CaP-coated Ti–40Nb;	7.6 (7.5–7.7)	139.0 (138.0–141.0)	411.0* (406.0–421.0)
group 3			P1 < 0.05
W–CaP coatings on Ti and Ti–40Nb			
Cells with W–CaP-coated Ti;	7.5 (7.5–7.8)	139.0 (137.0–142.0)	395.0 (376.0–412.0)
group 4			
Cells with W–CaP-coated Ti–40Nb;	7.7 (7.7–7.9)	140.0 (140.0–143.0)	416.0* (405.0–4171.0)
group 5			P1 < 0.05
Zn–CaP and Cu–CaP coatings on Ti and Ti–40Nb			
Cells with Zn–CaP-coated Ti;	7.4 (7.4–7.6)	137.0* (136.0–138.0)	395.0 (353.0–406.0)
group 6		P1 < 0.05	
Cells with Zn–CaP-coated Ti–40Nb;	7.5 (7.4–7.7)	137.0 (137.0–140.0)	405.0 (405–408)
group 7			
Cells with Cu–CaP-coated Ti;	7.5 (7.5–7.6)	137.0* (137.0–138.0)	410.0* (405.0–417.0)
group 8		P1 < 0.05	P1 < 0.05
Cells with Cu–CaP-coated Ti–40Nb;	7.5 (7.5–7.7)	138.0 (137.0–140.0)	411.0* (411.0–428.0)
group 9			P1 < 0.05

P0, statistically significant difference with the background group; P1, statistically significant difference with control group; *n*, the number of tested specimens.

the AMMSC culture, including their mobility in the interface of "implant/cells."

The highly proliferative Jurkat line of human leukemic T lymphoblast-like cells (Jurkat T cells) is widely used for the *in vitro* modeling of normal blood T lymphocyte reactions as well as those in acute T lymphoblastic leukemia and lymphoma reactions [125] to biomaterials [126]. This study was aimed to examine the death reaction of tumor Jurkat T cells to short-term *in vitro* exposure to CaP-coated, Zn–CaP-coated, and Cu–CaP-coated Ti specimens. From Table 8.10 it is seen that the CaP coatings have no significant effect on cell death compared to control cell culture on plastic wells. In contrast, Cu–CaP coatings and Zn–CaP coatings, to a greater extent, increased Jurkat T cell death two to three times by necrosis.

Thus, the developed coatings, irrespective of the metal substrate type (Ti or Ti–40Nb) and additional microelements (Zn, Cu, and Si), not only have no toxic effect on the functional status of *in vitro* bone marrow cells and HLPSC cultures, but also activate mesenchymal stromal cells. Bulk products and coatings on metals possessing both the regulator and antimicrobial activities formed on the basis of synthetic HA with incorporated Zn^{2+} and Cu^{2+} ions have wide prospects for application in osteosynthesis. The established cytotoxic activity against tumoral cells of the blood system rather than healthy MMSCs opens additional prospects for a study of the possibility of application of Zn–CaP and Cu–CaP coatings for implants and endoprosthesis intended for recovery of bone defects in oncopathology. In this case, the important requirements to such coatings are their

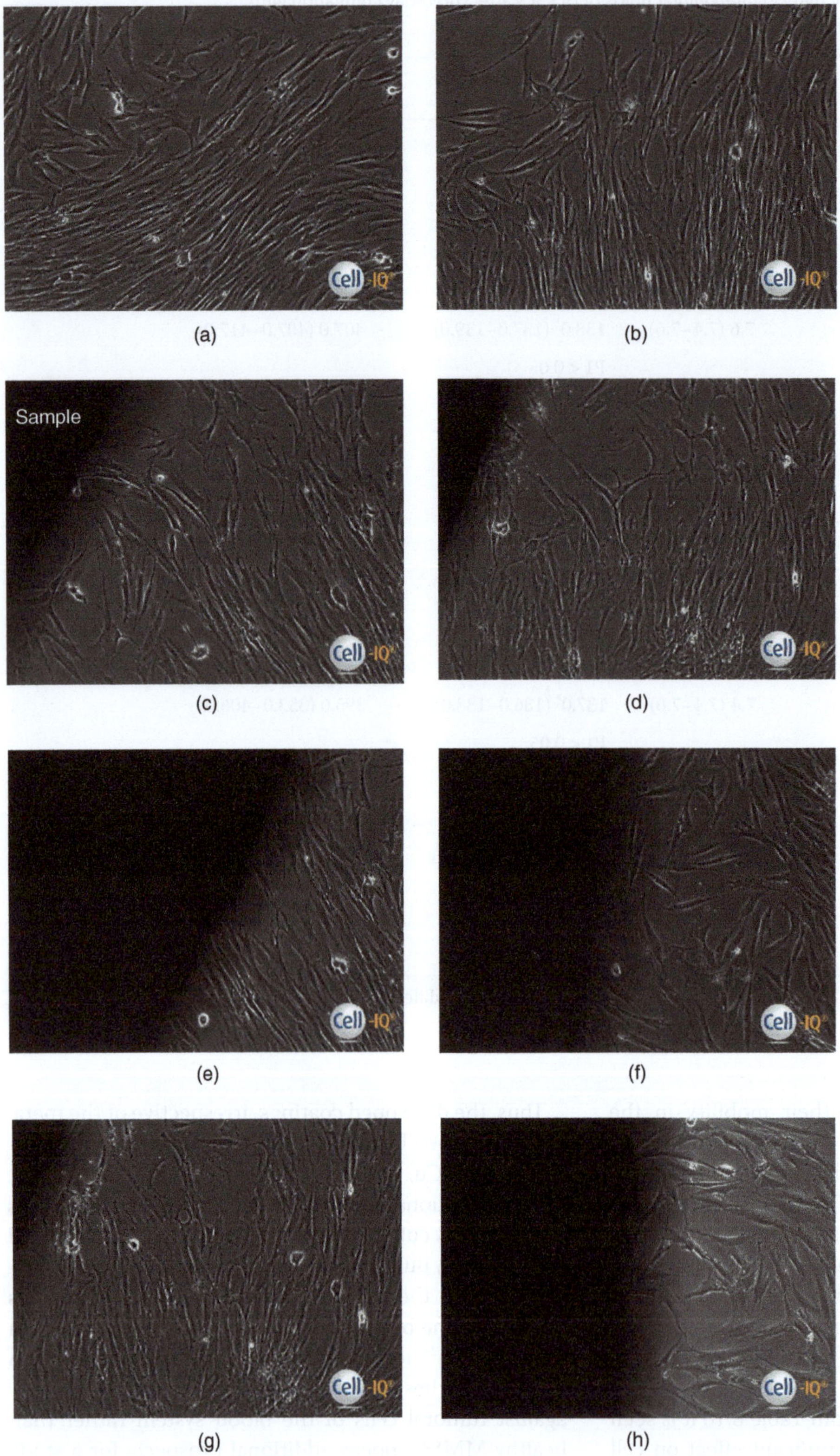

Figure 8.28 Phase-contrast microscopy images of AMMSCs adhered to plastic wells (control group) (a,b) in the interfaces between the cells and CaP-coated Ti (c,e,g,i) or coated Ti–40Nb (d,f,h,j) after seven days of cultivation; the dark field is a coated sample. Hence, (c,d) CaP coating; (e,f) W–CaP coating; (g,h) Zn–CaP coating; and (i,j) Cu–CaP coating.

Figure 8.28 (Continued)

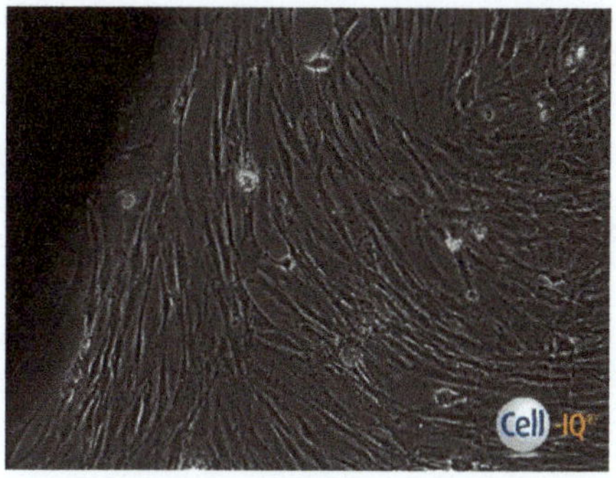

(i)

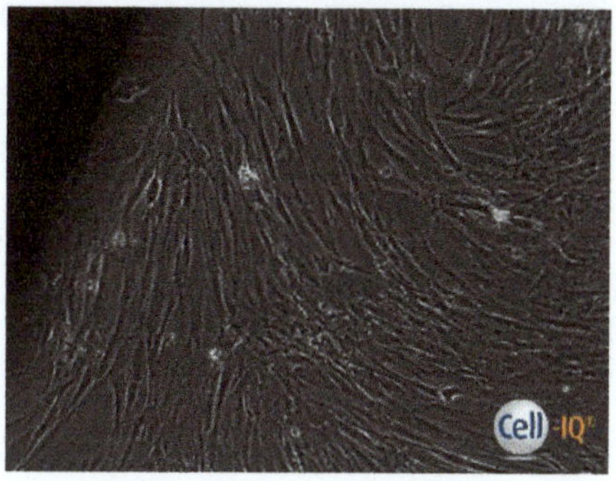

(j)

Table 8.10 Death indices of Jurkat T cells after 24 hours of cultivation with the titanium samples deposed by the different types of micro arc coatings, Me (Q1–Q3).

The number of died cells (%)	
Apoptosis	**Necrosis**
Group 1: Cell culture on the plastic culture plate surface (control), $n = 3$–15	
5.2 (5.2–8.9)	8.2 (8.1–14.2)
Group 2: Cell culture with CaP-coated specimens, $n = 3$–15	
5.5 (5.0–6.7)	12.0 (7.6–20.4)
Group 3: Cell culture with Zn–CaP-coated specimens, $n = 3$–15	
4.1 (3.3–4.7)	36.3 (16.2–38.0)
P1 < 0.01	P1 < 0.01
P2 < 0.001	P2 < 0.001
Group 4: Cell culture with Cu–CaP-coated specimens, $n = 3$–15	
6.1 (5.5–7.0)	21.2 (15.4–30.9)
	P1 < 0.02
	P2 < 0.005

n, The number of tested specimens; P1–P2, statistical significances in comparison with the corresponded groups according to the Mann–Whitney U test are shown.

osteogenic characteristics, which call for their further study *in vitro* and *in vivo*.

Preliminary results (see Table 8.11) have shown that for a seven-day culturing of AMMSCs with tested specimens of CaP coatings, they have no advantages in secretion of osteocalcin *in vitro*. The exception is the Cu–CaP coating in which the presence of the microelement in the coating structure on an average level of 0.1 at.% promotes strengthening of the cellular secretion of osteocalcin by 13–32% compared with the corresponding value for the CaP coating without calcium cation substitutes. However, statistically significant stimulating effect is manifested only for the Cu–CaP coating on the Ti substrate (see Table 8.11).

In vitro experiments [127] clearly demonstrate that Cu^{2+} ions releasing in trace amount from implants could promote the osteogenic differentiation by stimulating the ALP enzyme activity and the osteogenic gene expressions, and enhancing the adhesion and proliferation of osteoblasts cultured on its surface. In these investigations (see Table 8.9), Cu–CaP coatings also stimulate ALP secretion by HLPSC culture.

Thus, copper introduction in the CaP coating can yield potential antimicrobial properties and intensify the osteogenic processes. This double effect seems to be rather promising for the development of implants in cases of complicated osteosynthesis against the background of osteoporosis and infectious damage to the bone tissue. Nevertheless, questions on (i) optimal microelement concentration in the coating and (ii) dependences of the biological characteristics of the coatings on the composition of the metal substrate still remain open.

Table 8.11 Osteocalcin concentrations (ng/ml) in supernatants of seven-day adipose-derived MMSCs culture (control growth) with the presence of model implants with different CaP coatings, Me (Q1–Q3).

Groups ($n = 3$)	Surface roughness R_a (μm)	Osteocalcin concentration (ng/ml)
Plastic-adherent AMMSCs growth (control), $n = 8$	—	2.24 (2.18–2.41)
Ti substrate		
CaP coating	3.80 (2.80–4.50)	2.13 (2.07–2.47)
Zn–CaP coating	3.30 (3.30–5.50)	2.13 (1.72–2.93)
Cu–CaP coating	3.40 (3.30–5.50)	2.82* (2.59–3.79)
		<0.006
Ti–40Nb substrate		
CaP coating	3.40 (3.20–4.50)	1.95 (1.72–2.41)
Zn–CaP coating	3.30 (3.20–3.30)	2.30 (2.13–2.36)
Cu–CaP coating	3.0 (3.0–3.1)	2.41 (2.18–2.87)

*Statistical significance in comparison with the control according to the Mann–Whitney U test is shown; n, the number of tested specimens (wells).

8.8 Development and Medical Applications of Dental Implants Based on Nanostructured Titanium with Calcium Phosphate Coating

Dental implantology is considered one of the most promising fields in stomatology, having discovered new ways of aiding patients with a complete or partial edentia and providing a highly successful implant implementation. Hundreds of thousands of dental implants are installed annually worldwide. According to the Chicago Centre for Advanced Dentistry, in 2008 the world market of dental implants amounted to US $3.4 billion. The US implant market in 2009 was US $1.7–2.0 billion. The market of dental implants and abutments in Asian-Pacific region in 2008 amounted to US $480 million. According to the Association of Dental Dealers in Europe, comprising more than 900 companies and European Dental Industry with more than 500 enterprises in 10 European countries, the turnover of dental implants in Europe in 2001 was US $144.4 million, which was by 12.3% more than in 2000.

It is undoubtful that the choice of the material determines the functional reliability of dental implants. The material should be not only stable and flexible but also safe and biocompatible with a living organism. Since 1951, after Branemark [1] discovered the phenomenon of osseointegration, pure titanium has become the material used for implantation. Titanium corresponds completely to the implant requirements when it comes to biocompatibility, but only partially when it comes to mechanical requirements. Technically, pure titanium VT1-0 and VT1-00 is produced in Russia, and commercially pure titanium of four brands – Grade 1, 2, 3, and 4, which are different in composition and properties, is produced in the United States. Pure titanium has a relatively low wear resistance and yield point in comparison with the titanium alloys. However, these alloys have alloying components (A1, V, MO, etc.), toxic for a human being, especially during a long-term location in a human body. One of the promising applications of titanium in a high-strength nanostructured and ultra-fine grained state is dental implantology, where there is a little titanium needed to produce an implant at a moderate price, while the service temperature of the implant is the body temperature.

Over the past 10 years, biocomposites based on nanostructured titanium alloys and biological active CaP coatings have been developed in the Laboratory of Physics of Nanostructured Biocomposites at the Institute of Strength Physics and Materials Science of SB RAS (ISPMS SB RAS, Tomsk, Russia). During this time, there have been received patents of the Russian Federation [10, 83, 84, 128]. SPD methods allow to create nanostructured/ultrafine-grained homogeneous structure in the bulk of material with grain and sub-grain less than 100 nm (see Figure 8.29a). The developed nanostructured (ultrafine-grained) Ti VT1-0 has mechanical properties comparable to those of several titanium alloys and does not contain unhealthy alloying elements (A1, V, MO, etc.). These properties allow to apply successfully nanostructured Ti for medical applications [129]. Appropriate preparation of the titanium surface including mechanical treatment (See Figure 8.29b), sandblasting, and chemical etching (see Figure 8.29c) provides enhanced osseointegration, i.e. an attachment of the implant in the tooth tissue when there is no fibrous tissue between the implant and tooth tissue.

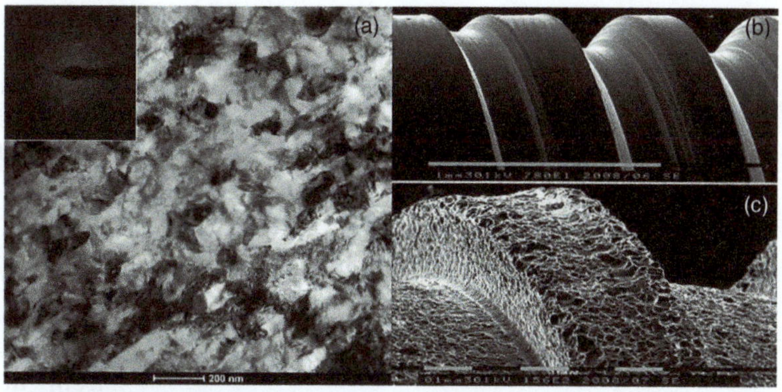

Figure 8.29 TEM image of microstructure of nanostructured/ultrafine-grained VT1-0 Ti (a); SEM images of implant surface after mechanical treatment (b) and after sandblasting and chemical etching (c).

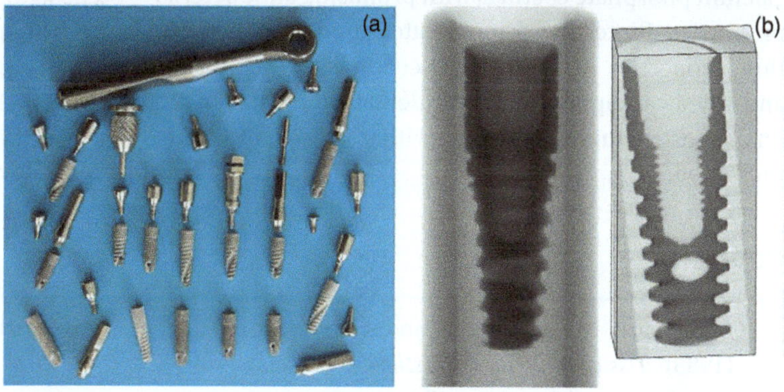

Figure 8.30 Set of dental screw intraosseous implants with instruments and implements (a); X-ray topographic images of the internal cross-sectional dental implants (b).

Meanwhile, the resorbed CaP coating provides successful osseointegration of the bone tissue to the implant. The deposition of CaP coating on nanostructured Ti dental implants is carried out using the Micro-arc-3.0 installation with a switch-mode power supply in electrolyte based on phosphoric acid, biological HA, and calcium carbonate that allowed to considerably increase the calcium content in the coating as compared with the traditionally used coatings. The coating has an adhesion to the base coat not less than 30 MPa [83, 84]. A biotesting carried out *in vitro* and *in vivo* has showed a high effectiveness of the coating produced [68, 110]. Thus, the implant surface has two-level roughness and resorbed amorphous CaP coating deposited by the MAO method, providing the stable osseointegration of the implant in the bone. The studies of the morphological features of the changes in bone tissue in the zone of implant implementation carried out on rabbits have showed that the dental implants based on nanostructured Ti have a better osseointegration [130].

The modern constructions of intraosseous screw dental implants of different modifications from the VT1-0 (VT1-00) nanostructured/ultrafine-grained titanium (they are characterized by the increased osseointegration) have been developed and patented at the ISPMS SB RAS in collaboration with Novokuznetsk State Institute of Advanced Medical Studies (Novokuznetsk, Russia), Siberian Chemical Plant (Seversk, Russia), and Siberian State Medical University (Tomsk, Russia). Instruments and implements necessary to perform surgical and orthopedic procedures with dental implants have been developed (Technical specifications No. 942422.001-10). Pilot sets of dental screw intraosseous implants, instruments, and implements have been produced (see Figure 8.30). The clinical tests of nanostructured titanium dental implants have been completed. They have confirmed that the implant constructions correspond to the modern state of implantology and their usage does not trigger any complications at the surgical and orthopedic stages of the treatment. Today, a designed set of the nanostructured titanium dental implants with instruments and implements (Technical specifications No. 942422.001–10) is recommended for the stomatological practice in Russian Federation and for the registration in Federal Supervisory Agency for Health Care and Social Development.

8.9 Conclusions

Bioinert alloys in nanostructured and ultrafine-grained states and bioactive calcium phosphate coatings are the main components for producing the effective biocomposites for medical applications. The more perspective metal materials for substrates are bioinert pure titanium and Ti–40Nb alloy. There are no harmful and toxic chemical elements. Moreover, Ti–Nb alloy has low elastic modulus closed to bone one. Ultrafine-grained and nanostructured states provide the high level of mechanical properties. MAO method is more convenient method for the production of bioactive calcium phosphate coatings on the surface of bioinert metals and alloys. This method allows to produce different CaP bioactive coatings on the bioinert valve metals. They are the hydrophilic calcium phosphate coatings with developed surface relief, porous morphology, and high rate of bioresorption; the wollastonite–calcium phosphate coatings with enhanced strength characteristic and high biological activity; the Zn- or Cu-incorporated calcium phosphate coatings with promising antibacterial properties. Biotesting demonstrates good osseointegration properties of MAO CaP coatings. Development and medical applications of dental implants based on nanostructured titanium with CaP coatings are presented.

Acknowledgments

The work has been partially financially supported by the Fundamental Research Program of the Siberian Branch of the Russian Academy of Sciences, Project Nos. III.23.2.5 and III.23.2.2; Project of Presidium of RAS, Program 35; the Russian Foundation for Basic Research, Grant No. 15-03-07659; and the Russian Science Foundation, Project Nos. 15-19-00191 and 16-15-10031 (in part of biological studies *in vitro*).

The authors are grateful to Prof. M.V. Chaikina from the Institute of Solid State Chemistry and Mechanochemistry SB RAS (Novosibirsk, Russia), Prof. Q. Zhu from General Research Institute Non-ferrous Metals (Beijing, China), Dr. E.V. Legostaeva, Dr. Zh. Kovalevskaya, A.I. Tolmachev, P.V. Uvarkin, T.V. Tolkacheva, I.A. Glukhov from Institute of Strength Physics and Materials Science SB RAS (Tomsk, Russia).

References

1 Branemark, P.I., Zarb, G.A., and Albrektsson, T. (1985). *Tissue-Integrated Prostheses: Osseointegration in Clinical Dentistry*. Chicago: Quintessence Publishing Co.

2 Esposito, M., Hirsch, J.M., Lekholm, U., and Thomsen, P. (1998). Biological factors contributing to failures of osseointegrated oral implants, (II). Etiopathogenesis. *Eur. J. Oral Sci.* **106** (3): 721–764.

3 Epple, M. (2003). *Biomaterialien und biomineralisation*. Stuttgart: Teubner Studienbücher Chemie.

4 Brown, A. and Lemons, J.E. (eds.) (1996). *Medical Applications of Titanium and Its Alloys: The Material and Biological Issues*. New York: ASTM Special Technical Publication.

5 Brunette, D.M., Tengvall, P., Textor, M., and Thomsen, P. (2001). *Titanium in Medicine*. Berlin: Springer-Verlag.

6 Niinomi, M., Nakai, M., and Hieda, J. (2012). Development of new metallic alloys for biomedical application. *Acta Biomater.* **8** (11): 3888–3903.

7 Gepreel, M.A.H. and Niinomi, M. (2013). Biocompatibility of Ti–alloys for long-term implantation. *J. Mech. Behav. Biomed. Mater.* **20**: 407–415.

8 Hanawa, T. (2004). Metal ion release from metal implants. *Mater. Sci. Eng., C* **24** (6–8): 745–752.

9 Sharkeev, Y.P., Legostaeva, E.V., Eroshenko, A.Y. et al. (2009). The structure and physical and mechanical properties of a novel biocomposite material, nanostructured titanium–calcium–phosphate coating. *Compos. Interfaces* **16** (4–6): 535–546.

10 Sharkeev, Y.P., Polenichkin, V.K., Belyavskaya, O.A. et al. (2012). Dental intraosseous implant and abutment for its. RU Patent 2,441,621.

11 Sharkeev, Y.P., Eroshenko, A.Y., Danilov, V.I. et al. (2014). Microstructure and mechanical properties of nanostructured and ultrafine–grained titanium and the zirconium formed by the method of severe plastic deformation. *Russ. Phys. J.* **56** (10): 1156–1162.

12 Sharkeev, Y.P., Eroshenko, A.Y., Glukhov, I.A. et al. (2015). Microstructure and mechanical properties of Ti–40 mass % Nb alloy after megaplastic deformation effect. In: *AIP Conference Proceedings*, vol. **1683**, 020206. New York: AIP Publishing LLC.

13 Valiev, R.Z., Semenova, I.P., Latysh, V.V. et al. (2008 Aug). Nanostructured titanium for biomedical applications. *Adv. Eng. Mater.* **10** (8): B15–B17.

14 Valiev, R.Z., Zhilyaev, A.P., and Langdon, T.G. (2014). *Bulk Nanostructured Materials: Fundamentals and Applications*. Hoboken, NJ: Wiley.

15 Kolobov, Y.R., Valiev, R.Z., Grabovetskaya, G.P. et al. (2007). *Grain Boundary Diffusion and Properties of Nanostructured Materials*. Cambridge: Cambridge International Science Publishing.

16 Salishchev, G.A., Zherebtsov, S.V., and Galeyev, R.M. (2003). Evolution of microstructure and mechanical behavior of titanium during warm multiple deformation. In: *Ultrafine Grained Materials II* (ed. Y.T. Zhu, T.G. Langdon and R.S. Mishra), 123–131. Warrendale, PA: TMS.

17 Stolyarov, V.V., Zhu, Y.T., Alexandrov, I.V. et al. (2001). Influence of ECAP routes on the microstructure and properties of pure Ti. *Mater. Sci. Eng., A* **229** (1–2): 59–67.

18 Segal, V.M. (1995). Materials processing by simple shear. *Mater. Sci. Eng., A* **197** (2): 157–164.

19 Langdon, T.G., Furukawa, M., Nemoto, M. et al. (2000). Using equal-channel angular pressing for refining grain size. *JOM* **52** (4): 30–33.

20 Sharkeev, Y., Kolobov, Y., Legostaeva, E. et al. (2006). The ultrafine–grained titanium–calcium–phosphate coating biocomposite material for medical applications. In: *Proceedings of 7th International Symposium of Energy and Environmental Aspects of Tribology*, Cracow, Poland (14–16 September 2006), 329–339.

21 Hon, Y.H., Wang, J.Y., and Pan, Y.N. (2003). Composition phase structure and properties of titanium–niobium alloys. *Mater. Trans.* **44** (11): 2384–2390.

22 Safronova, T.V. and Putlyaev, V.I. (2013). Medical nonorganic materials science in Russia: calcium phosphate materials. *Nanosist. Fiz. Khim. Matem.* **4**: 24–47.

23 Barinov, S.M. (2008). *Calcium Phosphate Based Bioceramics for Bone Tissue Engineering*. Stafa-Zurich: Trans Tech Publications.

24 Van Wazer, J.R. (1962). *Phosphorus and Its Compounds: Technology, Biological Functions, and Applications*, vol. **2**. New York: Interscience Publishers Inc.

25 Jolly, W.L. (1991). *The Synthesis and Characterization of Inorganic Compounds*. Prospect Heights, IL: Waveland Press.

26 Barinov, S.M. (2010). Calcium phosphate-based ceramic and composite materials for medicine. *Russ. Chem. Rev.* **79** (1): 13–29.

27 Evdokimov, P.V., Putlyaev, V.I., Merzlov, D.A. et al. (2013). Polymorphism of $Ca_3(PO_4)_2$. *Nanosist. Fiz. Khim. Matem.* **4**: 48–53.

28 Karlov, A.V. and Shakhov, V.P. (2001). *Systems of External Fixation and Regulatory Mechanisms of Optimal Biomechanics*. Tomsk: STT.

29 McConnell, D. (1974). The crystal chemistry of apatite. *Bull. Soc. Fr. Mineral. Cristallogr.* **97**: 237–240.

30 Lyasnikov, V.N., Lyasnikova, A.V., and Dmitrienko, T.G. (2011). *Materials and Coatings in Medical Practice*. Saratov: Science Book Publishing Ltd.

31 Chaikina, M.V., Bulina, N.V., Ishchenko, A.V., and Prosanov, I.Y. (2014). Mechanochemical synthesis of SiO_4^{4-}–substituted hydroxyapatite, Part I – kinetics of interaction between the components. *Eur. J. Inorg. Chem.* **2014**: 4803–4809.

32 Lu, Y.P., Li, M.S., Li, S.T. et al. (2004). Plasma-sprayed hydroxyapatite+titania composite bond coat for hydroxyapatite coating on titanium substrate. *Biomaterials* **25** (18): 4393–4403.

33 Beauvais, S. and Decaux, O. (2007). Plasma sprayed biocompatible coatings on PEEK implants. In: *Thermal Spray 2007: Global Coating Solutions* (ed. B.R. Marple and M.M. Hyland), 372–376. Materials Park, OH: ASM International.

34 de Sena, L.A., de Andrade, M.C., Rossi, A.M., and Soares, G.D.A. (2002). Hydroxyapatite deposition by electrophoresis on titanium sheets with different surface finishing. *J. Biomed. Mater. Res. Part A* **60** (1): 1–7.

35 Aves, E.P. and Estevez, G.F. (2009). Hydroxyapatite coating by sol–gel on Ti–6Al–4V alloy as drug carrier. *J. Mater. Sci.* **20** (2): 543–547.

36 Kim, H.W., Kim, H.E., and Knowles, J.C. (2005). Improvement of hydroxyapatite sol–gel coating on titanium with ammonium hydroxide addition. *J. Am. Ceram. Soc.* **88** (1): 154–159.

37 Zhang, E., Zou, C., and Zeng, S. (2009). Preparation and characterization of silicon-substituted hydroxyapatite coating by a biomimetic process on titanium substrate. *Surf. Coat. Technol.* **203** (8): 1075–1080.

38 Yanovska, A., Kuznetsov, V., Stanislavov, A. et al. (2012). Calcium–phosphate coatings obtained biomimetically on magnesium substrates under low magnetic field. *Appl. Surf. Sci.* **258** (22): 8577–8584.

39 Surmeneva, M.A., Surmenev, R.A., Nikonova, Y.A. et al. (2014). Fabrication, ultra-structure characterization and in vitro studies of RF magnetron sputter deposited nano-hydroxyapatite thin films for biomedical applications. *Appl. Surf. Sci.* **317**: 172–180.

40 López, E.O., Mello, A., Farina, M. et al. (2015). Nanoscale analysis of calcium phosphate films obtained by RF magnetron sputtering during the initial stages of deposition. *Surf. Coat. Technol.* **279**: 16–24.

41 Popova, A.A., Yakovlev, V.I., Legostaeva, E.V. et al. (2013). The effect of the granulometric composition of a hydroxyapatite powder on the structure and phase composition of coatings deposited by the detonation gas spraying technique. *Russ. Phys. J.* **55** (11): 1284–1289.

42 Nosenko, V., Strutynska, N., Vorona, I. et al. (2015). Structure of biocompatible coatings produced from hydroxyapatite nanoparticles by detonation spraying. *Nanoscale Res. Lett.* **10**: 464.

43 Legostaeva, E.V., Sharkeev, Y.P., Epple, M., and Prymak, O. (2014). Structure and properties of microarc calcium phosphate coatings on the surface

of titanium and zirconium alloys. *Russ. Phys. J.* **56** (10): 1130–1136.

44 Kazek-Kęsik, A., Krok-Borkowicz, M., Jakóbik-Kolon, A. et al. (2015). Biofunctionalization of Ti–13Nb–13Zr alloy surface by plasma electrolytic oxidation. Part I. Part II. *Surf. Coat. Technol.* **276**: 23–30, 59–69.

45 Sharkeev, Y.P., Sedelnikova, M.B., Komarova, E.G., and Khlusov, I.A. (2015). Titanium surface modification by the micro–arc oxidation in the electrolyte based on wollastonite and hydroxyapatite. In: *AIP Conference Proceedings*, vol. **1688**, 060002. New York: AIP Publishing LLC.

46 Ma, J., Karaman, I., Kockar, B. et al. (2011). Sever plastic deformation of $Ti_{74}Nb_{26}$ shape memory alloys. *Mater. Sci. Eng., A* **528** (25–26): 7628–7635.

47 Xu, Y.F., Yi, D.Q., Liu, H.Q. et al. (2012). Effect of cold deformation on microstructure, texture evolution and mechanical properties of Ti–Nb–Zr–Fe alloy for biomedical applications. *Mater. Sci. Eng., A* **547**: 64–71.

48 Kent, D., Wang, G., Zhentao, Y. et al. (2011). Strength enhancement of a biomedical titanium alloy through a modified accumulative roll bonding technique. *J. Mech. Behav. Biomed. Mater.* **4** (3): 405–416.

49 Aronso, C.R.M., Aleixo, G.T., Ramirez, A.J. et al. (2007). Influence of cooling rate on microstructure of Ti–Nb alloy for orthopedic implants. *Mater. Sci. Eng., C* **27** (4): 908–913.

50 Kim, H.Y., Ikehara, Y., Kim, J.I. et al. (2006). Martensitic transformation, shape memory effect and superelasticity of Ti–Nb binary alloys. *Acta Mater.* **54** (9): 2419–2429.

51 Wilkinson, W.D. (1970). *Fabrication of Refractory Metals*. New York: Gordon and Breach Science Publishers.

52 Colings, E.W. (1984). *Physical Metallurgy of Titanium Alloys*. Metals Park, OH: American Society for Metals.

53 Koneva, N.A., Kozlov, E.V., Trishkina, L.I., and Zhdanov, A.N. (2010). Hardening mechanisms and deformation stages in nanograined polycrystals. *Russ. Metall. (Met.)* **2010** (4): 264–267.

54 Park, H.K., Hong, Y.K., Lee, S.Q., and Kee, S. Development of a nanoindenter using a piezoelectric actuator. In: *Proceedings of the International Conference on Optomechatronic Sensors, Actuators, and Control*, Philadelphia, PA, USA (29 September 2004), Proceedings of SPIE, vol. **5602**, 115–121.

55 Mantani, Y. and Tajima, M. (2006). Phase transformation of quenched martensite by aging in Ti–Nb alloys. *Mater. Sci. Eng., A* **438–440**: 315–319.

56 Li, H.X., Rudnev, V.S., Zheng, Z.H. et al. (2008). Characterization of Al_2O_3 ceramic coatings on 6063 aluminum alloy prepared in borate electrolytes by micro–arc oxidation. *J. Alloys Compd.* **462** (1–2): 99–102.

57 Rao, K.P., Ram, G.D.J., and Stucker, B.E. (2008). Improvement in corrosion resistance of friction stir welded aluminum alloys with micro arc oxidation coatings. *Scr. Mater.* **58** (11): 998–1001.

58 Yerokhin, A.L., Nie, X., Leyland, A., and Matthews, A. (2000). Characterisation of oxide films produced by plasma electrolytic oxidation of Ti–6Al–4V alloy. *Surf. Coat. Technol.* **130** (2–3): 195–206.

59 Mayor, B., Arias, J., Chiussi, S. et al. (1998). Calcium phosphate coatings grown at different substrate temperatures by pulsed ArF–laser deposition. *Thin Solid Films* **317** (1–2): 363–366.

60 Wang, Y., Wang, L., Zheng, H. et al. (2010). Effect of frequency on the structure and cell response of Ca- and P–containing MAO films. *Appl. Surf. Sci.* **256** (7): 2018–2024.

61 Wei, D., Zhou, Y., Jia, D., and Wang, Y. (2007). Effect of heat treatment on the structure and in vitro bioactivity of microarc–oxidized (MAO) titania coatings containing Ca and P ions. *Surf. Coat. Technol.* **201** (21): 8723–8729.

62 Gupta, P., Tenhundfeld, G., Daigle, E.O., and Ryabkov, D. (2007). Electrolytic plasma technology: science and engineering – an overview. *Surf. Coat. Technol.* **201** (21): 8746–8760.

63 Dunleavy, C.S., Golosnoy, I.O., Curran, J.A., and Clyne, T.W. (2009). Characterization of discharge events during plasma electrolytic oxidation. *Surf. Coat. Technol.* **203** (22): 3410–3419.

64 Dunleavy, C., Curran, J., and Clyne, T. (2011). Self-similar scaling of discharge events through PEO coatings on aluminium. *Surf. Coat. Technol.* **206** (6): 1051–1061.

65 Suminov, I.V., Belkin, P.N., and Epelfeld, A.V. (eds.) (2011). *Plasma-electrolytic Modification of Metals and Alloys*, 1e, 2e. Moscow: Technosfera.

66 Liu, F., Song, Y., Wang, F. et al. (2005). Formation characterization of hydroxyapatite on titanium by microarc oxidation and hydrothermal treatment. *J. Biosci. Bioeng.* **100** (1): 100–104.

67 Li, Y., Lee, I.S., Cui, F.Z., and Choi, S.H. (2008). The biocompatibility of nanostructured calcium phosphate coated on micro–arc oxidized titanium. *Biomaterials* **29** (13): 2025–2032.

68 Sharkeev, Y.P., Psakhie, S.G., and Legostaeva, E.V. (eds.) (2014). *Biocomposites Based on Calcium–Phosphate Coatings, Nanostructured and*

Ultrafine-Grained Bioinert Metals, their Biocompatibility and Biodegradation. Tomsk: Publishing House of Tomsk State University.

69 Kim, H.S., Yang, Y., Koh, J.T. et al. (2009). Fabrication and characterization of functionally graded nano–micro porous titanium surface by anodizing. *J. Biomed. Mater. Res. Part B* **88B** (2): 427–435.

70 Puckett, S.D., Taylor, E., Raimondo, T., and Webster, T.J. (2010). The relationship between the nanostructure of titanium surfaces and bacterial attachment. *Biomaterials* **31** (4): 706–713.

71 Wei, D., Zhou, Y., Wang, Y., and Jia, D. (2007). Characteristic of microarc oxidized coatings on titanium alloy formed in electrolytes containing chelate complex and nano–HA. *Appl. Surf. Sci.* **253** (11): 5045–5050.

72 Abbasi, S., Bayati, M.R., Golestani-Fard, F. et al. (2011). Micro arc oxidized HAp–TiO_2 nanostructured hybrid layers – Part I: effect of voltage and growth time. *Appl. Surf. Sci.* **257** (14): 5944–5949.

73 Tian, Y., Ding, S., Peng, H. et al. (2012). Osteoblast growth behavior on porous-structure titanium surface. *Appl. Surf. Sci.* **261**: 25–30.

74 Kung, K.C., Yuan, K., Lee, T.M., and Lui, T.S. (2012). Effect of heat treatment on microstructures and mechanical behavior of porous Sr–Ca–P coatings on titanium. *J. Alloys Compd.* **515**: 68–73.

75 Farnoush, H., Mohandesi, J.A., Fatmehsari, D.H., and Moztarzadeh, F. (2012). A kinetic study on the electrophoretic deposition of hydroxyapatite– titania nanocomposite based on a statistical approach. *Ceram. Int.* **38** (8): 6753–6767.

76 Paitel, S.R. and Dahorte, N.B. (2009). Calcium phosphate coatings for bio-implant applications: materials, performance factors, and methodologies. *Mater. Sci. Eng., R* **66** (1–3): 1–70.

77 Huang, L., Ning, C.Q., Ding, D.Y. et al. (2010). Wettability and in vitro bioactivity of doped TiO_2 nanotubes. *J. Inorg. Mater.* **25** (7): 775–779.

78 Yu, S., Yu, Z., Wang, G. et al. (2011). Biocompatibility and osteoconduction of active porous calcium–phosphate films on a novel Ti–3Zr–2Sn–3Mo–25Nb biomedical alloy. Review. *Colloids Surf., B* **85** (2): 103–115.

79 Arrabal, R., Matykina, E., Hashimoto, T. et al. (2009). Characterization of AC PEO coatings on magnesium alloys. *Surf. Coat. Technol.* **203** (16): 2207–2220.

80 Sreekanth, D., Rameshbabu, N., and Venkateswarlu, K. (2012). Effect of various additives on morphology and corrosion behavior of ceramic coatings developed on AZ31 magnesium alloy by plasma electrolytic oxidation. *Ceram. Int.* **38** (6): 4607–4615.

81 Sun, J., Han, Y., and Huang, X. (2007). Hydroxyapatite coatings prepared by micro–arc oxidation in Ca– and P-containing electrolyte. *Surf. Coat. Technol.* **20** (9–11): 5655–5658.

82 Tsuchiya, H., Macak, J.M., Taveira, L. et al. (2005). Self-organized TiO_2 nanotubes prepared in ammonium fluoride containing acetic acid electrolytes. *Electrochem. Commun.* **7** (6): 576–580.

83 Shashkina, G.A., Sharkeev, Y.P., Kolobov, Y.R., and Karlov, A.V. (2007). Calcium–phosphate coating on titanium and titanium alloys and method for its production. RU Patent 2,291,918.

84 Legostaeva, E.V., Sharkeev, Y.P., Tolkacheva, T.V. et al. (2010). Bioactive coating on implant from titanium and method for its production. RU Patent 2,385,740.

85 Bulina, N.V., Chaikina, M.V., Andreev, A.S. et al. (2014). Mechanochemical synthesis of SiO_4^{4-}–substituted hydroxyapatite, part II – reaction mechanism, structure, and substitution limit. *Eur. J. Inorg. Chem.* **2014**: 4810–4825.

86 Lee, K.Y., Park, M., Kim, H.M. et al. (2006). Ceramic bioactivity: progress and perspectives. *Biomed. Mater.* **1** (2): 31–37.

87 Jones, J.R. (2013). Review of bioactive glass: from hench to hybrids. *Acta Biomater.* **9** (1): 4457–4486.

88 Hijo'n, N., Manzano, M., Salinas, A.J., and Vallet-Regi, M. (2005). Bioactive CaO–SiO_2–PDMS coatings on Ti6Al4V substrates. *Chem. Mater.* **17** (6): 1591–1596.

89 Dorozhkin, S.V. (2007). In vitro mineralization of silicon containing calcium phosphate bioceramics. *J. Am. Ceram. Soc.* **90** (1): 244–249.

90 Sedelnikova, M.B., Komarova, E.G., Sharkeev, Y.P., and Tolkacheva, T.V. (2015). Formation and properties of biocoatings based on wollastonite and calcium phosphates. In: *AIP Conference Proceedings*, vol. **1683**, 020202. New York: AIP Publishing LLC.

91 Shumakova, V.V., Pogrebenkov, V.M., Karlov, A.V. et al. (2000). Hydroxyapatite-wollastonite ceramics. *Stek. Keram.* **10**: 18–21.

92 Rudawska, A. and Jacniacka, E. (2009). Analysis for determining surface energy uncertainty by the Owens-Wendt method. *Int. J. Adhes. Adhes.* **29** (4): 451–457.

93 Legostaeva, E.V., Sharkeev, Y.P., Gnedenkov, S.V. et al. (2013). Micro arc calcium phosphate coatings on nanostructured titanium surface: morphology, physic–mechanical and electrochemical properties. *Materialovedenie* **4**: 48–56.

94 Nie, X., Leyland, A., and Matthews, A. (2000). Deposition of layered bioceramic hydroxyapatite/TiO_2 coatings on titanium alloys using a hybrid technique of micro–arc oxidation

and electrophoresis. *Surf. Coat. Technol.* **125** (1–3): 407–414.

95 Mohan, L., Durgalakshmi, D., Geetha, M. et al. (2012). Electrophoretic deposition of nanocomposite (HAp+TiO_2) on titanium alloy for biomedical applications. *Ceram. Int.* **38** (4): 3435–3443.

96 Komarova, E.G., Chebodaeva, V.V., Sharkeev, Y.P., and Sedelnikova, M.B. (2016). Effect of surface topography and chemical composition on wettability of calcium phosphate coatings formed on Ti–40Nb alloy. *Key Eng. Mater.* **683**: 370–376.

97 Khlusov, I.A., Dekhtyar, Y., Khlusova, M.Y. et al. (2013). Novel concepts of "niche–relief" and "niche–voltage" for stem cells as a base and hematopoietic tissues biomimetic engineering. In: *IFMBE Proceedings*, vol. **38**, 99–102. Berlin, Heidelberg: Springer-Verlag.

98 Cohen, A., Liu, S.P., Storey, D., and Webster, T.J. (2007). Decreased fibroblast and increased osteoblast functions on ionic plasma deposited nanostructured Ti coatings. *Nanoscale Res. Lett.* **2** (8): 385–390.

99 Puckett, S., Pareta, R., and Webster, T.J. (2008). Nano rough micron patterned titanium for directing osteoblast morphology and adhesion. *Int. J. Nanomed.* **3** (2): 229–241.

100 Yao, C., Slamovich, E.B., and Webster, T.J. (2008). Enhanced osteoblast functions on anodized titanium with nanotube-like structures. *J. Biomed. Mater. Res. Part A* **85** (1): 157–166.

101 Giavaresi, G., Fini, M., Cigada, A. et al. (2003). Mechanical and histomorphometric evaluations of titanium implants with different surface treatments inserted in sheep cortical bone. *Biomaterials* **24** (9): 1583–1594.

102 Sammons, R.L., Lumbikanonda, N., Gross, M., and Cantzler, P. (2005). Comparison of osteoblast spreading on microstructured dental implant surfaces and cell behaviour in an explant model of osseointegration: a scanning electron microscopic study. *Clin. Oral Impl. Res.* **16** (6): 657–666.

103 Elliot, J.C. (1994). *Structure and Chemistry of the Apatites and other Calcium Orthophosphates*. Amsterdam: Elsevier.

104 Ma, C., Nagai, A., Yamazaki, Y. et al. (2012). Electrically polarized micro–arc oxidized TiO_2 coatings with enhanced surface hydrophilicity. *Acta Biomater.* **8** (2): 860–865.

105 Dorozhkin, S.V. (2009). Calcium orthophosphates in nature, biology and medicine. Review. *Materials* **2** (2): 399–498.

106 Pan, Y.K., Chen, C.Z., Wang, D.G., and Lin, Z.Q. (2013). Preparation and bioactivity of micro–arc oxidized calcium phosphate coatings. *Mater. Chem. Phys.* **141** (2–3): 842–849.

107 Pan, Y.K., Chen, C.Z., Wang, D.G., and Zhao, T.G. (2013). Effects of phosphates on microstructure and bioactivity of micro–arc oxidized calcium phosphate coatings on Mg–Zn–Zr magnesium alloy. *Colloids Surf., B* **109**: 1–9.

108 Kazek-Kęsik, A., Krok-Borkowicz, M., Pamuła, E., and Simka, W. (2014). Electrochemical and biological characterization of coatings formed on Ti–15Mo alloy by plasma electrolytic oxidation. *Mater. Sci. Eng., C* **43** (1): 172–181.

109 Sharkeev, Y.P. and Kulyashova, K.S. (2014). Regularities of calcium phosphate coatings on zirconium from electrolytes based on synthesized and biological hydroxyapatite. *Russ. Phys. J.* **56** (10): 1170–1175.

110 Legostaeva, E.V., Kulyashova, K.S., Komarova, E.G. et al. (2013). Physical, chemical and biological properties of micro–arc calcium–phosphate biocoatings on titanium and zirconium. *Materialwiss. Werkstofftech.* **44** (2–3): 188–197.

111 Zou, Z., Xue, W., Jia, X. et al. (2013). Effect of voltage on properties of micro arc oxidation films prepared in phosphate electrolyte on Zr–1Nb alloy. *Surf. Coat. Technol.* **222**: 62–67.

112 Lin, X., Wang, X., Tan, L. et al. (2014). Effect of preparation parameters on the properties of hydroxyapatite containing micro–arc oxidation coating on biodegradable ZK 60 magnesium alloy. *Ceram. Int.* **40** (7): 10043–10051.

113 Rodionov, I.V., Butovskii, K.G., Beidik, O.V., and Surmenko, E.L. (2008). Oxide biocoatings with antiseptic and antithrombogenic properties on transosseous fixator in osteosynthesis devices. *Biomed. Radioelektr.* **8–9**: 98–101.

114 Hu, H., Zhang, W., Jiang, X. et al. (2012). Antibacterial activity and increased bone marrow stem cell functions of Zn–incorporated TiO_2 coatings on titanium. *Acta Bioamater.* **8** (2): 904–915.

115 Liu, X., Chu, P., and Ding, C. (2004). Surface modification of titanium, titanium alloys, and related materials for biomedical applications. *Mater. Sci. Eng., R* **47** (3–4): 49–121.

116 Lowe, N.M., Fraser, W.D., and Jackson, M.J. (2002). Is there a potential therapeutic value of copper and zinc for osteoporosis? *Proc. Nutr. Soc.* **61** (2): 181–485.

117 Tas, A.C., Bhaduri, S.B., and Jalota, S. (2007). Preparation of Zn–doped β–tricalcium phosphate (β–$Ca_3(PO_4)_2$) bioceramics. *Mater. Sci. Eng., C* **27** (3): 394–401.

118 Khlusov, I.A., Shevtsova, N.M., and Khlusova, M.Y. (2013). Detection in vitro and quantitative estimation of artificial microterritories which promote osteogenic differentiation and maturation of stromal stem cells. *Methods Mol. Biol.* **1035**: 103–119.

119 Zuk, P.A., Zhu, M., Mizuno, H. et al. (2001). Multilineage cells from human adipose tissue: implications for cell–based therapies. *Tissue Eng.* 7 (2): 211–228.

120 Kfoury, Y., David, T., and Scadden, D.T. (2015). Mesenchymal cell contributions to the stem cell niche. *Cell Stem Cell* **16** (3): 239–253.

121 Burtis, C.A., Ashwood, E.R., and Bruns, D.E. (eds.) (2001). *Tietz Fundamentals of Clinical Chemistry*, 5e. New York: W.B. Saunders Company.

122 Riggs, B.L. and Melton, L.J. III, (eds.) (1995). *Osteoporosis: Etiology, Diagnosis, and Management*, 2e. New York: Lippincott–Raven Publishers.

123 Karlov, A.V., Khlusov, I.A., Pozhen'ko, N.S., and Chaikina, M.V. (2004). In vitro regulation of cell behavior by calcium phosphates synthesized by the mechanochemical method. *Bull. Exp. Biol. Med.* **138** (3): 316–320.

124 Nepola, J.V. (1996). External fixation. In: *Rockwood and Green's Fractures in Adults*, 4e (ed. C.A. Rockwood Jr., and D.P. Green), 229–304. Philadelphia: Lippincott–Raven.

125 Chen, X., Su, J., Chang, J. et al. (2008). Inhibition of CD147 gene expression via RNA interference reduces tumor cell proliferation, activation, adhesion, and migration activity in the human Jurkat T–lymphoma cell line. *Cancer Invest.* **26** (7): 689–697.

126 Stevens, M.J., Donato, L.J., Lower, S.K., and Sahai, N. (2009). Oxide-dependent adhesion of the Jurkat line of T lymphocytes. *Langmuir* **25** (11): 6270–6278.

127 Ren, L., Wong, H.M., Yan, C.H. et al. (2015). Osteogenic ability of Cu–bearing stainless steel. *J. Biomed. Mater. Res. Part B* **103** (7): 1433–1444.

128 Sharkeev, Y.P., Belyavskaya, O.A., Polenichkin, V.K. et al. (2009). Dental intraosseous implant. RU Patent 2,376,955.

129 Sharkeev, Y.P. and Polenichkin, V.K. (2009). Prospects of ultrafine–grained titanium application in dentistry. *Perspekt. Mater.* **7**: 372–377.

130 Legostaeva, E.V., Khlusov, I.A., and Sharkeev, Y.P. (2006). Evolution of structure and properties of biocomposite based on nanostructured titanium and microarc calcium phosphate coatings in contact with biological medium. *Fizich. Mezomekh.* **9**: 205–208.

9

Engineering of Bioceramics-Based Scaffold and Its Clinical Applications in Dentistry

Ika D. Ana

Department of Dental Biomedical Sciences, Faculty of Dentistry, Universitas Gadjah Mada, Yogyakarta 55281, Indonesia

9.1 Introduction

9.1.1 Scaffold in Dentistry

Fundamentally, the body comprises of three elements. Those are cells, extracellular matrix (ECM) for cells to proliferate and differentiate, and signaling molecules [1]. Tissue engineering paradigm introduced the fact that tissue regeneration can be achieved by single or combined use of two or three elements in an appropriate way. When there is a defect in the body, tissue regeneration cannot happen only by a simple combination of the three elements. It needs biomedical orchestration to achieve tissue regeneration successfully.

The fundamental technology is through the preparation of biomaterials as an artificial scaffold, to act as synthetic ECM [2]. This concept is based on the natural function of the ECM that provides physical support to cells and natural environment for cell proliferation and differentiation [3–5]. Thus, when there is a defect in the body, both cells and ECM are lost. The scaffold or synthetic ECM induces tissue regeneration by providing three-dimensional structure as an artificially built environment to assist the remaining cells to attach, subsequently proliferate, and differentiate [2]. The remaining cells residing around the scaffold are expected to infiltrate into it, proliferate, and differentiate. In view of this, the first requirement for the scaffold to function as a synthetic ECM is it should be biologically compatible. The other requirements for the scaffold are to have a porous structure necessary for the cells to infiltrate as well as to facilitate oxygen and nutrient supply for cells. Besides, the scaffold should be biodegradable in a controllable manner at the defect site to induce long-term cell viability until ECM is produced naturally in the defect site. Adequate three-dimensional structure is also needed to be considered for a successful tissue regeneration, wherein scaffold should be able to maintain the tissue dimension, provide mechanical resistance to support *in vivo* stresses, and be mechanically compatible with surrounding tissues [6, 7].

In some cases, the tissue around the defect does not have inherent potential to regenerate. In this situation, scaffold should be used in combination with cells and/or signaling molecules [1, 2] that have potential to accelerate tissue regeneration. This can be provided by isolation, injection, protection, and/or transplantation of the cells, and/or growth factors or signaling molecules into the defect site wherein scaffold can function as a vehicle or delivery system to avoid cells and/or growth factors or signaling molecules to be diffused rapidly, enzymatically digested, or deactivated [8, 9].

Tissue engineering paradigm, which includes the fundamental technology of scaffolding system, has been a significant approach in dentistry. For example, in case of periodontal diseases (with a large proportion of the worldwide population up to 90%), which are caused either inherited or acquired disorder of the tissues surrounding and supporting the teeth [10], the traditional approach that is based solely upon infection control [11] has been shifted into periodontal tissue engineering. Tissue engineering approach through the application of periodontal ligament stem cells (PDLSC) and stem cells from apical papilla (SCAP) mixed in hydroxyapatite (HA)/tricalcium phosphate (TCP) scaffold allows reconstruction of a functional tooth with a root periodontal complex [12]. A periodontal stem cell–based therapy using HA/TCP scaffold can rapidly provide cells for the damaged diseased site and overcome the limited PDLSC in patients with periodontitis due to long-term inflammation [13].

In the area of implantology, the long-term implant success and survival rates are above 90% [14]. However, some conditions such as smoking, diabetes, radiotherapy, and postmenopausal estrogen therapy may compromise bone quantity and quality and lead to failure on bone healing [15]. Tissue engineering strategies enable bone

Bioceramics and Biocomposites: From Research to Clinical Practice, First Edition. Edited by Iulian Antoniac.

cell adhesion, modulate cell signaling, deliver growth factors, and promote osteoblast differentiation by matrix deposition and mineralization [16, 17]. Thus, it might be possible to place the implants even under less than ideal anatomical and biological circumstances [18].

One interesting strategy has also been applied in the area of implant dentistry wherein titanium implants were coated with ECM components, such as collagen, bone morphogenetic protein (BMP), transforming growth factor (TGF), or chondroitin sulfate [19, 20]. The BMP was coated on the implant surface because BMP is known to have the advantage of improving bone healing, inducing peri-implant bone formation, and enhancing osseointegration of endosseous implants [20]. Meanwhile, TGF was used since it is produced in response to factors that stimulate osteoclastic bone resorption, thus inhibit osteoclast formation and activity [21]. At the same time, TGF is also known to play a key role in osteoblastic formation [21]. Chondroitin sulfate has an anti-inflammatory effect while accelerating bone repair and regeneration [22]. Regarding the coating strategy, it is important to consider release kinetics and degradation rate of the growth factors to achieve maximum bone formation at proper crucial concentration to minimally reduce toxicity and side effects while providing affordable and clinically safe treatments [18]. To fulfill the requirements of optimum bone repair and regeneration in a controlled release and proper concentration of growth factors, biodegradable scaffold is the key point of the technology.

Regeneration of dentin pulp complex in a biological manner has been a challenging technique in the area of restorative dentistry. A lot of researches have been done to investigate the potential candidates of the techniques to do it. Sakai et al. [23] reported about the differentiation of stem cells from human exfoliated deciduous teeth (SHED) into odontoblast and generated tubular dentin *in vivo*. It was also found that SHED seeded in tooth slices containing scaffolds and implanted in immune-deficient mice are able to produce dental pulp tissue [24]. It is also found from the original work of Rosa et al. [18] that when SHED was mixed with nanofiber peptide scaffold and injected into full-length root canals, dental pulp was successfully generated, giving the support findings that cell-based therapy with scaffold as the fundamental technology is an achievable approach in dentistry.

In a review article by Nakashima and Akamine about the scaffold potential for pulp and dentin regeneration [25], it was also reported that synthetic ECM may also be a potential scaffold for reparative dentinogenesis [26]. Alginate hydrogel facilitates pulpal wound healing with hydration properties and tethering growth factors [27]. Torabinejad and Chivian [28] in a recent investigation found mineral trioxide aggregate (MTA) powder consisting of fine hydrophilic particles of tri-calcium silicate, tri-calcium aluminate, tri-calcium oxide, and silicate oxide as a potential alternative restorative material. It was known that MTA sets in the presence of moisture, prevents microleakage, promotes reparative dentin formation, and is biocompatible. Further progress in the scaffolds for regenerative endodontics depends on a three-dimensional microenvironment that promotes cell behavior including cell polarization and optimal delivery of morphogens such as BMPs. The three-dimensional microenvironment provided by scaffold as an artificial ECM can be designed and used as the culture substrate in tissue engineering concept [2]. Figure 9.1 shows the potential of scaffold-based tissue engineering in dentistry.

9.1.2 Ceramics and Composite Used as Scaffold in Dentistry

Because of the similarity of the human bone, so far calcium phosphate (CaP) ceramics are very popular materials for diverse clinical application in dentistry. Calcium phosphate ceramics are commonly used in dentistry since bone minerals are considered the version

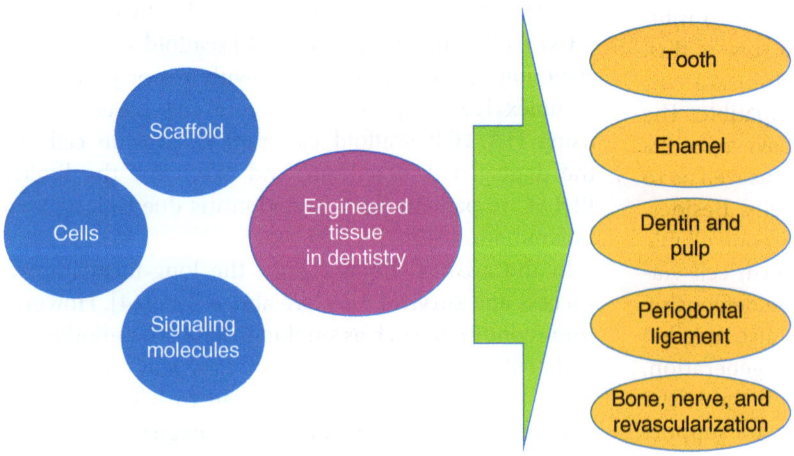

Figure 9.1 Enabling technology applied in dentistry by making use of scaffold as a synthetic ECM, in single or combination with cells and/or signaling molecules.

of calcium phosphate called calcium hydroxyapatite. Calcium hydroxyapatite contains $Ca_{10}(PO_4)_6(OH)_2$. Calcium hydroxyapatite minerals in bone are impure, with 4–6% of carbonate replacing the phosphate and making bone mineral a carbonated apatite (dahlite) [29, 30]. Extensive studies have been conducted on biological apatites, including bone apatites. It is known that biological apatite not only constitutes the inorganic and mineral phases of normal calcified tissues such as bone and teeth but is also found in some pathologic calcification such as dental calculus, heart calcification, urinary stones, soft tissues calcification [30].

Meanwhile, bioactive ceramics and bioglass have been in clinical use since 1985, based on the work of Larry Hench and colleagues in the University of Florida and was the first material seen to form an interfacial bond with host tissue after implantation [31]. Bioactive glass is an amorphous silicate-based material, which is compatible with human body. The basic component of the bioactive glass is SiO_2, Na_2O, CaO, and P_2O_5 and has been commercially available as bioglass. It can bind to bone and stimulate new bone growth while dissolving over time. Therefore, bioactive glass has the potential to restore diseased or damaged bone to its original state and function.

Thus, hydroxyapatite-based calcium phosphate compounds [32, 33] and bioactive glass [34] are considered as high potential scaffolds, especially for bone tissue engineering in dentistry due to their osteoconductive properties. However, some are regarded as slow degradable material that makes them not attractive for tissue engineering purposes. Besides, ceramics alone will raise problems on poor tensile strength and brittleness that also makes them difficult to provide a suitable scaffold.

On the other hand, calcium sulfate, or gypsum, or plaster of Paris (POP) has long history in regenerative dentistry, especially for the treatment of skeletal defects. It is a biocompatible and osteoconductive biomaterial [35]. Calcium sulfate is known as a self-setting material, has ability to deliver antibiotics, cells, or growth factors. However, calcium sulfate cements show a too fast resorption rate and are unable to provide a long-term 3D framework during the osteogenesis process. To solve this problem, a biocompatible and osteoconductive hydrogel calcium carbonate has been incorporated into calcium sulfate formulations [36, 37].

Thus, when it is combined with other materials such as collagen, carbohydrate, e.g. starch, chitosan, alginate, and other polymeric biomaterials such as poly lactic acid (PLA, PLLA, PDLLA), polyglycolic acid (PGA), ceramics is considered an ideal scaffold. This is because the combination of organic (polymer) and inorganic (ceramics) composite results in the tailored degradability and high release efficiencies of the polymer with the osteoconductivity and delayed/sustained release properties of the ceramic materials [38]. Polymer is also combined into the construct in order to compromise the brittleness of the ceramic material. The combination of organic/inorganic materials is also used to achieve the parameters for ideal scaffold in dentistry, and those are (i) A biodegradability that is enabling bone remodeling and tissue regeneration, (ii) A macroporosity that is enabling, (mechanical stability/ease of handling, in some cases (iii) Osteoconductivity to guide bone around/inside the implant, and (iv) Carrier for growth factors/cells [38].

Table 9.1 shows the list of calcium phosphate ceramics used as scaffold in the area of regenerative dentistry. Meanwhile, Table 9.2 shows polymer used in

Table 9.1 Calcium phosphate ceramics with corresponding chemical formula and Ca/P ratio [38–40].

Abbreviation	Name	Formula	Ca/P ratio	Log K_{sp}
ACP	Amorphous calcium phosphate	—	$1.25 < x < 1.57$	
BCP	Biphasic calcium phosphate	$Ca_3(PO_4)_2 + Ca_{10}(PO_4)_6(OH)_2$	$1.50 < x < 1.67$	
CA	Carbonated apatite, dahlite	$Ca_5(PO_4 \cdot CO_3)_3$	1.67	
CDHA	Calcium deficient hydroxyapatite	$Ca_{10-x}(HPO_4)_x(PO_4)_{6-x}(OH)_{2-x}$	$1.50 < x < 1.67$	
DCPA	Dicalcium phosphate anhydrous, moneteite	$CaHPO_4$	1.00	6.90
DCPD	Dicalcium phosphate dehydrate, brushite	$CaHPO_4 \cdot 2H_2O$	1.00	6.59
HA	Hydroxyapatite	$Ca_{10}(PO_4)_6(OH)_2$	1.67	116.8
MCPM	Monocalcium phosphate monohydrate	$Ca(H_2PO_4)_2 \cdot H_2O$	0.50	Highly soluble
OCP	Octacalcium phosphate	$Ca_8H_2(PO_4)_6 \cdot 5H_2O$	1.33	96.6
pHA	Precipitated hydroxyapatite	$Ca_{10-x}(HPO_4)_x(PO_4)_{6-x}(OH)_{2-x}$	$1.50 < x < 1.67$	
α-TCP	α-Tricalcium phosphate, Whitlockite	α-$Ca_3(PO_4)_2$	1.50	
β-TCP	β-Tricalcium phosphate, Whitlockite	β-$Ca_3(PO_4)_2$	1.50	28.9
TTCP	Tetracalcium phosphate, Hilgenstockite	$CaO \cdot Ca_3(PO_4)_2$	2.00	38–44

Table 9.2 Summary of polymers used in combination with ceramics, categorized in groups.

Group	Polymers
Polylactic/polyglycolic acid	Polylactic acid (PLA, PLLA, and PDLLA), polyglycolic acid (PGA), poly(lactic-*co*-glycolic acid) (PLGA), and poly-ε-caprolactone (PCL)
Proteins	Collagen, gelatin, fibrin, casein, and peptides
Carbohydrates	Chitin, chitosan, cellulose, starch, alginate, hyaluronan, hydroxymethylpropylcellulose (HPMC), and amylopectin
Other polymers	Poly(propylene fumarate) (PPF), polycarbonate, polyalkenoates, poly(1.8-octanediol-citrate) (POC), poly(ethylene glycol) (PEG), poly(ethylene imine) (PEI), poly(ethylene oxide) (PEO), prolypropylene (PP), nylon, aramide, and poly(allylamine hydrochloride) (PAH)

combination with ceramics, categorized in group, as adopted from the review paper by Habraken et al. [38].

Polylactic/polyglycolic acid–derived polymers are interesting and have already been investigated extensively due to their biocompatibility and tailor-made degradation properties by changing their molecular weight, ratio, or tactility. Protein-based polymers are used because when it is combined with ceramics, it can produce organic–inorganic composites that can be designed to mimic physical, mechanical, and biological properties of the human tissues, including bone. Carbohydrate-based polymers such as chitin, chitosan, alginate, hyaluronic acid, and cellulose are interesting for general use in biomedicine.

9.1.3 Engineering of Scaffold from Bioceramics and Its Application

Extensive research has been done to provide scaffold for tissue engineering in dentistry. There are a lot of methods applied to achieve ideal scaffold in terms of ideal architectural structure, physical and mechanical properties, and biodegradability of the scaffold, including its proper biological properties.

Dissolution and precipitation that leads to composition transformation method is one of the examples to provide CaP-based scaffold in dentistry. Phase transformation based on dissolution-precipitation reactions is one of the very useful methods for the fabrication of scaffold similar to bone apatite. Dissolution and precipitation reaction are based on the thermodynamic stabilities of calcium phosphate salts [40, 41]. The setting mechanism of gypsum or calcium sulfate or also known as POP in dentistry is the simplest example of dissolution and precipitation reaction. When calcium sulfate hemihydrate ($CaSO_4 \cdot ½H_2O$) is mixed with water, the calcium sulfate di-hydrate is formed, in a mild exothermic reaction [36] as follows:

$$CaSO_4 \cdot ½H_2O + 1½H_2O \rightarrow CaSO_4 \cdot 2H_2O + \text{Heat} \quad (9.1)$$

$$CaSO_4 \cdot ½H_2O + 1½H_2O \rightarrow Ca^{2+} + SO_4^{2-} + 2H_2O \quad (9.2)$$

$$Ca^{2+} + SO_4^{2-} + 2H_2O \rightarrow CaSO_4 \cdot 2H_2O \quad (9.3)$$

Once the hemihydrate dissolves, a two-phase suspension of hemihydrate particles in saturated aqueous solution is formed. When the dissolution becomes supersaturated with dehydrate, crystal nucleates in the suspension and forms a precipitate. Nucleation and crystal growth continue until the dissolution is no longer saturated, leading to further dissolution of the hemihydrate. Alternating dissolution and precipitation continues, with growth of existing crystal or nucleation of new crystals [36]. It was known that solubility of calcium sulfate hemihydrate at 20 °C is 0.82 [42]. Calcium and sulfate ions corresponding to 0.82 g $CaSO_4 \cdot ½H_2O$ are dissolved in water if there are no other phase in equilibrium. However, the solution is supersaturated with calcium sulfate di-hydrate ($CaSO_4 \cdot 2H_2O$) with its solubility as 0.20 at 20 °C [40]. Therefore, calcium sulfate di-hydrate crystal is precipitated, forming a set cluster.

In the case of α-TCP that is considered the simplest calcium phosphate cement (CPC) found by Monma and Kanazawa [43], it was known that α-TCP has an unstable phase in water. When α-TCP dissolves with water, it supplies calcium and phosphate ions into the solution. However, the solution is supersaturated with respect to apatite at neutral and alkaline pH [40]. Thus, calcium and phosphate ions will be precipitated as calcium-deficient apatite crystals, as reflected in Eqs. (9.4) and (9.5) [44]. The precipitated calcium deficient apatite crystals form a cluster with precipitated crystal interlock, thus to form hardened mass.

$$3Ca_3(PO_4)_2 \cdot H_2O \rightarrow 9Ca^{2+} + 6PO_4^{3-} + H_2O \quad (9.4)$$

$$9Ca^{2+} + 6PO_4^{3-} + H_2O \rightarrow Ca_9HPO_4(PO_4)_5(OH) \quad (9.5)$$

If there are various calcium phosphate salts in the solution, hardening mechanism becomes more complex, for example the cement consisting of tetracalcium phosphate (TTCP) and dicalcium phosphate anhydrous (DCPA). Both TTCP and DCPA are soluble calcium phosphate. Therefore, the reaction is as follows:

$$Ca_4(PO_4)_2O + H_2O \cdot 4Ca^{2+} + 6PO_4{}^{3-} + 2OH^- \quad (9.6)$$

$$2HPO_4 \cdot Ca^{2+} + H^+ + PO_4{}^{3-} \quad (9.7)$$

$$2Ca_4(PO_4)_2O + 2HPO_4 \rightarrow 10Ca^{2+} + 6PO_4{}^{3-} + 2OH^- \rightarrow Ca_{10}(PO_4)_6(OH)_2 \quad (9.8)$$

The solution is supersaturated with respect to HA, thus calcium and phosphate will be precipitated as HA crystals, form a cluster of precipitated crystals interlock, and then form a hardened mass.

Some investigations have been done to make use of the dissolution and precipitation method to fabricate ceramics scaffold. One requirement is the moderate instability, i.e. moderate solubility of the precursor when compared to the final block product. Due to the instability of the precursor, the precursor phase is dissolved in aqueous solution and supplies ions that are required for the precipitation of the final product [45]. Ishikawa and coworkers have been developing carbonate apatite monolith or block and 3D printing model from gypsum [46–50]. It was shown that gypsum monolith or block is able to be transformed into apatite using various ammonium phosphate solutions. The monolith was completely transformed into low crystalline β-type carbonated hydroxyl apatite during proper temperature, concentration, and type of phosphate solution without any change in its morphology. When 3D printing method was applied for fabrication of free-form apatite from gypsum, the use of additives such as binder ink should be considered carefully [49, 50], although 3D Printing is considered a potential candidate to form intended scaffold structure.

In 2010, Ana et al. [51] prepared macroporous carbonated hydroxyapatite (CHA) bone substitutes through composition transformation of gypsum and Ca-hydroxide, the abundant minerals in Indonesia. The work was directed to find low-cost technology to provide bone substitutes with proper mechanical and biological properties, based on the needs of reconstructive surgeon. The specimens were characterized in terms of chemical and physical properties, such as extent of transformation of $CaCO_3$ body into CHA body, type, and content of carbonate, and crystal morphology. Calcium sulfate hemihydrate ($CaSO_4 \cdot \frac{1}{2}H_2O$) was added by various weight% concentration of calcium hydroxide ($Ca(OH)_2$). The carbonation was applied by CO_2 gas to transform $Ca(OH)_2$ into calcium carbonate. It was found that after 72 hours of carbonation, treatment was continued by phosphatization of the composite by 1 M $Na_3PO_4 \cdot 12H_2O$ for 7 and 14 days. It was confirmed that hydroxyapatite (HA) phase was detected as a main reaction product regardless of the percentage of Ca-hydroxide added into gypsum.

References

1 Langer, R. and Vacanti, J.P. (1993). Tissue engineering. *Science* **260**: 920–926.

2 Tabata, Y., Nagano, A., and Ikada, Y. (1999). Biodegradation of hydrogel carrier incorporating fibroblast growth factor. *Tissue Eng.* **5** (2): 127–138.

3 Banerjee, I., Yekkala, K., and Borg, T.K. (2006). Dynamic interactions between myocytes, fibroblasts and extracellular matrix. *Ann. N Y Acad. Sci.* **1080**: 76–84.

4 Larsen, M., Artym, V.V., and Green, J.A. (2006). The matrix reorganized: extracellular matrix remodeling and integrin signaling. *Curr. Opin. Cell Biol.* **18**: 463–471.

5 Nelson, C.M. and Tien, J. (2006). Microstructured extracellular matrices in tissue engineering and development. *Curr. Opin. Biotechnol.* **17**: 518–523.

6 Kemppinen, J.M. and Hollister, S.J. (2010). Tailoring the mechanical properties of 3D-designed poly(glycerol sebacate) scaffolds for cartilage applications. *J. Biomed. Mater. Res. A* **94**: 9–18.

7 Saito, E., Kang, H., Taboas, J.M. et al. (2010). Experimental and computational characterization of designed and fabricated 50:50 PLGA porous scaffolds for human trabecular bone applications. *J. Mater. Sci. Mater. Med.* **21**: 2371–2383.

8 Langer, R. (1998). Drug delivery and targeting. *Nature* **392**: 5–10.

9 Ikada, Y. and Tabata, Y. (1998). Protein release from gelatin matrices. *Adv. Drug Delivery Rev.* **31**: 287–301.

10 Philstrom, B.L., Michalowicz, B.S., and Johnson, N.W. (2005). Periodontal diseases. *Lancet* **366**: 1809–1820.

11 Chen, F.M. and Jin, Y. (2009). Periodontal tissue engineering and regeneration: current approaches and expanding opportunities. *Tissue Eng. Part B* **16**: 219–255.

12 Sonoyama, W., Liu, Y., Fang, D. et al. (2006). Mesenchymal stem cell- mediated functional tooth regeneration in swine. *PLoS One* **1**: e76.

13 Liu, Y., Zheng, Y., Fang, D. et al. (2008). Periodontal ligament stem cells- mediated treatment for periodontitis in miniature swine. *Stem Cells* **26**: 1065–1073.

14 Melo, M.D., Shafie, H., and Obeid, G. (2006). Implant survival rates for oral and maxillofacial surgery residents: a retrospective clinical review with analysis of resident level of training on implant survival. *J. Oral Maxillofac. Surg.* **64**: 1185–1189.

15 Moy, P.K., Medina, D., Shetty, V., and Aghaloo, T.L. (2005). Dental implant failure rates and associated risk factors. *Int. J. Oral Maxillofac. Implants* **20**: 569–577.

16 Weir, M.D. and Xu, H.H. (2010). Culture human mesenchymal stem cells with calcium phosphate cement scaffolds for bone repair. *J. Biomed. Mater. Res. B Appl. Biomater.* **93**: 93–105.

17 Zhao, L., Weir, M.D., and Xu, H.H. (2010). An injectable calcium phosphate – alginate hydrogel – umbilical cord mesenchymal stem cell paste for bone tissue engineering. *Biomaterials* **31**: 6502–6510.

18 Rosa, V., Bona, A.D., Cavalcanti, B.N., and Nor, J.E. (2012). Tissue engineering: from research to dental clinics. *Dent. Mater.* **28**: 341–348.

19 Stadlinger, B., Pilling, E., Mai, R. et al. (2008). Effect of biological implant surface coatings on bone formation, applying collagen, proteoglycans, glycosaminoglycans and growth factors. *J. Mater. Sci. Mater. Med.* **19**: 1043–1049.

20 Liu, Y., Huse, R.O., de Groot, K., and Hunziker, E.B. (2007). Delivery mode and efficacy of BMP-2 in association with implants. *J. Dent. Res.* **86**: 84–89.

21 Nagai, M., Hayakawa, T., Fukatsu, A. et al. (2002). In vitro study of collagen coating of titanium implants for initial cell attachment. *Dent. Mater. J.* **21**: 250–260.

22 Stadlinger, B., Piling, E., Huble, M. et al. (2008). Evaluation of osseointegration of dental implants coated with collagen, chondroitin sulfate and BMP-4: an animal study. *Int. Oral Maxillofac. Surg.* **37**: 54–59.

23 Sakai, V.T., Zhang, Z., Dong, Z. et al. (2010). SHED differentiate into functional odontoblast and endhotelium. *J. Dent. Res.* **89**: 791–796.

24 Cordeiro, M.M., Dong, Z., Kaneko, T. et al. (2008). Dental pulp tissue engineering with stem cells from exfoliated deciduous teeth. *J. Endod.* **34**: 962–969.

25 Nakashima, M. and Akamine, A. (2005). The application of tissue engineering to regeneration of pulp and dentin in endodontics. *J. Endod.* **31** (10): 711–718.

26 Bohl, K.S., Shon, J., Rutherford, B., and Mooney, D.J. (1998). Role of synthetic extracellular matrix in development of engineered dental pulp. *J. Biomater. Sci. Polym. Ed.* **9**: 749–764.

27 Dobie, K., Smith, G., and Sloan, A.J. (2002). Effect of alginate hydrogels and TGF-β1 on human dental pulp repair in vitro. *Connect. Tissue Res.* **43**: 387–390.

28 Torabinejad, M. and Chivian, N. (1999). Clinical applications of mineral trioxide aggregate. *J. Endod.* **25**: 197–205.

29 Le Geros, R.Z. (1991). Calcium phosphate in oral biology and medicine. In: *Monograph in Oral Sciences*, vol. **15** (ed. H. Myers). Basel: Karger.

30 Young, R.A. and Elliot, J.C. (1966). Atomic scale bases for several properties of apatites. *Arch. Oral Biol.* **11**: 699–707.

31 Hench, L.L. (1991). Bioceramics – from concept to clinic. *J. Am. Ceram. Soc.* **74**: 1487–1510.

32 Block, J.E. and Thorn, M.R. (2000). Clinical indications of calcium-phosphate biomaterials and related composites for orthopedic procedures. *Calcif. Tissue Int.* **66**: 234–238.

33 Le Geros, R.Z. (2002). Properties of osteoconductive biomaterials: calcium phosphates. *Clin. Orthop. Rel. Res.* **395**: 81–98.

34 Thomas, M.V., Puleo, D.A., and Al- Sabbagh, M. (2005). Bioactive glass three decades. *J. Long Term Eff. Med. Implants* **15** (6): 585–597.

35 Thomas, M.V. and Puleo, D.A. (2008). Calcium sulfate: properties and clinical application. *J. Biomed. Mater. Res. B* **88**: 597–610.

36 Dewi, A.H., Ana, I.D., Wolke, J.G.C., and Jansen, J.A. (2015). Behavior of POP–calcium carbonate hydrogel as bone substitute with controlled release capability: a study in rat. *J. Biomed. Mater. Res. A* **103**: 3273–3283.

37 Dewi, A.H., Ana, I.D., and Jansen, J.A. (2016). Calcium carbonate hydrogel construct with cynnamaldehyde incorporated to control inflammation during surgical procedure. *J. Biomed. Mater. Res. A* https://doi.org/10.1002/jbm.a.35571.

38 Habraken, W.J.E.M., Wolke, J.G.C., and Jansen, J.A. (2007). Ceramics composite as matrices and scaffolds for drug delivery in tissue engineering. *Adv. Drug Delivery Rev.* **59** (4–5): 234–245.

39 Elliott, J.C. (1994). Structure and chemistry of the apatites and other calcium orthophosphate. In: *Studies in Inorganic Chemistry*, vol. **18**. Amsterdam: Elsevier Science.

40 Ishikawa, K. (2008). Calcium phosphate cement. In: *Bioceramics and their Clinical Application* (ed. T. Kokubo). Florida: CRC Press.

41 Ishikawa, K., Matsuya, S., Miyamoto, Y., and Kawate, K. (2003). Bioceramics. In: *Comprehensive Structural*

Integrity, vol. **9** (ed. I. Milne, R.O. Ritchie and B. Karihaloo). Philadelphia: Elsevier.

42 Ricci, J.L., Alexander, H., Nadkarni, P. et al. (2000). Biological mechanisms of calcium-sulfate replacement by bone. In: *Bone Engineering* (ed. J.E. Davies). Toronto: Em Squared Inc.

43 Monma, H. and Kanazawa, T. (1976). The hydration of a-tricalcium phosphate. *Yogyo-Kyokai-Shi* **84**: 209–213. View at Google Scholar.

44 Tsuru, K., Maruta, M., Ruslin, M.S., and Ishikawa, K. (2015). Effects of the method of apatite seed crystals addition on setting reaction of α-tri calcium phosphate based apatite cement. *J. Mater. Sci. Mater. Med.* **26** (10): 244. https://doi.org/10.1007/s10856-015-5570-8.

45 Ishikawa, K. (2010). Bone substitute fabrication based on dissolution- precipitation reactions. *Materials* **10**: 1138–1155.

46 Ishikawa, K., Matsuya, S., Suzuki, Y. et al. (2005). Fabrication of apatite monolith from calcium sulfate. *Key Eng. Mater.* **288–289**: 533–536.

47 Ishikawa, K., Matsuya, S., Suzuki, Y. et al. (2006). Effects of pH on the transformation of gypsum to carbonate apatite in the presence of ammonium hydrogen phosphate. *Key Eng. Mater.* **309–311**: 199–202.

48 Suzuki, Y., Matsuya, S., Suzuki, Y. et al. (2005). Fabrication of hydroxyapatite block from gypsum block based on $(NH_4)_2HPO_4$ treatment. *Dent. Mater. J.* **24** (4): 515–521.

49 Lowmunkong, R., Sohmura, T., Takahashi, J. et al. (2007). Transformation of 3DP gypsum model to ha by treating in ammonium phosphate solution. *J. Biomed. Mater. Res. Part B* **80**: 386–393.

50 Lowmunkong, R., Sohmura, T., Takahashi, J. et al. (2009). Fabrication of freeform bone- filling calcium phosphate ceramics by gypsum 3D printing method. *J. Biomed. Mater. Res. Part B* **90**: 531–539.

51 Ana, I.D., Matsuya, Y., and Ishikawa, K. (2010). Engineering of carbonate apatite bone substitute based on composition transformation of gypsum and calcium hydroxide. *J. Eng.* **4**: 344–352.

10

Bioceramics in Endodontics

Alexandru A. Iliescu[1], *Paula Perlea*[2], *Gabriel Tulus*[3], *Mihaela G. Iliescu*[2], *Irina M. Gheorghiu*[2], *and Horia O. Manolea*[1]

[1] Department of Oral Rehabilitation, University of Medicine and Pharmacy of Craiova, Craiova, Romania
[2] Department of Endodontology, "Carol Davila" University of Medicine and Pharmacy, Bucharest, Romania
[3] European Society of Endodontology, Viersen, Germany

10.1 Introduction

Bioceramics are frequently used in endodontics in indirect or direct pulp capping, pulpectomy, root perforation repair, apexification, and retrograde fillings and as root canal sealers.

Gartner and Dorn [1] and Damas et al. [2] claimed that the prerequisites of an ideal bioceramic endodontic material should be quick setting, sufficient working time, excellent sealing quality to dentin, undisturbed setting by blood and tissue fluids, dimensional stability, adequate compressibility, insolubility, antimicrobial effect, acceptable radiopacity, biocompatibility, and noncarcinogenic and nonstaining properties.

Endodontic bioceramics should also have trouble-free handling properties and consider the particle size, which affects the early strength and ease of clinical manipulation. According to Parirokh and Torabinejad [3], Lovato and Sedgley [4], Modareszadeh et al. [5], Parirokh and Torabinejad [6], Zhang et al. [7], and Öncel Torun et al. [8], the main requirement, based on their bioactivity, is to promote dentinogenesis, cementogenesis, and apical bone healing.

The susceptibility of microorganisms to an endodontic material depends on their different existence phases, which can be stationary, exponential growth, or starvation. Lovato and Sedgley added that in case of calcium hydroxide, the most used endodontic antiseptic, its high pH, hydrophilicity and active diffusion in dentinal tubules of hydroxyl ions are other differentiating factors of antimicrobial effect [4].

Modareszadeh et al. classify the bioceramics used in dentistry in four classes: bioinert (alumina and zirconia), resorbable (tricalcium phosphate), porous (hydroxyapatite-coated metals and alumina), and bioactive (hydroxyapatite, bioactive glasses, and glass ceramics) [5].

Shokouhinejad et al. affirm that the root-end filling can be considered a bioactive material if it is able to form a layer of apatite at the interface with the periapical tissue [9]. Sarkar et al. [10] and Tay et al. [11] also argue that the bioactivity of ceramics already used as root-end filling was proved *in vitro* by the presence of hydroxyapatite or carbonated apatite at the surface of mineral trioxide aggregate (MTA) after its contact with phosphate-containing liquids.

Modareszadeh et al. showed that bioactive ceramics stimulate both the tissue mineralization and the strong biomaterial–bone interface creation since they directly adhere at the bone tissue that surrounds the tooth root [5].

In endodontic surgery, Johnson et al. stimulated a cementogenesis process that covers the root-end filling material due to the deposition of hydroxyapatite on bioceramic [12]. Ma et al. also describe the occurrence of a biological bond between the resected surface of tooth root and surrounding periapical tissues, which generates a new periodontal ligament [13].

Recently, Öncel Torun et al. called MTA cements alkalinizing materials that release bio-interactive ions [8]. As Shokouhinejad et al. proved, during the hydration mechanism of MTA result a precipitate of calcium hydroxide (portlandite) and a hydrogel of calcium silicate hydrate, which afterwards in the presence of phosphorus ions provided by tissue fluids, generate a precipitate of hydroxyapatite crystals [9].

Shokouhinejad et al. also demonstrated that the volume of newly formed apatite crystals, after immersion of some bioactive ceramic materials such as MTA, EndoSequence Root Repair Material (ERRM), and BioAggregate

Bioceramics and Biocomposites: From Research to Clinical Practice, First Edition. Edited by Iulian Antoniac.

in phosphate-buffered saline (PBS), is directly related to their exposure time in phosphate fluids [9].

10.2 Portland Cement

Portland cement is very common, inexpensive hydraulic cement that is obtained from a mix of lime, silica, and alumina. Parirokh and Torabinejad and Berzins think that there are 10 types of Portland cement admitted according to ASTM Standard C150/C150M, but their chemical purity is almost impossible to assess as they are delivered by many different companies [6, 14].

Type I Portland cement represents the main component of MTA in which the composition is present up to 75%. However, Berzins emphasizes that the Portland component of MTA is present in a purer form, since heavy metals like Cu, Mn, and Sr are in lower amount compared to common Portland cements (Figure 10.1) [14].

Despite the basic similarities of Portland cements to white and gray ProRoot MTA, and low price advantage as well, some chemical and physical properties do not make it suitable to be used without risk for endodontic treatments in humans. In this line, Parirokh and Torabinejad [6] and Berzins [14] remind that unlike Portland cements, MTA is manufactured respecting all medical requirements.

10.2.1 Chemical Composition

Type I Portland cement contains tricalcium silicate (Ca_3SiO_5), dicalcium silicate (Ca_2SiO_4), and tricalcium aluminate ($Ca_3Al_2O_6$). Parirokh and Torabinejad [6] and Berzins [14] consider that roughly, excepting the radiopacifier bismuth oxide, the chemical composition of Portland cement is comparable to MTA. The main components are tricalcium silicate and dicalcium silicate that are estimated to be up to 75–80%. Minor components such as tricalcium aluminate and tetracalcium aluminoferrite represent 10% of the cement's composition.

Berzins [14] showed that the content of Portland cements in tricalcium aluminate and also in calcium sulfate is more elevated compared to MTA. There is also reported in MTA the lack of potassium. However, according to Parirokh and Torabinejad [6], compared to white and gray ProRoot MTA, both white and gray Portland cements have a significantly higher amount of arsenic.

Parirokh and Torabinejad also underscore that gray Portland cement has more lead, cadmium, chromium,

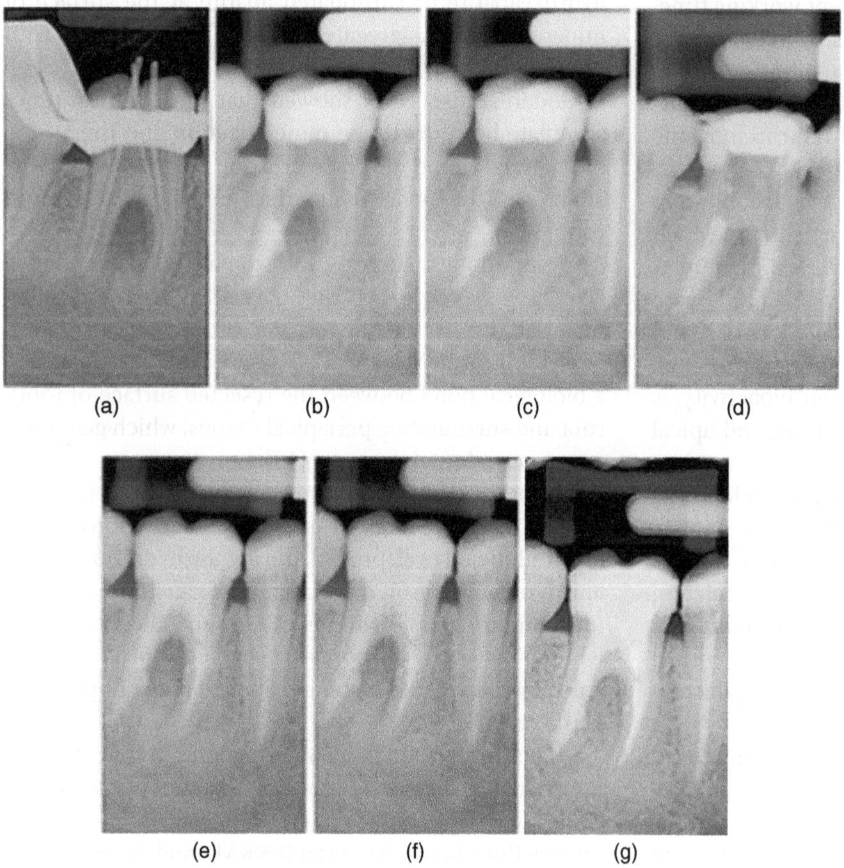

Figure 10.1 Healing of periradicular bone in case of root perforations, regardless of their etiology: (a) internal resorption-related perforation in mesial wall of distal, (b) repair of root perforation with MTA, (c) finishing the distal root canal filling with MTA and strip perforation in mesial root of lower right first molar, (d) final radiographic control of repair with MTA in mesial and distal root perforations, (e) control at 2 months, (f) control at 8 months and furcation healing in progress, (g) control at 20 months and furcation remineralization.

copper, manganese, and zinc than white Portland cement and both white and gray ProRoot MTA [6].

Excepting for bismuth that is present in MTA formulation, regarding other 14 elements, no differences were recorded between Portland cement and ProRoot MTA by Funteas et al. [15]. However, Dammaschke et al. reported that PC CEM 1 (calcium-enriched mixture) (Teutonia Zementwek, Hanover, Deutschland) and CEM II (Spenner Zement, Erwitte, Deutschland) contain a higher level of aluminum and toxic heavy metals [16].

It was also emphasized by Lee et al. that, in the composition of Portland cements, depending on the source of rough materials used in the production process, there may be found a lot of some other toxic ingredients such as arsenic, beryllium, boron, cadmium, chromium, cobalt, dioxins, lead, manganese, mercury, molybdenum, polycyclic aromatic hydrocarbon, selenium, strontium, thallium, and vanadium [17].

10.2.2 Physical Parameters

Concerning the particle size in the powder of common industrial Portland cements, Berzins considers they are in range from less than 1 to 30–50 µm; but, as components of white MTA (WMTA) powder, they are smaller and of more uniform shape (Figure 10.2) [18]. Accordingly, after hydration, the particles of white ProRoot MTA are also smaller compared to white Portland cement as was shown by Parirokh and Torabinejad [6].

Ordinary Portland cement revealed a compressive strength similar to MTA and higher than two experimental Portland cements when used in pulp capping or as material for root perforations repair. However, lower resiliency and tensile strength of Portland cement may result due to carbonation while setting in contact with body-inflamed tissues. Parirokh and Torabinejad highlighted that another clinical failure could be produced by initiating root cracks after root-end resection if the cement is placed as retrograde filling [6].

Portland cements have a reduced resistance to displacements due to the particle size. Thus, according to Parirokh and Torabinejad, the push-out strength of Portland cement is substantially lower compared to ProRoot MTA and MTA Angelus [6]. Similar results were found by Dregger et al. in case of MTA Bio and MTA Branco [19].

Portland cement is acid-soluble. Though earlier studies showed a higher solubility of Portland cement compared to MTA, later Parirokh and Torabinejad reported a lower solubility of Portland cement compared to white ProRoot MTA and MTA Angelus [6].

In vitro the sealing ability of Portland cement is superior to white and gray ProRoot MTA in root perforation repair, but used as retrograde root filling proved to be similar. However, Parirokh and Torabinejad observed it occurs a high risk of its degradation that facilitates microleakage, when the tissue liquids around the margins of the filling become acidic [6].

Parirokh and Torabinejad also reported that due to the release of calcium hydroxide, called *portlandite* after hydration process, Portland cement exhibits an alkaline pH [6]. During the first three hours after setting, the pH values of white Portland cement, combined with the radiopacifier calcium tungstate, were higher than that of WMTA. However, Hungaro Duarte et al. proved after seven days substantially reduced records of pH, probably due the superior solubility of MTA [20].

The radiopacity of Portland cement is lower than MTA and, because it does not fulfill the requirements of ANSI/ADA Specification 57/2000 and ISO 6876/2001, it needs an additional radiopacifying agent. Parirokh and Torabinejad mention investigations are in progress to improve this parameter by introducing different radiopacifiers in formulation of Portland cements (Table 10.1) [6].

The additional effect of radiopacifiers may alter the physical properties of bioceramics. It was observed that bismuth oxide, calcium tungstate, and zirconium oxide increased the setting time of white Portland cement. This issue is highly disadvantageous in endodontic surgery because, as observed by Hungaro Duarte et al. in this manner, it facilitated the retrograde filling dissolution [20].

Regrettably, there were observed an extended setting time, lower compressive strength, and cytotoxic effects when combining Portland cement with bismuth oxide, the radiopaque component of MTA. However, it is claimed that excellent radiopacifiers such as calcium tungstate and zirconium oxide, components of AH Plus sealer, are potential radiopacifying agents for Portland cement because, according to Hungaro Duarte et al., they already proved to be not cytotoxic in combination with Portland cement [20].

Portland cement induces a lower risk of tooth discoloration than gray ProRoot MTA. However, Parirokh and Torabinejad claim that there is a high risk of tooth discoloration after endodontic treatments when Portland cement or white ProRoot MTA is contaminated with blood [6].

10.2.3 Biological Properties

Portland cement is a bioactive endodontic material but not to the same extent as white ProRoot MTA, due to its lower release of portlandite up to one year after setting. Though Portland cement showed calcium ion release and subsequent precipitation of apatite crystals, according to Parirokh and Torabinejad the process of

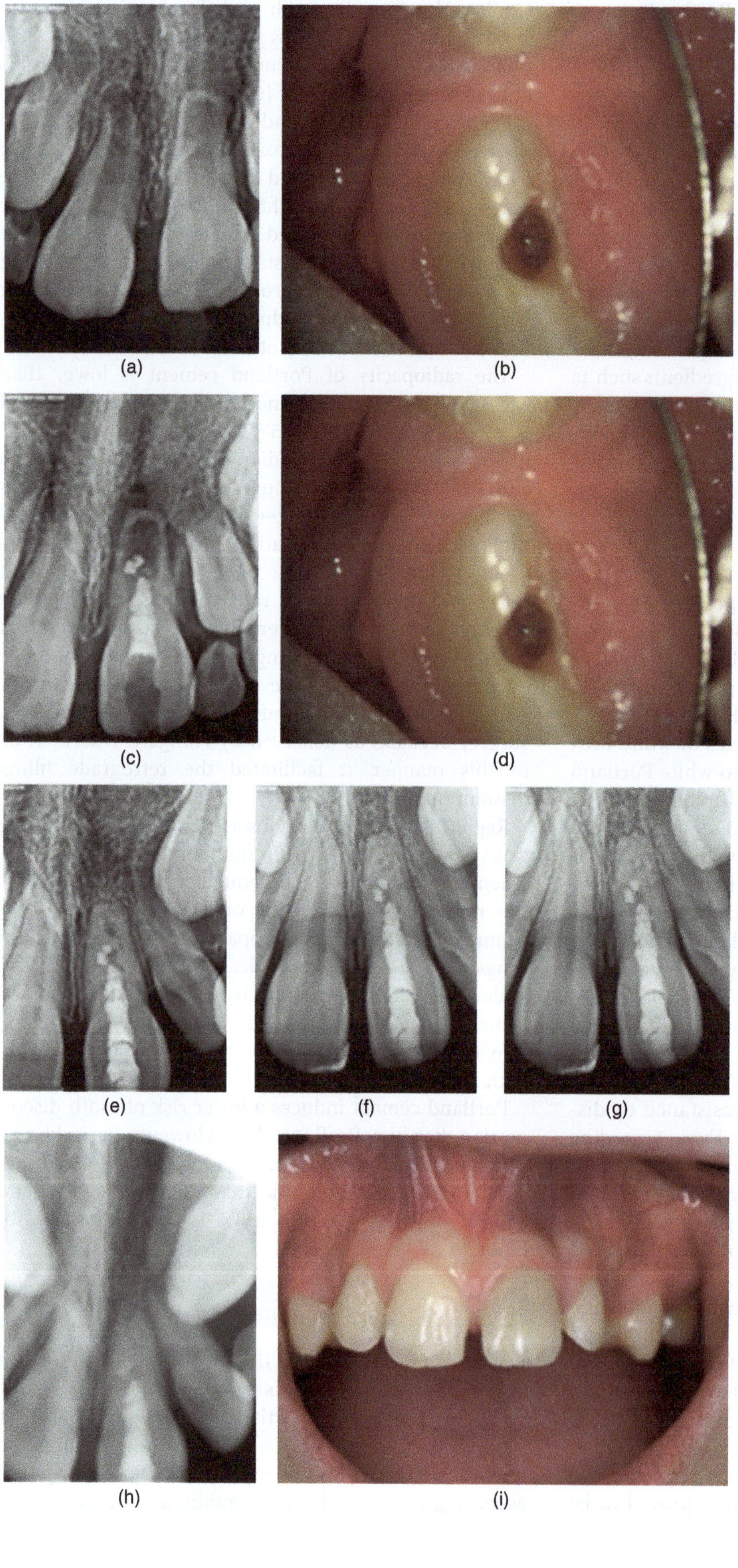
(a) (b) (c) (d) (e) (f) (g) (h) (i)

Figure 10.2 Healing of periradicular bone in case of root perforations, in regenerative procedures: (a) traumatic necrosis in upper left central incisor, (b) microscopic view after necrotic pulp removal, (c) pulp revitalization and apical blood clot covered with MTA, (d) MTA sealing of blood clot inside the canal after three weeks dressing with triple antibiotic paste, (e) root development after 20 months, (f) root development after 26 months, (g) root development after 42 months, (h) root development after 51 months, (i) crown darkening of left upper central incisor due to a possible associated adverse effect of minocycline from triple antibiotic paste and MTA.

Table 10.1 Radiopacifiers used in endodontic bioceramics.

Bioceramic material	Radiopacifier	Equivalent mm Al
BioAggregate	Tantalum pentoxide	Unspecified
Biodentine	Zirconium oxide	4.8
Calcium silicate	Bismuth oxide	Unspecified
Capasio	Unspecified	4.2
CEM	Unspecified	2.27 (under ISO standard)
Ceramicrete-D	Cerium oxide	3.2
Cimento Endodontico Rapido (CER)	Barium sulfate	Unspecified
DiaRoot BioAggregate	Tantalum pentoxide	Unspecified
EndoBinder	Bismuth oxide	Similar to gray MTA
Endocem MTA	Bismuth oxide	Unspecified
Endo-CPM Sealer	Barium sulfate 10%	Unspecified
EndoSequence BC Sealer	Zirconium oxide	3.83
EndoSequence Root Repair Material (ERRM)	Zirconium + tantalum oxide	Unspecified
Generex A	Unspecified	6.8
iRoot BP	Zirconium + tantalum oxide	Unspecified
iRoot BP Plus	Zirconium + tantalum oxide	Unspecified
Light-cured MTA	Barium sulfate	Under ISO standard
MM-MTA	Bismuth oxide	>3
MTA Angelus	20% Bismuth oxide	5.6–6.9
MTA Bio	20% Bismuth oxide	3.93
MTA Fillapex	Bismuth oxide	7.06
MTA Obtura	Bismuth oxide	Unspecified
MTA Plus	Bismuth oxide	Unspecified
Nano-modified MTA	20% Bismuth oxide	<8.5
Nanosized bioactive glasses	Bismuth oxide up to 50 wt%	4.94
OrthoMTA	Bismuth oxide	Unspecified
Portland cement	20% Bismuth oxide	5.93
Portland cement	20% Calcium tungstate	3.11
Portland cement	20% Zirconium oxide	3.41
ProRoot Endo Sealer	Bismuth oxide	Unspecified
Radiopaque dicalcium silicate cement (RDSC)	20% Bismuth oxide	7.3
TechBiosealer endo	Bismuth oxide	Unspecified
Theracal	Unspecified	Under ISO standard
White/gray MTA	20% Bismuth oxide	7.17
White ProRoot MTA	20% Bismuth oxide	8.5

Source: References [6, 21–29].

calcium hydroxide (portlandite) formation and dissociation in calcium and hydroxyl ions is running much slower compared to MTA [6].

Min et al. mention that over the last 10 years, the cytotoxicity and genotoxicity of Portland cements were investigated *in vitro* on numerous types of cell lines such as mouse lymphoma cells, Chinese hamster ovary cells, Saos-2 osteosarcoma cells, human endothelial cells, and human osteosarcoma cells [30].

Commonly in various cell culture tests, by modifying the chemical and physical parameters of experimental environment, may be encountered different results despite the use of same materials. However, it was concluded by Parirokh and Torabinejad that several cytotoxicity tests on cell cultures showed pretty similar effects of both Portland cements and MTA [6]. Using the reverse transcription polymerase chain reaction (RT-PCR) in human dental pulp cell (hDPC) culture,

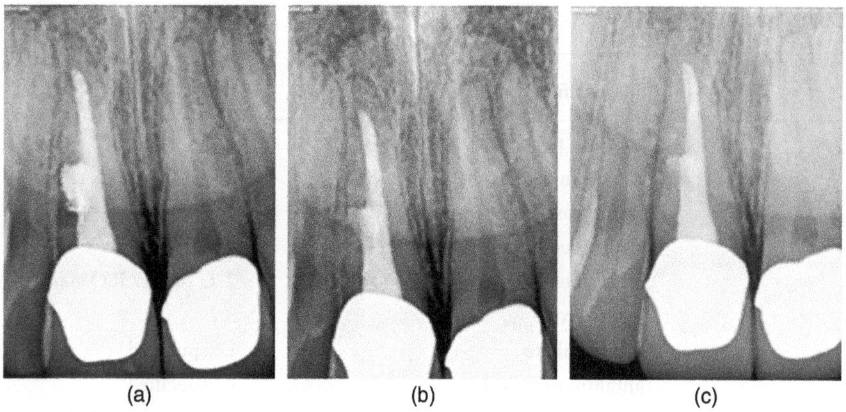

Figure 10.3 (a) Resorption-related perforation in right upper central incisor. Root canal filling with guttapercha and EndoSequence BC Sealer, (b) radiographic control after two weeks, (c) radiographic control after seven months, favorable outcome.

there was recorded for Portland cements and MTA a comparable expression of osteonectin, a dentin and bone protein involved in tissue mineralization, and dentin sialophosphoprotein (DSPP), a protein synthesized and released by differentiated odontoblasts to form the mineralizing matrix of dentin. Min et al. also revealed by scanning electron microscope (SEM) analysis that Portland cement is not cytotoxic and allows cell attachment on the material surface and subsequent growth and proliferation [30]. Parirokh and Torabinejad cite equivalent results *in vitro* regarding fibronectin, collagen I, and TGF-β1 growth factor when used Portland cements and ProRoot MTA in cell cultures of human periodontal ligament fibroblasts [6].

Another *in vitro* research studied, by confocal laser scanning microscopy (CLSM), the comparative potential of white Portland cement and white ProRoot MTA to stimulate the adhesion, proliferation, and locomotion of human bone marrow stem cells. D'Antò et al. observed that cells seeded on white Portland cement displayed a reduced proliferation and migration ability compared to cells cultured on ProRoot MTA both initially, after 24 hours, and at the completion of this 28-day investigation [31]. Starting from previous reports, which revealed similar biocompatibility of bismuth oxide (Bi_2O_3) containing Portland cement to pure Portland cement, an *in vitro* investigation on hDPCs included in the formulation the radiopacifier in ratio cement $Bi_2O_3 = 4 : 1$. Using simultaneously simvastatin and Emdogain, Lee et al. found even an improved cell growth and differentiation compared to unmodified Portland cement (PC Ssangyong, Seoul, Korea) [17].

The higher alkaline phosphatase (ALP) activity and Type I collagen synthesis, the increased expression either of odontogenic gene DMP-1 (dentin matrix protein 1) and DSPP or osteoblastic gene OPN (osteopontin) and OC (osteocalcin) suggested to Lee et al. that the differentiation of odontoblast-like phenotype was induced by bismuth oxide-containing Portland cement [17].

Lee et al. also demonstrated that when simvastatin and Emdogain were added in the cell's culture medium at days 7 and 14 of the experiment, there was revealed an up-regulation of the essential transcription factors for osteoblasts and bone formation Runx2 and Osterix, proving their involvement in mineralization process induced by bismuth oxide-containing Portland cement [17].

A study of Dregger et al. investigated the integration of Portland cement in living tissues following the experimental subcutaneous implantation, starting from a hypothesis that a bioactive material induces precipitates of carbonated apatite on implanted cement [19].

Using dentin tubes filled with Portland cement, which were implanted in subcutaneous tissue of Wistar rats, Dregger et al. found that between the cement and the tube wall (dentinal tissue) was formed a mineralized layer. Moreover, this interfacial layer also penetrated in the interior of dentinal tubules resembling mineralized tag-like structures [19].

After 30 and 60 days MTA Bio and MTA Branco, which induced an increased mineral deposition in experimental dentin tubes, Dregger et al. proved a higher potential of biomineralization compared to Portland cements, since last ones release fewer calcium ions and contain particles of significantly greater size [19].

Numerous conventional histological studies highlighted the subsequent acute inflammation accompanying the application of a direct pulp capping material, which paves the way for future tissue healing. Reyes-Carmona et al. proved that the biomineralization mechanism aforementioned by Dregger et al. is running in parallel with the evolution of acute inflammatory process [32].

According to this research of Reyes-Carmona et al., during the first three days after placing subcutaneous implants of white ProRoot MTA in Swiss mice, there was observed an up-regulation of proinflammatory cytokines TNF-α and IL-1β. Parallel with subsequent inflammation resolution, it starts simultaneously an over-expression of cytokine IL-10, which in turn down-regulates TNF-α and IL-1β activity [32].

A bulk of previous studies showed the close relationship between pulp inflammation and healing process and coparticipation of several molecular mediators as well. It may be assumed that biomaterials enable several signaling pathways to suppress the acute inflammatory phase and to stimulate the healing of local tissue lesion correlated with the procedure of direct pulp capping.

Reyes-Carmona et al. proved that the biomineralization mechanism aforementioned by Dregger et al. is running in parallel with the evolution of acute inflammatory process [19, 32].

On the other hand, Shahi et al. noticed that the subcutaneous connective tissue response to surgically implanted white and gray MTA in Sprague-Dawley rats showed a higher biocompatibility of these endodontic materials compared to similar implants of white and gray Portland cements [33].

According to Shahi et al., all investigated materials elicited after 7–15 days a dense infiltration of chronic inflammatory cells, tissue edema, and vascular congestion without significant differences either between WMTA and white Portland cement or between gray MTA and gray Portland cement [33].

Despite the general decrease in inflammation severity with time, Shahi et al. ascertained that after a 90-day interval both Portland cements similarly showed the trend of preserving sporadic infiltrations of chronic inflammatory cells without tissue edema, whereas around white and gray MTA implants healing occurred [33].

This issue was explained by Shahi et al. relying on the higher release of calcium ions and lower content in potassium and sulfur of MTA after setting, as compared to the presence of lead and arsenic in Portland cements [33].

Using baboons as animal model in a comparative study of three direct pulp capping materials (calcium hydroxide, white ProRoot MTA, and white Portland cement), Al-Hezaimi et al. observed that the reparative hard tissue formation (mineralized barrier) differed only in thickness. In pulp capping with calcium hydroxide, the histomorphometric analysis revealed a minimal and incomplete reparative hard tissue apposition of 0.22 ± 0.024 mm in contrast to the thickness either of 0.43 ± 0.053 mm after white ProRoot MTA or pretty similar 0.4 ± 0.058 mm barrier induced by white Portland cement [34].

All abovementioned pulp capping materials created atubular hard tissue barrier presenting porosities and ingrown granulation tissue in its tunnel defects. Though there was no qualitative difference among the reparative hard tissue, Al-Hezaimi et al. concluded that unfortunately this new induced mineralized barrier is not alike neither to secondary nor to tertiary dentin [34].

10.2.4 Clinical Studies

A few comparative studies investigated the human pulp response to Portland cements. However, a histological analysis of dental pulp reaction, undertaken by Oliveira et al. who used Portland cement as capping agent in pulpotomies of human primary teeth, showed the formation of hard tissue barrier and calcification of radicular pulp [18].

Though the follow-up studies of pulpotomies in carious primary molars using Portland cement described a high ratio of clinical and radiographic success, it was reported by Sakai et al. that another capping agent, gray MTA Angelus, induced less frequently a complete calcification of the root canal [35].

In another investigation focused on direct capping with Portland cement, Barbosa et al. confirmed that dental pulp remained vital as the formation of mineralized barrier is an evident sign of active tissue repair [36].

The pulp tissue response in pulpotomies of human primary molars was also studied by associating to Portland cement different radiopacifiers such as iodoform and zirconium oxide. By evaluating up to 24 months the treatment outcome, Marques et al., suggests a satisfactory biological effect of Portland cement combined with radiopacifiers as microscopically was observed that pulp repair and hard tissue barrier formation occurs despite the frequent dystrophic calcification developed in the radicular pulp [37].

10.3 Mineral Trioxide Aggregate (MTA)

According to USA Patent #5,415,547 and #5,769,638 MTA is a bioceramic aggregate comprised primarily of Portland cement [14].

10.3.1 Chemical Composition

Wang [21], Yan et al. [38], and Lee et al. [39] consider that MTA is a mixture of fine hydrophilic particles of tricalcium silicate, tricalcium aluminate, dicalcium silicate, tetracalcium aluminoferrite, calcium sulfate, and bismuth oxide that sets in the presence of water.

The first formula of marketed MTA was gray MTA. In order to avoid the dentin discoloration Wang mentions that later on it was introduced in dental practice WMTA, since as compared to gray MTA contains a reduced amount of iron, aluminum, and magnesium [21]. The oxides of late transitional elements such as Fe, Mn, and Cu exhibit strong colors since their free d-electrons are readily excited in the visible spectrum of light. Conversely, as explained Asgary et al., the oxides of Ca, Mg, Al, Si, and S that do not have easily excited electrons are white or colorless [40].

WMTA contains 75% Portland cement, 5% calcium, and 20% bismuth oxide. Though initially Damas et al. [2] thought that bismuth oxide was introduced exclusively as radiopacifer, later on Wang [21] and Saghiri et al. [22] observed that it also was a promoter of better physical properties.

10.3.2 Physical Parameters

For clinical use, MTA is prepared on a dry mixing pad by manually spatulating the powder with sterile water in a 3 : 1 ratio. Wang cites a setting time of about 165 minutes [21]. Gray MTA has a longer setting time than WMTA, including both initial and final set. Regrettably, as observed by Camilleri et al., the attempts to eliminate its drawbacks by adding hydration accelerators adversely affected the biocompatibility and physical properties [41]. The setting time of the initial set for white ProRoot MTA (Dentsply Tulsa Dental, Tulsa, USA) is 40 ± 2.9 minutes and for the final set is 140 ± 2.6 minutes. In case of gray MTA, the total setting time is reported up to 165 ± 5 minutes by Lovato and Sedgley and Funteas et al. [4, 15]. Another study, of Choi et al., measured for white ProRoot MTA an initial setting time of 78 ± 5 minutes [42]. The final setting time was 261 ± 21 minutes.

Wang also underlined that the MTA microhardness, its basic physical parameter of clinical success, is adversely influenced by porosity, low humidity during setting, acidic environment, chelating agents, and high condensation forces [21].

A real concern is also provoked by the solubility of MTA. Wang mentions that the debate between the low and increased solubility is still running [21]. The solubility and long setting time of MTA cement may have in root-end resection an extremely unfavorable outcome that threatens the apical seal, the wash out of the retrofilling. As observed Choi et al., this is an important risk of treatment failure because surrounding blood and tissue fluid adversely interact with an insufficiently set dental material [42].

Manipulating difficulties of the cement may be encountered by filling the root-end cavity. The use of operative microscope and syringe-type carrier definitely facilitates the proper placement of MTA (Figure 10.2).

The compressive strength of MTA depends on the storage conditions, powder and liquid composition, the pH of the liquid, and condensation pressure. MTA exhibits a higher compressive strength than MTA Angelus. During the first day of setting, the compressive strength of MTA is lower than of older endodontic retrofilling materials such as IRM (polymer-resin-reinforced zinc oxide-eugenol material), amalgam, or Super EBA (ortho-ethoxy benzoic acid). However, according to Wang, in three weeks, the values of compressive strength statistically become almost the same [21].

Tricalcium silicate (Ca_3SiO_5) is the main constituent of MTA and Portland cement. Though as single-phase component proved excellent bioactivity and biocompatibility, Liu et al. observed that tricalcium silicate also exhibits disadvantages such as long setting time (similar to complex compound MTA) and reduced initial compressive strength [43].

Tricalcium aluminate ($Ca_3Al_2O_6$) is the most reactive component of Portland cements and accelerates their hydration reaction. When added to Ca_3SiO_5 cements, it does not modify their original structure and enhances the short-term compressive strength of the newly formed $Ca_3SiO_5/Ca_3Al_2O_6$ mixture. Liu et al. revealed that such a cement mixture with at least 10% $Ca_3Al_2O_6$ is also more compact since it has less porosities [43].

Regarding the flexural strength of MTA, a proper moisture environment is beneficial during the first 24 hours of setting. However, Wang mentions that some reports proved an unwelcome decreased flexural strength of root dentin after a couple of months from MTA application [21].

The push-out strength of MTA depends on environmental pH values. At neutral pH the push-out strength records a stable range of values (7.28–7.68 MPa). Wang concluded that the maximal values of push-out strength are encountered at alkaline pH 8.4, in contrast to the minimal ones recorded at acidic pH 5.4 [21].

The study of Reyes-Carmona et al. showed that the push-out strength might be explained by the biomineralization ability of several MTA-based endodontic materials, capable to generate tags-like micro-retentions in dentinal tubules [44].

The radiopacity of MTA is at 7.17 mm equivalent thickness of aluminum. Wang considers WMTA more radiopaque than gray MTA [21].

10.3.3 Biological Properties

MTA developed a high success in endodontic treatments and rapidly gained widespread use. Zhang et al. [7], Wang [21], Yan et al. [38], and Khalil and Eid [45] suggested that MTA biocompatibility is based on intimate mechanism of setting reaction and discharge of calcium ions in surrounding tissues.

It is worthy to remind that even the $Ca_3SiO_5/Ca_3Al_2O_6$ mixture preserves the common MTA-based cements' capability to form a layer of hydroxyapatite on their surface, as any bioactive material in contact with biologic tissue fluids containing phosphates, when, according to Liu et al., the amount of $Ca_3Al_2O_6$ is less 10% [43].

Wang explains the biocompatibility of an endodontic material depending on its low cytotoxicity, the ability to stimulate cell differentiation and induce the mineralization of dentin, bone, and root cementum [21]. D'Antò et al. mention previous *in vitro* studies concerning the MTA action in cells' cultures [31]. All experiments proved that MTA allowed the attachment, multiplication, and migration of different types of cells seeded on the material surface, such as mouse MC3T3-E1 pre-osteoblasts, rat bone marrow cells, human bone marrow stem cells, Saos-2 human osteoblast-like cells, human osteoblasts, and human alveolar bone cells. First of all, MTA is regarded as the most biocompatible current endodontic cement since the studies of Damas et al. [2], Hansen et al. [46], Lee et al. [39], Choi et al. [42], and Kim et al. [47] attested it has the least cytotoxicity. Moreover, Modareszadeh et al. [5], Zhang et al. [7], and Öncel Torun et al. [8] demonstrated that MTA up-regulates the expression of mineralization-related genes involved in periradicular healing. It was also mentioned by Parirokh and Torabinejad that MTA also secures a tight seal of damaged dentin [3].

Even though Wang comments some dissimilarities between white and gray MTA, it is recognized that the biocompatibility of MTA is higher than of older root-end filling materials (amalgam, IRM, glass ionomers, and even Super EBA) and akin as newcomers ERRM, iRoot BP Plus, and Biodentine [21].

Using the methyl-thiazol-tetrazolium (MTT) assay in an *in vitro* study on mouse fibroblast cell line L929, Liu et al. revealed a stimulatory effect of $Ca_3SiO_5/Ca_3Al_2O_6$ mixture on cell growth, similar to that on pure tricalcium silicate Ca_3SiO_5, when trialuminum silicate proportion $Ca_3Al_2O_6$ was 5–10% [43]. Liu et al. also suggested that $Ca_3SiO_5/Ca_3Al_2O_6$ mixture with 10% trialuminum silicate would be "the best compromise between setting time, compressive strength and *in vitro* bioactivity and biocompatibility" of MTA [43].

Referring to the improvement of regenerative treatments of dental pulp, Wang highlighted the ability of MTA, already demonstrated by numerous investigations, to trigger the proliferation of stem cells of dental pulp and subsequent odontoblast-like cells differentiation and mineralization [21]. The materials for root-end filling in use proved to be biocompatible both *in vitro* and *in vivo*. However, their performance to positively influence the cell biological behavior is versatile. Even though both MTA and BioAggregate contain calcium silicate, the amount and release rate of calcium and silicate might be different. Moreover, Yan et al. [38] and Khalil and Eid [45] proved that MTA release toxic ions of aluminum, bismuth, and arsenic, which could suppress the growth of periodontal ligament fibroblasts. It seems that chemical composition of biocompatible ceramic cement may have a key role in preserving the cellular vitality in cell cultures. WMTA elicits a higher level of an isoform of heme oxygenase (HO-1) than iRoot BP in cultures of hDPCs. Öncel Torun et al. revealed that this enzyme is activated in oxidative stress as a defensive mechanism and has a cytoprotective effect against the initial toxicity of MTA, which gradually decreases after a 48-hour period of cell culture [8].

It was also proved by Hung et al. that MTA restrain the differentiation and activity of osteoclasts, giant multinucleated cells, mediating the inflammatory bone resorption such as chronic apical periodontitis [48]. Zhang et al. underline that MTA in high concentration strongly diminishes the (receptor activator of nuclear factor-κB ligand) RANKL-induced osteoclastogenesis and osteoclast viability, and even triggers cell apoptosis [7].

All dental materials are in a way irritant, even though the subcutaneous tissue response to MTA consists in a mild-to-moderate inflammation that returns to a milder one after 30–60 days. However, Khalil and Eid also described a systemic response since it was observed that during periradicular surgery arsenic from WMTA Angelus root-end filling was transferred to blood red cells and afterward carried and laid down in the liver and kidney [45].

The systemically induced lesions in liver and kidney still persisted after 7–21 days of WMTA Angelus subcutaneous implantation. The local tissue damage in both internal body organs were illustrated by vascular congestion, inflammatory cells infiltration, tissue degeneration, and steatosis. Khalil and Eid suggest that the endodontic materials able to elicit systemic lesions at a distance from their placement could act either by their composition in traces of heavy metals and arsenic or by locally elaborated cytokines IL-1 and IL-6 [45].

Parirokh and Torabinejad outline the utmost importance of immediate high alkaline value of MTA (12.5), which explains its expanded antibacterial activity after setting [3]. Wang reported a freshly mixed MTA pH value of 10.2, which during the following three hours achieved the level of 12.5. He also mentioned that the pH of WMTA rose faster than the pH of gray MTA during the first one hour after spatulating [21].

According to Zhang et al. [49] the real antimicrobial potential of MTA, considered to be enhanced by dentine, presently is under debate because Torabinejad et al. [50], Miyagak et al. [51], Parirokh and Torabinejad [3], and Wang [21] showed no inhibitory effect on strictly anaerobic usually found in the infected root canals.

10.3.4 Clinical Studies

In Wang's opinion, MTA is often regarded as the gold standard of endodontic repair materials because, based on calcium hydroxide formation and constant release of calcium ions, it displays important advantages in both pulp and hard tissues healing [21].

Since this biomaterial demonstrated a reliable osteo-inductive activity, Yan et al. [38], Khalil and Eid [45], Zhang et al. [7], and Wang [21] support its current use in root-end fillings, direct pulp capping, pulpotomy, apexification, root perforation repair, and regenerative endodontic procedures (Tables 10.2 and 10.3).

The endodontic practice of last 10 years proved that MTA or MTA-based bioceramics are the material of choice either to achieve the healing of periradicular bone in case of root perforations, regardless of their etiology (Figure 10.1) or in regenerative procedures (Figure 10.2).

Despite the biocompatibility and lack of genotoxicity of MTA, Khalil and Eid [45], Choi et al. [42], and Kim et al. [47] underline some disadvantages that can result in treatment failure, such as prolonged setting time, risk of washing out under bleeding, manipulating difficulties, traces of heavy metals, increased risk of tooth crown discoloration (gray ProRoot MTA), and high cost.

Shi et al. explain the grayish discoloration as the interaction result of bismuth oxide with dentin matrix collagen, and manganese and iron presence as well [62]. However, the WMTA can also change the dentin color. In a study regarding the diffusion of hydroxyl ions through dentin after the placement of white ProRoot MTA into the root canal, Hansen et al. observed at the 24-hour examination that some samples had discolored. After one week, discoloration of WMTA treated teeth involved all samples [46].

10.4 MTA Angelus

MTA Angelus (Angelus, Londrina, Brazil), a newcomer bioceramic material with shorter setting time, opened the opportunity for being a competitive alternative to MTA. On the market, it is delivered as white and gray MTA Angelus.

Table 10.2 Clinical application of bioceramics in vital pulp therapy.

Vital pulp therapy	Bioceramic material	Manufacturer
Direct pulp capping	Gray ProRoot MTA	Dentsply, Tulsa
	White ProRoot MTA	Dentsply, Tulsa
	White Portland cement	Votorantim Cimentos
	MTA Angelus	Angelus, Londrina
	MTA Plus	Avalon Biomed
	Endocem MTA	Maruchi, Wonju
	Biodentine	Septodont, Saint-Maur-des-Fosses
	iRoot BP	Innovative Bioceramix, Vancouver
	iRoot BP Plus	Innovative Bioceramix, Vancouver
	CEM	Bionique Dent, Tehran
	Quick-Set	Avalon Biomed, Bradenton
Pulpotomy in primary teeth	Gray ProRoot MTA	Dentsply, Tulsa
	White ProRoot MTA	Dentsply, Tulsa
	White Portland cement	Votorantim Cimentos
	Endocem MTA	Maruchi, Wonju
	Biodentine	Septodont, Saint-Maur-des-Fosses
Partial pulpotomy in immature teeth	White ProRoot MTA	Dentsply, Tulsa
	MTA Plus	Avalon Biomed
	Endocem MTA	Maruchi, Wonju
	Biodentine	Septodont, Saint-Maur-des-Fosses
	CEM	Bionique Dent, Tehran
Pulp capping and partial/full pulpotomy in reversible pulpitis	White ProRoot MTA	Dentsply, Tulsa
	CEM	Bionique Dent, Tehran

Source: References [3, 6, 21, 47, 52–58].

Table 10.3 Clinical application of bioceramics in nonvital teeth.

Root canal therapy	Bioceramic material	Manufacturer
Apexification	ProRoot MTA	Dentsply, Tulsa
	MTA Angelus	Angelus, Londrina
	MTA Plus	Avalon Biomed
Pulp chamber perforation	White ProRoot MTA	Dentsply, Tulsa
Furcation repairs	Gray MTA	Dentsply, Tulsa
	ProRoot MTA	Dentsply, Tulsa
Root perforation repair	ProRoot MTA	Dentsply, Tulsa
	OrthoMTA	BioMTA, Seoul
	MTA Plus	Avalon Biomed
	DiaRoot BioAggregate	Diadent Group International, Burnaby
	iRoot BP	Innovative Bioceramix, Vancouver
Internal/external resorption-related root perforations	ProRoot MTA	Dentsply, Tulsa
	MTA Angelus	Angelus, Londrina
	MTA Plus	Avalon Biomed
1. Current root canal fillings 2. Root canal fillings in dental anomalies: – dens invaginatus – dens evaginatus – germination – fusion – C-shaped canals	MTA Fillapex	Angelus, Londrina
	BioRoot RCS	Septodont, Saint-Maur-des-Fosses
	OrthoMTA	BioMTA, Seoul
	MTA Plus	Avalon, Biomed
	MTA Bio	Angelus, Londrina
	MTA Sealer	
	iRoot BP	Innovative Bioceramix, Vancouver
	iRoot BP Plus	Innovative Bioceramix, Vancouver
	iRoot SP	Innovative Bioceramix, Vancouver
	EndoSequence BC Sealer	Brasseler, Savannah
	Endo-CPM Sealer	Egeo, Buenos Aires
	White MTA (preferable versus gray MTA)	Dentsply, Tulsa
Gutta-percha cones with bioceramic nanoparticles	EndoSequence BC Points	Brasseler, Savannah
Retreatment with MTA (improved outcome)	ProRoot White MTA	Dentsply, Tulsa
	OrthoMTA	BioMTA, Seoul
Root-end fillings	Gray MTA/White MTA	Dentsply, Tulsa
	MTA Angelus	Angelus, Londrina
	MTA Bio (Angelus)	Angelus, Londrina
	EndoSequence BC RRM	Brasseler, Savannah
	OrthoMTA	BioMTA, Seoul
	Endocem MTA	Maruchi, Wonju
	MTA Plus	Avalon, Biomed
	E-MTA	Innovative Bioceramix, Vancouver, Canada

(Continued)

Table 10.3 (Continued)

Root canal therapy	Bioceramic material	Manufacturer
	MM-MTA	Micromega, Besançon
	BioAggregate	Innovative Bioceramix, Vancouver
	DiaRoot BioAggregate	Diadent Group International, Burnaby
	iRoot BP Plus	Innovative Bioceramix, Vancouver
	Endo-CPM Sealer	Egeo, Buenos Aires
	ProRoot Endo Sealer	Dentsply, Tulsa
Pulp regeneration	ProRoot White MTA	Dentsply, Tulsa

Source: References [3, 6, 21, 38, 47, 52, 59–61].

10.4.1 Chemical Composition

MTA Angelus is an MTA-based bioceramic that is composed of 80% Portland cement and 20% bismuth oxide. Wang deems that the higher content in calcium carbonate, calcium silicate, and barium zinc phosphate of Portland cement ameliorates the handling properties and shortens the setting time compared to traditional MTA [21].

10.4.2 Physical Parameters

Unlike MTA, the MTA Angelus has a decreased setting time (under 15 minutes) because it does not contain calcium sulfate. The particle size of WMTA Angelus is smaller than gray MTA (from 30 μm to less than 1 μm). However, Parirokh and Torabinejad [3] and Wang [21] showed that the size of MTA Angelus particle exhibits a higher variation.

Parirokh and Torabinejad and Wang allege there is still not a consent regarding the pH values and calcium ions release after setting. On the other hand the differences between MTA Angelus and gray MTA do not seem to be significant [3, 21].

However, Wang affirms that the microhardness depends on the technique of mixing and increases over time [21].

The sealing ability of MTA Angelus as root-end filling and perforations repair material compared with other materials with same clinical indications such as Super EBA or Vitremer is not proved to be definitely better. Wang insists there is no conclusion regarding sealing value of MTA Angelus opposite to gray MTA [21].

According Wang the radiopacity of MTA Angelus is lower compared to both white and gray MTA cements [21].

10.4.3 Biological Properties

Conflicting results are reported concerning the cytotoxicity of MTA Angelus. Some studies such as showed favorable results on Chinese hamster ovary cells (Ribeiro et al. [63]), L929 cell line (Miranda et al. [64]) or transfected human pulp cells (Camargo et al. [65]). Some other investigations concluded that MTA Angelus has a variable degree of cytotoxicity. De Deus et al. observed an initial lowered viability of ECV 304 endothelial cell but not later on [66]. A cytotoxic effect similar to MTA was found by Souza et al. on V79 fibroblasts line [67] and by Guven et al. on human gingival fibroblasts [68].

It was shown that MTA Angelus and ProRoot MTA release from human fibroblasts transforming growth factor beta-1 (TGF-β1) and bone morphogenetic protein (BMP-2) that may induce odontoblasts differentiation and maturation. However, Guven et al. found that the synthesis of TGF-β1 is bioceramic material dependent [68]. While MTA Angelus was subcutaneous implanted in an animal model occurred a tissue dystrophic mineralization. Wang underscores that both light-cured and non-light-cured MTA Angelus exhibited in rat bone comparable pattern and intensity of inflammatory response, and bone healing as well, compared to Portland cement [21].

It was demonstrated by Sipert et al. that MTA Angelus and Portland cement were active on numerous bacteria including the *Enterococcus faecalis* that is resistant to calcium hydroxide, the currently used root canal antiseptic, but both bioceramic cements were inefficient against *Escherichia coli* [69]. The antimicrobial potential of MTA Angelus compared to MTA is disputable. According to Wang even though some studies would indicate that MTA Angelus is a weaker antimicrobial, some other investigations consider both materials to be equivalent [21].

10.4.4 Clinical Studies

Studying in parallel on human premolars the effects of MTA Angelus and calcium hydroxide in pulp capping Wang observed after two months a favorable outcome, with low pulp inflammation and hard tissue bridge configuration beneath the former exposure [21].

In clinical use of MTA Angelus in internal inflammatory resorption it was reported after 20 months a beneficial effect. Wang also reported favorable results in temporary teeth after two years of pulp capping with MTA Angelus [21].

10.5 OrthoMTA

OrthoMTA (BioMTA, Seoul, Korea) is an easy-to-manipulate, bioactive material, cheaper than MTA. Kim et al. recommend it for conventional orthograde root canal fillings, retrofillings and as root repair material [47].

10.5.1 Chemical Composition

OrthoMTA consists of tricalcium silicate, dicalcium silicate, tricalcium aluminate, tetracalcium aluminoferrite, gypsum, free calcium oxide, and bismuth oxide as radiopacifier. Kim et al. also reports that OrthoMTA has fewer traces of heavy metals [47].

10.5.2 Physical Parameters

The setting time of OrthoMTA cement, longer than five hours (324.3 ± 2.1 minutes), is pretty similar to ProRoot MTA (318.0 ± 56.0 minutes). According to Lee et al. [39] and Kim et al. [47] it has to be considered that the prolonged setting time of OrthoMTA is not clinically encouraging [39]. Kim et al. found that the pH of storage water was still high alkaline (11.42) after preserving the cement seven days in water [47]. Lee et al. and Kim et al. claim that OrthoMTA efficiently annihilates the microleakage by a layer of newly induced hydroxyapatite between the root filling and the canal wall.

10.5.3 Biological Properties

By releasing calcium ions, OrthoMTA proved to generate an interfacial layer of hydroxyapatite in contact with periapical tissues, which according to Lee et al. [39] and Kim et al. [47] is supporting its bioactivity.

In an *in vitro* study on murine osteoblast precursor cell line MC3T3-E1 Kim et al., also found that the cytotoxicity exhibited by OrthoMTA was significantly higher than ProRoot MTA and Endocem MTA [47].

Same *in vitro* study of Kim et al. revealed that, at least during the first three days, OrthoMTA down-regulated OPN (a glycophosphoprotein found in mineralized and nonmineralized tissues), which has an inhibitory effect in modulating the growth of bone hydroxyapatite crystals [47]. However, this result might be controversial as the investigation of Lee et al. claimed that OPN is up-regulated by OrthoMTA [39].

According to XTT assay, the relative viability of human osteosarcoma cell-line MG-63 following cells exposure to OrthoMTA and ProRoot MTA was similar after one day. However, Lee et al. showed that after four and seven days of experiment the viability of OrthoMTA exposed cells significantly decreased compared to ProRoot MTA [39].

Regardless the type of investigated cement (OrthoMTA, ProRoot MTA, or Fuji II glass ionomer cement), SEM images of MG-63 line cells cultured on aforementioned endodontic materials showed in the first 24-hours growing, adhesion and spreading in intimate contact with cement surface of confluent, dense ,and elongated cells with anchoring processes, having normal morphology. Lee et al. noticed matching features in 48- and 72-hour cell cultures [39].

10.6 MTA Fillapex

MTA Fillapex (Angelus, Londrina, Brazil) is a newcomer among calcium silicate-based bioceramic materials used in root canal fillings. Faria-Junior et al. [70] and Wang [21] revealed that this ceramic cement was imagined to join the properties of a resin promoting adhesion (Epiphany/Resilon system) with the biologic activity of MTA.

10.6.1 Chemical Composition

Sagsen et al. [71], Faria-Junior et al. [70], Silva et al. [72], and Wang [21] proved that MTA Fillapex is a bioceramic sealer, basically made up by mineral trioxide aggregate, salicylate resin, natural resin, nanoparticulated silica, diluting resin, pigments, and bismuth trioxide as radiopacifier. Since according to Sagsen et al. actually MTA Fillapex sealer is both salicylate resin- and calcium silicate-based sealing cement, Zhou et al. [73] claims that its appurtenance to the true bioceramic cements becomes controversial.

10.6.2 Physical Parameters

The delivery syringe of MTA Fillapex facilitates its correct mixing. Wang ascertained that the bioceramic material is also easy to manipulate and has an appropriate working time [21].

According to the value of flow test (31.09 ± 0.67 mm) significantly greater than of AH Plus (25.80 ± 0.83 mm), the widely used endodontic sealer in root canal fillings, MTA Fillapex is compliant to ISO 6786/2001 recommendations of minimum 20 mm. Being facilitated a deeper penetration of a bioceramic sealer into the ramifications of the endodontic system, Silva et al. suggest as very attractive the use of MTA Fillapex in order to improve periradicular healing [72].

SEM examination of set MTA Fillapex showed a homogenous and compact surface, compared to iRoot SP, an aluminum-free, calcium silicate root cala sealer, which even initially presented some porosity. After the solubility test the surface morphology of MTA Fillapex changed since porosities and cracks were formed in the resin matrix. In both bioceramics were exposed the filler particles due to matrix loss. However, Borges et al. found that the iRoot SP surface appeared more porous and irregular since allowed a greater ingress of water [74].

The differences in surface morphology between MTA Fillapex and iRoot SP may be explained by the size of polymer chain that is formed during setting. Before the solubility test the energy-dispersive X-ray spectroscopy (EDX) analysis revealed carbon peaks of MTA Fillapex similar to AH Plus and higher compared to iRoot SP. SEM analysis done by Borges et al. also demonstrated similar images of MTA Fillapex and AH Plus [74].

Sagsen et al. found an oscillating bonding strength to dentin of bioceramic sealers. Both newer MTA-based sealers ProRoot Endo and Endo-CPM developed higher bond strength than AH Plus [71]. Though iRoot SP was similar to AH Plus, Amin et al. observed the lowest value of push-out test in MTA Fillapex [75].

The push-out bond strength of MTA Fillapex was also studied in cold lateral compaction of gutta-percha in contrast with iRoot SP and AH Plus sealers and no differences were found among them in the coronal third of root canal. Sagsen et al. showed that all materials properly bonded to the dentin of root canal walls and no dislodgement of the filling occurred [71].

However, in the middle and apical third of the root the push-out values of iRoot SP and AH Plus were significantly higher than MTA Fillapex. Sagsen et al. claim that the lower bond strength of MTA Fillapex to the dentin might be the result of reduced adhesion of its interfacial layer of tag-like structures [71].

Jainaen et al. suggest that it is more correct to consider that the push-out bond strength of a sealer depends also on the obturation technique, since the bond developed by a sealer alone is significantly higher than with a matching single-cone technique [76]. This could explain the similar bond strength values of AH Plus and bioceramic sealer iRoot SP in the cold lateral condensation technique of gutta-percha, found by Amin et al., though when used alone AH Plus demonstrated higher records [75].

In a comparative study of Amin et al. regarding three root canal sealers MTA Fillapex, iRoot SP, and AH Plus, it was revealed that the latest reached the highest push-out strength values and so that the dislodgement resistance of both bioceramic sealers MTA Fillapex and iRoot SP was significantly lower than AH Plus [75].

Silva et al. observed that the radiopacity value of MTA Fillapex (7.06 mm Al) is in agreement with ISO 6876/2001 recommendations, since is higher than minimal radiopacity equivalent to 3.00 mm aluminum (Al) required by international standards [72].

Though the radiopacity of MTA Fillapex claimed by the producer proved to be higher than the standard of 3-mm aluminum thickness, actually according to Xuereb et al., it is lower than of EndoSequence BC Sealer, Septodont Sealer, and Apexit Plus [77]. Therefore, Wang recommends to consider in current practice that the radiopacity of MTA Fillapex is lower than of frequently used AH Plus [21].

The maximum pH value of MTA Fillapex, recorded by Silva et al. at 3 hours (9.68 ± 0.08), also remained in alkaline range in all following periods, i.e. at 24 hours (9.34 ± 0.32), 48 hours (8.25 ± 0.27), 72 hours (8.02 ± 0.31), and 168 hours (7.76 ± 0.28). Altogether the pH of MTA Fillapex at 168 hours was higher up to one week than the 6.92 ± 0.06 pH of AH Plus [72].

Silva et al. consider that the high pH value of MTA Fillapex, though disadvantageous for cell viability, is a favorable parameter for its antimicrobial activity, ALP stimulation and neutralization effect of acids released in periapical bone by local inflammatory processes [72].

Using agar diffusion test, Morgental et al. revealed that MTA Fillapex is a sealer with antibacterial activity against *E. faecalis* [78]. Another study, of Faria-Junior et al., also proved *in vitro* that MTA Fillapex, both freshly mixed and after seven days, has an antibiofilm activity against *E. faecalis*, which could be explained by its high pH, calcium ions release and solubility [70].

Faria-Junior et al. also observed that the *E. faecalis* biofilm could not be completely eliminated, even though the solubility of MTA Fillapex after seven days from setting was higher compared to other sealers such as Epiphany SE, AH Plus, or Sealapex [70].

However, for favorable clinical outcome in endodontic treatment, is above all of utmost importance the low solubility of root-filling material and less its antibacterial activity, in order to avoid the microleakage and ingress of biofilms into the root canals system. Borges et al. showed that unfortunately MTA Fillapex and two other sealers, such as iRoot SP and Sealapex, demonstrated a higher solubility than the requirements of ANSI/ADA Specification 57/2000 [74].

Investigating by MTT assay the viability of Balb/c 3T3 cells exposed to various extracts of MTA Fillapex, Silva et al. revealed a high cytotoxic effect immediately after mixing and during four succeeding weeks [72].

As compared to EndoSequence BC Sealer on a cell culture of human fibroblasts, MTA Fillapex showed a constant cytotoxicity over the whole experimental period. Zhou et al. proved that initially, when freshly mixed, the MTA Fillapex cytotoxicity was explained by the resinous component and later on by lead released from the material after setting [73].

Studying the comparative cytotoxicity of MTA Fillapex versus three other sealers (Sealapex, Pulp Canal Sealer EWT, and Real Seal SE) on a cell line of primary human osteoblasts by a multiparametric assay, Scelza et al. found that all root canal sealers displayed a strong cytotoxicity at the 24-hours period after mixing. Though at the seven days period after mixing the pattern of cytotoxicity changed for the other sealers, as proved by mitochondrial dehydrogenase activity (XTT assay), membrane integrity (neutral red uptake test), and cell density (crystal violet dye exclusion test), MTA Fillapex preserved its highly cytotoxic effect on cell viability [79].

In the same study, Scelza et al. observed that after mixing Sealapex gradually allowed cell survival. Real Seal SE also exhibited higher survival rates than MTA Fillapex, whereas Pulp Canal Sealer EWT had even a superior cell-stimulating effect than all other materials involved in this study, equivalent to the control [79].

Bin et al. observed that AH Plus has a satisfactory biocompatibility despite the early mild inflammation induced by two proven cytotoxic substances, initially by bisphenol A and later by formaldehyde, that is secondary released during the polymerization reaction [80].

However, using MTT, a quick and accurate assay using the 3-(4,5-dimethylthiazol-2-il)-2,5-diphenyl tetrazolium bromide, that displays the number of viable cells and the activity of succinyl dehydrogenase as indicator of the level of the cell's metabolic activity, Bin et al. showed that WMTA is less cytotoxic and genotoxic than commonly used AH Plus sealer and newly introduced bioceramic MTA Fillapex [80].

It is well documented that the genotoxicity tests display gene mutation, chromosomal and DNA breaks or alterations in DNA repair ability. Accordingly another kind of test, MNT (micronucleus assay), was used by Bin et al. to detect chromosomal mutations, clastogenicity, and aneugenicity [80].

Compared to control at 48-hours period Bin et al. demonstrated that both sealers investigated *in vitro*, bioceramic cement MTA Fillapex and epoxy-resin AH Plus in 1 : 4 dilution, triggered in V79 cells culture an eight times higher formation of micronuclei [80].

The cytotoxic study on Chinese hamster fibroblasts (V79 cells) showed that WMTA displayed cell viability rates for all dilutions above 70%, whilst MTA Fillapex at dilutions up to 1 : 8 was significantly more cytotoxic. At 48 hours, MTA Fillapex, in dilution 1 : 2, reduced V79 cells viability to less than 23% and control sealer AH Plus, in the same dilution, was also highly cytotoxic.

Bin et al. think that initially MTA Fillapex is strongly cytotoxic probably do to its composition in resin salicylate. However, after 48 hours even in dilution of 1 : 2 and 1 : 4 allowed an increased survival conditions to V79 cell culture [80].

Regarding widely used sealer in root canal fillings AH Plus, Bin et al. consider that the toxic effect is based on the epoxy resin, which is also mutagenic, and on its curing accelerator, an amine component. The AH Plus cytotoxicity is evident in V79 cell culture a period of 24–48-hours after setting up to dilutions of 1 : 4, whereas at one month allowed a nondisturbed cell proliferation [80].

An *in vitro* investigation also using MTT assay on a monolayer culture of human osteoblast cells, Saos-2 line ATCC HTB-85, revealed that MTA Fillapex, Epiphany SE, and EndoFill substantially decreased cell viability a period of three days after setting. However, Salles et al. noticed at seven days following setting that the adverse activity of MTA Fillapex diminished [81].

According to Salles et al., the unfavorable effect of MTA Fillapex may be related to its resin component and release of some contaminants, like arsenic. The resin is also involved in MTA Fillapex antibacterial activity, this time together with its suspension pH range of 10.14–10.5 [81].

Salles et al. also demonstrated initially in all mentioned sealers a reduced activity of ALP, the pivotal enzyme in the mechanism of hydroxyapatite nucleation. After seven days only MTA Fillapex, started to be involved in mineralization, as it enhanced twofold this enzyme synthesis [81].

Accordingly, based on ALP stimulation, Salles et al. explain why at 21 days a significantly larger number of mineralized nodules were detected in MTA Fillapex cell culture by alizarin red staining, compared to Epiphany SE [81].

After setting, MTA Fillapex developed a suitable bioactivity level, enabling the crystal nucleation of hydroxyapatite in Saos-2 cells. At 21 days SEM analysis, Salles et al. revealed hydroxyapatite-like crystals attached to the cell membrane and irregularly smooth surface of compact spherical nanoparticles, while EDX highlighted peaks of Ca, P, O, and Si indicating calcium phosphate deposition [81].

The identification of Si in newly formed hydroxyapatite crystallites is explained by Salles et al. as either due to silicate coprecipitation with apatite or to substitution of silicon for phosphorus in the apatite lattice of already-formed apatite [81].

According to Salles et al., the high Si/Ca ratio found in hydroxyapatite crystallites, by incorporating the silicon ions released from MTA Fillapex, definitely evokes the real biologic potential of this ceramic sealer, as it was proved that silicon is an essential element in connective tissue and bone turnover [81].

As a rule, excepting the studies on cells cultures, the biocompatibility of a sealer is also investigated in animal models using implants in subcutaneous connective tissue or direct in bone. However, exploring the literature, Wang frequently found versatile results concerning the tissue reactions to endodontic materials, including root canal sealers such as MTA Fillapex [21].

In a histological study Assmann et al. compared the effect of bioceramic sealer MTA Fillapex and epoxy resin-based sealer AH Plus, both placed in direct contact with bone tissue in femurs of Wistar rats. They scored the neutrophils, lymphocytes, plasma cells, macrophages, multinucleated foreign-body giant cells, eosinophils, collagen fibers condensation, and hard tissue barrier from 7 days period up to 90 days [82].

Assmann et al. found differences between sealers only when scoring neutrophils, lymphocytes, and plasma cells. At seven days period, due the initial acute inflammatory response, neutrophils were predominant cells, considerably higher in MTA Fillapex than in AH Plus [82].

The scores of chronic inflammatory cells, lymphocytes and plasma cells, in MTA Fillapex group diminished over all time periods, in contrast to AH Plus and control group, that also significantly decreased only from the 30- to 90-days period, when became almost absent.

After 90 days, Assmann et al. concluded that both sealers succeeded to induce a good repair of osseous tissue, though in control rats the complete formation of mineralized barrier that proves bone healing occurred much earlier, at only 30 days [82].

Overall, at the end of the three-month observation period, no histological differences were displayed among both sealers and control groups. According to Assmann et al., it seems that the issue regarding the biological role of MTA introduced by producer in MTA Fillapex sealer in order to improve bone tissue repair remains still questionable [82].

In white male Wistar rats Zmener et al. evaluated the response to Fillapex sealer when implanted in subcutaneous connective tissue. At 10 days, a dense granulomatous tissue was observed. At 30 days, the granulomatous tissue was surrounded by fibrous tissue and a severe feature of granulomatous reaction persisted even after 90 days. Moreover, numerous particles of unresorbed sealer occurred around the implant and within the macrophages and multinucleated foreign-body giant cells [83].

Currently, the implantation of filling materials into the subcutaneous connective tissue in rats is regarded as a screening test for biocompatibility. Zmener et al. noticed that the solubility of 3.95% that exceeds the ADA recommendations is controlling the long-term toxicity of Fillapex implant due to its further leaching, even at 90 days after setting [83].

By comparing the reaction of subcutaneous connective tissue to three endodontic materials, bioceramic sealer MTA Fillapex, epoxy resin-based sealer AH Plus, and zinc oxide eugenol-based sealer EndoFill, Tavares et al. concluded that none facilitated an ideal outcome [84].

At seven days, inflammatory cells infiltrates of neutrophils, lymphocytes, and macrophages were scored higher around sealers than around control. Tavares et al. observed that the protective tissue response against spreading of inflammation, expressed by fiber condensation, was even lower in case of bioceramic sealer MTA Fillapex than to irritant eugenol containing EndoFill [84].

The score of connective tissue responses to MTA Fillapex concerning the inflammatory cells and abscesses at seven days was a little lower compared to eugenol containing sealer EndoFill. However, to Tavares et al. was evident that both sealers recorded higher scores for multinucleated foreign-body giant cells and abscesses. Later on, after 60 days, around MTA Fillapex and EndoFill implants there were noticed more frequently lymphocytes and macrophages than in control specimens [84].

Altogether, the connective tissue expressed a stronger and longer-lasting inflammatory response to MTA Fillapex than it was thought for a bioceramic sealer. Moreover, Tavares et al. found a similar outcome to recognized one of irritant zinc oxide eugenol-based sealers, such as EndoFill.

The same study revealed that at present time the widely used in endodontics epoxy resin-based AH Plus displayed at 7 days a moderate inflammation, whereas at 60 days the inflammatory response became mild and well limited by fibrous condensation [84].

According to Tavares et al. it seems that bioceramic sealer MTA Fillapex has no advantage of biocompatibility compared to zinc oxide eugenol- or epoxy resin-based sealers, so that AH Plus might be still considered as the gold standard in root canal fillings [84].

10.7 MTA Plus

According to Gandolfi et al., MTA Plus (Avalon Biomed, Bradenton, USA) is a bioceramic recommended in cavity lining, pulp capping, pulpotomy, root canal obturation in pulpectomy, root resorption, perforation repair, apexification, and root-end filling [52].

10.7.1 Chemical Composition

In the opinion of Gandolfi et al. [52] and Wang [21], though similar in composition to white (tooth-colored)

ProRoot MTA, the MTA Plus is finer powder and lower-cost bioceramic material.

MTA Plus is delivered with two mixing liquids, a salt-free polymer gel and water. Gandolfi et al. [52], Eid et al. [85], Wang [21], and DeLong et al. [86] underline that the gel increases the wash-out resistance, while powder improves the handling properties of mixed cement.

10.7.2 Physical Parameters

Gandolfi et al. [52], Eid et al. [85], Wang [21], and DeLong et al. [86] found that, due to the stoichiometric properties of MTA plus, varying powder to gel ratio when spatulating may be obtained different setting times and flow characteristics.

Gandolfi et al. also observed that if mixed with gel, MTA Plus creates in three hours a high alkaline pH (12.0) that decreases after 28 days, though it remains more elevated compared to pH value of white ProRoot MTA. MTA Plus displays higher porosity (39–40%) and solubility (18.5%), compared to 29.36% porosity and 14.7% solubility of white ProRoot MTA [52].

The calcium ions release is initially maximal for MTA Plus mixed with gel (119 ppm), intermediary for MTA Plus mixed with water (43 ppm) and minimal for white ProRoot MTA (24 ppm). However, Gandolfi et al. mention that after 28 days the value of calcium ions release of MTA Plus mixed with gel, though considerably decreased, remains still higher than 16 ppm value of white ProRoot MTA [52].

The newcomer bioceramic material MTA Plus, due its prolonged apatite-forming ability at the interface with dentinal walls of the root canal, and to some extent also into the dentinal tubules, may be considered as an useful alternative to currently used calcium silicate cements. However, Gandolfi et al. think that the clinical relevance of MTA Plus is hard to establish because, despite its solubility, white ProRoot MTA proved to be still reliable material in endodontic treatments [52].

The suitable explanation may be the quick deposition of a calcium phosphate layer due to intimate contact of MTA with tissue fluids. Since white ProRoot MTA and MTA Plus stimulate thick precipitates whose Ca/P ratio is higher than 1.67, Gandolfi et al. suggest that both bioceramic cements are inducing a coprecipitation of calcium carbonate [52].

MTA Plus may be used in root canal filling either as filling material alone or as sealer with gutta-percha cones. It has to be underlined that the producers recommend MTA Plus in single-cone obturation technique of root canals, due its dimensional stability and excellent flowability. However, an *in vitro* study of DeLong et al., evaluating the push-out bonding strength developed in single-cone obturation technique, showed lower values for MTA Plus than for EndoSequence BC Sealer [86].

DeLong et al. consider it to be very useful for practitioners to understand that the value of push-out strength in single-cone obturation technique using MTA Plus is higher compared to the value recorded by the same sealer in continuous wave vertical condensation, which is the most popular technique among endodontists worldwide [86].

Since continuous wave condensation is a thermoplasticized technique for root canal obturation, DeLong et al. mention that to some extent there occurs the risk of mechanically removing the sealer by the heat source and to facilitate the consecutive mixed or cohesive interfacial failures when testing push-out bond strength [86].

It is also worthy to consider that, depending on chemical composition of sealers, the heat may differently modify their adhesive properties. In this line, DeLong et al. proved that MTA Plus displayed the lowest push-out bond strength compared to other sealers, such as AH Plus and EndoSequence BC Sealer [86].

Similarly, the heating procedures change the porosity of sealers used in root canal obturation. Viapiana et al. found that initial disadvantageous porosity of AH Plus is later substantially improved by heating the gutta-percha cones during the root canal filling [87].

Viapiana et al. remind that, by overheating the external surface of the root, in clinical practice the heat generated by pluggers during warm vertical compaction of gutta-percha is a real concern mainly regarding the risk to cause irreversible bone and periodontal ligament lesions [87].

However, Viapiana et al. observed that the electronically controlled tip end of heat source System B commonly used in warm vertical compaction developed much lower temperature values than the temperature of 200 °C set on its LCD display. Actually the recorded temperature of the external root surface, after the necessary 30 seconds of heat application during clinical procedure of warm gutta-percha condensation, roused only up to 79.7 °C. When stopping the heat source, after no more than 30 seconds, the external root temperature dropped to 36.4 °C. Moreover, both investigated sealers, MTA Plus and AH Plus, reduced heat spreading inside the root canal so that recorded temperature of external root surface was only 37–41 °C, which biologically is a harmless value [87].

Viapiana et al. also affirm that shear bond strength of an epoxy resin sealer is not different with or without heating. Even though it is not proved yet to what extent might be clinical relevant, the temperature generated by warm vertical compaction affected the polymers matrix structure of AH Plus sealer, while MTA Plus bioceramic sealer was not chemically modified [87].

10.7.3 Biological Properties

Investigating on mitochondrial dehydrogenase activity-base the cellular viability of rat odontoblast-like cells MPDC-23, Eid et al. found by XTT assay that in the first weekly cycle white and gray MTA Plus and respectively white and gray ProRoot MTA exhibited a significant cytotoxicity. In the second cycle excepting gray MTA Plus, that was equivalent to unexposed control, the other three sealers preserved the cytotoxicity. For the third cycle, gray MTA Plus accompanied by gray ProRoot MTA showed no difference compared to control [85].

A significantly higher percentage of vital cells versus apoptotic/necrotic cells were revealed in the same study by flow cytometry and CLSM in white and gray MTA Plus compared to white and gray ProRoot MTA. However, Eid et al. found no difference between white and gray versions either for MTA Plus or ProRoot MTA [85].

MPDC-23 exposed to gray ProRoot MTA and both MTA Plus cements (white and gray) showed significantly lower level of intracellular reactive oxygen species (ROS) than untreated control cells. It was argued by Eid et al. that the bioceramics may be involved by inducing the elevation of extracellular pH [85].

The cytotoxic effects of MTA Plus on MDPC-23 cells are time and concentration dependent. Apparently, the initial irreversible damage is extracellularly located. Accordingly, the cytotoxicity of MTA Plus and ProRoot MTA is preferentially expressed by an apoptotic mechanism and not by a necrotic one. In line with biologic effects, Eid et al. forwarded the opinion that white versions of both bioceramic cements seem to be more cytotoxic than their gray versions [85].

A capping agent in pulpotomy performed on male Sprague-Dawley rats by Kramer et al. MTA Plus proved to be successful by lowering the secretion of proinflamatory cytokines IL-1β and IL-1βα and stimulating of reparative dentinal bridging [53].

10.8 MTA Bio

MTA Bio (Angelus, Londrina, Brazil) is considered by Parirokh and Torabinejad a bioactive endodontic cement [6].

10.8.1 Chemical Composition

MTA Bio contains 80% Portland cement and 20% bismuth oxide, while in the formulation of ProRoot MTA Portland cement is only up to 75%. However, Gonçalves et al. [88] and Parirokh and Torabinejad [6] underline that the main distinction is considered the content in gypsum, which is 5% higher in ProRoot MTA.

According to Parirokh and Torabinejad [6] there is still a dispute regarding its content in arsenic. Evaluating in MTA Bio the trivalent arsenic (As III), the most toxic form of this metalloid, Gonçalves et al. found a safe concentration (below 2 μg/l), at least according to the Brazilian regulation of Environment Council that admit a maximal concentration of 0.05 mg/l in drinking water [88].

10.8.2 Physical Parameters

The initial setting time was noted at 11 minutes and the final one at 23.33 minutes from mixing. Parirokh and Torabinejad noticed that MTA Bio exhibits an alkaline value of pH, similar to ProRoot MTA but higher than light-cured MTA [6].

The variable concentrations of calcium hydroxide released during the hydration reaction result in different pH values. According to Gonçalves et al., since white and gray Portland cements are rich in clinker commonly they also have a higher pH than white and gray MTA [88].

However, Gonçalves et al. found that the average pH of MTA Bio (11.81 ± 0.11), after immersing in distilled water at a pH of 5.6, was not different from ProRoot MTA and gray Portland [88].

Parirokh and Torabinejad observed a higher level of calcium ions released by MTA Bio than that of ProRoot MTA and MTA Angelus [6]. The same releasing potential of calcium ions, higher than ProRoot MTA, was proved by Gonçalves et al. [88]. Additionally, it was also found in this last study that the amount of calcium ions released by MTA Bio was similar to that of white nonstructural Portland cement, but different from white structural Portland, gray Portland, and ProRoot MTA [88].

The solubility of MTA Bio is theoretically more reduced compared to ProRoot MTA due to its higher amount of Portland cement. Evaluating the electrical conductivity, which is directly related to the cement solubility, Gonçalves et al. proved that statistically the conductivity of MTA Bio, ProRoot MTA, white nonstructural Portland cement, white structural Portland, and gray Portland was similar [88].

However, in this study the lowest value was found for MTA Bio (1294.4 ± 407.3 μS/cm) and the highest for white nonstructural Portland cement (1677.5 ± 1563.4 μS/cm). ProRoot MTA recorded an intermediate value of $1{,}388 \pm 263.5$ μS/cm [88].

The push-out strength of MTA Bio was found by Parirokh and Torabinejad comparable to ProRoot MTA and MTA Angelus, but higher than Portland cements [6].

MTA Bio satisfies the requirements of ANSI/ADA Specification 57/2000 and ISO 6876/2001 for radiopacity of root canal sealers. According to Parirokh and Torabinejad, its radiopacity corresponds to the value of

3.93 ± 0.22 mm Al, which is similar to white and gray ProRoot MTA, but higher than light-cured MTA and lower than MTA Angelus [6].

10.8.3 Biological Properties

Parirokh and Torabinejad found no differences *in vitro* between MTA Bio and WMTA Angelus concerning the cytotoxic effects on cultures of odontoblast-like cells MDPC-23, though the contact surface of MTA Bio specimens was less homogenous and had more porosity [6].

Parirokh and Torabinejad related a study *in vivo* regarding the subcutaneous connective tissue response to MTA Bio implants, which proved the material was able to successfully induce a process of biomineralization [6].

10.9 MTA Sealer (MTAS)

Parirokh and Torabinejad mention two MTA sealers better known until now, one introduced by Camilleri's team and the other produced in Brazil [6].

10.9.1 Chemical Composition

According to Parirokh and Torabinejad, the powder of MTA Sealer introduced by Camilleri is a mixture of 80% white Portland cement and 20% bismuth oxide. Concerning the Brazilian MTA Sealer, it contains Portland cement, calcium chloride, and zirconium oxide as radiopacifier and a resinous vehicle [6].

10.9.2 Physical Parameters

Compared to current endodontic materials used as root canal sealers, Parirokh and Torabinejad found no differences in the sealing ability of Camilleri's MTA Sealer [6].

While mixing the Brazilian MTA Sealer, the recommended powder/liquid ratio is 5 : 3. According to Parirokh and Torabinejad, the duration of initial setting is up to 535 ± 29.5 minutes and the final setting is achieved in 982.5 ± 53.46 minutes [6].

Compared to WMTA Angelus, Parirokh and Torabinejad observed that Brazilian MTA Sealer develops up to 48 hours a higher alkaline pH. Also, they found that, following mixing, the calcium ions release from Brazilian MTA Sealer was higher up to 28 days than that of WMTA Angelus [6].

10.9.3 Biological Properties

Camilleri's MTA Sealer is deemed bioactive since it proved to generate crystals of calcium phosphate that gradually cover the sealing material [6].

Parirokh and Torabinejad also say the connective tissue reaction of subcutaneous implants of Brazilian MTA Sealer in rats is similar to either Portland cement or WMTA Angelus [6].

10.10 E-MTA

E-MTA (Innovative Bioceramix, Vancouver, Canada) is an experimental Bis-EMA/MTA dual-cure, root-end filling material.

10.10.1 Chemical Composition

E-MTA contains bisphenol A ethoxylate dimethacrylate/mineral trioxide aggregate. For clinical use, Jacinto et al. recommend E-MTA to be prepared by mixing equal parts of Paste 1 and Paste 2 [89].

Jacinto et al. say Paste 1 contains MTA, Bis-EMA 10, Bis-EMA 30, camphorquinobe, DHEPT, and EDAB whereas Paste 2 is composed of ytterbium fluoride, Bis-EMA 10, Bis-EMA 30, and benzoyl peroxide [89].

10.10.2 Physical Parameters

E-MTA is a fast setting material (less than one minute) but according to Jacinto et al., by incorporating 2% chlorhexidine (CHX) it remains unset at least one week [89]. Accordingly, the addition of CHX to E-MTA cannot be useful in a clinical setting. A similar compromising effect was also observed while mixing chlorhehidine with resins or glass ionomer cements.

However, a previous study of Stowe et al. showed a setting time of only one to two minutes for tooth-colored ProRoot MTA mixed with 0.12% CHX gluconate, compared to five to six minutes required by the same MTA blend mixed with distilled water [90].

Jacinto et al. found that throughout the first 30 days after mixing E-MTA exhibited fluctuant values of pH. The initial alkaline pH of 9.32 turned to acidic during the first 15 days. Despite its gradual increase up to neutral value of 7.04 after an one month period, the pH did not come back to alkaline range. However, when mixed with 2% CHX the pH values of E-MTA remain alkaline at least 15 days, and after 30 days, it turned acidic [89].

It was also shown by Jacinto et al. that E-MTA released a significantly lower amount of calcium ions compared to WMTA the whole measuring period of 30 days, while E-MTA mixed with 2% CHX proved to increase the calcium ions discharge even more than WMTA [89].

10.10.3 Biological Properties

Since the very beginning of its use, Torabinejad et al. observed that pure MTA-based endodontic materials proved to be biocompatible with human tissues [91]. However, according to an *in vitro* study on mouse fibroblasts and macrophages cell cultures, white ProRoot MTA mixed with cationic antimicrobial agent 0.12% CHX gluconate of Hernandez et al. increased the cytotoxicity of pure white ProRoot MTA. Previous *in vitro* and *in vivo* reports also found that the toxic potential of chlohexidine to human tissues is dose and time dependent [92].

Using flow cytometry, Hernandez et al. also observed that when exposed to white ProRoot MTA fresh mixed with 0.12% CHX gluconate apoptosis occurred as response in mouse fibroblasts and macrophages cell cultures [92].

The same flow cytometry study highlighted the decrease of fibroblasts and macrophages proportion during the G_1 phase of cell cycle when exposed to both fresh and set white ProRoot MTA mixed with CHX. Usually in order to improve the resolution and regenerative potential a root canal medication has to be at least bacteriostatic if not bactericidal. Unfortunately Hernandez et al. showed that the ProRoot MTA/CHX mix exhibits a cellular antiproliferative effect due to the inhibition of DNA replication in S phase of cell cycle [92].

If extrapolating these *in vitro* findings to the clinical relevance of possible use of ProRoot MTA/CHX mix it appears a high risk of healing delay in periapical tissue after endodontic surgery [92].

The subcutaneous implantation tests are commonly used on animal models to evaluate biocompatibility of an endodontic material. Using this method, Sumer et al. found that ProRoot MTA mixed with a cationic antimicrobial agent (0.12% CHX gluconate) implanted subcutaneously in Wistar albino rats elicited an initial severe inflammatory response that gradually subsided to a moderate one after 60 days. Around the inflammatory tissue there was formed around a fibrous connective tissue capsule, increasing in thickness with time and proving the biocompatibility of experimental material MTA/CHX-based [93].

Since the CHX was previously introduced in the formulation of other dental materials, a microbiological *in vitro* study was designed to test its efficacy against some bacteria of infected root canals. Using the agar-diffusion test, Stowe et al. found that a mix up of tooth-colored ProRoot MTA with 0.12% CHX gluconate had an enhanced antimicrobial potential on *Fusobacterium nucleatum*, *E. faecalis*, and *Candida albicans* as compared to pure tooth-colored ProRoot MTA mixed with sterile water [90].

10.11 MM-MTA

MM-MTA (Micromega, Besançon, France) is a novel MTA delivered in predosed capsules that following activation requires mechanical mixing. Khalil et al. say it has the advantage of correct proportioning the ratio powder/liquid and homogenous mixing as well [23].

10.11.1 Chemical Composition

MM-MTA contains primarily Portland cement and bismuth oxide, but additionally also calcium carbonate and a chloride accelerator. Khalil et al. revealed by X-ray diffraction analysis that MM-MTA has tricalcium silicate, bismuth oxide, and calcium carbonate. The energy dispersive spectroscopy also detected chloride [23].

Unlike MM-MTA and Bioentine, MTA Angelus and ProRoot MTA do not have in their formulation calcium carbonate and chloride. Khalil et al. mention that calcium carbonate is added to Portland cement to accelerate the hydration of tricalcium silicate, whereas calcium chloride is shortening the setting time [23].

10.11.2 Physical Parameters

Though tricalcium silicate is the main MM-MTA cementation phase, Khalil et al. did not detect *portlandite* by usually used X-ray diffraction analysis since calcium carbonate impeded its crystallization. However, MM-MTA releases elevated levels of calcium ions that could be based on calcium carbonate decomposition [23].

According to Khalil et al., MM-MTA has a similar setting time to MTA Angelus but shorter than ProRoot MTA [23].

The same study of Khalil et al. showed that the MM-MTA surface porosity, lower than ProRoot MTA, is actually negligible due to the low water/powder ratio and to the effect of automatic mixing [23].

The radiopacity of MM-MTA is greater than the 3 mm aluminum thickness required by ISO 6876 specification, but Khalil et al. underline it is significantly lower than MTA Angelus and ProRoot MTA due to its lower level of bismuth [23].

10.12 Fluoride Containing MTA Cements

10.12.1 Chemical Composition

1. Parirokh and Torabinejad say fluoride-doped MTA cement consists of Portland cement, anhydrite and bismuth oxide, as radiopacifier, mixed with sodium fluoride to confer expansion capability and enhanced retention [6].
2. Calcium fluoro-aluminate cement (Italcementi SPA, Bergamo, Italy) is a mixture of Portland cement

and fluoro-aluminate containing as main elements tricalcium silicate and calcium fluoro-aluminate. Actually according to Camilleri [94] and Camilleri [95] this product is Portland-based cement is similar to MTA due to the presence of tricalcium silicate as the main constituent phase its chemical composition.

10.12.2 Physical Parameters

Camilleri observed that calcium fluoro-aluminate cement is fast-setting cement exhibiting an initial set of 1.83 ± 0.29 minutes and final set of 3.08 ± 0.14 minutes, which is clinically adequate [94].

However, despite the presence in high proportion of calcium silicate, another study of Camilleri demonstrated that calcium fluoro-aluminate cement has a different hydration reaction to that of original Portland cement because no calcium hydroxide is resulting as final by-product [95].

Verifying by fluid filtration test the sealing capability of fluoride-doped MTA cement in root canal fillings Parirokh and Torabinejad observed that, spatulated with articaine solution in a ratio powder/liquid 2.8 : 1, the result was as good as of AH Plus sealer used with warm gutta-percha technique [6].

Parirokh and Torabinejad say fluoride-doped MTA cement is a bioactive material since its content in sodium fluoride in concert with calcium fluoride facilitates calcium ions release and fluoroapatite crystals while the material contacts tissue fluids [6].

Calcium fluoro-aluminate cement has sufficient amount of tricalcium silicate to result in high early compressive strength even though Camilleri proved that the formation of the main by-product of hydration reaction, ettringite, is slower compared to other experimental cement containing tricalcium silicate such as the sulfo-silicate cement [94].

Parirokh and Torabinejad mention that fluoride-doped MTA cement is a root canal sealer that at least 28 days after mixing has an alkaline pH [6]. Camilleri found that calcium fluoro-aluminate cement has immediately after mixing a high pH, between 11 and 12. The high pH values were preserved roughly constant around 11.4 throughout 58 days [95].

10.12.3 Biological Properties

Even though during the hydration of the tricalcium silicate is released calcium hydroxide, this reaction by-product is immediately depleted by further reaction with calcium fluoro-aluminate, resulting in ettringite production. Accordingly, Camilleri thinks that the absence of calcium hydroxide cannot render to calcium fluoro-aluminate cement the characteristic of a proper bioactive ceramic [95].

Using MTT assay, which reveals the activity of mitochondrial enzyme succinate dehydrogenase, an *in vitro* study of Camilleri on human osteosarcoma cells P68 found that seven days the elution of calcium fluoro-aluminate cement induced higher cell activity rather than the cement itself. However, after 28 days the cell growth stimulation diminished since ettringite formation interfered with calcium hydroxide release [96].

The presence of calcium hydroxide as by-product of the hydration mechanism is of paramount importance to support the bioactivity of calcium fluoro-aluminate cement. Therefore, Camilleri underlines that changes resulting in calcium hydroxide production adversely affect the biocompatibility [96].

10.13 Nano-modified MTA

10.13.1 Chemical Composition

Saghiri et al. mention that the cement powder is composed of $2CaO{\cdot}SiO_2$, $3CaO{\cdot}SiO_2$, $3CaO{\cdot}Al_2O_3$, Bi_2O_3, gypsum, $SrCO_3$, zeolite, $CaSO_4$, and Na_2HPO_4 [22].

Parirokh and Torabinejad [6] and Saghiri et al. [22] say that nano-modified MTA is similar in composition to white ProRoot MTA, excepting the nanoscale of powder particles ranging from 40 to 100 nm and the presence of strontium, which was introduced to increase the resistance to acidic environments.

Saghiri et al. [22] remind that strontium, like zeolite and carbonate, is also a stabilizer agent. Moreover, in another study, Saghiri et al. proved that strontium salts do not have a deleterious effect on the physical properties of MTA-based cements and are claimed to upgrade the bioactivity and bioconductivity of bone substitute materials [97].

10.13.2 Physical Parameters

Based on the smaller particles size of the powder, leading to an increased surface area, usually nanomaterials have improved properties compared to traditional ones. According to Saghiri et al. [97] and Parirokh and Torabinejad [6], nano-modified MTA exhibits an ameliorated and faster process of hydration that reduces the setting time.

Later, Saghiri et al. showed that nano-modified MTA is also definitely more homogenous than ProRoot MTA, since the distribution of its nano-size radiopacifier particles results in an enhanced uniform orientation of ettringite crystals [22].

It was also demonstrated by Saghiri et al. [97] and Parirokh and Torabinejad [6] a mean surface area of $7.8 \pm 1.2\,m^2{}_{/}g$ for nano-WMTA crystals compared of those of merely $1.8 \pm 0.2\,m^2/g$ for white ProRoot MTA. The significantly reduced setting time of nano-WMTA is 6 ± 1 minutes while white ProRoot MTA showed an extended time interval up to 43 ± 2 minutes [97].

Saghiri et al. [97] and Parirokh and Torabinejad [6] proved that the higher surface microhardness and lower porosity than white ProRoot MTA confer to nano-modified MTA a better stability in acidic environments. However, Saghiri et al. underline that it has to consider the adverse lowering effect of acidic pH on both materials. At pH 7.4 there were found Vickers microhardness values of 81.53 ± 2.62 for nano-WMTA and 51.31 ± 1.14 for white ProRoot MTA. When pH turned to acidic range (pH 4.4) the Vickers microhardness values diminished to 54.59 ± 1.08 for nano-WMTA and respectively 16.10 ± 2.84 for white ProRoot MTA [97].

There was also described by Saghiri et al. a mean number of open porosities over the surface of white ProRoot MTA about twofold higher compared to nano-WMTA samples (88 ± 24 and 44 ± 13, respectively). Grater porosity has a definite adverse effect on microhardness since it increases the acid penetration into the depth of material and subsequent crack propagation [97].

Saghiri et al. [97] and Parirokh and Torabinejad [6] showed that the push-out strength and wash-out resistance of nano-WMTA are also higher than other bioceramic cements, such as white ProRoot MTA or MTA Angelus.

A subsequent study of Saghiri et al. proved that excepting the radiopacity, which is lower than that of white ProRoot MTA, the nano-modified MTA exhibits the highest values for push-out strength, compressive strength, and surface microhardness [22].

10.13.3 Biological Properties

Though nano-modified WMTA stimulates the bone healing, it was observed by Saghiri et al. that also the mixture C_3S/C_3A of tricalcium silicates with tricalcium aluminate resulting by addition of nano-tricalcium aluminate (nano-C_3A) enhances the already proved effect of nano-WMTA in bone regeneration [98].

As bone substitute, calcium aluminate allows accelerated healing due it fast degradation and proved efficacy in promoting the new hard tissue formation. Moreover, Saghiri et al. showed that C_3S/C_3A mixtures may stimulate the hydroxyapatite formation on their surface that substantiates a strong bond with bone tissue [98].

Using serial dual-energy X-ray absorptiometry method to measure the bone mass, Saghiri et al. demonstrated that, partly due to its better and faster hydration rate, nano-WMTA mixed with nano-C_3A promoted after implantation in Dutch rabbits an accelerated bone regeneration due to higher release of calcium ions [98].

10.14 Light-Cured MTA

10.14.1 Chemical Composition

Parirokh and Torabinejad mention that light-cured MTA (Bisco, Itasca, USA) has in its composition MTA (44.5%), resin (42.5%), AeroSil (8.0%), and barium sulfate (5.0%) as radiopacifier [6].

Theracal (Bisco, Schamburg, USA) is another light-cured MTA. Parirokh and Torabinejad say it has Type III Portland cement, fumed silica as hydrophilic thickening agent, resin, and a radiopaque material [6].

10.14.2 Physical Parameters

In both initial and final setting times, light-cured MTA is higher than MTA Bio. Parirokh and Torabinejad underline that regrettably its radiopacity does not correspond to requirements of ISO 6876/2001 and is considerably lower compared to MTA Bio, MTA Angelus, and Clinker PC [6].

Parirokh and Torabinejad say that Theracal exhibits a lower solubility and less water uptake than white ProRoot MTA [6].

The radiopacity of Theracal is similar to light-cured MTA but Parirokh and Torabinejad showed that does not correspond to ISO 6876/2001 requirements and is lower compared to white ProRoot MTA [6].

According to Parirokh and Torabinejad, Theracal is recommended as pulp capping agent due to alkaline value of pH and to the higher amount of calcium ions released than Dycal and white ProRoot MTA [6].

10.14.3 Biological Properties

The connective tissue reaction to subcutaneous implants of light-cured MTA after 60 days observation period, excepting the lack of calcification, is mentioned by Parirokh and Torabinejad to be alike to MTA Angelus, though initially the chronic inflammatory response was stronger [6].

Parirokh and Torabinejad noted no difference in bone reaction between light-cured MTA and MTA Angelus when implants of these materials were introduced into the socket immediately after tooth extraction [6].

10.15 Endocem MTA

Endocem MTA (Maruchi, Wonju, Korea) is MTA-derived pozzolan cement.

10.15.1 Chemical Composition

According to Choi et al. [42] and Kim et al. [47] Endocem MTA consists of 46.7% CaO, 5.43% Al_2O_3, 12.80% SiO_2, 3.03% MgO, 2.32% Fe_2O_3, 2.36% SO_3, 0.21% TiO_2, 14.5 H_2O/CO_2, and 11% Bi_2O_3 as radiopacifier.

10.15.2 Physical Parameters

Its fast-setting mechanism is running like an acid–base reaction and does not require chemical accelerators due to the content in small particles of pozzolan cement. Choi et al. proved calcium hydroxide decreases that as much as the setting progresses. Subsequently it follows the formation of calcium silicate hydrate and calcium aluminate hydrate stable crystals [42].

Endocem MTA has a shorter working time compared to other silicate-based cements, oscillating between 4 ± 0.5 minutes recorded by Miyagak et al. [51] and 15.3 ± 0.5 minutes measured by Liu et al. [43].

An *in vitro* investigation of Choi et al. recorded different values: 2 minutes $\pm$ 30 seconds for initial setting time and 4 minutes $\pm$ 30 seconds for the final setting time [42].

Choi et al. claim that the fast-setting reaction of Endocem is a guarantee of its wash out resistance, as compared to ProRoot MTA, which after 24 hours had marginal gaps and achieved a high wash out score [42].

Kim et al. found that the pH of storage water (11.33) was even lower than ProRoot MTA pH (11.90) [47]. However, alkaline is still high after preserving the cement seven days in water, and Hansen et al. [46] underline that it might be bactericidal and efficient in inhibiting the inflammatory external root resorption.

10.15.3 Biological Properties

In an *in vitro* study Endocem MTA proved a higher affinity for the cells of murine osteoblast precursor cell line MC3T3-E1 and a lower cytotoxicity than OrthoMTA. However, the expression of OPN was comparable. Even though in clinical practice Kim et al. proved that Endocem MTA has better manipulating properties and an acceptable setting time, as compared to ProRoot MTA, biologically is yet inferior [47].

In a SEM evaluation of three-days seeded MG63 cells on Endocem Choi et al. revealed attached flat cells with multiple well-defined cytoplasmic extensions to neighboring cells. This morphological feature, akin to ProRoot MTA, suggests that Endocem sustain the cell growth, proliferation, and differentiation to the same extent as the already proved biocompatible material [42].

Using the real time polymerase chain reaction (PCR) analysis, Choi et al. also found that between Endocem and ProRoot MTA the expression of the osteogenic differentiation markers such as bone sialoprotein, OPN, and OC was not substantially different [42].

10.15.4 Clinical Studies

The main clinical indications of Endocem MTA are vital pulp therapies since it proved biocompatibility and antibacterial activity. Kim et al. [47] and Parirokh and Torabinejad [6] mention that Endocem MTA also exhibits a reduced risk of tooth discoloration.

10.16 Biodentine

According to Wang [21], Biodentine (Septodont, Saint-Maur-des-Fosses, France) is calcium silicate-based cement, suitable as dentin substitute for endodontic use.

10.16.1 Chemical Composition

Wang specifies that Biodentine is delivered as a powder of tricalcium silicate, calcium carbonate, zirconium oxide (radiopacifier), and a water solution of calcium chloride (setting accelerator) [21].

10.16.2 Physical Parameters

Biodentine is a fast-setting material (10–12 minutes). In clinical manoeuvres it has to be used a wet mixed cement because, as Wang mentions, a drier one does not properly adhere to dentin and might compromise the treatment [21].

According to Nowicka et al. [54] and Wang [21], Biodentine fulfills the esthetic requirements for proper clinical use in anterior teeth with superior effects than the pioneer bioceramic cement MTA.

Other worthy characteristics of Biodentine in clinical applications, specified by Wang, are the high microhardness, compressive strength, push-out strength, and sealing ability that strongly recommend this bioceramic cement as intermediate base in coronal restoration as well [21].

Grech et al. found that after 24 hours the measured pH *in vitro* of Biodentine leachate was as high as 11.7 and remained unchanged at least four weeks [99].

Biodentine is recommended by Nowicka et al. [54] and Wang [21] in direct pulp capping, pulpotomy, root perforation repair, and as root-end filling material because it has dentin-like mechanical properties and releases a higher amount of calcium ions promoting the local healing than other bioceramics such as MTA, BioAggregate, or EndoSequence BC Sealer.

Wang mentions that Biodentine also has a proper radiopacity, greater than 3 mm thickness of aluminum recommended by ISO norms 6876/2001 [21].

In clinical use, Elnaghy suggests to also consider that the microhardness, compressive strength and push-out resistance of Biodentine decrease insofar as pH values descend. However, compared to WMTA Branco, the Biodentine physical properties were less affected [100].

Elnaghy found that when used as root-end filling, repair material of root and furcation perforations or apical plug in immature teeth with chronic apical periodontitis, Biodentine is often exposed to an acidic pH induced by the turnover of local bacterial biofilms or of surrounding pre-existing inflamed tissues, which may weaken its chemical and physical properties [100].

In an *in vitro* investigation of the outcome of Biodentine exposure to a possible clinical acidic environment, by reproducing a range of intermediary acidic pH levels between pH 7.4 and 4.4, Elnaghy depicted a substantial change in microstructure [100].

While at 7.4 pH value the SEM analysis displayed the structure of an amorphous superficial gel poorly crystallized with globular aggregate particles and microchannels, when reducing the pH to the value of 6.4 Elnaghy observed only needle-shaped and cubic crystals. Selective loss of matrix preserving needle-like structure was present at pH value of 5.4 and finally, at the lowest value of 4.4, the cement surface appeared more eroded, characterized by laminated cross-stratified and honeycomb-shaped structures, pores and microchannels [100].

Biodentine has higher push-out strength than MTA due to the smaller particle dimension. Its push-out strength can be diminished by previous removing of smear layer. Sodium hypochlorite and CHX solutions for root canal irrigation almost do not modify the push-out strength of Biodentine. However, in case of MTA Wang mentions that the value of push-out strength is reduced after the contact with CHX [21].

10.16.3 Biological Properties

Biodentine proved to be biocompatible preserving a high level of cell viability in various studies on cells culture. Depending on type of cell culture in some lines of cells, as pseudo-odontoblastic cells MDPC-23, Biodentine exhibited according to Wang a lower level of viability than MTA but in other pulp cell-line, OD-21, the viability level was as low as in MTA samples [21].

After an initial decrease of vitality during the first 6 hours of contact *in vitro* with cells belonging to mouse embryo fibroblast cell line 3T3, in the following time period up to 72 hours Corral Nuñez et al. noticed a recovering of cell vitality so that Biodentine and ProRoot MTA displayed similar toxicity. At SEM analysis the cells that were seeded on Biodentine samples resembled the normal fibroblast spindle shape and covered most of the material surface compared to fewer and more retracted cells, without cellular processes, attached to ProRoot MTA [101].

At 24 hours, Corral Nuñez et al. found by semi-quantitative RT-PCR a similar pattern of IL-1α mRNA expression for both bioceramic cements unlike the IL-6 mRNA expression. At 3 hours its value was higher in ProRoot MTA and later, up to 24 hours, equalized the Biodentine level. The initial and transient stimulation of potent proinflammatory cytokines IL-1α and IL-6 induced in pulp tissue by capping materials might be considered, within acceptable limits, a prerequisite of reparative process [101].

Wang claims Biodentine is able to induce odontoblasts differentiation by MAPK and CaMKII pathways. There was revealed a higher expression of *Runx2*, *Msx2*, *Osx*, and *Dix5* genes during the odontoblasts differentiation from pulp stem cells and alizarin red-stained nodules of mineralization as well [21].

Wang also underlines that Biodentine stimulates osteoblasts differentiation in different stem cells and promotes the mineralization by increasing the expression of ALP, bone sialoprotein, and OC osteogenic-related genes [21].

An *in vitro* study of Chang et al. on immortalized hDPC line showed that the level of cell viability, their potential to differentiate into odontoblasts, and inflammatory response exhibited by Biodentine was similar to MTA Angelus and OrthoMTA. Moreover, the high mRNA expression of differentiation markers genes, increased level of ALP activity and formation of mineralized nodules suggest that the phenotype of differentiated cells resembles the odontoblast [102].

Over time, the calcium and silicate ions released from Biodentine assist the dentin remineralization. Even though it could have some adverse effect on the dentin collagen, Wang says it seems to be clinically acceptable because it occurs only on the contact surface [21].

Wang concluded that in vital pulp therapy, i.e. direct pulp capping and pulpotomy, it was clearly demonstrated that the Biodentine succeeded to induce in rat model a good pulp healing, similar to MTA, due to the formation of a continuous and homogenous dentin bridge on day 14 [21].

10.16.4 Clinical Studies

Clinical studies of Tran et al. [103] and Wang [21] demonstrated that Biodentine successfully preserved the pulp vitality in indirect pulp capping if the therapeutic protocol was appropriately respected. Histological, clinical, and radiographic performances of Biodentine used in human teeth for direct pulp capping are similar to MTA.

A clinical and histological comparative study on 28 intact human molars of Nowicka et al. showed that the efficacy of Biodentine, used as direct pulp capping, was similar to white ProRoot MTA after six weeks of experiment. There was no clinical complaint of spontaneous pain or radiolucencies on periapical radiographs and all teeth preserved their vitality [54].

A dentinal bridge was formed in direct contact with both capping materials. Underneath the mineralized barrier closing the exposure site, in juxtaposed pulp tissue, Nowicka et al. noticed no inflammation, abscesses, or necrosis [54].

Next to the complete dentinal bridge, the morphologic studies of Nowicka et al. [54] and Wang [21] also revealed tubular dentin and odontoblasts or odontoblast-like cells with polarized nuclei, columnar-placed beneath the new-generated osteodentin, suggesting that Biodentine might be an alternative to white ProRoot MTA in vital pulp treatments.

10.17 BioAggregate

BioAggregate (Innovative Bioceramix, Vancouver, Canada) is, according to Zhang et al., aluminum-free, calcium silicate-based bioceramic produced as nanoparticles [104].

Yan et al. [38] and Zhang et al. [7] think that this white hydraulic cement used as root-end filling material in surgical endodontics could be a potential alternative to MTA, because over recent years the nanostructured bioceramics proved to be very promising in regenerative medicine.

10.17.1 Chemical Composition

Its most significant ingredients are tricalcium silicate, dicalcium silicate, and calcium phosphate monobasic. Tantalum pentoxide is mentioned by Zhang et al. to be introduced as radiopacifier [104]. Yan et al. [38] and Zhang et al. [7] also consider calcium silicate, calcium hydroxide, and hydroxyapatite as important ingredients.

10.17.2 Biological Properties

As compared to MTA, BioAggregate has a lower tissue toxicity because it is aluminum free, contains tantalum pentoxide that substitutes as radiopacifier the bismuth oxide, and its nanocrystals of hydroxyapatite proved to stimulate the fibroblastic proliferation in human periodontal ligament. Yan et al. [38] and Zhang et al. [7] observed that BioAggregate also exhibits acceptable biocompatibility, good quality sealing, high push-out bond strength, antiseptic action, high fracture and acidic resistance, but lower microhardness.

In endodontic surgery, the proper osseous wound healing after root-end resection is definitely dependent of regenerative potential of root-end filling. The periodontal ligament fibroblasts are obviously the main cells of periradicular tissues in direct and long-lasting contact with a root-end filling material. If in these circumstances the fibroblasts preserve their potential to differentiate in osteoblasts the outcome will be a good local healing.

Evaluating the ALP gene expression (bone turnover marker of osteoblasts) in cell cultures by quantitative real-time PCR, it was demonstrated that on day 7 BioAggregate significantly enhanced the osteogenic differentiation of human periodontal ligament fibroblasts. A simultaneous assessment of COLI gene (collagenous protein marker of osteoblast-like cell) also revealed an expression peak on days 5 and 7, induced by calcium silicate and hydroxyapatite content of same root-end filling material. Finding out the aforementioned changes in metabolic activity of viable fibroblasts, Yan et al. claimed that BioAggregate is a real inducer of their differentiation in osteoblasts [38].

On the other side, BioAggregate is also involved in suppressing the osteoclastic activities resulting in the inflammatory process of chronic apical periodontitis, the major indication for surgical endodontics if the conventional root canal treatment fails. The occurrence of differentiated osteoclasts among chronic inflammatory cells in periapical area is based on monocyte-macrophage lineage vehiculated by blood circulation from the bone marrow.

Various types of cytokines are involved into the differentiation of precursors and function of mature osteoclasts. However, Zhang et al. observed that only some of them, such as M-CSF (macrophage colony stimulating factor) and RANKL might be critical [7].

Zhang et al. investigated in a mouse calvarial model of LPS (lipopolysaccharides)-induced inflammatory bone resorption the BioAggregate effect in osteoclastogenesis on RANKL-stimulated mouse bone marrow macrophages and found that the number of osteoclasts diminished in a dose-dependent way [7].

BioAggregate decreased simultaneously the number of activated monocytes and macrophages expressing some osteoclast-related factors which elicit inflammatory reactions, such as cathepsin K and its upstream regulators NFATc1 and c-Fos [7].

Cathepsin K is an extremely active enzyme involved in bone resorption, with highly deleterious effect on collagen and tissue extracellular matrix. Since this enzyme was clearly suppressed, investigated concluded that

NFATc1 and c-Fos are molecular targets of bioceramic materials such MTA and BioAggregate [7].

According to the same study it seems that are also involved other downstream regulators of osteoclastogenesis, because calcium silicate-based bioceramics release in periapical tissue fluids numerous silicon ions that are potent osteoclast inhibitors [7].

Yuan et al. [105] and Zhang et al. [7] observed that the osteo-conductive effect of BioAggregate in osteoblasts and periodontal ligament fibroblasts is the consequence of upregulating the mineral-associated gene expression of these periapical cells.

An *in vitro* study of Shokouhinejad et al. showed after one-week exposure to PBS a homogenous layer covered the immersed root sections containing BioAggregate in their canals, as root canal fillings. SEM analysis after two-months immersion in PBS revealed spherical precipitates of apatite [9].

10.18 DiaRoot BioAggregate

Khalil and Eid mention DiaRoot BioAggregate (Diadent Group International, Burnaby, Canada) among the newer, aluminum-free bioceramics used in endodontics [45].

10.18.1 Chemical Composition

It is also claimed by Khalil and Eid that, as compared to MTA, DiaRoot BioAggregate contains tantalum oxide (radiopacifier) and hydroxyapatite [45].

10.18.2 Physical Parameters

According to Khalil and Eid, DiaRoot BioAggregate is an easy-to-handle bioceramic cement displaying an optimum working time [45].

10.18.3 Biological Properties

DiaRoot BioAggregate has *in vitro* a comparable biocompatibility to MTA and Khalil and Eid also proved it is an antifungal bioceramic [45].

A comparative study of systemic biocompatibility with the liver and kidney concerning DiaRoot BioAggregate and MTA was done by Khalil and Eid introducing subcutaneously in male albino rats sterile Teflon tubes filled with freshly spatulated root-end filling material. It was found at 7–30 days of experiment that the severity of lymphocytes inflammatory response in the liver and kidney was substantially higher in MTA than in DiaRoot BioAggregate rats [45].

Morphometric study of periportal and pericentral areas of the liver on day 7 showed in DiaRoot BioAggregate subgroup of rats enhanced inflammatory cells infiltration, increased number of Kupffer cells, congestion of sinusoidal spaces, and highly dilated and distorted portal vein with disrupted endothelial lining. On day 30 Khalil and Eid observed that the central vein was still dilated and the nuclei of some hepatocytes came to be pyknotic. However, the collagen fibers seemed to be normal [45].

Due to a morphometric study of renal cortex, Khalil and Eid revealed on day 7 in the same DiaRoot BioAggregate subgroup some glomeruli-free Malpighian's corpuscles, debris of degenerated glomeruli, collagen deposits, pyknotic nuclei of Bowman's capsule, and vacuolated cytoplasm of the distal convoluted tubules. On day 30, some areas of cortex hemorrhage were still present and the collagen fibers returned to normal [45].

As compared to DiaRoot BioAggregate, in the liver of the sMTA subgroup of rats on day 7 was noted a substantial increase of inflammatory cells associated with dilated bile ducts, interlobular lymphocytes infiltrate, Kupffer cells degeneration, and hepatocytes vacuolation. On day 30 were observed focal leucocytes infiltrations around dilated sinusoids and portal vein, with disrupted epithelial lining of the central vein and pyknotic nuclei of Kupffer cells and hepatocytes. Khalil and Eid underline that the inflammatory cells were much more numerous than in the DiaRoot BioAggregate subgroup [45].

Morphometric study of renal cortex on day 7 revealed in MTA subgroup some malformed glomeruli and debris of destroyed distal convoluted tubules but Khalil and Eid noticed no difference concerning collagen depositions. On day 30 thin Bowman's capsules were observed around glomeruli. The number of inflammatory cells noticeably decreased and the lymphocytes infiltrate was located around the glomeruli and tubules. Some of the tubules were obliterated by hyaline depositions and collagen fibers were thicker [45].

Khalil and Eid concluded that the systemic induced hepatocellular injury was also reflected by significant increase of serum alanine aminotransferase (ALT) and aspartate aminotransferase (AST) [45].

10.19 EndoSequence Root Repair Material (ERRM)

Lovato and Sedgley [4], Hansen et al. [46], Shokouhinejad et al. [9], Alsalleeh et al. [106], Wang [21], and Shinbori et al. [59] claim that ERRM (Brasseler, Savannah, USA) is a biocompatible, chemically stable, antibacterial (pH 12.4), insoluble, and radiopaque bioceramic material that does not provoke tooth discoloration.

10.19.1 Chemical Composition

ERRM, according to Lovato and Sedgley [4], Hansen et al. [46], Shokouhinejad et al. [9], Alsalleeh et al. [106], Wang [21], and Shinbori et al. [59], is composed of calcium silicates, calcium phosphate monobasic, zirconium oxide, tantalum oxide, thickening agents, and proprietary fillers.

10.19.2 Physical Parameters

According to Hansen et al. [46], Shokouhinejad et al. [9], and Wang [21] ERRM is delivered as a ready-to-use, premixed, firm and moldable putty or flowable preloaded syringeable paste and sets in moisture environment in round four hours [9, 21, 46].

Öncel Torun et al. underline that calcium silicate of ERRM requires moisture to set [8]. Lovato and Sedgley say that, as the manufacturer claims, the moisture delivered by dentinal tubules would permit the setting reaction [4]. However, Damas et al. revealed that ERRM needed up to 168 hours to achieve the complete set [2]. Lovato and Sedgley insist upon the need of further studies to precisely assess its setting time in periradicular biological environment [4].

ERRM is superior to MTA due its uniform consistency and sufficient working time for placement (30 minutes). The far-achieving reduction in particle size compared to MTA improved the clinical handling. Damas et al. [2], Lovato and Sedgley [4], Shokouhinejad et al. [9], and Wang [21] observed that acidic pH decreases the microhardness and the material becomes porous because its crystalline structure is adversely affected [2, 4, 9, 21].

ERRM does not shrink upon setting and maintain a tight seal. Lovato and Sedgley [4], Hansen et al. [46], Ma et al. [39], Shokouhinejad et al. [9], Alsalleeh et al. [106], Wang [21], and Shinbori et al. [59] found a compressive strength similar to gray MTA.

The composition of ERRM is different to MTA that contains tricalcium silicate, dicalcium silicate, bismuth oxide, tricalcium aluminate, and calcium sulfate. However, Ma et al. proved that the ERRM Putty and ERRM Paste surface crystallographic structure is similar to gray MTA since it contains mainly calcium, carbon, and oxygen [13].

The mineral component of MTA acicular crystals is ettringite, a hydrated calcium–aluminum–sulfate, generated by chemical reaction between calcium sulfate and calcium aluminate hydrate. Regarding the needle-like crystals found in a study after ERRM exposure to PBS Shokouhinejad et al. say they definitely cannot be ettringite, as ERRM is an aluminum-free bioceramic [9]. When MTA, BioAggregate, or ERRM come in contact with PBS calcium ions from these bioceramics react with phosphate from PBS and results in hydroxyapatite or carbonated apatite. Shokouhinejad et al. demonstrated that even though a precipitate can be detected in one week, it takes two months to be generated between bioceramic and dentin a mineral interfacial layer proving the material bioactivity [9].

Following the placement of ERRM and white ProRoot MTA in root canals, an *in vitro* study of Hansen et al. measured the pH values in 0.7-mm deep cavities on the root surface simulating an external inflammatory root resorption. The diffusion of hydroxyl ions through dentin from canal lumen to the cavities carved at 2 and 5 mm from the apex revealed a higher pH in white ProRoot MTA filled samples that were time and root level dependent [46]. During the first 20 minutes of setting and at 3-hours time-point, at both levels of 2 and 5 mm, no pH differences occurred between ERRM and white ProRoot MTA. Evenly pH values were also recorded at 24 hours at the 5-mm level. Hansen et al. observed that all later evaluations at one-, two-, and three-weeks exhibited a significantly higher pH in white ProRoot MTA compared to ERRM, depending on their setting time proved in previous studies [46].

The steeper decline of ERRM than MTA pH during the first week might be explained by the time that ERRM required achieving the complete set. However, at the four-week time point, Hansen et al. reported a similar pH in both experiment materials, ERRM and white ProRoot MTA [46].

10.19.3 Biological Properties

It seems, according to Wang, that ERRM develops by biomineralization a micromechanical adhesion mechanism to dentin because beneath the bioceramic material tag-like structures were depicted in dentinal tubules [21]. ERRM is recommended in endodontic surgery by Modareszadeh et al. as retrofilling and root perforation repair material [5].

After one-week immersion in PBS of root sections containing ERRM in their canals as root canal fillings Shokouhinejad et al. observed on the bioceramic material surface a limited precipitate consisting in smooth aggregates of individual and fused globular particles. SEM analysis at two-months exposure to PBS revealed a thicker precipitate of spherical acicular particles grouped in clusters and an intermediary mineral layer between ERRM and root dentin [9].

Energy dispersive analysis by X-ray showed that the main component of crystals precipitated on the surface of bioceramic materials was calcium carbonate. However, SEM analysis of Ma et al. proved that these crystals allowed the cell adhesion [13].

Ma et al. [13] and Damas et al. [2] claim that ERRM has comparable biocompatibility to mineral trioxide aggregate. Testing the root repair materials on cell cultures of human dermal fibroblasts by standard method MTT-based colorimetric assay, it was found out that EndoSequence RRM had similar cytotoxicity to white ProRoot MTA and WMTA Angelus. Actually, according to Damas et al., the cell viability was ≥91.8% [2]. Another study, of Lovato and Sedgley showed that ERRM cytotoxicity seems to be similar to WMTA, gray MTA, and MTA Angelus [4].

In a human osteoblast-like cells culture belonging to the cell-line MG-63, ERRM Putty, and ERRM flowable paste showed negligible cytotoxicity, similar to ProRoot MTA. Using RT-PCR Ciasca et al., noticed that all materials induced a comparable expression of the inflammatory cytokines IL-1β, IL-6, and IL-8 [107].

Even though the ERRM Putty and MTA demonstrated a minimal cytotoxicity level in all samples, ERRM proved to be insignificantly more cytotoxic. The highest levels of cytokines were recorded at the 24-hour time point. However, Ciasca et al. detected a minor difference between the cytokines levels owing to their increased value at 24 hours in ERRM Putty group of study [107].

The biocompatibility of ERRM Putty and ERRM Paste was also tested on human gingival fibroblasts. The cell viability depended on the type of material, setting time, and contact time with cultured cells. The MTT assay, measuring mitochondrial dehydrogenase activity as marker of cell viability, demonstrated at each time interval up to seven days that fresh ERRM Paste displayed a slightly lower cell viability compared to gray ProRoot MTA. However, Ma et al. proved that the set ERRM Paste and ERRM Putty showed *in vitro* the same biocompatibility as gray ProRoot MTA [13].

After seven days, Ma et al. demonstrated that the gingival fibroblasts seeded on ERRM Putty and ERRM Paste preserved their attachment and reached 100% confluence on the cement surface forming a matrix-like overlay, similar to gray ProRoot MTA [13].

Ciasca et al. showed that in contrast to fibroblasts cell lines, that proved to be low cost, easy and rapidly growing, and very resistant in cultures as well, osteoblast-like cells MG-63 have the advantage to create a proper clinical and histological setting to investigate the periradicular tissues reaction to a root-end bioceramic material [107].

In another study Modareszadeh et al. investigated the effect of ERRM on days 1, 3, and 7 in a different type of osteoblast-like cells culture, the widely used human osteosarcoma cell line Saos-2. Using a colorimetric method with the tetrazolium compound MTS, it was found that both undiluted and 50% diluted ERRM samples substantially decreased cell viability at each time-point [5].

In case of ERRM simultaneous assessment of ALP, a cellular marker of differentiated osteoblasts after a bone injury, Modareszadeh et al. also proved a decline in releasing this enzyme and the resulting tissue biologic mineralization [5].

Using ERRM Putty as root-end filling material in an experimentally induced chronic apical periodontitis in dogs, despite the comparable biocompatibility and sealing ability, Chen et al. found histologically at six months after surgery a better periradicular healing than gray MTA even though the remaining root canal was still infected [108].

When ERRM was used, a greater area of mineralized cementum-like tissue covered both the resected root-dentin surface and retrograde filling. The newly formed mineralized tissue resembling either cementum or bone also extended on the lateral root surface and appeared to be in continuity with the original radicular cementum. In addition, Chen et al. observed microscopically dense fibrous tissue suggesting periodontal ligament-like tissue regeneration and in few cases a complete reconstitution of bone buccal and lingual lamina dura [108].

Though after surgery no histological differences were observed in the local inflammatory response, unlike the usual periapical radiography, ERRM Putty induced a better healing on CBCT and micro CT images compared to gray MTA. However, despite the better inductive or conductive properties of ERRM, Chen et al. could not detect a regenerated bone cortical plate [108].

ERRM demonstrated antibacterial properties due to its highly alkaline pH developed during setting. In a study using 10 clinical strains of *E. faecalis* both delivery forms of ERRM, putty and flowable, and white ProRoot MTA exhibited similar antimicrobial activity. According to Lovato and Sedgley, out of investigated clinical strains of *E. faecalis* the most susceptible to root-end filling materials were GS9, followed by GS7, GS25, GS33, and GS4 [4].

Baumgartner et al. revealed that the root canal biofilms may also harbor fungi like *C. albicans*, which may be found in up to 21% of infected root canals [20]. Alsalleeh et al. concluded that it would be extremely advantageous for a root repair material to also exert an antifungal activity, especially in persistent periapical lesions where *Candida* species are frequently present [106].

Recently, it was found that ERRM Putty, WMTA and gray MTA, allowed to set 3 or 24 hours before to come in contact with *C. albicans* wild-type SC5314 (CA42) strain, have comparable antifungal activity. However, the materials tested by Alsalleeh et al. had higher antifungal efficiency after 3 hours than those tested at 24 hours. Both bioceramic materials set for 24 hours preserved their antifungal activity within the basic range of pH values, MTA at pH 8.5, and ERRM at pH 8 [106].

10.19.4 Clinical Studies

According to Setzer et al. [109], Johnson et al. [12], and Shinbori et al. [59] the high success rate of modern endodontic surgery (over 90%), compared with the traditional one (60%), is based on the microsurgical technique using operating microscope, ultrasonic root-end cavity preparation and bioceramic material as retrofilling.

Using EndoSequence BC Root Repair Material as root-end filling, Shinbori et al. found the overall success rate in 113 teeth was as high as 92% one year after endodontic microsurgery. The recorded clinical and radiographic findings demonstrated that EndoSequence BC Root Repair Material provided the guarantee of biocompatibility, antimicrobial activity, hermetical apical seal, and bioactivity as well [59].

10.20 iRoot BP

iRoot BP (Innovative Bioceramix, Vancouver, Canada) is an injectable, premixed paste used as root repairing material or root canal filling. Parirokh and Torabinejad mention that it actually is one of the three forms of dental products launched on the market by same manufacturer, namely iRoot Sp, iRoot BP, and iRoot BP Plus [6].

10.20.1 Chemical Composition

According to Zhang et al. [55] and Shi et al. [62], iRoot BP is an aluminum-free bioceramic similar in composition to MTA.

10.20.2 Physical Parameters

Parirokh and Torabinejad claim that iRoot BP needs moisture to harden, does not shrink after setting, it is insoluble and radiopaque [6].

10.20.3 Biological Properties

The *in vitro* cytotoxicity of iRoot BP (Innovative Bioceramix, Vancouver, Canada) and white mineral trioxide aggregate (Angelus, Londrina, Brazil) was investigated after 24-, 48-, and 72-hour incubation periods. The evaluation was performed by Öncel Torun et al. using a standard spectrophotometric quantification (XTT assay) in hDPCs exposed to various dilutions (1 : 1, 1 : 2, 1 : 5, and 1 : 10) [8].

Except 1 : 10 dilutions after 24-hour period, Öncel Torun et al. observed in both ceramic cements a pretty similar cellular proliferation and viability of hDPCs with an acceptable cell survival level (>90%) according to ISO 2009 international standard [8].

In the same study of Öncel Torun et al. mineralizing-related gene expression (dentin sialophosphoprotein, BMP, bone sialoprotein, OPN, osteonectin, collagen Type 1) measured by quantitative real-time polymerase chain reaction (qRT-PCR) revealed the biocompatibility of iRoot BP and white mineral trioxide aggregate [8].

Even though their degree of involvement may differ someway, Öncel Torun et al. agree that both aforementioned bioceramic cements are facilitating the odontoblasts differentiation and pulp tissue mineralization [8].

10.21 iRoot BP Plus

Zhang et al. [55] and Shi et al. [62] claim that iRoot BP Plus (Innovative Bioceramix, Vancouver, Canada), also labeled as EndoSequence RRM Putty (Brasseler, Savannah, USA) and TotalFill RRM Putty (FKG, La-Chaux-de-Fonds, Switzerland) is an aluminum-free bioceramic similar in composition to MTA.

10.21.1 Chemical Composition

According to Zhang et al. [55] and Shi et al. [62] the principal components of iRoot BP Plus are tricalcium silicate, dicalcium silicate, calcium phosphate, zirconium oxide, and tantalum oxide as radiopacifier.

10.21.2 Physical Parameters

Parirokh and Torabinejad [6] and Liu et al. [110] specify that iRoot BP Plus is a premixed putty material having the setting time of approximately 2 hours 30 minutes.

Shi et al. found that iRoot BP Plus has 31.73–58.92 N/mm^2 microhardness, 2.2% solubility, and 0.02% dimensional change following setting [62].

iRoot BP Plus is successfully used as root-end filling material because it has superior sealing quality and is insoluble, biocompatible, osteo-conductive, regenerative, and radiopaque. Zhang et al. [55], Parirokh and Torabinejad [6], and Liu et al. [110] mention that iRoot BP Plus might also be used as root-repairing material, in root canal filling, or in pulp capping.

10.21.3 Biological Properties

Zhang et al. proved that iRoot BP Plus increased hDPCs proliferation, triggered the odontoblast differentiation and induced mineralization, similar to BioAggregate [55].

According to Liu et al. the biocompatibility of iRoot BP Plus was proved by various *in vitro* studies either on fibroblasts and osteoblasts cell lines or on periodontal ligament cells and hDPCs [110].

As compared to MTA, in long-time cultures of hDPCs, iRoot BP Plus induces higher expression of odontoblast-specific markers such as DSPP and DMP-1. Zhang et al. proved that the presence of these two proteins involved in mineralization, DSPP (noncollagenous protein) and DMP-1 (regulator of mineralization) is an evidence of already differentiated mature and functional odontoblasts [55].

The bioceramic root-end fillings also increase some other molecular markers involved in mineralization such as ALP and OC, but these factors are not odontoblast-specific. ALP was detected in early stages of hDPCs differentiation and iRoot BP Plus showed a higher ALP activity than MTA. Zhang et al. specify that in contrast to ALP, OC is produced only by mature cells like osteoblasts, cementoblasts, and odontoblast [55].

Using qRT-PCR Zhang et al. also revealed that both iRoot BP Plus and BioAggregate have higher mineralization potential and induce more powerful odontoblast-related gene expression of DSPP, DMP-1, and OC in dental pulp cells than MTA [55].

Evaluating the cell density, membrane integrity and mitochondrial activity on primary human osteoblasts exposed to iRoot BP Plus and white ProRoot MTA by multiparametric cell viability assay (XTT, NR, CVDE) De-Deus et al. observed that in the first 24 hours the cytocompatibility pattern looked similar [111].

However, after 48 hours of exposure occurred a cytotoxicity pattern difference between the two cements. The osteoblasts viability in iRoot BP Plus specimens significantly decreased compared to white ProRoot MTA even though it was still higher than 70% [111].

It was concluded by De-Deus et al. that iRoot BP Plus did not trigger critical cytotoxic effects. Actually it is considered that iRoot BP Plus has a substandard cytotoxic pattern only at the metabolic level of mitochondrial dehydrogenases (XTT assay), since the integrity of cell membrane (NR assay) and cell density (CVDE assay) remained unaffected [111].

Using MTT assay it was observed by Liu et al. on a cell culture of hDPCs that iRoot BP Plus developed an earlier and enhanced cell proliferation than MTA [110].

In direct pulp capping of healthy dental pulps in beagle dogs Shi et al. noticed at three months on postoperative radiographs a complete mineralized bridge, as a sign of healing, directly underneath the iRoot BP Plus capping material as in MTA control specimens. MTA was used as a reference material since it is currently considered the gold standard in vital pulp treatments [62].

This newly generated bridge by both cements, iRoot BP Plus and MTA, at the interface of pulp experimental exposure was underlined by healthy pulp tissue. Shi et al. concluded that histologically this bridge had a changeable appearance that did not depend on capping material. There were displayed regular and irregular dentin tubules and osteodentine-resembling amorphous eosinophilic morphological structures as well [62].

The formation of an earlier and stronger reparative dentin bridge after pulp capping with iRoot BP Plus, as compared to MTA, was substantiated by another study of Liu et al. on Wistar rats. In case of iRoot BP Plus even after one week was observed mild hard tissue deposition within a newly generated matrix. After four weeks, the exposure site was effectively sealed by a thick and continuous dentin bridge with homogenous dentinal tubule-like appearance. In the adjacent pulp tissue underneath the newly formed mineralized barrier were situated in direct contact polarized odontoblast-like cells [110].

As compared to MTA iRoot BP Plus also recorded similar better results in pulpotomies. After one week no inflammatory cells were found in the majority of radicular dental pulps and a layer of hard tissue already appeared at all root canal orifices. At four weeks time interval, Liu et al. found the same proportion of specimens capped with iRoot BP Plus showing a complete seal of root canal, no inflammation within the remaining radicular pulp tissue and polarized odontoblast-like cells juxtaposed to newly formed dentin bridge [110].

10.22 iRoot SP

Wang mentions that iRoot SP (Innovative BioCeramix, Vancouver, Canada) is also known as EndoSequence BC Sealer (Brasseler, Savannah, USA) [21].

10.22.1 Chemical Composition

Concerning the chemical components Wang specifies that iRoot SP is a sealer similar to ERRM [21].

10.22.2 Physical Parameters

According to the opinion of Wang, the bond strength of iRoot AP, compared to MTA Fillapex, Epiphany, and AH Plus, is still controversial. Regarding the debates, it has to compare the methods of study because is a difference between the push-out strengths of a core material when used alone and of a sealer used with gutta-percha cones in cold lateral condensation [21].

Nagas et al. found that the expected value of clinically efficient bonding strength between conventional and resin-based sealers and dentin after root canal obturation may be diminished by pre-existent residual moisture [112]. In this line Zhang et al. proved a low contact angle to water of iRoot SP [49].

However, a moisture status would facilitate a proper setting of hydrophilic bioceramic sealers, as iRoot SP. Regrettably even such sealers, as Nagas et al. proved, are never able to completely absorb water in a wet canal so that the sealer-dentin interface can be disrupted by residual water [112].

Nagas et al. recommend that regardless of sealer composition, currently it would preferably to preserve the root canal slightly moist before obturation and to avoid the extreme clinical conditions of completely dry or wet canal [112].

On a four-steps scale of intracanal moisture conditions, starting from a dry dentin (step 1) up to a wet one (step 4), MTA Fillapex developed significant higher push-out bond strength on moist dentin (step 3) than on dry dentin or normal moisture (step 2). Nagas et al. showed that in wet canals (step 4) sealer adhesion failed [112].

iRoot SP sealer achieved highest bond strength in dry, normal moisture and moist intracanal conditions and lowest values in wet canals. The epoxy resin-based sealer AH Plus displayed bond strength of similar value in normal moisture and moist conditions. iRoot SP proved to develop in all moist conditions higher bond strength than MTA Fillapex, AH Plus, and Epiphany/Resilon. Moreover, according to Nagas et al. the push-out test revealed increased levels of resistance when gutta-percha cones were used for cold lateral condensation [112].

The stability of sealer-intracanal dentin interface depends on a range of parameters such as chemical bond, micromechanical retention, and frictional resistance. Nagas et al. underline that additional improving factors might be the small particle size, preferentially nanoparticulates, enhanced sealer flow, and minimal or no setting shrinkage [112].

10.22.3 Biological Properties

As advantages of iRoot SP, Wang [21] claims the adequate apical sealing after placement whereas Lovato and Sedgley [4] highlight mild cytotoxicity, comparable to AH Plus, and the prolonged antibacterial activity up to one week in contact with periradicular tissues.

The cytotoxicity may be time and concentration dependent. Wang mentions that even though freshly mixed iRoot SP is slightly cytotoxic as set cement it loses its adverse effect in high dilutions or after one week [21].

Zhang et al. observed that during the first three days after mixing iRoot SP proved to be very efficient against *E. faecalis* due to its hydrophilicity, high pH value, and active release of calcium hydroxide [49]. Wang et al. claim that dentin is also involved in enhancing the antibacterial effect of endodontic sealers [113].

The high hydrophilicity of iRoot SP is also facilitating its antibacterial activity in the depth of dentinal tubules. According to Wang it was demonstrated that this bioceramic was able to kill *E. faecalis* in rates of 18% at one day, 35% at one week, and 45% at one month [21].

10.23 iRoot FS

Wang claims that iRoot FS (Brasseler, Savannah, USA) has a setting time of one hour at body temperature in 100% humidity environment and improved handling properties [21].

10.24 EndoSequence BC Sealer

Wang mentions that EndoSequence BC Sealer (Brasseler, Savannah, USA) is a premixed and injectable bioceramic root canal sealer [21].

10.24.1 Chemical Composition

According to Wang, EndoSequence BC Sealer is made up by tricalcium silicate, dicalcium silicate, colloidal silica, calcium silicates, calcium phosphate monobasic, calcium hydroxide, and zirconium oxide as radiopacifier [21].

Loushine et al. specifies that EndoSequence BC Sealer differs from ERRM-putty and ERRM-flowable only by the amount of additional water-free thickening agent [114].

10.24.2 Physical Parameters

According to Loushine et al. [114] and Wang [21], the setting reaction is induced by the moisture from dentinal tubules and results in a calcium silicate hydrate phase. Additional water is released from the reaction of calcium phosphate and calcium hydroxide to support this hydrate formation. Simultaneously, hydroxyapatite coprecipitates within the hydrate phase and generates between root canal wall and sealer a mineral composite-like structure.

The producer claimed the setting time is around four hours. However, Wang underlines that the sclerosis of dentinal tubules, presence of smear layer and overly dried canals, postpone the final setting to more than 10 hours [21]. Later on, it was proved that the initial set occurs at 72 hours and the final one is observed after 240 hours. Loushine et al. proved that the flow values and pH of EndoSequence BC Sealer before setting are higher than AH Plus sealer [114].

Wang says that EndoSequence BC Sealer exhibits lower release of calcium ions compared to another bioceramic material, Biodentine [21]. It was also proved by Loushine et al. that the microhardness and setting time of EndoSequence BC Sealer are negatively influenced by the changes in environmental water [114].

Unfortunately, Wang underlines that its radiopacity value is equivalent to only 3.83 mm Al, around twice lower than frequently used root canal sealer AH Plus [21].

10.24.3 Biological Properties

Investigating the succinic dehydrogenase (SDH) activity as profile of cytotoxicity on MC3T3-E1 mouse osteoblasts, Loushine et al. demonstrated that EndoSequence BC Sealer, AH Plus and Pulp Canal Sealer EWT showed at 24 hours the same high cytotoxicity. Compared to AH Plus that lost its cytotoxicity in three weeks, EndoSequence BC Sealer was assessed as mild cytotoxic only after six weeks [114].

However, Wang says that human gingival fibroblasts spread after 24 hours over samples of EndoSequence BC Sealer set for three days [21].

Studying by flow cytometry the viability of human gingival fibroblast exposed to various concentrations of sealer-derived extracts of freshly mixed and set MTA Fillapex and EndoSequence BC Sealer over a period of four weeks Zhou et al. observed that, regardless of extract concentrations, fresh and set EndoSequence BC Sealer reached a higher level of cell viability than MTA Fillapex [73].

A parallel cell adhesion assay described, after 24 hours of culture, numerous fibroblasts with typical spindle-shaped morphology attached on samples surface of EndoSequence BC Sealer. During the following days Zhou et al. found an increasing number of spreading fibroblasts, connected with each other, while the cells that covered MTA Fillapex samples were round and weakly attached [73].

10.25 Ceramicrete-D

Ceramicrete-D (Tulsa Dental Specialties, Argonne, USA) is according to Porter et al. magnesium–potassium–phosphate ceramic containing calcium silicate and hydroxylapatite, that is potential bioactive and has better sealing ability than ProRoot MTA.

10.25.1 Chemical Composition

Tay et al. introduces Ceramicrete-D as a version for dental use that contains additional calcium silicate whiskers in order to improve the mechanical properties, hydroxyapatite to enhance biocompatibility, and cerium oxide as radiopacifier. X-ray diffraction analysis of the set Ceramicrete-D showed the formation of reaction phases, $KMgPO_4{\cdot}6H_2O$ and $CaHPO_4{\cdot}2H_2O$ [18, 24, 25, 34].

According to Tay et al., the main components of Ceramicrete-D powder are MgO, KH_2PO_4, $CaSiO_3$ whiskers, hydroxyapatite powder, and cerium oxide radiopaque fillers. When mixing with deionized water in a powder/liquid ratio of 1.85 : 1 the initial setting time is of 6 minutes and the final one of 12 minutes [24].

10.25.2 Physical Parameters

Compared to white ProRoot MTA mixing ratio powder to liquid of 3 : 1, the mixing ratio recommended by Porter et al. for Ceramicrete-D is 2 : 1. Ceramicrete-D sets in 2.5 hours and has an acidic pH (2.2) [25].

Tay et al. claim that basically Ceramicrete-D is a self-setting phosphate ceramic that sets by acid–base reaction between KH_2PO_4 (acidic phosphate) and MgO (basic oxide) and forms the ceramic matrix phase of potassium–magnesium–phosphate–hexahydrate $KMgPO_4{\cdot}6H_2O$ [24].

Porter et al. noticed that Ceramicrete-D requires thorough mixing in order to achieve after setting a notable wash-out resistance and higher adhesiveness than MTA. The resulting cement mix is nonporous and easy to manipulate and has a proper minimal wash-out resistance [25]. Tay et al. found that during setting Ceramicrete-D releases calcium and phosphate ions, so that it may be suggested it exhibits bioactive properties while in direct contact with tissue fluids [24].

After a week of setting, Porter et al. noticed that it exhibits a chalky consistency since its compressive strength does not overpass the value of 6.6 MPa [25].

In case of already set Ceramicrete-D, Tay et al. depicted a significantly lower value of leakage compared to white ProRoot MTA, i.e. 0.025 ± 0.004 and 0.109 ± 0.022 µl/min, respectively. When immersed in deionized water, Ceramicrete-D produced in 12 hours from setting a pH elevation of the solution to the value of 10.85. After 72 hours the pH rose to the value of 11.31 [24].

Though the subsequent calcium phosphate crystals formation seems to be common to calcium silicates, the reactivity of wollastonite, the calcium silicate constituent of Ceramicrete-D, is lower than tricalcium and dicalcium silicates constituents of Portland cements. Accordingly, Tay et al. underline that it would be beneficial to replace the wollastonite in the formula of Ceramicrete-D with tricalcium or dicalcium silicates, in order to increase the calcium and phosphate ions release [24].

Porter et al. showed that whenever the local tissue pH exceeds the value of 9.25 Ceramicrete-D enables the formation and deposition of hydroxylapatite crystals on its surface, suggesting that might be considered bioactive cement [25].

For clinical use Ceramicrete-D obviously requires a higher radiopacity than 3.2 mm of Al equivalent, which was measured. Tay et al. recommend that a more elevated value could be obtained by increasing the amount of radiopacifier fillers, either of cerium or of bismuth oxide [24].

Porter et al. underline that is required an improvement of chemical formula in order to reach higher compressive strength and radiopacity, when comparatively considering the clinically accepted compressive strength of WMTA (27 MPa) and its radiopacity (8.5 mm Al) [25].

10.25.3 Biological Properties

Though the study of Porter et al. revealed that after 72 hours of setting its pH became clearly alkaline (about pH value of 11), is not recommended to use an endodontic material in either an acute vital pulp or an acute apical inflammation that initially could aggravate the already acidic pH of the pathologic condition [25].

10.26 Generex A

10.26.1 Chemical Composition

Porter et al. claim that Generex A (Dentsply Tulsa Dental Specialties, Tulsa, USA) is a calcium silicate-based material [25].

10.26.2 Physical Parameters

According to Porter et al., Generex A has finer powder components than WMTA, a shorter working time and improved manipulating properties [25].

The mixing ratio powder to gel of Generex A is 4 : 1 compared to white ProRoot MTA ratio of 3 : 1. Porter et al. underline that Generex A requires thorough mixing in order to achieve after setting a notable wash-out resistance and higher adhesiveness than MTA [25].

Porter et al. proved that Generex A sets in 1.25 hours and has an alkaline pH (10.8). The compressive strength achieved 39 MPa. Its radiopacity is equivalent to 6.8 mm of Al [25].

Though the final pH value of Generex A is not high alkaline as the pH of MTA (12.6), these cements are also able to release during setting calcium hydroxide, due to their content in calcium silicates. Accordingly, by subsequently precipitating hydoxylapatite on its surface, Porter et al. concluded that Generex A might be considered bioactive cement [25].

10.27 Capasio

10.27.1 Chemical Composition

Porter et al. claim that Capasio (Primus Consulting, Bradenton, USA) is calcium-phospho-aluminosilicate-based cement [25].

10.27.2 Physical Parameters

Capasio mixing ratio powder to gel is 4 : 1 compared to white ProRoot MTA ratio powder/water of 3 : 1. When adequately mixed Porter et al. observed that a proper wash-out resistance and even higher adhesiveness than MTA can be obtained [25].

According to Porter et al. [25], Capasio set in 2.5 hours and has an alkaline pH (10.3). It has shorter working time and higher resistance in acidic environment than MTA. The compressive strength is 31 MPa [25].

Though the radiopacity of Capasio is only equivalent to 4.2 mm of Al, Porter et al. specify that it is still higher than that of EndoSequence BC Sealer [25].

The final pH value of Capasio is not high alkaline as the pH of MTA (12.6). However, Porter et al. mention that due to the content in calcium silicates, it is able to release calcium hydroxide during setting and afterwards, by precipitating hydoxylapatite on its surface, Capasio proves to be bioactive cement [25].

According to SEM and energy dispersive X-ray analysis in chemical composition and structure these crystals were similar to those precipitated on MTA. Additionally, Bird et al. confirmed by X-ray diffraction technique that the crystals are corresponding to hydroxyapatite [115].

These precipitates of apatite crystals gradually induced by Capasio were found in an *in vitro* study of Bird et al. on the filling material surface, in interfacial layer between dentin and root-filling material, as globules forming a lattice, and in the surrounding synthetic tissue fluid, a PBS solution with pH value of 7.2 [115].

A comparative SEM analysis investigated the penetration of bioceramic cements into dentinal tubules in root-end cavities. Capasio exhibited a penetration depth ranging from 18 to 264 μm unlike ProRoot MTA, which did not penetrate into the dentinal tubules. By comparison, considering the common diameter of dentinal tubules ranging between 2.0 and 3.2 μm, Bird et al. found a mean particle size of 10 μm for ProRoot MTA and 5.3 μm for Capasio, which also presented 5% particles finer than 1 μm [115].

10.28 Geristore

Modareszadeh et al. define Geristore (Den-Mat LLC, Santa Maria, CA, USA) as a resin-modified glass ionomer [5].

10.28.1 Biological Properties

In a study using human osteosarcoma cell line, Saos-2 Modareszadeh et al. found that the full strength concentration of Geristore reduced the cells bioactivity on days 1 and 3. This diminishing effect occurred only on day 1 at the 50% elute concentration. However, using a chromogenic phosphatase substrate (para-nitrophenylphosphate), it was established that both concentrations of Geristore elute did not affect at all the mineralization activity of ALP [5].

10.29 Radiopaque Dicalcium Silicate Cement (RDSC)

Radiopaque dicalcium silicate cement is quick-setting, aluminum-free calcium silicate cement prepared by a sol–gel method. Chen et al. claim that this method confers a better chemical and structural homogeneity than conventional manufactured ceramic cements [116].

10.29.1 Chemical Composition

According to Chen et al., the powder consists mainly of β-dicalcium silicate (β-Ca_2SiO_4). The phase evolution is dependent on the Si/Ca ratio of its precursors SiO_2 and CaO. It was suggested that β-dicalcium silicate is both a biocompatible and bioactive material since its components are similar to MTA and SiO_2–CaO-based bioactive glass [116].

Chiang et al. proved that by incorporating the radiopacifier (Bi_2O_3), the dicalcium silicate is preserving the biocompatibility and its high bioactivity as well [26].

10.29.2 Physical Parameters

Chiang et al. observed that when mixed with distilled water at liquid/powder ratio 0.5 ml/g, β-dicalcium silicate (β-Ca_2SiO_4) sets within 15–16 minutes. The more rapid set compared to MTA is beneficial due to the diminished risk of blood or tissue fluids contamination or dislodgement [26].

Another study accomplished by Chen et al. showed that the setting time of β-dicalcium silicate cements is inversely proportional to Si/Ca ratio and calcium silicate hydrate formed as final product of hydration reaction. Whenever the amount of calcium silicate hydrate is more elevated the setting time becomes shorter [116].

The setting time of dicalcium silicate may be modified by changing the molar ratio of SiO_2 : CaO in its formulation. Ranging the ratio from 5 : 5 to 3 : 7, Chen et al. found setting times decreasing from 24 ± 2 minutes (ratio 5 : 5) to 16 ± 2 minutes (ratio 4 : 6) and finally to 12 ± 2 minutes (ratio 3 : 7) [116].

Since the SiO_2 : CaO ratios of 4 : 6 (16 ± 2 minutes) and 3 : 7 (12 ± 2 minutes) have shorter setting times, Chen et al. consider these formulations to be useful in cavity lining, direct pulp capping, coronal amputation, and root-end filling [116].

Though higher, the diametrul tensile strength of bismuth oxide-containing β-dicalcium silicate is close to that of the pure formulation (2.1 versus 1.8 MPa). However, Chiang et al. observed that this mechanical property is substantially reduced compared to WMTA (7.4 MPa), due to the same deficient content of calcium silicate hydrate [26].

The compressive strength of aluminum-free calcium silicates is dependent on SiO_2 : CaO molar ratio. Chen et al. proved that the highest value (15.2 MPa) is achieved by equimolar ratio 5 : 5 and the lowest (0.3 MPa) by SiO_2 : CaO ratio of 7 : 3 [116].

It was also observed by Chen et al. that calcium silicate hydrate, the main phase of the hydration reaction of β-dicalcium silicate, in contact with simulate body fluids quickly may form bone-like apatite spherulites that are an indicator of bioactivity because it achieves a chemical bond with human living tissues [116].

Using SEM analysis and energy dispersive spectroscopy, after one hour immersion of radiopaque dicalcium silicate cement in a simulated body fluid similar to human blood plasma, Chen et al. found clusters of precipitated spherulites on pure β-dicalcium silicate surface, having Ca/P and Ca/Si ratios of 1.98 and respectively 6.19 [117]. Another study of SEM analysis accomplished by Chiang et al. also described a more porous surface of both β-dicalcium silicates, with and without radiopacifier bismuth oxide [26].

Chen et al. underline that apatite precipitation represents the outcome of two synergistic factors, the calcium–silicate–hydrate gel structure with its Si–OH functional groups that play the role of nucleation centers and calcium ions as precipitation accelerator [117].

Chiang et al. remind that the pure β-dicalcium silicate has an insufficient radiopacity, of only 1.1 mm aluminum thickness, that is much below the value required by ISO Specification 6876/2001 [26].

In MTA family of cements the successfully used radiopacifier is the bismuth oxide (Bi_2O_3). However, Chiang et al. highlight that when mixed with Portland cement in order to improve the radiopacity, bismuth oxide proved to increase the porosity, extend setting time and lessen the compressive strength [26].

When 20 wt% bismuth oxide is added to β-dicalcium silicate, the radiopacity is enhanced and according to Chiang et al. becomes equivalent to 7.3 mm aluminum thickness but regrettably the setting time is extended up to 24 minutes [26].

Commonly, at pH measurements, Chen et al. found values ranging from an initial 11 up to 13. Since the releasing mechanism of calcium ions is similar to MTA, at one hour after mixing the Bi_2O_3-containing β-dicalcium silicate displays an alkaline pH of 12.7, which is an intermediate value between pure β-dicalcium silicate (pH 13.5) and WMTA (pH 12.5). Chiang et al. [26] showed that the radiopacifier somewhat lowers pH value compared to pure β-dicalcium silicate since during the hydration reaction occurs decreased calcium silicate hydrate [117].

10.29.3 Biological Properties

Chiang et al. found that β-dicalcium silicate increases MG63 human osteoblast-like cell viability. A possible reason might be the lack of aluminum oxide (Al_2O_3) that is neurotoxin acting by disruption of cellular homeostasis and promoting cellular oxidation [26].

Though initially at one day the cell viability was stronger stimulated by WMTA, after seven days the viability of cells seeded on bismuth oxide-containing β-dicalcium silicate cement was significantly more elevated than that cultured on WMTA specimens [26].

Another study, of Chen et al., found that the viability of MG63 human osteoblast-like cells BCRC 60279 seeded on pure β-dicalcium silicate increased up to 23% after seven days incubation. The cells preserved their intact flat morphology, attached, proliferated, and spread on the cement surface [117].

Incubating radiopaque dicalcium silicate cement and white ProRoot MTA with L929 mouse fibroblast cells (BCRC 60279), Wu et al. proved that either the absence of cytotoxicity or cell attachments after seeding the fibroblasts on freshly mixed and set cements was comparable [118].

In a comparative *in vitro* study of radiopaque dicalcium silicate cement and white ProRoot MTA on hDPCs sampled from caries-free, intact premolar, Chen et al. investigated the cell cycle phases of subG1 (cell death), G1 (interval between mitosis and initiation of DNA synthesis), S (DNA replication), and G2 (protein synthesis and preparation for mitosis) using the propidium iodide flow cytometric assay. In all four phases of cell cycle, there was no significant difference between the two bioceramic cements [119].

Accordingly, the results mirroring the subG1 phase (cell death) too, it might be suggested that similar to white ProRoot MTA the newly radiopaque dicalcium silicate cement did not provoke the apoptosis of pulp cells [119].

The immune response of hDPCs to radiopaque dicalcium silicate cement was found by Chen et al. less intense than to white ProRoot MTA, though no significant differences were demonstrated regarding proinflammatory IL-1 (interleukin-1) and iNOS (inducible nitric oxide synthase) [119].

IL-1 is controlling the bone turnover and activates iNOS pathway in bone cells. Initially, radiopaque dicalcium silicate cement and white ProRoot MTA, when incubated with dental pulp cells, triggered more elevated values of IL-1 and iNOS while later their expression gradually diminished [119].

In cell cultures of hDPCs Chen et al. noticed that the expression of ALP, bone sialoprotein, and OC did not exhibit a difference between radiopaque dicalcium silicate cement and white ProRoot MTA. Nevertheless especially the time-depending values of bone sialoprotein and OC were higher compared to control, suggesting the stimulating activity of bioceramic cements [119].

The antibacterial activity of fresh-mixed radiopaque dicalcium silicate cement is high enough to inhibit the growth of *E. faecalis* ATCC 29212. Although the ProRoot MTA had a stronger inhibitory effect, Wu et al. could not prove a significant difference between these two cements. Moreover, both of them did not demonstrate to be fully effective against this pathogenic strain [118].

10.30 Calcium-enriched Mixture (CEM) Cement

10.30.1 Chemical Composition

Asgary et al. mention that CEM cement (Bionique Dent, Tehran, Iran) contains lime as a major constituent and the other components, excepting some trace elements, are greatly different in concentration from those in WMTA [120].

According to Asgary et al. and Parirokh and Torabinejad [6], lime (51.81%), SO_3 (9.48%), P_2O_5 (8.52%), Na_2O (0.35%), and H&C (22.2%) are present in higher proportion compared to WMTA, while some other components such as SiO_2 (6.28%), Al_2O_3 (0.95%), MgO (0.23%), and Cl (0.18%) are in lower concentration [120].

By using electron probe microanalysis, Asgary et al. found that phosphorus is a CEM major component, in contrast to Portland cements and MTA, where its presence is situated at the detection limit. The X-ray intensity maps showed the absence of phosphorus in surrounding dentin when MTA retrograde filling was investigated, while in case of CEM the same chemical element was almost even distributed both in the filling material and neighboring radicular dentin [40].

10.30.2 Physical Parameters

Asgary et al. claim that ranging from 0.075 to 0.085 mm (setting expansion changes), 4.5 to 5 minutes (working time), and 10.71 to 10.61 (pH), the CEM and WMTA values are not significantly different [120].

Conversely, differences were encountered in setting time being shorter for CEM (50 minutes) versus WMTA (70 minutes), CEM film thickness of 174 µm compared to 452 µm in WMTA, or better flow of CEM (14 mm) than WMTA (10 mm) due to more elevated frequency of small particles (0.5–2.5 µm diameter) in CEM composition [120].

Different *in vitro* investigating methods such dye leakage, fluid filtration, and bacterial penetration proved that CEM is a reliable material for retrograde filling. Due to reasonable film thickness, flow and push-out strength, and its sealing ability, Parirokh and Torabinejad consider CEM comparable to white ProRoot MTA and MTA Angelus [6].

However, Parirokh and Torabinejad agree that an explicit drawback of CEM is its inadequate radiopacity (2.227 mm Al), lower than ProRoot MTA (5.009 mm Al) or MTA Angelus (5.589 mm Al), that does not correspond to 3 mm Al requirements of ANSI/ADA Specification 57/2000 and ISO 6876/2001 for root canal sealers [6].

10.30.3 Biological Properties

When mixing, Asgary et al. found that CEM develops a high alkalinity (pH 10.71) due to generated calcium hydroxide that dissociates into calcium and hydroxyl ions. The presence of elevated calcium and phosphate ions in CEM, following interaction with surrounding tissue fluids, stimulates interfacial formation and deposition of coarse crystals, comparable to hydroxyapatite, on filling surface [120].

Later on was proved that CEM endogenous source of calcium and phosphate ions actually induced a hydroxyapatite precipitate, which gradually covered and sealed the endodontic material in a biologic way. Asgary et al. [40] and Nosrat and Asgary [121] noticed that since hydroxyapatite is the main component of dentin and the surface composition of set CEM cement was found similar to dentin, whenever CEM is used the healing process in periradicular surgery might be regarded as having a natural course.

Investigating the cell viability of different cell cultures as L929 mouse fibroblast cells or human gingival fibroblasts after interacting with CEM or ProRoot MTA, despite some not significant discrepancies, both materials displayed less toxicity compared to the traditional IRM used since many years in periradicular surgery. However, according to Parirokh and Torabinejad, CEM and ProRoot MTA might act suppressive on neural cell excitability [6].

Since subcutaneous implantation is recognized as one of the most suitable local *in vivo* biocompatibility tests, Parirokh et al. compared the connective tissue reaction of Wistar albino rats to implants of CEM and white and gray MTA at 7-, 30-, and 60-days intervals [122].

After one week, there were no significant differences regarding the spreading and severity of inflammatory process between CEM and both MTA cements. However, as opposed to MTA, in CEM specimens, there was not signaled tissue necrosis [122].

The absence of necrosis around CEM as compared to MTA specimens might be explained by lower pH, setting temperature, and down streamed IL-1 and IL-6 proinflammatory cytokine production as well [122].

At 30-days period in all tested cements was still present a substantially diminished inflammation and the CEM implants were surrounded by a thinner connective tissue capsule. Despite the lowest extension of inflammation in CEM specimens, no significant differences were found after 60 days among CEM and gray and WMTA regarding the thickness of connective tissue capsule and intensity of inflammation.

Since dystrophic calcification occurred at 33% in CEM and gray MTA, and 22% in WMTA, Parirokh et al. suggested that these cements are potentially osteoinductive [122].

Pulpotomy is another kind of vital therapy that aims to preserve a healthy and uninflamed dental pulp in immature permanent teeth in order to allow apexogenesis.

Studying the histological pulp response to CEM after two months in cervical pulpotomy in dogs, Tabarsi et al. observed that pulp vitality, calcified bridge formation and lack of pulp tissue inflammation were equivalent in teeth capped with either CEM or MTA and significantly more frequent in those teeth capped with calcium hydroxide, the former traditional material used in vital pulpotomies [123].

The alkalinity of CEM is also supporting its antibacterial effect. Parirokh and Torabinejad claim that CEM had higher activity on *Staphylococcus aureus*, *E. coli*, *Pseudomonas aeruginosa*, and *E. faecalis* than white and gray ProRoot MTA, while the fungicidal effect on *C. albicans* was similar to white ProRoot MTA [6].

10.30.4 Clinical Studies

In vital treatments of dental pulp in order to avoid the filling displacement, akin to ProRoot MTA, Parirokh and Torabinejad recommend caution in adhesive restorations to protect CEM with resin-modified glass ionomer before acid etching [6].

Since a smoother surface of an endodontic cement placed in direct contact with vital tissues is less irritating, Asgary et al. underline that the small size of CEM particles is critical to avoid an adverse response of surrounding periradicular morphological structures [40].

According to Zarrabi et al., the mineralized dentinal barrier, induced either by former traditional material calcium hydroxide, used in pulp capping or modern MTA and the new-comer CEM, is still a contentious issue in vital pulp therapy since this pulp tissue response of reparative dentin could be both a healing and an irritating one. Moreover, when presenting tunnel defects and insufficient thickness the newly formed dentinal bridge does not protect the pulp from permanent risk of microbial challenges [56].

Since CEM displayed the same biocompatibility, but better handling parameters and shorter setting time, it was suggested to be considered a possible clinical alternative of MTA. Zarrabi et al. reported that when experimentally used as pulp capping material in first humans' premolars scheduled for extractions for orthodontic reasons, CEM showed a favorable response in preserving a vital pulp and no significant differences compared to MTA, currently considered the gold standard in vital treatments [56].

However, compared to MTA, Zarrabi et al. underline that after two months in CEM capped pulps there was less inflammation and was formed a thicker and more tubular reparative dentinal bridge with adequate thickness, bordered by palisade pattern of columnar odontoblast-like cells [56].

It seems that the mechanism of reparative dentin production resembles the primary dentinogenesis. After two weeks, in pulp capping of human premolars, Zarrabi et al. proved that CEM and MTA induce at their direct contact with dental pulp a thin layer of fibrodentine that closes the exposure site. Two months later, the fibrodentine matrix is replaced by a tubular mineralized bridge, but a very thin layer is still present at interface with the juxtaposed new differentiated odontoblast-like cells [56].

During first two weeks of regenerative dentin formation after pulp capping with CEM, Zarrabi et al. noticed that the extracellular matrix of dental pulp is highly enriched in fibronectin, a glycoprotein belonging to adhesive proteins, which is involved in recruitment, growth, and differentiation of odontoblasts, and further in their polarization and migration [56].

Tenascin, another glycoprotein found in extracellular matrix of dental pulp, which is produced by fibroblasts and stimulates odontoblasts differentiation, showed also a comparable elevated level at two weeks after using CEM in capping [56].

Zarrabi et al. [56] and Zarrabi et al. [124] concluded that the high expression of fibronectin and tenascin has substantiated the role of both pulp capping materials MTA and CEM in stimulating fibrodentinal matrix formation, which on its turn is pivotal for cells recruitment and odontoblasts differentiation.

At two months time period of pulp capping with CEM, when the fibrodentin barrier turns to a calcified one, there was reported a decrease in secretion of both glycoproteins. It was underlined by Zarrabi et al. that these noncollagenous proteins, fibronectin and tenascin, are highly expressed in dental pulp only during cell migration and differentiation. Later on, they gradually diminishing as the fibrodentin matrix turns into mineralized dentinal bridge and finally are restricted to the unmineralized border of the calcified barrier of reparative dentin [56].

A successful outcome was also obtained by Asgary et al. using direct pulp capping with CEM cement in a mature molar with symptomatic pulpitis associated with symptomatic apical periodontitis. After 15 months follow-up, the tooth preserved its vitality without any acute or chronic inflammatory symptoms. The radiograph displayed a normal width of periodontal ligament space and no signs of periapical radiolucency [57].

Nosrat and Asgary also recommend the use of CEM in pulp pathology of permanent immature teeth. After completing pulpotomy in a mandibular second molar with immature roots, due to a history of lingering pain, the radicular pulp was capped with CEM. The final assessment at 12 months revealed the complete root development and formation of a mineralized bridge underneath the capping material [58].

Since the tooth preserved the vitality and clinical and radiographic examinations showed no signs and symptoms of either acute or chronic pulpitis, Nosrat and Asgary suggested that CEM may be successfully used in immature symptomatic teeth to achieve apexogenesis [58].

Nosrat and Asgary also proved that CEM, due to its biocompatibility, sealing ability, high alkalinity, and tight bacterial seal is a reliable pulp capping material for apexogenesis in traumatized immature teeth, even with a delay up to one month after dental pulp exposure [58].

At 12 months recall after such pulpotomy performed in an upper central incisor using CEM, Nosrat and Asgary ascertained radiographically the completion of root development, apex formation, and a continuous calcified bridge with no tunnel defects or irregularities underneath the capping agent [58].

10.31 Calcium Silicate

Parirokh and Torabinejad mention Calcium Silicate as an experimental sealer [6].

10.31.1 Chemical Composition

According to Parirokh and Torabinejad the powder of Calcium Silicate contains tricalcium silicate, dicalcium silicate, tricalcium aluminate in small amount, calcium sulfate, and bismuth oxide as radiopacifier. The liquid is an aqueous solution of a polymer [6].

Based on X-ray diffraction study, Chen et al. claim that basically Calcium Silicate and ProRoot MTA are the same materials. Calcium Silicate contains CaO, SiO_2, and Al_2O_3 as matrices and ZnO, MgO, and Fe_2O_3 as additives [125].

10.31.2 Physical Parameters

Though still unsettled, the physical properties of Calcium Silicate are considered acceptable or similar to MTA. However, Chen et al. proved that the setting time is definitely shorter than MTA [125].

Parirokh and Torabinejad showed Calcium Silicate release after setting calcium and hydroxyl ions. The apatite precipitates observed on the material surface after contacting phosphate ions in surrounding fluids proves its expected bioactivity [6].

Loading the Calcium Silicate cement with 25% atomized gold (Sigma-Aldrich, Gillingham, UK) and 20% powdered silver/tin alloy (Degussa Dental, Hanau, Germany), without to modify the hydrated microstructure typical for Portland cement, Camilleri noticed that the radiopacity becomes equal to ProRoot MTA. Moreover, the included heavy metals gold, silver, and tin are just fillers so they are not involved in the hydration mechanism like MTA radiopacifier bismuth oxide [27].

10.31.3 Biological Properties

Using tetrazolium bromide colorimetric assay as cell viability test Chen et al. found that Calcium Silicate was biocompatible with MG63 cells up to 15 days of cell culture and also promoted cellular proliferation to the same extent as ProRoot MTA [125].

The ALP activity stimulated by Calcium Silicate is comparable to white ProRoot MTA. In a comparative study on cell cultures, Parirokh and Torabinejad revealed that one week after setting Calcium Silicate exhibited less cytotoxicity than AH Plus, broadly used root canal sealer in dental practice [6].

Ding et al. observed accomplishing an accurate genotoxicity test based on DNA precipitation that Calcium Silicate and white ProRoot MTA are cytocompatible with MG63 cells and, despite the low percentage of DNA breakage, both endodontic cements did not show a significant genotoxicity in order to be considered cancer-causing materials [126].

An *in vitro* study by Bryan et al., investigating the cytotoxicity and osteogenic potential of experimental Calcium Silicate-based sealer (Dentsply Tulsa Dental Specialties), showed that in direct contact with osteogenic mouse preosteoblast cell line MC3T3-E1 did not interfere with bone regeneration and exhibited minimal tissue toxicity [127].

Searching for SDH activity by MTT assay, Bryan et al. noticed after two weeks a mild cytotoxicity in case of Calcium Silicate and AH Plus sealers. The toxicity of both sealers decreased over time but it took three weeks to completely move out [127].

Chen et al. found that both Calcium Silicate and ProRoot MTA appear to be osteoconductive despite their different patterns of bone markers expression in human osteosarcoma MG63 cell, which is a cell line with proved remodeling potential. Type I collagen showed a time-dependent increase up to 15 days for both materials in contrast to bone sialoprotein, which started decreasing at day 15, whereas ALP and OC expression was higher in case of Calcium Silicate [125].

According to Bryan et al., in osteogenic medium AH Plus induced a higher expression of ALP activity compared to similar values of Calcium Silicate sealer and white ProRoot MTA. This issue suggests that both Calcium Silicate and white ProRoot MTA down-regulate the differentiation of preosteoblast without to suppress MC3T3-E1 cell growth. Accordingly, Calcium Silicate sealer requires an extended time period to stimulate osteoblasts differentiation and subsequent bone formation [127].

Chen et al. proved that Calcium Silicate-based sealers and white ProRoot MTA showed short-term and long-term biocompatibility with primary cultured hDPCs, which are more sensitive to test than established cell lines. However, both sealers proved to induce pulp cell inflammation by increasing cyclooxygenase-2 (COX-2) expression [128].

Using RT-PCR, Chen et al. also observed in short term (three days) that the proinflammatory cytokines stimulated a high COX-2 production, unlike the long-term experimental period (seven days) when the value of the same inflammatory marker decreased [128].

10.32 EndoBinder

10.32.1 Chemical Composition

Aguilar et al. claim that EndoBinder (Binderware, São Carlos, Brazil) is prepared by calcining Al_2O_3 and $CaCO_3$ at temperatures between 1315 and 1425 °C. From the resulted calcium aluminate are eliminated oxides that induce undesired expansion (MgO and CaO) or color darkening of the tooth (Fe_2O_3) and is added a radiopacifier (bismuth oxide) [129].

According to Oliveira et al. in a similar product Secar-71 (Kerneos, Neuilly sur Seine, France) the proportion of CaO (62.40%) and Al_2O_3 (4.40%) met within WMTA Angelus is completely changed in the calcium aluminate cement (CAC), as follows: Al_2O_3 68.5% and CaO 29.5% [130].

Oliveira et al. also say that calcium aluminate product is made up by two main compounds, Al_2O_3 (68.5%) and CaO (29.5%) and broadly comprises two phases, calcium aluminate ($CaO{\cdot}Al_2O_3$) and calcium dialuminate ($CaO{\cdot}2Al_2O_3$), that in contact with water release Ca^{2+}, OH^-, and $Al(OH)_4{}^-$ ions [130].

Using a more detailed stoichiometric analysis, Oliveira et al. noticed that actually there are involved in hydration reaction three main phases in following proportion: $CaO{\cdot}Al_2O_3$ (40–70%), $CaO{\cdot}2Al_2O_3$ (>25%), and $12CaO{\cdot}7Al_2O_3$ (about 10%) [130].

During hydration reaction a precipitate of calcium aluminate hydrate and aluminum hydroxide is formed:

$$3(CaO \cdot 2Al_2O_3) + 12H_2O \rightarrow Ca_3[Al(OH)_4]_2(OH)_4 + 4Al(OH)_3$$

10.32.2 Physical Parameters

Compared to MTA, Oliveira et al. found a shorter setting time, close to 20 minutes, due to lithium carbonate (Li_2CO_3) added in proportion 1 : 1 to CaO to accelerate the hydration. The Li^+ ions initiate the formation of $LiAl(OH)_4$, an insoluble compound, and elevates Ca^{2+} concentration at interface to tissue fluids [28]. The $LiAl(OH)_4$ crystals deposition plays the role of precipitation nuclei for calcium aluminate hydrates [130].

A shorter setting time is clinically extremely advantageous since it reduces the solubility and disintegration of the endodontic material in tissue fluids. Oliveira et al. has also underlined that while setting the temperature of calcium aluminates cement increases with 20 °C [130].

A comparative *in vitro* study of Garcia et al. showed that EndoBinder had significantly higher shear bond strength to dentin (2.99 ± 0.17 MPa) than WMTA (2.51 ± 0.38 MPa). It was concluded that this cement might be an alternative to MTA [131].

Oliveira et al. proved that the pH values of CACs exhibit slower increase than MTA cements because aluminum hydroxide is insoluble in water and calcium aluminate hydrate is releasing at a slower rate Ca^{2+} and OH^- ions [130].

Calcium aluminates cements exhibit improved fluidity and handling properties than WMTA Angelus. According to Oliveira et al. they also proved reduced porosity and a compressive strength almost 2.5 times greater than MTA by addition of dispersant, plasticizer, and radiopacifier [130].

Aguilar et al. [132] and Oliveira et al. [28] noticed that calcium aluminates cements in the presence of bismuth oxide respects ISO 6876 recommendations, exhibiting a radiopacity similar to gray MTA.

After introducing bismuth oxide in its initial formulation, Aguilar et al. found that EndoBinder demonstrated an adequate radiopacity because the attained values were greater than 3 mm of the aluminum scale, the minimal standard required by ISO 6876 recommendations [132].

10.32.3 Biological Properties

A novel CAC+, similar to EndoBinder, and composed mainly by 68.5% Al_2O_3 and 29.5% CaO was found in a study of Castro-Raucci et al. that stimulated *in vitro* a stronger differentiation of preosteoblastic MC3T3-E1 cells than WMTA Angelus. The same higher values were recorded for cells density, total protein content and ALP activity too [133].

Castro-Raucci et al. say that the better biological performance of CAC+ might be explained by lower releasing potential of calcium hydroxide compared to MTA Angelus. Accordingly, an attractive hypothesis suggests that various level of calcium hydroxide release would provide adequately designed materials for a more differentiate pH-based endodontic use [133].

At seven days after surgery in a subcutaneous implant study on male Wistar rats, Oliveira et al. observed in EndoBinder a moderate inflammatory infiltrate formed by neutrophils, mononuclear phagocytes, fibroangioblastic proliferation, collagen synthesis, blood vessel neoformation, and some inflammatory giant cells [130].

Additionally, congested blood vessels, edema, and necrotic residue occurred in gray MTA Angelus specimens. After three weeks the inflammatory cell infiltrate diminished, excepting gray MTA Angelus still surrounded by discrete mononuclear phagocytes and inflammatory giant cells infiltrate [130].

The final microscopic analysis, at 42-days period, showed around EndoBinder implants a reduced number of mononuclear cells as opposed to gray MTA Angelus implants that were surrounded by discrete fibroangioplastic proliferation, some mononuclear phagocytes, and foreign body giant cells. Oliveira et al. also observed that the dimension of inflammatory capsule decreased in both materials, particularly in EndoBinder specimens [130].

To assess the biocompatibility of an endodontic material, much more important than the initial irritant effect is the duration of its activity in the intimate contact with tissues. Oliveira et al. explain the persistence of chronic inflammation in case of gray MTA Angelus implants by its well-known prolonged release of hydroxyl ions. Conversely, EndoBinder is less irritant and cytotoxic without losing its antimicrobial efficiency since it releases slowly a reduced quantity of irritant ions [130].

Both MTA and CACs proved to be bioactive in contact with phosphorus in liquid environment. However, according to Oliveira et al., MTA preferentially stimulates the precipitation of carbonated apatite that might be used in filling the bone defects since it is bioresorbable material, as opposed to calcium aluminate that generates hydroxyapatite, a recognized osteoconductive material [28].

10.33 Quick-Set

10.33.1 Chemical Composition

Kramer et al. claim that Quick-Set (Avalon Biomed, Bradenton, USA) is bioactive calcium aluminosilicate cement [53].

10.33.2 Physical Parameters

According to Kramer et al., Quick-Set has lower pH (10.9 ± 0.5) than MTA (11.6 ± 0.5) but unlike MTA showed deeper penetration in dentinal tubules [53].

10.33.3 Biological Properties

Kramer et al. affirm that Quick-Set improves the inflammatory response after capping. It has equivalent properties to MTA in pulp-capping (viable option) [53].

10.34 Bioceramic Gutta-percha

Wang presents EndoSequence BC Points (Brasseler, Savannah, USA) as a new product of stiffened gutta-percha cones, impregnated and coated with bioceramic nanoparticles [21].

It is also claimed by Wang that the use of EndoSequence BC Points with EndoSequence BC Sealer guarantees three-dimensional root canal fillings of monobloc-type [21].

10.35 Bioactive Glasses

Gong et al. mention bioactive glasses as a category of calcium silicate-based highly biocompatible dental materials that exhibit osteoinductive and osteoconductive functions [134].

10.35.1 Chemical Composition

According to Zehnder et al., the common composition of bioactive glasses that are studied as alternative of traditional antiseptic medication is based mainly on the system SiO_2–Na_2O–CaO–P_2O_5. The powder of S53P4 bioactive glass (Abmin Technologies, Turku, Finland) is composed of 53% SiO_2, 23% Na_2O, 20% CaO, and 4% P_2O_5 [135].

Gong et al. underlined that the chemical formulation may also depend on manufacturing procedure. Thus sol–gel 58S bioactive glass is composed of 58% SiO_2, 33% CaO, and 9% P_2O_5 whereas the traditional melt 45S5 contains 45% SiO_2, 24.5% Na_2O, 24.5% CaO, and 6% P_2O_5 [134].

Gubler et al. mention that there are also bioactive glasses in nanoparticulate form with varying formulation, depending on their content of sodium, such as 28S5, 45S5, and 77S. Bioactive glass 28S5 has a higher percent of Na_2O (42%) than bioactive glass 45S5 (24.5%), but lowers SiO_2 (27.5% versus 45%). Both glasses contain CaO and P_2O_5 to the same extent as the powder of S53P4. The bioactive glass 77S has no sodium and a reduced proportion of CaO (16.3%) and P_2O_5 (4%) [136].

In addition to polyisoprene or polycaprolactone, Mohn et al. specify that the nanosized bioactive glass 45S5 can also be used to synthesize composite systems of sealers for root canal filling that preserve the high bioactivity of bioglasses and develop an improved immediate sealing efficacy [137].

10.35.2 Physical Parameters

The previous traditional bioglasses had micron-sized particles regardless the manufacturing process, either by melting (1–10 μm) or by sol–gel procedure (2–20 μm). Gong et al. noticed that the novel nano-sized 58S sol–gel particles of bioglass have more regular size (10–100 nm), a higher specific reactive area, and improved bioactivity [134].

Based on sodium oxide release after S53P4 bioactive glass wetting and the incorporation of protons into the corroding glass, Zehnder et al. [135] and Gubler et al. [136] mentioned that the aqueous suspension achieves pH value of 11, which does not differ from that of its combination with dentin powder. Unlike the pH values of 28S5 and 45S5 bioactive glasses, which is similar to calcium hydroxide, the pH of sodium-free 77S formulation is lower than value of 10.

While existing in suspension an excess of calcium and phosphates, which can be also delivered by dentin, Zehnder et al. noticed that there occurs Ca/P precipitates on bioactive glass surfaces extended around even up to 2 mm [135].

Nanometric bismuth oxide-containing bioactive glass can form slowly on its surface a layer of hydroxyapatite which was found by Mohn et al. to be thinner and less apparently structured than that of original bioglass [138].

According to Mohn et al. novel flame spray-derived nanosized bioactive glass including bismuth oxide up to 50 wt% exhibited a radiopacity equivalent to 4.94 mm of aluminum thickness, which corresponds to ISO 6876/2001 specification for clinical use [138].

Adding to original formulation of nanometric bioactive glass 20% bismuth oxide, Mohn et al. observed no difference in alkaline capacity. However, increasing the same radiopacifier up to 50% the alkaline capacity decreased though remained higher than that of mechanically prepared mixture [138].

The nanosized bioactive glass with bismuth oxide preserved the *in vitro* alkaline capacity and bioactivity of pure material. Mohn et al. proved that a densely packed material demonstrated a higher alkaline capacity than an uncompressed one, which is of clinical relevance because the high level of pH suggests an antibacterial potential of bioactive glasses [138].

Mohn et al. also observed that unlike the homogenous dispersion of 30 wt% glass in combination with polycaprolactone, the incorporation of 30 wt% nano-sized particles of 45S5 bioactive glass in a composite compound based on polyisoprene creates a rough surface [138].

After 30 days of immersion in simulate body fluid, mature apatite crystals completely covered the polyisoprene composite, whereas the apatite structures on polycaprolactone composite were still growing [138].

The bioglass content of composite material can also induce an interfacial hydroxyapatite layer between composite sealer and dentin wall of the root canal. Accordingly, Mohn et al. presume that the clinical outcome might be ideal because the bioactive glass, with its initial disinfection activity, is gradually transformed in inert calcium phosphate that completely seal the endodontic system [138].

10.35.3 Biological Properties

Mohn et al. claim that bioactive glasses release calcium, silica, phosphate, and sodium [138]. Gong et al. explains the enhanced bioactivity of nano-sized 58S based on higher concentration of calcium and silicon ions release, in a short time, than former micron-sized bioactive glasses [134].

An *in vitro* study on hDPCs showed that all investigated bioactive glasses promoted on days 1–3 the mRNA expression of DMP1, DSPP, Type I collagen, and ALP genes. However, assessing after 21 days of culture the matrix mineralization, Gong et al. found that the nano-58S bioglass stimulated a higher rate of mineralized nodules formation, compared to traditional 58S and 45S5. The same increased efficacy of nano-58S bioglass was demonstrated in inducing pulp cells differentiation [134].

In a comparative study *in vitro* on standardized bovine dentin blocks, seeded with *E. faecalis* strain ATCC 29212, Zehnder et al. showed that a fresh suspension in sterile water of S53P4 bioactive glass proved a stronger antibacterial efficacy in dentinal tubules than commonly used medication of infected root canals with calcium hydroxide [135].

Zehnder et al. mention that the aqueous suspension of S53P4 bioactive glass is not acting immediately against bacteria, because similar to calcium hydroxide, it possesses a late-onset effect that is long-lasting too [135].

Moreover, the antimicrobial efficacy of S53P4 bioactive glass is enhanced *in vitro* by preincubation with powder of dentin. The bacteria might be also destroyed by mineralized Ca/P deposition on their cell surface [135].

Zehnder et al. proved that Ca/P precipitation is initiated by the increased release of silica ions in surrounding environment [139]. Gubler et al. underline that the nanoparticulate bioactive glasses 28S5, 45S5, and 77S also form precipitates of apatite crystals on their surface and on bacteria as well [136].

Compared to calcium hydroxide that almost eradicated the *E. faecalis* strain ATCC 29212 seeded in root canals of mature premolars, Zehnder et al. found that S53P4 bioactive glass exhibited merely a mild antibacterial efficacy [139]. Later on, Gubler et al. proved that nanoparticulate glasses 45S5 and 28S5 have a stronger antibacterial activity on *E. faecalis* strain ATCC 29212 than 77S bioactive glass [136].

However, Zehnder et al. [139] and Gubler et al. [136] recommend to consider the issue of balance between the beneficial antiseptic potential and deleterious outcome to the dentin stability of long-lasting calcium hydroxide root canal dressing because, due its proteolytic action on dentin collagen matrix, this strong antibacterial agent is producing the increase of elasticity module (risk of cracks and fracture of tooth root) and dentin erosions in root canal wall as well.

Mainly the antibacterial alkaline pH is based on sodium release. Another antimicrobial effect depends on continuous release of some other ions species such as calcium and silicon. Compared to 77S, Gubler et al. found that

28S5 and 45S5 bioactive glasses showed higher concentration of silicon ions in aqueous suspensions but no calcium release. Though the bioactive glass 77S achieved a calcium ions concentration of 100–200 ppm, this value is at least five times more reduced than that of traditional calcium hydroxide [136].

As treatment technique it seems that clinically of utmost importance is the consistency of endodontic dressing, since in case of the calcium hydroxide a thinner suspension is more efficient against *E. faecalis* than a thicker one. It was proved by Zehnder et al. that when mixed to thin slurries, both calcium hydroxide and S53P4 bioactive glass, showed a proper antimicrobial efficiency in an infected root canal [139].

10.36 Cimento Endodontico Rapido (CER)

10.36.1 Chemical Composition

Santos et al. [140], Gomes-Filho et al. [141], and Parirokh and Torabinejad [6] claim that Cimento Endodontico Rapido (CER) is composed of Portland cement powder and a gel including water, barium sulfate, and an emulsifier, for better manipulating properties.

10.36.2 Physical Parameters

According to Santos et al. [140] and Santos et al. [142], CER has a faster setting time (7 ± 1 minutes) than MTA Angelus (15 ± 1 minutes). The CER linear coefficient of thermal expansion measured by Santos et al. ($\alpha = 11.76$ μstrain/°) is not significantly different to MTA Angelus (10.90 μstrain/°) and dentin (10.59 μstrain/°).

The extreme temperatures recorded in oral cavity by drinking cold or hot liquids are in the range of 0–67 °C. Santos et al. proved that the thermal expansion of CER, similar to dentin, is a paramount requirement for an ideal sealer to decrease the microleakage between the repair material and root dentin, since the gaps formation, which open the way to microleakage, depends on coefficient of thermal expansion [142].

Santos et al. [140] and Gomes-Filho et al. [141] noticed that similar to MTA and Portland cement, CER in contact with tissue fluids release hydroxyl ions promoting alkalinization, pH increase, and antimicrobial action. Simultaneously, the delivery of calcium ions stimulates the formation of an adjacent calcified tissue barrier.

Santos et al. proved that the hydroxyl and calcium ions release of CER in first 24 hours is higher compared to MTA Angelus, but the difference diminishes during following 24–96 hours and subsequent values become comparable [140].

10.36.3 Biological Properties

Assessing the connective tissue response to CER subcutaneous implants on Wistar albino rats, Gomes-Filho et al. observed that after initial moderate inflammation at 30 and 60 days the chronic inflammatory cell infiltration gradually diminished [141].

The cell density of lymphocytes and macrophages and the reduced thickness of fibrous capsule surrounding the implant were similar to MTA Angelus implants, a material already used in clinical practice. Moreover, the birefringent granulations located in close contact with CER implants suggest the stimulation of mineralization within the connective tissue [141].

Calcium ions release is pivotal not only for inducing the local carbonate apatite formation by interfering with carbon dioxide, which is a nucleus for calcification. Gomes-Filho et al. confirmed that the cell migration and differentiation during the healing process is also calcium dependent [141].

10.37 Endo-CPM Sealer

Parirokh and Torabinejad [3] and Scarparo et al. [143] claim that Endo-CPM Sealer (Egeo srl, Buenos Aires, Argentina) belongs to MTA-based sealers; it is also considered as a white modified Portland cement. Da Silva et al. underline that this cement was synthesized with the aim of combining the biological properties of mineral trioxide aggregate with the clinical requirements of root canal sealer [144].

10.37.1 Chemical Composition

According to Gomes-Filho et al. [145], Parirokh and Torabinejad [3], Scarparo et al. [143], and Parirokh and Torabinejad [6] the hydrophilic powder is formed from MTA 50% (tricalcium silicate, tricalcium oxide, tricalcium aluminate, and other oxides), SiO_2 7%, calcium carbonate 10%, Bi_2O_3 10%, $BaSO_4$ 10%, sodium citrate 1%, propylene glycol 1%, and propylene glycol alginate 1%. The liquid components are saline solution and calcium chloride 10%.

10.37.2 Physical Parameters

Scarparo et al. say that Endo-CPM Sealer powder mixed with its liquid forms a colloidal gel that sets in one hour. It has adequate flow rate and adhesion to root canals walls. The apical sealing properties are similar to gray MTA Angelus [143].

Tanomaru-Filho et al. add that Endo-CPM Sealer may be mixed either with the consistency of a sealer for root canal obturation or in higher proportion powder/liquid to obtain a proper consistency as a retrograde filling in apical resection [146].

Gomes-Filho et al. [145], Scarparo et al. [143], and da Silva et al. [144] proved that Endo-CPM Sealer release hydroxyl and calcium ions by a mechanism similar to MTA, developing an alkaline pH. However, the release of calcium ions is increased compared to Portland cements due to its large amount of calcium carbonate.

Tanomaru-Filho et al. found at three hours after setting that the pH values of Endo-CPM Sealer were between 9.386 and 9.496, depending on lower (sealer) or increased (retrograde filling) consistency of initial mixed paste. After one week the pH values diminished to 8.028 for sealer, respectively 8.098 for retrograde filling. For both consistency pH were still above values of 8 after two weeks and at the end of the study, at four weeks, the recorded values were of 7.745 for sealer and 7.904 for retrograde filling [146].

No significant differences were found by Tanomaru-Filho et al. between pH values of WMTA Angelus and Endo-CPM Sealer, though the addition of calcium chloride to the last one as setting reaction accelerator may increase the pH immediately after manipulation [146].

According to Tanomaru-Filho et al. the calcium ions release of both mixing consistency of Endo-CPM Sealer, especially as sealer and less as retrograde filling, is significantly higher than of WMTA Angelus, demonstrating an obvious potential of bioactivity in almost all periods of the study, up to four weeks [146].

Assmann et al. noticed that the dentin bond strength of Endo-CPM Sealer is significantly higher than other sealers in clinical use, such as MTA Fillapex and AH Plus. Though the push-out test values are elevated, Endo-CPM Sealer is potentially permissive to microleakage compared to resin-based sealers, due to the voids and gaps radiographically detected in root canal filling [147].

The bond failure of Endo-CPM Sealer is mixed, both adhesive and cohesive, in contrast to the other bioceramic sealer MTA Fillapex, which fails at interface with dentin. However, due to the high dentin bond strength Assmann et al. recommend the use of Endo-CPM Sealer when the objective of endodontic treatment involves a post preparation [147].

10.37.3 Biological Properties

Various studies proved the good biocompatibility and biologic potential of Endo-CPM Sealer. Subsequent to subcutaneous implants in Wistar rats, Parirokh and Torabinejad [3], Gomes-Filho et al. [145], Scarparo et al. [143] found mild to moderate inflammatory reaction of connective tissue equivalent with that induced by MTA, including the formation of the protective fibrous capsule, which limits the extension of inflammatory tissue damage.

The addition of calcium carbonate reduces the pH typical value of 12.5 belonging to MTA to 10.00. Gomes-Filho et al. [145], Scarparo et al. [143], and da Silva et al. [141] observed that the surface necrosis of the tissue contacting the set cement is limited, allowing an improved healing. Simultaneously calcium carbonate stimulates the deposition of mineralized tissue by activating ALP.

The Endo-CPM Sealer is also inducing mineralization in soft tissues. In a study on Wistar rats, at 90 days after subcutaneous implantation, Gomes-Filho et al. observed birefringent granulations to polarized light, which surrounded the material. It was found that these granulations were actually calcium carbonate displayed as calcite crystals. The subsequent formation of carbonate apatite is an evidence of bioactivity developed by bioceramic cement in direct contact with rat connective tissue [145].

Despite the mild cytotoxic effect after 24 hours, another *in vitro* study of Gomes-Filho et al. also proved that Endo-CPM Sealer, similar to MTA Angelus, is a biocompatible dental material since it did not inhibit the cell viability of L929 mouse fibroblasts cell line [148].

Endo-CPM Sealer, like MTA Angelus, induces *in vitro* in L929 mouse fibroblasts the release of proinflammatory cytokines IL-1β and IL-6. It has to be mentioned that when IL-1β release of MTA Angelus is significant, the IL-6 secretion is comparable for both cements [148].

Investigating *in vivo* on animal model (Holtzman rats) the biological response of periodontium to Endo-CPM Sealer, when used to repair a furcation perforation in molars, da Silva et al. found at 60 days an adequate biocompatibility and re-establishment of experimentally induced tissue damage [144].

Compared to MTA, the Endo-CPM Sealer showed at 60 days significantly reduced density of chronic inflammatory cells and osteoclasts. It was also observed a continuous layer of osteoblasts on the surface of previous bone injury [144].

The width of the periodontal space in MTA-treated perforations (0.24 mm) was significantly higher than in Endo-CPM Sealer group (0.19 mm) up to 30 days due to the inflammatory process initially induced by MTA in the periodontal ligament. Though compared to healthy control (0.05 mm) the periodontal space remained widened, at the end of observation period (60 days) occurred a similar decrease in width (0.16 mm) for both cements.

It is claimed by Parirokh and Torabinejad that Endo-CPM Sealer exhibits an antimicrobian effect comparable to WMTA Angelus and white ProRoot MTA [3]. Unlike MTA Fillapex, Morgental et al. found that before setting Endo-CPM Sealer showed no antibacterial activity *in vitro* on *E. faecalis* strain ATCC 29212.

However, despite their high pH, seven days after setting neither Endo-CPM Sealer nor MTA Fillapex exhibit an antimicrobial effect on the same strain of *E. faecalis* [78].

10.38 ProRoot Endo Sealer

Weller et al. [60], Camilleri [149], Huffman et al. [61], Parirokh and Torabinejad [6], and Shen et al. [29] claim that ProRoot Endo Sealer (Dentsply, Tulsa, USA) is a calcium silicate bioceramic sealer based on ProRoot MTA.

10.38.1 Chemical Composition

According to Parirokh and Torabinejad, the powder of ProRoot Endo Sealer contains mainly tricalcium silicate, dicalcium silicate, calcium sulfate, bismuth oxide, and tricalcium aluminate. The liquid is a mix of water and a viscous water-soluble polymer [6].

10.38.2 Physical Parameters

Camilleri [149] and Parirokh and Torabinejad [6] mention that the mixing ratio powder/liquid of ProRoot Endo Sealer is 2 : 1.

Weller et al. observed that after setting ProRoot Endo Sealer displayed similar sealing properties to an epoxy resin-based sealer and forms interfacial apatite-like depositions in the apical two thirds of root canals [60]. Huffman et al. found that these mineral deposits consist in spherical amorphous calcium phosphate-like phases, which after immersion in a simulated body fluid are spontaneously transformed in apatite-like phases [61].

Weller et al. [60] and Huffman et al. [61] ascertained that the sealing ability of ProRoot Endo Sealer in conjunction to a gutta-percha cone as core material was similar to epoxy resin-based sealers. Weller et al. also proved that after immersion in a phosphate-containing fluid ProRoot Endo Sealer sealed better the root canals than an usual zinc oxide eugenol-based sealer, Pulp Canal Sealer (SybronEndo, Orange, USA) [60].

When used on its own, without gutta-percha cone, Huffman et al. found that the push-out strength of ProRoot Endo Sealer is almost four times higher compared to epoxy resin-based sealer AH Plus Jet (Dentsply Caulk, Milford, USA) and its failure is of cohesive-type. However, the same study revealed that both ProRoot Endo Sealer and AH Plus Jet achieve a more elevated resistance to dislodgement after immersion in a simulated body fluid [61].

A study using the water-soluble polymer Glenium (Degussa Construction Chemicals, Manchester, UK) mixed with WMTA (Dentsply, Tulsa, USA) Camilleri found that polymer did not affect the hydration mechanism of MTA, because the main typical final products were the calcium–silicate–bismuth hydrate and calcium hydroxide [149].

10.38.3 Biological properties

Huffman et al. observed that ProRoot Endo Sealer is not only a biocompatible ceramic but also a bioactive one, due to the deposition of calcium phosphate crystals on its surface and to subsequent transformation into apatite-like phases [61]. Moreover, Camilleri et al. [41] and Camilleri [96] also demonstrated the biocompatibility of the polymer mixed with other calcium silicate-based formulations.

10.38.4 Clinical Studies

According to Weller et al. [60] and Huffman et al. [61], ProRoot Endo Sealer is recommended in clinical practice for root canal fillings using gutta-percha as core material, regardless the method of obturation, either cold lateral and warm vertical compaction or carrier-based technique.

10.39 Concluding Remarks

Over the past 20 years, mineral trioxide aggregate and similar bioceramic cements revealed superior physicochemical and biological properties to traditional materials used in common endodontic practice.

In the present, bioceramics, due to their high clinical success rate that amazingly rose in recent years, are the material of choice for various endodontic treatments such as pulp capping, pulp amputation, apexification, root-end fillings, root perforation repair, and pulp regeneration.

Moreover, based on their bioactivity, the bioceramics opened an encouraging perspective in controlling the periradicular tissue healing and pulp regeneration. Actually, conservative vital pulp therapy, endodontic surgery, and recently, the regenerative endodontics are the main beneficiaries of new acquisitions in bioceramics technology.

However, since the balance between clinical and histological outcomes is pivotal in both vital pulp therapy and regenerative procedures in nonvital teeth, proper treatment protocols and rigorous long-term clinical studies to confirm the worth of the bioceramics use in endodontics are still required.

Another attractive and extremely practical issue is related to promotion of bioceramic as materials for root canal fillings. Ongoing research seems to be optimistic in proving an efficient bond between bioceramic sealers and root canal walls, able to impede the risk of interfacial microinfiltration that facilitates the treatment failure.

The expectations to eliminate some still-existing shortcomings of endodontic bioceramics could be settled by the newcomers in the family. Nanotechnologies seem to further guarantee the improvement of their physical, chemical, and biological properties.

References

1 Gartner, A.H. and Dorn, S.O. (1992). Advances in endodontic surgery. *Dent. Clin. North Am.* **36**: 357–378.

2 Damas, B.A., Wheater, M.A., Bringas, J.S., and Hoen, M.M. (2011). Cytotoxicity comparison of mineral trioxide aggregates and EndoSequence bioceramic root repair materials. *J. Endod.* **37**: 372–375.

3 Parirokh, M. and Torabinejad, M. (2010). Mineral trioxide aggregate: a comprehensive literature review - Part I: Chemical, physical, and antibacterial properties. *J. Endod.* **36**: 16–27.

4 Lovato, K.F. and Sedgley, C.M. (2011). Antibacterial activity of EndoSequence root repair material and ProRoot MTA against clinical isolates of *Enterococcus faecalis*. *J. Endod.* **37**: 1542–1546.

5 Modareszadeh, M.R., Di Fiore, P.M., Tipton, D.A., and Salamat, N. (2012). Cytotoxicity and alkaline phosphatase activity evaluation of EndoSequence root repair material. *J. Endod.* **38**: 1101–1105.

6 Parirokh, M. and Torabinejad, M. (2014). Calcium silicate-based cements. In: *Mineral Trioxide Aggregate. Properties and Clinical Applications* (ed. M. Torabinejad), 281–332. Oxford: Wiley Blackwell.

7 Zhang, J., Zhu, L., and Peng, B. (2015). Effect of BioAggregate on osteoclast differentiation and inflammatory bone resorption in vivo. *Int. Endod. J.* **48**: 1077–1085.

8 Öncel Torun, Z., Torun, D., Demirkaya, K. et al. (2015). Effects of iRoot BP and white mineral trioxide aggregate on cell viability and the expression of genes associated with mineralization. *Int. Endod. J.* **48**: 986–993.

9 Shokouhinejad, N., Nekoofar, M.H., Razmi, H. et al. (2012). Bioactivity of EndoSequence root repair material and BioAggregate. *Int. Endod. J.* **45**: 1127–1134.

10 Sarkar, N.K., Caicedo, R., Ritwik, P. et al. (2005). Physicochemical basis of the biological properties of mineral trioxide aggregate. *J. Endod.* **31**: 97–100.

11 Tay, F.R., Pashley, D.H., Rueggeberg, F.A. et al. (2007). Calcium phosphate phase transformation produced by the interaction of the Portland cement component of white mineral trioxide aggregate with a phosphate-containing fluid. *J. Endod.* **33**: 1347–1351.

12 Johnson, B.R., Fayad, M.I., and Witherspoon, D.E. (2011). Periradicular surgery. In: *Pathways of the Pulp*, 10e (ed. S. Cohen and K. Hargreaves), 720–776. St. Louis, MO: Mosby Elsevier.

13 Ma, J., Shen, Y., Stojicic, S., and Haapasalo, M. (2011). Biocompatibility of two novel root repair materials. *J. Endod.* **37**: 793–798.

14 Berzins, D.W. (2014). Chemical properties of MTA. In: *Mineral Trioxide Aggregate. Properties and Clinical Applications* (ed. M. Torabinejad), 17–35. Oxford: Wiley Blackwell.

15 Funteas, U.R., Wallace, J.A., and Fochtman, E.W. (2003). A comparative analysis of mineral trioxide aggregate and Portland cement. *Aust. Dent. J.* **29**: 43–44.

16 Dammaschke, T., Gerth, H.U., Zuchner, H., and Schafer, E. (2005). Chemical and physical surface and bulk material characterization of white ProRoot MTA and two Portland cements. *Dent. Mater.* **21**: 731–738.

17 Lee, S.Y., Min, K.S., Choi, G.W. et al. (2012). Effects of simvastatin and enamel matrix derivative on Portland cement with bismuth oxide-induced growth and odontoblastic differentiation in human dental pulp cells. *J. Endod.* **38**: 405–410.

18 Oliveira, T.M., Moretti, A.B., Sakai, V.T. et al. (2013). Clinical, radiographic and histologic analysis of the effects of pulp capping materials used in pulpotomies of human primary teeth. *Eur. Arch. Paediatr. Dent.* **14**: 65–71.

19 Dregger, L.A.S., Fellipe, W.T., Reyes-Carmona, J.F. et al. (2012). Mineral trioxide aggregate and Portland cement promote biomineralization in vivo. *J. Endod.* **38**: 324–329.

20 Hungaro Duarte, M.A., Minotti, P.G., Rodrigues, C.T. et al. (2012). Effect of different radiopacifying agents on the physicochemical properties of white Portland cement and white mineral trioxide aggregate. *J. Endod.* **38**: 394–397.

21 Wang, Z. (2015). Bioceramic materials in endodontics. *Endod. Top.* **32**: 3–30.

22 Saghiri, M.A., Gutmann, J.L., Orangi, J. et al. (2015). Radiopacifier particle size impacts the physical properties of tricalcium silicate-based cements. *J. Endod.* **41**: 225–230.

23 Khalil, I., Naaman, A., and Camilleri, J. (2015). Investigation of a novel mechanically mixed mineral trioxide aggregate (MM-MTA™). *Int. Endod. J.* **48**: 757–767.

24 Tay, K.C.Y., Loushine, B.A., Oxgord, C. et al. (2007). In vitro evaluation of a ceramicrete-based root-end filling material. *J. Endod.* **33**: 1438–1443.

25 Porter, M.L., Bertó, A., Primus, C.M., and Watanabe, I. (2010). Physical and chemical properties of new-generation endodontic materials. *J. Endod.* **36**: 524–528.

26 Chiang, T.Y. and Ding, S.J. (2010). Comparative physicochemical and biocompatible properties of radiopaque dicalcium silicate cement and mineral trioxide aggregate. *J. Endod.* **36**: 1683–1687.

27 Camilleri, J. (2010). Hydration characteristics of calcium silicate cements with alternative radiopacifiers used as root-end filling materials. *J. Endod.* **36**: 502–508.

28 Oliveira, I.R., Andrade, T.L., Jacobovitz, M., and Pandolfelli, V.C. (2013). Bioactivity of calcium aluminate endodontic cement. *J. Endod.* **39**: 774–778.

29 Shen, Y., Peng, B., Yang, Y. et al. (2015). What do different tests tell about the mechanical and biological properties of bioceramic materials? *Endod. Top.* **32**: 47–85.

30 Min, K.S., Kim, H.I., Park, H.J. et al. (2007). Human pulp cells response to Portland cement in vitro. *J. Endod.* **33**: 163–166.

31 D'Antò, V., Di Caprio, M.P., Ametrano, G. et al. (2010). Effect of mineral trioxide aggregate on mesenchymal stem cells. *J. Endod.* **36**: 1839–1843.

32 Reyes-Carmona, J.F., Santos, A.S., Figueiredo, C.P. et al. (2010). Host-mineral trioxide aggregate inflammatory molecular signaling and biomineralization ability. *J. Endod.* **36**: 1347–1353.

33 Shahi, S., Rahimi, S., Yavari, H.R. et al. (2010). Effect of mineral trioxode aggregate and Portland cements on inflammatory cells. *J. Endod.* **36**: 899–903.

34 Al-Hezaimi, K., Salameh, Z., Al-Fouzan, K. et al. (2011). Histomorphometric and micro-computed tomography analysis of pulpal response to three different pulp capping materials. *J. Endod.* **37**: 507–512.

35 Sakai, V.T., Moretti, A.B., Oliveira, T.M. et al. (2009). Pulpotomy of primary molars with MTA and Portland cement: a randomised controlled trial. *Br. Dent. J.* **207**: 128–129, E5 discussion.

36 Barbosa, A.V., Sampaio, G.C., Gomes, F.A. et al. (2009). Short-term analysis of human dental pulps after direct capping with Portland cement. *Open Dent. J.* **3**: 31–35.

37 Marques, N., Lourenço Neto, N., Fernandes, A.P. et al. (2015). Pulp tissue response to Portland cement associated with different radiopacifying agents on pulpotomy of human primary molars. *J. Microsc.* **260**: 281–286.

38 Yan, P., Yuan, Z., Jiang, H. et al. (2010). Effect of BioAggregate on differentiation of human periodontal ligament fibroblasts. *Int. Endod. J.* **43**: 1116–1121.

39 Lee, B.N., Son, H.J., Noh, H.J. et al. (2012). Cytotoxicity of newly developed ortho MTA root-end filling materials. *J. Endod.* **12**: 1627–1630.

40 Asgary, S., Eghbal, M.J., Parirokh, M. et al. (2009). Comparison of mineral trioxide aggregate's composition to Portland cements a new endodontic cement. *J. Endod.* **35**: 243–250.

41 Camilleri, J., Montesin, F.E., Di Silvio, L., and Pitt Ford, T.R. (2005). The chemical constitution and biocompatibility of accelerated Portland cement for endodontic use. *Int. Endod. J.* **38**: 834–842.

42 Choi, Y., Park, S.J., Lee, S.H. et al. (2013). Biological effects and washout resistance of a newly developed fast-setting pozzolan cement. *J. Endod.* **39**: 467–472.

43 Liu, W.N., Chang, J., Zhu, Y.Q., and Zhang, M. (2011). Effect of tricalcium aluminate on the properties of tricalcium silicate-tricalcium alumiate mixtures: setting time, mechanical strength and biocompatibility. *Int. Endod. J.* **44**: 41–50.

44 Reyes-Carmona, J.F., Felippe, M.S., and Felippe, W.T. (2010). The biomineralization ability of mineral trioxide aggregate and Portland cement on dentin enhances the push-out strength. *J. Endod.* **36**: 286–291.

45 Khalil, W.A. and Eid, N.F. (2013). Biocompatibility of BioAggregate and mineral trioxide aggregate on the liver and kidney. *Int. Endod. J.* **46**: 730–737.

46 Hansen, S.W., Marshall, J.G., and Sedgley, C.M. (2011). Comparison of intracanal EndoSequence root repair material and ProRoot MTA to induce pH changes in simulated root resorption defects over 4 weeks in matched pairs of human teeth. *J. Endod.* **37**: 502–506.

47 Kim, M., Yang, W., Kim, H., and Ko, H. (2014). Comparison of the biological properties of ProRoot MTA, OrthoMTA, and Endocem MTA cements. *J. Endod.* **40**: 1649–1653.

48 Hung, C.J., Kao, C.T., Chen, Y.J. et al. (2013). Antiosteoclastogenic activity of silicate-based materials antagonizing receptor activator for nuclear factor kappa B ligand-induced osteoclast differentiation of murine macrophages. *J. Endod.* **39**: 1557–1561.

49 Zhang, H., Shen, Y., Ruse, N.D., and Haapasalo, M. (2009). Antibacterial activity of endodontic sealers by modified direct contact test against Enterococcus faecalis. *J. Endod.* **35**: 1051–1055.

50 Torabinejad, M., Hong, C.U., Pitt Ford, T.R., and Kettering, J.D. (1995). Antibacterial effects of some root end filling materials. *J. Endod.* **21**: 403–406.

51 Miyagak, D.C., de Carvalho, E.M., Robazza, C.R. et al. (2006). In vitro evaluation of the antimicrobial activity of endodontic sealers. *Braz. Oral Res.* **20**: 303–306.

52 Gandolfi, M.G., Siboni, F., Primus, C.M., and Prati, C. (2014). Ion release, porosity, solubility, and bioactivity of MTA Plus tricalcium silicate. *J. Endod.* **40**: 1632–1637.

53 Kramer, P.R., Woodmansey, K.F., White, R. et al. (2014). Capping a pulpotomy with calcium aluminosilicate cement: comparison to mineral trioxideaggregates. *J. Endod.* **40**: 1429–1434.

54 Nowicka, A., Lipski, M., Parafiniuk, M. et al. (2013). Response of human dental pulp capped with biodentine and mineral trioxide aggregate. *J. Endod.* **39**: 743–747.

55 Zhang, S., Yang, X., and Fan, M. (2013). BioAggregate and iRoot BP Plus optimize the proliferation and mineralization ability of human dental pulp cells. *Int. Endod. J.* **46**: 923–929.

56 Zarrabi, M.H., Javidi, M., Jafarian, A.H., and Joushan, B.J. (2010). Histologic assessment of human pulp response to capping with mineral trioxide aggregate and a novel endodontic cement. *J. Endod.* **36**: 1778–1781.

57 Asgary, S., Nosrat, A., and Homayounfar, N. (2012). Periapical healing after direct pulp capping with calcium-enriched mixture cement: a case report. *Oper. Dent.* **37**: 571–575.

58 Nosrat, A. and Asgary, S. (2010). Apexogenesis of a symptomatic molar with calcium enriched mixture: a case report. *Int. Endod. J.* **43**: 940–944.

59 Shinbori, N., Grama, A.M., Patel, Y. et al. (2015). Clinical outcome of endodontic microsurgery that uses EndoSequence BC Root Repair Material as the root-end filling material. *J. Endod.* **41**: 607–612.

60 Weller, R.N., Tay, K.C.Y., Garrett, L.V. et al. (2008). Microscopic appearance and apical seal of root canals filled with gutta-percha and ProRoot Endo Sealer after immersion in a phosphate-containing fluid. *Int. Endod. J.* **41**: 977–986.

61 Huffman, B.P., Mai, S., Pinna, L. et al. (2009). Dislocation resistance of ProRoot Endo Sealer, a calcium silicate-based root canal sealer, from radicular dentine. *Int. Endod. J.* **42**: 34–46.

62 Shi, S., Bao, Z.F., Liu, Y. et al. (2016). Comparison of in vivo dental pulp response to capping with iRoot BP Plus and mineral trioxide aggregate. *Int. Endod. J.* **49**: 154–160.

63 Ribeiro, D.A., Sugui, M.M., Matsumoto, M.A. et al. (2006). Genotoxicity and cytotoxicity of mineral trioxide aggregate and regular and white Portland cements on Chinese hamster ovary (CHO) cells in vitro. *Oral. Surg. Oral Med. Oral Pathol. Oral Radiol. Endod.* **101**: 258–261.

64 Miranda, R.B., Fidel, S.R., and Boller, M.A. (2009). L929 cell response to root perforation repair cements: an in vitro cytotoxicity assay. *Braz. Dent. J.* **20**: 22–26.

65 Camargo, S.E., Camargo, C.H., Hiller, K.A. et al. (2009). Cytotoxicity and genotoxicity of pulp capping materials in two cell lines. *Int. Endod. J.* **42**: 227–237.

66 De Deus, G., Ximenes, R., Gurgel-Filho, E.D. et al. (2005). Cytotoxicity of MTA and Portland cement on human ECV 304 endothelial cells. *Int. Endod. J.* **38**: 604–609.

67 Souza, N.J., Justo, G.Z., Oliveira, C.R. et al. (2006). Cytotoxicity of materials used in perforation repair tested using the V79 fibroblast cell line and the granulocyte-macrophage progenitor cells. *Int. Endod. J.* **39**: 40–47.

68 Guven, G., Cehreli, Z.C., Ural, A. et al. (2007). Effect of mineral trioxide aggregate cements on transforming growth factor beta1 and bone morphogenetic protein production by human fibroblasts in vitro. *J. Endod.* **33**: 447–450.

69 Sipert, C.R., Hussne, R.P., Nishiyama, C.K., and Torres, S.A. (2005). In vitro antimicrobial activity of Fill Canal, Sealapex, Mineral Trioxide Aggregate, Portland cement and EndoRez. *Int. Endod. J.* **38**: 539–543.

70 Faria-Junior, N.B., Tanomaru-Filho, M., Berbert, F.L., and Guerreiro-Tanomaru, J.M. (2013). Antibiofilm activity, pH and solubility of endodontic sealers. *Int. Endod. J.* **46**: 755–762.

71 Sagsen, B., Ustun, Y., Demirbuga, S., and Pala, K. (2011). Push-out bond strength of two new calcium silicate-based endodontic sealers to root canal dentine. *Int. Endod. J.* **44**: 1088–1091.

72 Silva, E.J., Rosa, T.P., Herrera, D.R. et al. (2013). Evaluation of cytotoxicity and physicochemical properties of calcium silicate-based endodontic sealer MTA Fillapex. *J. Endod.* **39**: 274–277.

73 Zhou, H.M., Du, T.F., Shen, Y. et al. (2015). In vitro cytotoxicity of calcium silicatecontaining endodontic sealers. *J. Endod.* **41**: 56–61.

74 Borges, R.P., Sousa-Neto, M.D., Versiani, M.A. et al. (2012). Changes in the surface of four calcium silicate-containing endodontic materials and an epoxy resin-based sealer after a solubility test. *Int. Endod. J.* **45**: 419–428.

75 Amin, S.A., Seyam, R.S., and El-Samman, M.A. (2012). The effect of prior calcium hydroxide intracanal placement on the bond strength of two calcium silicate-based and an epoxy resin-based endodontic sealer. *J. Endod.* **38**: 696–699.

76 Jainaen, A., Palamara, J.E., and Messer, H.H. (2007). Push-out bond strengths of the dentine-sealer interface with and without a main cone. *Int. Endod. J.* **40**: 882–890.

77 Xuereb, M., Vella, P., Damidot, D. et al. (2015). In situ assessment of the setting of tricalcium silicate-based sealers using a dentin pressure model. *J. Endod.* **41**: 111–124.

78 Morgental, R.D., Vier-Pelisser, F.V., Oliveira, S.D. et al. (2011). Antibacterial activity of two MTA-based root canal sealers. *Int. Endod. J.* **44**: 1128–1133.

79 Scelza, M.Z., Linhares, A.B., da Silva, L.E. et al. (2012). A multiparametric assay to compare the cytotoxicity of endodontic sealers with primary human osteoblasts. *Int. Endod. J.* **45**: 12–18.

80 Bin, C.V., Valera, M.C., Camargo, S.E. et al. (2012). Cytotoxicity and genotoxicity of root canal sealers based on mineral trioxide aggregate. *J. Endod.* **38**: 495–500.

81 Salles, L.P., Gomes-Cornélio, A.L., Guimarães, F.C. et al. (2012). Mineral trioxide aggregate-based endodontic sealer stimulates hydroxyapatite nucleation in human osteoblast-like cell culture. *J. Endod.* **38**: 971–976.

82 Assmann, E., Bottcher, D.E., Hoppe, C.B. et al. (2015). Evaluation of bone tissue response to a sealer containing mineral trioxide aggregate. *J. Endod.* **41**: 62–66.

83 Zmener, O., Martinez Lalis, R., Pameijer, C.H. et al. (2012). Reaction of rat subcutaneous connective tissue to a mineral trioxide aggregatebased and a zinc oxide and eugenol sealer. *J. Endod.* **38**: 1233–1238.

84 Tavares, C.O., Bottcher, D.E., Assmann, E. et al. (2013). Tissue reactions to a new mineral trioxide aggregate-containing endodontic sealer. *J. Endod.* **39**: 653–657.

85 Eid, A.A., Gosier, J.L., Primus, C.M. et al. (2014). In vitro biocompatibility and oxidative stress profiles of different hydraulic calcium silicate cements. *J. Endod.* **40**: 255–260.

86 DeLong, C., He, J., and Woodmansey, K.F. (2015). The effect of obturation technique on the push-out bond strength of calcium silicate sealers. *J. Endod.* **41**: 385–388.

87 Viapiana, R., Baluci, C.A., Tanomaru-Filho, M., and Camilleri, J. (2015). Investigation of chemical changes in sealers during application of the warm vertical compaction technique. *Int. Endod. J.* **48**: 16–27.

88 Gonçalves, J.L., Viapiana, R., Miranda, C.E.S. et al. (2010). Evaluation of physico-chemical properties of Portland cements and MTA. *Braz. Oral Res.* **24**: 277–283.

89 Jacinto, R.C., Linhares-Farina, G., Sposito, O.S. et al. (2015). Influence of 2% clorhexidine on pH, calcium release and setting time of a resinous MTA-based root-end filling material. *Braz. Oral Res.* **29**: 1–6.

90 Stowe, T.J., Sedgley, C.M., Stowe, B., and Fenno, J.C. (2004). The effect of chlorhexidine gluconate (0.12%) on the antimicrobial properties of tooth-colored ProRoot mineral trioxide aggregate. *J. Endod.* **30**: 429–431.

91 Torabinejad, M., McDonald, F., and Pitt Ford, T.R. (1995). Physical and chemical properties of a new root-end filling material. *J. Endod.* **21**: 349–353.

92 Hernandez, E.P., Botero, T.M., Mantellini, M.G. et al. (2005). Effect of ProRoot MTA mixed with chlorhexidine on apoptosis and cell cycle of fibroblasts and macrophages in vitro. *Int. Endod. J.* **38**: 137–143.

93 Sumer, M., Muglali, M., Bodrumlu, E., and Guvenc, T. (2006). Reactions of connective tissue to amalgam, intermediate restorative material, mineral trioxide aggregate, and mineral trioxide aggregate mixed with chlorhexidine. *J. Endod.* **32**: 1094–1096.

94 Camilleri, J. (2008). Modification of mineral trioxide aggregate. Physical and mechanical properties. *Int. Endod. J.* **41**: 843–849.

95 Camilleri, J. (2008). Characterization and chemical activity of Portland cement and two experimental cements with potential for use in dentistry. *Int. Endod. J.* **41**: 791–799.

96 Camilleri, J. (2008). The biocompatibility of modified experimental Portland cements with potential for use in dentistry. *Int. Endod. J.* **41**: 1107–1114.

97 Saghiri, M.A., Asgar, K., Lotfi, M., and Garcia-Godoy, F. (2012). Nanomodification of mineral trioxide aggregate for enhanced physicochemical properties. *Int. Endod. J.* **45**: 979–988.

98 Saghiri, M.A., Orangi, J., Tanideh, N. et al. (2014). Effect of endodontic cement on bone mineral density using serial dual-energy x-ray absorptiometry. *J. Endod.* **40**: 648–651.

99 Grech, L., Mallia, B., and Camilleri, J. (2013). Characterization of set Intermediate Restorative Material, Biodentine, BioAggregate and a prototype calcium silicate cement for use as root-end filling materials. *Int. Endod. J.* **46**: 632–641.

100 Elnaghy, A.M. (2014). Influence of acid environment on properties of Biodentine and white mineral trioxie aggregate: a comparative study. *J. Endod.* **40**: 953–957.

101 Corral Nuñez, C.M., Bosomworth, H.J., Field, C. et al. (2014). Biodentine and mineral trioxide aggregate induce similar cellular responses in a fibroblast cell line. *J. Endod.* **40**: 406–411.

102 Chang, S.W., Lee, S.Y., Ann, H.J. et al. (2014). Effects of calcium silicate endodontic cements on biocompatibility and mineralization-inducing potentials in human dental pulp cells. *J. Endod.* **40**: 1194–1200.

103 Tran, X.V., Gorin, C., Willig, C. et al. (2012). Effect of calcium-silicate-based restorative cement on pulp repair. *J. Dent. Res.* **91**: 1166–1171.

104 Zhang, H., Pappen, F.G., and Haapasalo, M. (2009). Dentin enhances the antibacterial effect of mineral trioxide aggregate and BioAggregate. *J. Endod.* **35**: 221–224.

105 Yuan, Z., Peng, B., Jiang, H. et al. (2010). Effect of BioAggregate on mineral-associated gene expression in osteoblast cells. *J. Endod.* **36**: 1145–1148.

106 Alsalleeh, F., Chung, N., and Stephenson, L. (2014). Antifungal activity of EndoSequence root repair material and mineral trioxide aggregate. *J. Endod.* **40**: 1815–1819.

107 Ciasca, M., Aminoshariae, A., Jin, G. et al. (2012). A comparison of the cytotoxicity and proinflammatory cytokine production of EndoSequence Root Repair Material and ProRoot Mineral Trioxide Aggregate in human osteoblast cell culture using reverse-transcriptase polymerase chain reaction. *J. Endod.* **38**: 486–489.

108 Chen, I., Karabucak, B., Wang, C. et al. (2015). Healing after root-end microsurgery by using mineral trioxide aggregate and a new calcium silicate-based bioceramic material as root end filling materials in dogs. *J. Endod.* **41**: 389–399.

109 Setzer, P.C., Shah, S.B., Kohli, M.R. et al. (2010). Outcome of endodontic surgery: a meta-analysis of the literature - Part 1: Comparison of traditonal root-end surgery and endodontic microsurgery. *J. Endod.* **36**: 1757–1765.

110 Liu, S. and Wang, S. (2015). Evaluation of a bioceramic as a pulp capping agent in vitro and in vivo. *J. Endod.* **41**: 652–657.

111 De-Deus, G., Canabarro, A., Alves, G.G. et al. (2012). Cytocompatibility of the ready-to-use bioceramic putty repair cement iRoot BP Plus with primary human osteoblasts. *Int. Endod. J.* **45**: 508–513.

112 Nagas, E., Uyanik, M.O., Eymirli, A. et al. (2012). Dentin moisture conditions affect the adhesion of root canal sealers. *J. Endod.* **38**: 240–244.

113 Wang, Z., Shen, Y., and Haapasalo, M. (2014). Dentin extends the antibacterial effect of endodontic sealers against *Enterococcus faecalis* biofilms. *J. Endod.* **40**: 505–508.

114 Loushine, B.A., Bryan, T.E., Looney, S.W. et al. (2011). Setting properties and cytotoxicity evaluation of a premixed bioceramic root canal sealer. *J. Endod.* **37**: 673–677.

115 Bird, D.C., Komabayashi, T., Guo, L. et al. (2012). In vitro evaluation of dentinal tubule penetration and biomineralization ability of a new root-end filling material. *J. Endod.* **38**: 1093–1096.

116 Chen, C.C., Ho, C.C., Chen, C.H.D., and Ding, S.J. (2009). Physicochemical properties of calcium silicate cements for endodontic treatment. *J. Endod.* **35**: 1288–1291.

117 Chen, C.C., Ho, C.C., Chen, C.H.D. et al. (2009). In vitro bioactivity and biocompatibility of dicalcium silicate cements for endodontic use. *J. Endod.* **35**: 1554–1557.

118 Wu, B.C., Wei, C.K., Hsueh, N.S., and Ding, S.J. (2015). Comparative cell attachment, cytotoxicity and antibacterial activity of radiopaque dicalcium silicate cement and white-coloured mineral trioxide aggregate. *Int. Endod. J.* **48**: 268–276.

119 Chen, C.C., Shie, M.Y., and Ding, S.J. (2011). Human dental pulp cell responses to new calcium silicate-based endodontic materials. *Int. Endod. J.* **44**: 836–842.

120 Asgary, S., Shahabi, S., Jafarzadeh, T. et al. (2008). The properties of a new endodontic material. *J. Endod.* **34**: 990–993.

121 Nosrat, A. and Asgary, S. (2010). Apexogenesis treatment with a new endodontic cement: a case report. *J. Endod.* **36**: 912–914.

122 Parirokh, M., Mirsoltani, B., Raoof, M. et al. (2011). Comparative study of subcutaneous tissue responses to a novel root-end filling material and white and grey mineral trioxide aggregate. *Int. Endod. J.* **44**: 283–289.

123 Tabarsi, B., Parirokh, M., Eghbal, M.J. et al. (2010). A comparative study of dental pulp response to several pulpotomy agents. *Int. Endod. J.* **43**: 565–571.

124 Zarrabi, M.H., Javidi, M., Jafarian, A.H., and Joushan, B.J. (2011). Immunohistochemical expression of fibronectin and tenascin in human tooth pulp capped with mineral trioxide aggregate and a novel endodontic cement. *J. Endod.* **37**: 1613–1618.

125 Chen, C.L., Huang, T.H., Ding, S.J. et al. (2009). Comparison of calcium and silicate cement and mineral trioxide aggregate biologic effects and bone markers expression in MG63 cells. *J. Endod.* **35**: 682–685.

126 Ding, S.J., Kao, C.T., Chen, C.L. et al. (2010). Effects of mineral trioxide aggregate and calcium silicate cements. *J. Endod.* **36**: 1158–1162.

127 Bryan, T.E., Khechen, K., Bracket, M.G. et al. (2010). In vitro osteogenic potential of an experimental calcium silicate-based root canal sealer. *J. Endod.* **36**: 1163–1169.

128 Chen, C.L., Kao, C.T., Ding, S.J. et al. (2010). Expression of the inflammatory marker cyclooxygenase-2

in dental pulp cells cultured with mineral trioxide aggregate or calcium silicate cements. *J. Endod.* **36**: 465–468.

129 Aguilar, F.G., Roberti Garcia, L.F., and Panzeri Pires-de-Souza, F.C. (2012). Biocompatibility of new calcium aluminate cement (EndoBinder). *J. Endod.* **38**: 367–371.

130 Oliveira, I.R., Pandolfelli, V.C., and Jacobovitz, M. (2010). Chemical, physical and mechanical properties of a novel calcium aluminate endodontic cement. *Int. Endod. J.* **43**: 1069–1076.

131 Garcia, L.F.R., Rossetto, H.L., and Pires-de-Souza, F.C.P. (2014). Shear bond strength of novel calcium aluminate-based cement (EndoBinder) to root dentine. *Eur. J. Dent.* **8**: 498–503.

132 Aguilar, F.G., Roberi Garcia, L.F., Rossetto, H.L., and Pardini, L.C. (2011). Radiopacity evaluation of calcium aluminate cement containing different radiopacifying agents. *J. Endod.* **37**: 67–71.

133 Castro-Raucci, L.M.S., Oliveira, I.R., Teixeira, L.N. et al. (2011). Effects of a novel calcium aluminate cement on the early events of the progression of osteogenic cell cultures. *Braz. Dent. J.* **22**: 99–104.

134 Gong, W., Huang, Z., Dong, Y. et al. (2014). Ionic extraction of a novel nano-sized bioactive glass enhances differentiation and mineralization of human dental pulp cells. *J. Endod.* **40**: 83–88.

135 Zehnder, M., Söderling, E., Salonen, J., and Waltimo, T. (2004). Preliminary evaluation of bioactive glass S53P4 as endodontic medication in vitro. *J. Endod.* **30**: 220–224.

136 Gubler, M., Brunner, T.J., Zehnder, M. et al. (2008). Do bioactive glasses convey a disinfecting mechanism beyond a mere increase in pH? *Int. Endod. J.* **41**: 670–678.

137 Mohn, D., Bruhin, C., Luechinger, N.A. et al. (2010). Composites made of flame-sprayed bioactive glass 45S5 and polymers: bioactivity and immediate sealing properties. *Int. Endod. J.* **43**: 1037–1046.

138 Mohn, D., Zehnder, M., Imfeld, T., and Stark, W.J. (2010). Radio-opaque nanosized bioactive glass for potential root canal aplication: evaluation of radiopacity, bioactivity and alkaline capacity. *Int. Endod. J.* **43**: 210–217.

139 Zehnder, M., Luder, H.U., Schätzle, M. et al. (2006). A comparative study on the disinfection potentials of bioactive glass S53P4 and calcium hydroxide in contra-lateral human premolars ex vivo. *Int. Endod. J.* **39**: 952–958.

140 Santos, A.D., Moraes, J.C.S., Araújo, E.B. et al. (2005). Physico-chemical properties of MTA and a novel experimental cement. *Int. Endod. J.* **38**: 443–447.

141 Gomes-Filho, J.E., Rodrigues, G., Watanabe, S. et al. (2009). Evaluation of the tissue reaction to fast endodontic cement (CER) and Angelus MTA. *J. Endod.* **35**: 1377–1380.

142 Santos, A.D., Araújo, E.B., Yukimitu, K. et al. (2008). Setting time and thermal expansion of two endodontic cements. *Oral Surg. Oral Med. Oral Pathol. Oral Radiol. Endod.* **106**: e77–e79.

143 Scarparo, R.K., Haddad, D., Acasigua, G.A.X. et al. (2010). Mineral trioxide aggregate-based sealer: analysis of tissue reactions to a new endodontic material. *J. Endod.* **36**: 1174–1178.

144 da Silva, G.F., Guerreiro-Tanomaru, J.M., Sasso-Cerri, E. et al. (2011). Histological and histomorphometrical evaluation of furcation perforations filled with MTA, CPM and ZOE. *Int. Endod. J.* **44**: 100–110.

145 Gomes-Filho, J.E., Watanabe, S., Bernabé, P.F.E., and Moraes Costa, M.T. (2009). A mineral trioxide aggregate sealer stimulated mineralization. *J. Endod.* **35**: 256–260.

146 Tanomaru-Filho, M., Faleiros, F.B.C., Saçaki, J.N. et al. (2009). Evaluation of pH and calcium ion release of root-end filling materials containing calcium hydroxide or mineral trioxide aggregate. *J. Endod.* **35**: 1418–1421.

147 Assmann, E., Scarparo, R.K., Böttcher, D.E., and Grecca, F.S. (2012). Dentin bond strength of two mineral trioxide aggregate-based and one epoxy resin-based sealers. *J. Endod.* **38**: 219–221.

148 Gomes-Filho, J.E., Watanabe, S., Gomes, A.C. et al. (2009). Evaluation of the effects of endodontic materials on fibroblast viability and cytokine production. *J. Endod.* **35**: 1577–1579.

149 Camilleri, J. (2009). Evaluation of selected properties of mineral trioxide aggregate sealer cement. *J. Endod.* **35**: 1412–1417.

11

Extending the Concept of Hemopoietic and Stromal Niches as an Approach to Regenerative Medicine

Igor A. Khlusov[1,2] *and Marina Yu. Khlusova*[1,2]

[1] *Department of Morphology and General Pathology, Siberian State Medical University, 634050, Tomsk, Russia*
[2] *National Research Tomsk Polytechnic University, Research School of Chemistry & Applied Biomedical Sciences, 634050, Tomsk, Russia*

11.1 Introduction

The nature of the stem cell niche and its interaction with stem cells is one of fundamental questions in stem cell biology [1]. According to our analysis of Ion Channel Media Group Ltd. data, in the year 2007 more than 10% of papers in scientific journals with high impact factor were devoted to the problems of physiology and pathology of stem cell niche.

Bone marrow is the major and well-known site of hematopoiesis in mammals. Nevertheless, the exact location, cellular composition, and associated molecular signals of the hematopoietic niche have remained elusive until recently [2]. Current trends lead to asking the question: What does the concept of the stem cell niche really mean today? [3].

Here, we summarized our point of view connected with the historic development (see Figure 11.1), recent studies, concepts and controversies of the hematopoietic and mesenchymal stem cells niches in mammals, and their prospects for the tissue bioengineering and regenerative medicine.

11.2 Postulated Stage (a Hypothesis) of the Niche Concept

Upon division of the hematopoietic stem cells (HSCs), at least one daughter cell retains the stem state. This capacity was called "self-renewal." Symmetric divisions expand the number of HSCs, whereas asymmetric divisions retain HSC potential in one daughter cell, generating further differentiated progeny in the other daughter cell. Divisions that generate two differentiated progeny daughter cells delete the HSCs potential [4–6].

The probability of the HSCs dividing either symmetrically, asymmetrically, or fully differentiating is believed to vary [7], as well as structures and signals in the bone marrow environment to influence the type of the HSCs division are else discussed. Both environmental regulatory signals and intrinsic genetic program are required to maintain stem cell properties and to direct the stem cell proliferation and differentiation [8].

In 1978, Schofield put forward the "niche" hypothesis to describe the physiologically limited microenvironment that supports long-term stem cell activity. In addition to hierarchical organized microenvironments, there was also a specific HSC niche, which "fixed" the stem cells in place and prevented their maturation, allowing the stem cell to proliferate and retain its stemness (self-renewal capacity). Once the stem cell progeny left the stem cell niche they proceeded to differentiate [9]. As such, the niche would provide a mechanism to precisely balance the production of stem cells and their progenitors to maintain tissue homeostasis [10]. However, the problems of the exact niche location, its structure and functioning haven't been resolved, because some difficulties of stem cell niches locating and identifying in mammals existed [8]. Morphofunctional features of the hemopoietic inductive microenvironment (HIM) are still spreading to specialized microenvironment of HSCs. Numerous definitions of HSCs niche emphasize this trend, such as:

(1) Li and Xie consider the stem cell niche as a group of cells in a special tissue location for the maintenance of stem cells. The niche's overall structure is variable, and different cell types can provide the niche environment [8]. It postulates an existence of niche hierarchy because of HIM heterogeneity in the different sites of the bone marrow.
(2) Wilson and Trumpp define niches in the bone marrow as the cellular and molecular microenvironment that regulates HSCs function [11].

Bioceramics and Biocomposites: From Research to Clinical Practice, First Edition. Edited by Iulian Antoniac.

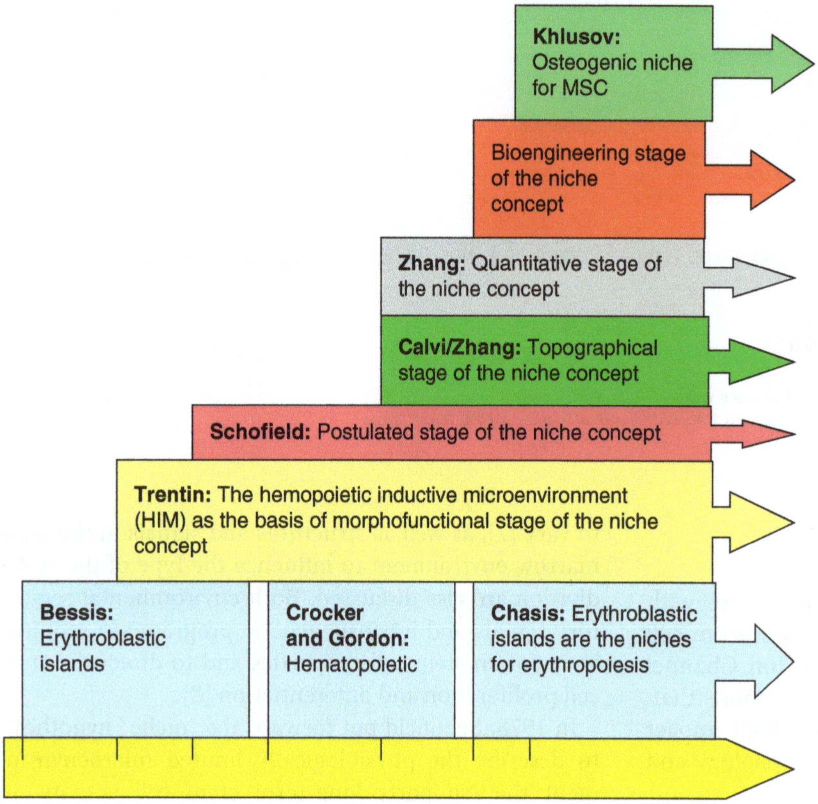

Figure 11.1 A timeline representation of major points that extended our understanding of hemopoietic and stromal niches.

(3) "Niche" is composed of the cellular components of the microenvironment surrounding stem cells as well as the signals emanating from the support cells. Scientific community maintains such point of view. For example, the niche is the specific microenvironment surrounding stem cells, and playing a vital role in the regulation of the stem cell activity [12].

(4) The niche is a restricted region in an organ that supports the self-renewal divisions of stem cells [6] and is composed of both localized signaling cells and an extracellular matrix (ECM) that controls the stem cell fate [13].

(5) Niche is a highly specialized complex instructive microenvironment [14] that physically localizes stem cells and maintains their stem cell fate [15].

11.3 Morphofunctional Stage of the Niche Concept

Bone marrow is the first tissue for revealing and studying the stem cells. The bone trabeculae, arterioles, and venules form the structural framework of the bone marrow, around which hematopoiesis develops in the intersinusoidal spaces [16]. The hematopoietic cells have their own stromal microenvironment named as HIM [17]. The microenvironment structure of the bone marrow can be subdivided into mobile components (T-lymphocytes, hormones, neurotransmitters, etc.) and resident stromal elements, which are fixed in certain regions of the hemopoietic organs to form their "meshwork." Hormones control every stage of the stem cell life, including establishment, expansion, maintenance, and differentiation. The effects can be cell autonomous or non-cell autonomous through the niche [18]. Morphological components of HIM were defined by Tavassoli [19] as follows: (i) blood vessels; (ii) tissue component consisting of resident and migrating cells penetrating the ECM with fibers and soluble molecules; and (iii) nerve terminals. HIM components control the HSCs fate via direct (cell–cell and cell–matrix) and indirect (soluble molecules) manners.

The concept of HIM has developed from the need to answer the basic questions about migration, control of proliferation, and differentiation of lymphohematopoietic cells; e.g. how are cells with the same genes induced to express different sets of these genes which lead to differentiation; what regulates the proliferation and differentiation of these cells and why do they home to different sites in different stages of development? [20].

11.3.1 Blood Vessels

The bone marrow (including the endosteal surface) is highly vascularized [21] and the character of the local blood flow influences the hematopoiesis. The arterial blood supply of the bone marrow comes from two major sources: nutrient artery penetrated the cortex with radial branches to inner bone surface; muscular arteries [22]. In fine, a concentration of HSCs pool diminishes from mouse endosteum toward the center of femoral cavity [23].

In addition to the ability of the vasculature to provide key nutrients, and circulating regulators (cytokines, etc.) that control stem cells and/or the niche, it would provide a mechanism to coordinate the stem cell activity in dynamic fashion in response to metabolic factors, such as oxygen. There are the bone marrow sites where milieu is hypoxic in nature [24]. Vascular niche is considered to be more oxygenic site relative to osteoblastic niche [25]. Jang and Sharkis proposed that HSCs moving to a more oxygenic HIM within the niche reflects the physiologic capacity of quiescent cells to self-renew and differentiate [26]. Thus, higher oxygen concentration gradients as the cells progress from the osteoblastic niche to the vascular niche might play a role in recruitment, proliferation, and differentiation of HSCs and their progenitor cells [2].

After transferring human mesenchymal stromal cells (MSCs) from atmospheric oxygen levels from 21% down to 1%, stromal cells did not proliferate *in vitro* as rapidly as under 21% oxygen and accumulated in G_1 phase. Reduced oxygen tension severely impaired adipogenic and osteogenic differentiation of MSCs. Elevation of oxygen from 1% to 3% restored MSCs osteogenic differentiation. Physiological hypoxia may keep a proportion of MSCs in a resting state [27] to be regulating factor of quiescent state of the HSCs niche.

Vascularization of the cartilage template is a crucial process during the formation of embryonic bone by endochondral ossification, and the vasculature is highly important in the ongoing process of bone and marrow remodeling [28, 29].

The essential role of vascular endothelial growth factor (VEGF) in the recruitment of vascular precursors required for blood vessel invasion of the bone analog, chondrocyte apoptosis, and the migration of the incoming HSCs occurs. Furthermore, there are direct effects on HSCs and their niches [2, 30, 31].

The bone marrow vasculature is being actively studied as the HSCs niche as well as a potential therapeutic target for hematologic and/or orthopedic diseases [32].

11.3.2 Nerve Terminals

Anatomically, the bone marrow is highly innervated tissue [33] with both myelinated and nonmyelinated nerve fibers [34]. Argentophilic nerve terminals are located near arterioles and on reticular cells [35], and minority is connected with marrow parenchyma [36].

It was speculated by Purton and Scadden [37] that a part of MSCs in humans could be identical to the CXCL12-abundant reticular (CAR) cells that are associated not only with the efferent nerves [35], but also with the perivascular and osteoblastic niches for HSCs [38, 39].

In turn, Mendez-Ferrer et al. [40] specified CAR cells as part of nestin-expressing stromal cell population that contains functional MSCs. Of interest is a fact that non-myelinating Schwann cells of the sympathetic nervous system (SNS) belong to the nestin-positive stromal subset and can mediate SNS negative signals on the activity of nestin$^+$ MSCs [3].

The SNS has an important role in regulating the HSCs niche [41, 42]. Despite an existence of cholinergic terminals in the bone marrow [43], the participation of acetylcholine in the HSCs, HIM and niche regulation is still unclear because of its fast utilization by cholinesterase.

Catecholaminergic neurotransmitters play the roles in HSCs (CD34$^+$ cells) mobilization, proliferation, and differentiation [32, 44].

The cyclical release of HSCs from their niche and expression of CXCL12 chemokine ([C-X-C motif] ligand 12; stromal cell derived factor-1 SDF-1) in the bone marrow HIM was regulated by circadian neurotransmitter norepinephrine (NE) secretion by the SNS [42]. When a β2-adrenergic agonist was administered to both control and NE-deficient mice, HSCs egress from the bone marrow was enhanced [45].

Adrenergic agonists stimulated the hemopoietic progenitors and HIM function in conditions of immobilization stress [46]. On the contrary, SNS stimulation caused by an administration of high dose of cytostatics (5-fluorouracil [5-FU] or cyclophosphamide) was capable of prolonging postcytostatic hemopoiesis recovery, in particular by means of depression of DNA-synthesizing colony-forming units of granulomonocytopoiesis (CFU-GM) and colony-forming units of erythropoiesis (CFU-E) damaged by cytostatics and diminishing the number of hematopietic islets (HIs) [47, 48]. For all this, we consider HIs as one of the type of the bone marrow niches for committed precursor cells and migrating HSCs (see below).

11.3.3 Cellular Components of the HSCs Niche

HIM studies based on either microscopy investigations (light and ultrastructural; [22]) or *ex vivo* culture systems (the Dexter long-term bone marrow cultures, etc.; [49]) identified fibroblasts, reticular cells, endothelial and advential cells, adipocytes, osteoclasts (OCLs), and osteoblasts (OBLs). Niche cell types and their functions are presented, in particular, by Smith and Calvi [32].

However, the exact identity of the cell type(s) comprising the HSCs niche remained unknown [37].

Bone marrow stromal cells (BMSCs) include MSCs and a lot of other cell types (macrophages, endothelial cells [ECs], fibroblasts, reticular cells, adipocytes, OBLs, and OCLs) [5, 50], each of which, in principle, may play a crucial role in hematopoiesis. Stromal cells modulate hematopoiesis through the remodeling of ECM, secretion of cytokines, chemokines, and hematopoietic diffusible factors, direct stromal cell-hematopoietic cell contact, and intercellular gap junctions.

The putative functions expected to be performed by the stroma are as follows: (i) osteogenesis, (ii) control of lineage-specific differentiation, (iii) expression of differentiation inducers, (iv) localized presentation of inducers, and (v) support of stem cell renewal. BMSCs inhibit the differentiation induced by colony stimulating factor, promote accumulation of myeloid progenitor cells, and create conditions favorable for their self-renewal. Direct contact inhibition of hemopoietic cells having a corresponding restrictins (receptor molecules) on the stromal cells, as hypothesized by Zipori [51], underlies, apparently, the systemic HIM as well its specific sites ("quiescent" HSC niches).

MSCs have potential to differentiate into at least four orthodox phenotypes confirmed *in vivo*: OBLs, chondrocytes, fibroblasts, adipocytes, and stromal support cells [52, 53]. They also produce OCL-supportive cells with preosteoblastic origin, mainly [54].

Live imaging within the mouse calvarium provided by elegant intravital microscopy studies using two-photon video imaging and high-resolution confocal optics [55, 56], indicated that hematopoietic stem/progenitor cells reside within perivascular sites near OBLs in close contact with endothelial vasculature [10].

In this connection, we reviewed shortly these types of stromal cells as known components of both systemic HIM and the HSCs niche.

11.3.3.1 Mesenchymal Stem Cells

A subset of colony-forming units of fibroblast-like cells (CFU-Fs), stromal stem cells [57] or MSCs [58] were first identified in the bone marrow, where they are presented with about 10-fold higher concentrations than the circulation and can be obtained from all tissues with varying frequencies [59, 60]. They have been recently named skeletal stem cells [61].

The International Society for Cellular Therapy (ISCT) to issue a nomenclature clarification restricted the use of the term MSCs for cells that meet the stem cell criteria and recommended the term "multipotent mesenchymal stromal cells" (MMSCs) for the fibroblast-like plastic adherent cells regardless of the tissue of origin [62] because of their opportunity to differentiate into multiple cell types [60, 63]. The differentiation potential of MSCs into standard four mesenchymal lineages (OBLs, chondroblasts, adipocytes, hematopoiesis-supportive stromal cells with a vascular smooth muscle-like phenotype) is known as the orthodox differentiation [60].

There is heterogeneity of MSCs population [5, 62, 64]. MSCs are diversely distributed *in vivo*. There are central (bone marrow) and regional tissue-resident (amnion, placenta, adipose tissue, periostium, synovial membrane, skeletal muscle, dermis, pericytes, blood, trabecular bone, human umbilical cord, lung) pools of MSCs [62, 65, 66] that respond to injury by cell homing and paracrine regulation.

Cells having CFU-Fs nature and multi-lineage *in vitro* differentiation capacity were demonstrated to be present in many tissues (bone marrow, adipose tissue, cartilage, umbilical cord, placenta, amniotic fluid, dental pulp, skeletal muscle, tendons and synovial membrane, breast milk, etc.) [60, 67, 68]. The origin of MSCs in different tissues could be pericytes [69] associated with vasculature.

MSCs pool is a rare population (approximately 0.001–0.01%) of adult human bone marrow [70]. The number and differentiation potential of putative MSCs decreases markedly in aging [71].

Minimal criteria for MSCs defining required by ISCT are the following: (i) an adherence to plastic surface; (ii) the expression of CD105, CD73, and CD90 antigens; (iii) the lack of expression of CD45, CD34, CD14 or CD11b, and CD79a or CD19; (iv) human leukocyte antigen – DR isotype (HLA–DR) surface molecules; and (v) the ability to differentiate *in vitro* into the osteogenic, chondrogenic, and adipogenic lineages (reviewed in [62]). Today, it is clear that the cluster determinants of MSCs *in vitro* are not indicative of their *in vivo* function.

The primary role of MSCs as the HIM component is support of HSCs survival, maintenance of quiescence and differentiation, and reparation of tissue injury [72] providing growth factors, cell–cell interactions, and matrix proteins. It has potential utility in regenerative medicine.

Mesenchymal cells have putative roles in maintaining tissue homeostasis and are increasingly recognized as components of the stem cell niches [62]. It appears that more immature mesenchymal progenitor or stem cells are the regulators of the HSCs niche. Nestin-expressed MSCs are spatially associated with HSCs and adrenergic nerve fibers, highly express HSC maintenance genes and constitute an essential HSCs niche component. Purified HSCs home near nestin$^+$ MSCs in the bone marrow of lethally irradiated mice, whereas *in vivo* nestin$^+$ cell depletion significantly reduces bone marrow homing of haematopoietic progenitors [40]. Subendothelial CD146$^+$ osteoprogenitor stromal cells with CFU-Fs capability from adult human bone marrow stroma residing on the sinusoidal wall can generate *in vivo* both bone and HIM and produce angiopoietin-1 (Ang-1, a pivotal molecule of the HSCs niche) [38]. Mesenchymal precursor cells expressing Osterix transcriptional factor have possible significance in HSCs maintaining in adult organism [73].

Overall historical background and current understanding of the MSCs and the HIM are precisely presented by Kfoury et al. [62]. A long list of biologically important paracrine and autocrine molecules produced by the MSCs occurs [60, 74]. Besides, they seem to reside in their own bone marrow niche, where stromal stem cells are able to self-renew and generate mature conjunctive/stromal cell types [74].

11.3.3.2 Osteoblasts

Hematopoietic foci arise in close connection with the bone tissue. A part of hematopoietic cells can be found to connect tightly with the endosteal bone surface, which is lined primarily by OBLs. This anatomic arrangement suggests a potential role for OBLs (responsible for bone growth) in regulating the HSCs (responsible for blood formation) [31].

Nearly 50% of human marrow stromal fibroblasts formed bone when they were transplanted *in vivo*. More important, these fibroblast-derived clones recruit circulating host hematopoietic progenitors to reestablish a fully functional marrow of recipient's origin [63].

OBLs are usually found in a layer along the endosteum (internal surfaces of bone) at the interface between bone and marrow. The osteoblastic pool includes (from most primitive to most mature) MSCs, osteoprogenitor cells, OBLs, and osteocytes [75, 76]. Different subtypes of OBLs may play a role in regulating the hematopoietic progenitor cells (HPCs) [2].

OBLs themselves are heterogeneous cell population with trabecular and endosteal spindle-shaped endosteal lining cells and the oval-shaped cells, which are the direct precursors of osteocytes [77]. Among the osteoblastic lining cells, only N-cadherin positive/CD45 negative osteoblastic cells (SNO) interact directly with HSCs [78] and provide "quiescence" signaling [77].

OBLs express and secrete a lot of molecules known for modulation of hematopoiesis *in vitro* and *in vivo* reflected in review of Taichman, in particular. OBL-expressed regulatory components that influence stem cell function are likely to include cell–cell receptors, soluble and cell surface–associated cytokines, and growth factors. Each of these factors – those known and those yet to be determined – are likely influenced by mechanical, systemic (e.g. parathyroid hormone; PTH), and local (e.g. bone morphogenic proteins; BMPs), Ang-1 signals that regulate osteoblastic function [31].

The number of OBL products has positive regulation of the HSCs niche (e.g. Ang-1, thrombopoietin [THPO], and Jagged-1), whereas OBL-associated negative regulators of the HSCs niche include osteopontin (OPN), for instance [37]. The OPN-null microenvironment was sufficient to increase the number of stem cells associated with increased stromal Jagged1 and Ang-1 expression and reduced primitive hematopoietic cell apoptosis [79].

The wide spectrum of presented and secreted molecules that mediate HSC–OBL interactions is described in [31]. At the same time, evidence against a direct effect on HSCs for osteoblastic cells in favor of MMSCs is now considerable [62]. MSCs are considered to be a determining component for HSCs controlling [80]. Most likely, direct HSCs contact with MSCs and OBLs leads to their inactivation [11, 81].

11.3.3.3 Osteoclasts

OCLs are generated from $CD34^+$ hematopoietic cells of the monocyte/macrophage lineage and are essential for mineralized bone resorption [82]. During embryogenesis, rapid formation of primitive marrow occurs in bone resorption centers [83] via medullary cavities formed by OCLs. In turn, blood precursors migrate and colonize spaces carved out of embryonic bone and cartilage [31].

In adults, OCLs promote post-transplantation hematopoietic recovery and the mobilization of hematopoietic progenitors into the circulation as reviewed by Frisch et al. [77]. However, the role of OCLs in HSCs maintenance remains controversial. According to [32] opinion, neither normal bone marrow cavities nor OCLs are required for maintenance and mobilization of functional hematopoietic stem and progenitor cells and that in fact they may negatively regulate hematopoiesis.

There is a close structural–functional interconnection of OBLs and OCLs to regulate the size of the HSCs niche. OBLs and stromal cells express receptor activator of nuclear factor kappa B ligand (RANKL), macrophage colony-stimulating factor (M-CSF), and osteoprotegerin (OPG), while early OCL precursors express c-Fms (M-CSF receptor) and RANK (a receptor for RANKL) [84, 85]. RANKL (OPG ligand, tumor necrosis factor [TNF]-related cytokine) and M-CSF stimulate OCLs differentiation. However, OPG, as an inhibitor of RANKL, competes with RANKL for RANK [86].

Possibly, OCLs can itself initiate the MMSCs or HSCs niche formation. Short-term *in vitro* contact of human lung prenatal stromal cells (the cells of regional MMSCs pool) with smooth (roughness index $R_a < 1\ \mu m$) calcium phosphate (CP) surface mimicking cortical bone matrix, led to activation of the acid phosphatase (ACP) positive cells with OCL-like function versus intact alkaline phosphatase (ALP) OBL-like cells. Nevertheless, smooth CP materials were capable to induce the bone/marrow system recovery in conditions of ectopic subcutaneous test [87]. MMSCs culture has macrophages additive [60].

Thus, osteoresorptive cells have a function to prepare the bone matrix for MMSCs and OBLs colonization.

In addition to OCLs, endosteal monocytes and macrophages are also capable of modulating the endosteal HSCs niche via hematopoietic cells mobilization in response to granulocyte colony-stimulating factor (G-CSF). Multiple pharmacologic strategies are currently used to inhibit OCLs for the treatment of osteoporosis; therefore, cells of the monocyte–macrophage lineage remain a very feasible therapeutic target for the HSCs niche manipulation and bioengineering [32].

Blin-Wakkach et al. integrated the main role of bone-resorbing OCLs in HSC niches regulation as follows [88]: (i) carving space for HSCs homing; (ii) providing signals and cytokines that affect the molecular and cellular niche components [75, 89]; (iii) formatting the HSC niches; (iv) maintaining the HSCs in these niches; and (v) mobilizing the HSCs from the bone marrow. At the same time, their exact role in the HSCs niche remains unclear.

11.3.3.4 Vascular Cells

Endothelial cells (ECs) are the site of cell entrance into the bone marrow from bloodstream and its emigration to circulation. ECs of various tissues can support HSCs and progenitors *in vitro* [90, 91].

The sites of embryonic hematopoiesis contain endothelial cells closely associated with self-renewing HSCs in absence of OBLs [92, 93]. Indeed, HSCs seem to originate from a perivascular progenitor (hemangioblast) during embryonic development. There is a strong embryologically interdependence between HSCs and endothelial cells of bone marrow sinusoids and indicate that these cells hold distinct functional characteristics from endothelial cells present in other tissues [94].

Primitive hematopoietic cells as revealed by supravital imaging in animals persisted or increased in number in the specific subsets of the marrow vasculature [95]. Endothelial-derived CXCL12 (SDF-1) and FGF-4 (fibroblast growth factor-4) induce upregulation of adhesion molecules, including very late antigen (VLA4)/vascular cell adhesion molecule (VCAM1), facilitating localization of HSCs to the vascular niche [96].

A number of studies proposed HSCs/HPCs niche function for endothelial cells in the bone marrow [97]. Recently, Smith and Calvi [32] discussed that HSCs frequency and function were only impaired by the absence of stem cell factor (SCF) from Tie2+ ECs and Leptin receptor (Lepr)-expressing perivascular cells ($Lepr^+$ cells) of mesenchymal and stromal origin, respectively.

However, ECs have not yet been shown to be a necessary regulatory component of the adult HSCs microenvironment *in vivo* [77]. The perivascular location of MMSCs raises the issue of whether ECs effects on HSCs are in part mediated by their interaction with MMSCs pool. Indeed, $Lepr^+$ MSCs is determined as the main source of bone formed by adult bone marrow [98].

An important hallmark of many adult stem cell niches is their proximity to the vasculature *in vivo*, a feature common to neural stem cells (NSCs), MSCs from bone marrow, adipose, and other tissues, HSCs, and many tumor stem cells [99]. When the exact role of ECs and perivascular cells will be tightly examined, hope of the vascular/perivascular niche design will appear.

11.3.3.5 Chondrocytes

Little is known about the chondrocytes participation in a formation of niches and local micro-environments required for the stem cell maintenance. Jacenko et al. [100] and then Chan et al. suggest that endochondral ossification is necessary for the HSCs niche formation *in vivo*. Collectively, their data implicates endochondral ossification, bone formation that proceeds through a cartilage intermediate, as a requirement for adult HSCs niche formation.

$CD105^+Thy1.1^-$ skeletal progenitors isolated from fetal limb bones and injected underneath the renal capsule of mice were able to initiate ectopic HSCs niche formation [29]. According to authors' opinion, skeletal progenitors gave rise to donor-derived chondrocytes, which recruited host-derived vasculature into the center of the developing bone graft. As endochondral ossification proceeded, the recruited vasculature facilitated the filling of the niche with host-derived hematopoietic cells: first erythroid and myeloid, then c-kit^+ progenitors, and finally the HSCs. HSC–niche interactions have to be further investigated at the cellular level because of obligatory role of OCLs and osteogenic cells in hemopoiesis remodeling.

In conditions of biomechanical loading caused by subcutaneous implantation of the bone marrow on scaffolds with CP coating, donor bone/recipient marrow system repopulated through the stage of endochondral ossification only on implants with marked topography [101, 102]. Overhead ectopic output of the bone with marrow tissue was observed by us at the surface roughness index R_a in the range of 2–3 μm [103]. As approximation of *in situ* results, bone mineral matrix remodeling it seems to switch over MMSCs/osteoblastic niche for HSCs from quiescent to active position (it will be discussed below).

11.3.3.6 Adipocytes

Adipocytes are heterogenic cellular population including MMSCs, ECs and macrophages-derived subsets. For all this, latest cells form possible niche for adipocyte development [104, 105].

MMSC-derived [24] adipocytes are very abundant in the bone marrow [77], especially, in the fatty marrow of the diaphyseal region. Preadipocytes and adipocytes which probably derived from transformed reticular cells may be candidates for structural-functional involvement in the HIM [22, 35].

The most well-known adipocytokines are leptin, adipsin, adiponectin, and TNFα [106]. Adiponectin elevates *in vitro* undifferentiated HSCs proliferation via its receptor AdipoR1 on HSCs, as reviewed in [77].

During the past few years a steadily increasing number of cell types have been proposed to regulate the HSCs function. These include osteomacs (specific macrophages combined with OBLs), CAR cells, Nestin$^+$ MSCs, Nestin$^+$ Schwann cells, at least [3]. First, these investigations have only started to be concluded. Second, a lot of HIM and HSCs subsets could not form one to two niches. Apparently, multiple microterritories for HSCs have to exist in the bone marrow cavity.

11.3.4 HSCs Niche Hierarchy

A stem cell niche is a specific site in adult tissues where stem cells reside and undergo self-renewal and produce large numbers of progeny (differentiation) [2]. On the one hand, niches as specific sites suggest their topographical distribution in the bone marrow space. On the other hand, a variety and hierarchy of hematopoietic cells in the HSCs pool supposes a variety and the hierarchy of HSCs niches in the bone marrow. In turn, there is well-recognized HIM mosaicism.

HSCs are not a homogeneous population of stem cells. They are hierarchically organized based on their functional properties and repopulating potential. Long-term HSCs self-renew throughout the body life span, while short-term HSCs maintain their proliferative capacity for about eight weeks [107]. This suggests that both hematopoietic populations are maintained by the different niches.

These evidences led to many as yet unanswered questions, such as [37]: Are all niches equal? Are one or more niches? Are the niches for quiescent and activated HSCs the same or do they differ?

11.3.4.1 Structural Hierarchy of the Niches

Different kinds of niche and the regulatory mechanisms occur [108]. Here, Morrison and Spradling [109] proposed two general classes of the stem cell niches based on the physical relationship of stem cells with possible niche components. Stromal niches are discrete anatomical sites containing niche support cells that physically contact with stem cells and influence their behavior via close range signaling and soluble molecules. In contrast, epithelial niches have a lack of specific support cells and typically consist of stem cells directly contacted both with a basement membrane and more mature cells of the cell lineage.

Most HSCs reside in the bone marrow at or near the inner bone surface (endosteum). Many HSCs localize adjacent to specialized blood vessels (sinusoids) [109]. It has proposed at least the existence of two structurally distinct HSC niches formed by OBL or/and endothelial cells [2] and named the "hard" and the "soft" niches, respectively [110].

Perivascular microenvironments in the bone marrow confer distinct vascular niches, regulating HSCs quiescence and the supply of lineage-committed progenitors [111].

MSCs may be stromal components of HSCs niche. On the contrary, MMSCs niche has been steady suggested only [24].

Besides, HIs are the structural–functional units of medullar tissue where transitory HSCs have a possibility to proliferate and differentiate into committed and mature forms [112]. HIs can also be considered as specific niches with final sizes for stem and progenitor cell proliferation and differentiation [113]. HIs have diverse central stromal elements (macrophages, fibroblast-like reticular cells) surrounded by hematopoietic cells [112, 114].

Human embryonic stem cells (hESCs) create *in vitro* heterogeneous microenvironments (niches) that influence the fate of themselves [115]. Embryonic stem cells (ESCs) are regularly used as models for early developmental events.

11.3.4.2 Functional Hierarchy of the Niches

Issues from [116] show that the niche can maintain two controversial evidences: HSCs self-renewal and production of differentiated daughter cells. Some recent studies have proposed the existence of two distinct HSC niches that support quiescent or activated HSCs. The OBL-containing niche represents a niche in which HSCs remain quiescent, mainly. In contrast, the perivascular niche has been proposed to represent a niche in which the HSCs are in a more activated state [37].

The early lymphoid progenitor (ELP) cells are located on the endosteal surface of the bones suggest that HPCs may directly [117] and indirectly (through the interleukin IL-7/IL-7R) [118] interact with OBLs. HSCs and B cell progenitors is unclear to reside the same niche or use different OBL subsets.

There was revealed three types of HIs named erythroblastic [119], granulocytic, and erythro-granulocytic clusters [112] in accordance with the lineages of hemopoietic progenitors differentiation. In this regard, erythroid HIs have been proposed by Chasis [120] to be the erythroid niche.

Vascular wall of adipose tissue capillaries may serve as regional adipogenic niche, and ECs give rise to white and brown adipocytes [104].

In pathology, the molecular mechanisms for maintaining quiescence of normal HSCs may also facilitate a survival of leukemia stem cells [94], which are mostly in a quiescent state and are responsible for the maintenance of the neoplasm [121]. Moreover, leukemic cells design own niches that disrupt normal HSCs and HIM [122].

During the progression of cancer and formation of metastasis, cancer cells are self-sufficient to bring their own niche material to the distant site and produce the components of a supportive metastatic niche. These components can be various growth factors, chemokines or secreted enzymes, and ECM [3]. Tumor stem cell-like characteristics of β-catenin accumulating cell clusters in adamantinomatous craniopharyngioma may represent a tumor stem cell niche and might contribute to tumor recurrence [123].

11.3.4.3 Quiescent Niches as an Evidence of Functional Hierarchy of the Niches

The bone marrow HSCs reside in the osteoblastic niche (located near the endosteum) [78, 124] and/or the vascular niche (located in the sinusoidal vasculature) [125].

The signaling lymphocytic activation molecule (SLAM) marker ($CD48^{-}CD150^{+}LKS^{+}$) associated HSCs do not express N-cadherin, an adhesion molecule that maintains quiescent state of HSCs in the OBL niche [126, 127]. More than 70% of SLAM positive HSCs express CD34 antigen [128], a marker that is normally associated with activated (non-quiescent) or short-term repopulating HSCs [129, 130].

Niches or niche cells for quiescent stem cells are located in hypoxic regions of tissues not rich in vasculature, such as the trabecular zone of bone for HSCs [26]. Yin and Li reviewed the osteoblastic niche as a "hypoxic" niche to maintain HSCs in a quiescent (slow cycling or G_0) state [2].

Almost 75% of HSCs are quiescent (G_0 phase in cell cycle) in intact bone marrow [131]. In this regard, osteoblastic niche might serve as a reservoir for HSCs storage [94].

The vascular niche (an "oxygenic" niche) supports short-term stem/progenitor hematopoietic cells that are actively proliferating [2], differentiating and mobilizing [132].

Postnatal HSCs self-renewal is closely related to the slow cell cycling or quiescence. Sub-populations of adult long-term HSCs are in the quiescent state, and quiescence is critical for long-term sustaining stem cell compartment [12]. Quiescent HSCs are resistant to 5-FU-induced myelosuppression, suggesting that the quiescence of HSCs is closely associated with the protection of the HSCs pool from the various myelotoxic stresses [133], and hemopoietic progenitors restoration after 5-FU administration [48].

Cell cycle regulation by the niche is critical for the fate of HSCs [25]. A change in environment leads to the transition between quiescent and cycling HSCs. For instance, the disruption of the osteoblastic niche induces the proliferation of HSCs and their transition to the vascular niche area [134].

We have recently established an existence and certain size of an artificial endosteal niche to promote MMSCs osteogenic potential. Rough (roughness index $R_a > 2\,\mu m$) CP surface with artificial microregions named as "niche – relief" is capable of activating the human MMSCs maturation and differentiation into OBLs *in vitro* [135] and promoting mouse bone and marrow growth in ectopic test [136]. Intriguingly, we hypothesized the sites with smooth bone surface as the microterritories where the quiescent niches may be distributed not only for HSCs but MMSCs, too.

11.3.4.4 Age-related Hierarchy of the Niches

There is evidence that the HSCs population has an "age-structure" [9]. Stem cell number and/or their activity decreases during aging. According to [26] point of view, in the aged mice, a 25% decrease in the low expressing the reactive oxygen species (ROS^{low}) population rather than slight increase (approximately 5%) in the ROS^{high} subset could be responsible for the declined repopulating activity of the HSCs [26].

Aging of the niche has also been proposed to contribute to the decline in stem cell function. Quiescent muscle and liver stem cells of aged mice were rejuvenated when exposed to the circulating blood of younger animals [137]. Factors from the young stem cell niche enhance the neural progenitor cell proliferation *in vivo* in old age mice [138].

Maintenance of young-equivalent levels of stem cell function in older individuals (e.g. in conditions of tissue regeneration) could increase the risk of cancer [139] because of an ability of normal niches to promote the proliferation and maintenance of cancer cells [140]. In addition, leukemic cell proliferation resulted in the generation of malignant niches that downregulated CXCL12 (SDF-1) production and negatively affected normal hematopoietic progenitor ($CD34^{+}$) cells [122].

Drummond-Barbosa speculated four hypothetic models of how stem cell function affects and is affected during aging [141]: (i) intrinsic stem cell aging model: intrinsic stem cell aging may be a predominant factor leading to aging of the organism; (ii) niche aging model: aging of the niches may significantly contribute to aging by affecting the stem cell activity; (iii) systemic aging model: aging of the systemic environment may drive aging of stem cells;

and (iv) multidirectional aging model: complex interactions are likely to drive aging. It is possible that different stem cells age at different rates and via different mechanisms and that the impact that their aging has on the aging of the organism as a whole varies according to their specific function.

Recovery of niche function can prevent aging-related changes in stem cell behavior [137], indicating that rejuvenation and/or expansion the niche number may promote stem cell-based strategies in regenerative medicine.

11.3.5 Cue Molecules of the HSCs Niche

Inter- and intracellular signal pathways seem to be booming area of niche research. Nevertheless, it is unclear whether and how all of the molecules and pathways are present in the niches along or belong to systematic HIM, because niche outlines are still unclear. The analysis of the signals generated by the niche has begun via gene expression in HSCs and stromal cells [62].

A variety of distant and local signaling molecules and a lot of pathways could be involved in the niche regulation, including [2, 6, 8, 31, 32, 37, 62, 142, 143]:

(1) SCF/c-Kit (v-kit Hardy-Zuckerman 4 feline sarcoma viral oncogene homolog) signaling, human homologs of the *Drosophila* proteins Jagged/Notch, Ang-1/Tie2 (a tyrosine kinase receptor), Wnt (mammalian homolog of *Drosophila* wingless) ligands/β-catenin, and Ca^{2+}-sensing receptor (CaR).
(2) Matrix-bound and soluble cytokines and secreted growth factors (BMP, THPO, IL-3, IL-6, SCF, granulocyte-macrophage colony-stimulating factor [GM-CSF], transforming growth factor [TGF]), VEGF, TNFα, etc.) are playing the roles in stem cell regulation. More details for several cytokines that affect the HSCs fate are discussed, in particular, by Zhang and Lodish [144]. The growth factors for oligo- and unipotent hematopoietic precursors (e.g. erythropoietin) are more than the simple survival factors and might dynamically modify the erythroblast cell surface and its microenvironment [145].
We believe, TNFα, pleiotropic cytokine commonly produced by monocytes and macrophages [60] has an essential regulatory significance for ECM and bone remodeling [89], can switch quiescent/active status of the stem cell niche. TNF has been known to show preferential ability to inhibit some hemopoietic targets more efficiently than others restrictins [142].
(3) Membrane-bound factors, including VCAM and intracellular cell adhesion molecule (ICAM) and integrins of cells and ECM (N-cadherin/β-catenin; OPN/β1 integrin; VLA-4[α4β1]/VCAM-1; etc.).
(4) Chemokines for HSCs and HPCs homing and mobilization: SDF-1 (also called CXCL12) and its receptor CXCR4; FGF-4 and its receptors fibroblast growth factor receptor (FGFR), and G-CSF. Endothelial cells, OBLs, and other stromal cells constitutively express SDF-1, while HSCs express CXCR4.
(5) Prostaglandin E_2 (PGE_2) locally secreted by OBLs is considered a potential mediator of the PTH-dependent HSCs development [77].
(6) Systemic PTH/parathyroid hormone-related peptide receptor (PPR) [124] regulate the size of the HSCs osteoblastic niche in mouse models [146].
(7) The network of ECM (collagen, reticulin, fibronectin, laminin, tenascin, hemonectin, proteoglycans, glycosaminoglycans [GAGs], etc.) is produced by BMSCs [51]. A matrix glycoprotein, OPN is a negative regulatory element of the stem cell niche that limits the size of the stem cell pool and may provide a mechanism for restricting excess stem cell expansion under conditions of the niche stimulation [79].

Some of these regulating molecules and pathways are defined below.

11.3.5.1 Niche Signaling for Quiescent Stem Cells

Understanding the structural-functional signals in the niche that keep HSCs in a quiescent state is of much interest. In 1992, Zipori assumed that quiescent state and slow renewal of HSCs are maintained by stromal factors of a nature yet undefined [142]. Today the following perspectives are proposed:

(1) Quiescence or slow cell cycling of HSCs is induced by Tie2 expressed by HSCs and endothelial cells. Its ligand Ang-1 signaling is expressed by osteoblastic cells in endosteum. It contributes to the maintenance of long-term repopulating ability of HSCs and for the protection of the HSCs compartment from various cellular stresses. The mechanisms of Tie2/Ang-1 signaling may be connected with activating the β1-integrin and N-cadherin in LSK (Lineage–Sca-1^+c-Kit^+)-$Tie2^+$ cells and promoting the HSC structural interactions (adhesion) with ECM and cellular components of the niche [133]. Ang-1 is expressed in human BMSCs [38], suggesting that mesenchymal progenitor cells provide the niche for human HSCs.
Tie2/Ang-1 pathway is needed to increase angiogenesis (the formation of new blood vessels) and reduce vascular permeability [147, 148]. As a fact, diverse niches interact closely.
(2) Mpl protooncogene (THPO receptor) and its ligand THPO regulate megakaryopoiesis. On the other hand, Mpl expression in long-term HSCs was closely correlated with cell cycle quiescence, and Mpl^+

HSCs are in close contact with THPO producing osteoblastic cells at the endosteal surface in trabecular bone area [149].

(3) Wnt ligands are a key-signaling pathway in stem cell self-renewal [150] and negatively affects quiescence of adult stem cells [151, 152]. For all this, Wnt ligands activate a β-catenin-dependent pathway (canonical pathway), or β-catenin-independent (noncanonical) pathway, such as the Wnt/planar cell polarity pathway and Wnt/Ca^{2+} pathway [12].

(4) Cell adhesion molecules (N-cadherin, β1-integrin, and OPN) might not only be required for HSC anchoring to the niche, but also involved in the regulation of cell cycle of HSCs. β1-integrin and N-cadherin are the key downstream targets of Tie2/Ang-1 and Mpl/THPO signaling in HSCs. N-cadherin expression levels regulate the localization of HSCs between the osteoblastic and vascular niche because of osteoblastic niche has higher level of N-cadherin than those in the vascular niche [12]. OPN negatively regulates HSCs number in the bone marrow niche [153].

(5) TGFβ/TGFβ type 2 receptor expressed by HSCs maintains their dormant status [3].

(6) c-Myc protooncogene (v-myc avian myelocytomatosis viral oncogene homolog) controls the balance between the cell self-renewal and differentiation by adjusting the adhesion between HSCs and the niche. Its overexpression led to the loss of self-renewal activity and augmented differentiation of HSCs [154].

(7) According to a metabolic point of view, quiescent HSCs with more self-renewal potential associated with the low-oxygenic osteoblastic niche have the low level of ROS expression. For all this, CaR, N-cadherin, Notch1 (a member of the type 1 transmembrane protein family), p21, p53, and telomerase reverse transcriptase (TERT) attributes are higher in the ROS^{low} population of primitive (long-term self-renewing) HSCs. They exhibit a higher G_0 activity and might be more enriched for the quiescent HSCs and physically located in the osteoblastic niche. ROS^{high} subset expressed higher mTOR (mammalian target of rapamycin) and activated h38 MAPK (mitogen-activated protein kinase) and may be accumulated in more oxygenic vascular niche [26].

11.3.6 Extracellular Matrix

Key niche components and interactions include soluble factors, cell–cell contacts, and cell–matrix adhesions. ECM tightly regulates growth factors distribution in space and time by binding and limiting their diffusion, modulating the effects of matrix and cell contacts [155].

ECM is an extremely compound substance and consists of complex, spatially and temporally controlled mixtures of soluble biochemical factors (e.g. ions, dissolved gases, nutrients, cell excrements, chemokines, cytokines and growth factors, etc.), as well as insoluble transmembrane receptor ligands and fibers. In general, ECM components include the following:

(1) Fibrillar proteins contain collagen, the reticulin fibers, fibronectin, laminin, tenascin, hemonectin, and some other components of the filamentous network. The extracellular substance of hematopoietic tissue includes collagen of five types: the types I, II, and III collagens are secreted by fibroblasts, while type IV collagen (a protein of basal membrane) and type V collagen are produced by endotheliocytes. Collagen is considered to play a key role among the proteins in ECM by providing its mechanical stability [156]. At the same time, in physiologic conditions, HIM in healthy bone marrow contains sparse collagen. Therefore, collagen fibers are not considered to be standard components of the bone marrow stroma [60]. Fibrous ECM (e.g. fibronectin and laminin) binds cell transmembrane integrins through the arginine-glycine-aspartic acid (RGD) sequences. This event promotes integrins interaction with the cytoskeleton at focal adhesion complexes (protein aggregates that include vinculin, α-actinin, and talin). In turn, it initiates the production of intracellular messengers, or can directly mediate nuclear signals. Collectively, changes in cytoskeletal tension and cytosol components lead to shape transformation, locomotion, cell growth, and differentiation [89, 157].
Adhesive, anchorage, binding, and epigenetic nuances of ECM glycoproteins and their integrin receptors are presented in details in [31, 65, 89, 158].

(2) GAGs, primarily, hyaluronic acid (HyA), are one of the key components of the ECM. Hydroxyapatite (HA) (40% of all GAGs in the bone marrow) [156] is a prominent ECM polymer in supporting human ESCs growth in undifferentiated masses (i.e. embryoid bodies) [159]. HA plays a role as a modulator of supportive function of the bone marrow niche via its receptor, CD44 (a multifunctional transmembrane protein) expressed by a wide variety of cells, including MSCs [60], HSCs, and the hematopoietic progenitors [108]. Chung and Burdick demonstrated the ability of hydrogels of HA to promote chondrogenic differentiation of encapsulated human MSCs [160].
The remodeling of plasma membrane glycocalyx with synthetic heparan sulfate proteoglycans may be applicable to promote ESCs differentiation [161].

Salchert et al. reconstituted fibrillar collagen from mixtures of monomeric tropocollagen and the GAGs (heparin or HA). Migration rates of HSCs on fibrillar structures were significantly lower than on tropocollagen indicating a more intimate contact of cells to the fibrillar assemblies [162].

(3) Multiple soluble factors in ECM (e.g. cytokines, growth factors, ions) by means of their membrane receptors, ion channels start intracellular signal pathways (see above).

No specific matrix components have been yet identified that help to maintain MSCs in their naïve state, as a niche matrix would do [24].

However, MSCs constitute a specific niche composed of ECM proteins with unique features. Djouad et al. hypothesized that the induction of MSCs differentiation toward chondrocytes in articular cartilage might be induced and/or influenced by molecules from the microenvironment. Therefore, a cross talk between ECM components of the microenvironment and MSCs within the cartilage is responsible for the differentiation of MSCs into chondrocytes [163].

ECM left by OBLs on titanium scaffolds after decellularization increased osteogenesis markers, such as ALP and calcium deposition, in MSCs [164]. ECM deposited by microvascular endothelial cells enhances MSCs endotheliogenesis [24].

Bone-like ECM structure alone can regulate MSCs differentiation into OBLs (see below). On this basis, ECM properties underlie the MSCs and HSCs niche development, hierarchy, and function, with potential applications for tissue engineering. More quantitative and molecular information on ECM–MSCs interaction is currently needed.

In pathology, ECM provides a structural scaffold for migrating cancer cells and is actively involved in modulating cellular signaling in cancer [165]. Thus, the ECM protein tenascin C produced by myofibroblasts was recently noted to play an important role in metastatic breast cancer [3]. Besides, myofibroblast-derived periostin, another ECM protein recently identified as a component of the metastatic niche [166].

11.3.7 Bone Matrix as a Specialized Extracellular Matrix

It is poor estimated component of the niches. There is evidence that ECM alone can regulate MSCs differentiation, with potential applications for tissue engineering. Mineralization of synthetic scaffolds has been well known to be an effective technique to promote cell adhesion, stimulate differentiation of MSCs into osteogenic lineage, and improve osseointegration of implant materials [167].

The increasing ionic calcium concentration immediately arises surrounding the region where OBLs and OCLs actively remodel bone. Bone cells (BCs), particularly OBLs, chondrocytes and OCLs, exhibit functional responses to ionic calcium (Ca^{2+}). Scadden hypothesized that the stem cell may be able to recognize extracellular calcium content [14]. The CaR has been recently found to facilitate retention of HSCs on the endosteal bone surface. CaR [168] is a member of family C of G protein-coupled membrane receptors that does not serve as a channel to transport calcium, but recognizes extracellular calcium. It responds to multiple extracellular cations (gadolinium, aluminum), with calcium as its major ligand [169].

The absence of CaR in knockout mice (null mouse model) leads to HSCs release into the bloodstream. The stem cells were unable to engraft at the endosteal surface in a competitive setting [170]. Based on these findings, the intricacy of the interactions between bone and bone marrow was noted by Scadden [14].

Indeed, Liu et al. established *in vitro* significant effect of both extracellular Ca^{2+} and inorganic phosphate (Pi) levels on the growth and osteogenic differentiation of rabbit bone-marrow-derived MSCs. Their results showed that the optimal extracellular Ca^{2+} and Pi concentrations for the cell proliferation and differentiation were 1.8 and 0.09 mM, respectively, which are the concentrations supplied in many commonly used culture media such as Dulbecco's modification of Eagle medium (DMEM) and α-minimum essential medium (α-MEM). Greater Ca^{2+} concentrations did not change cell proliferation but significantly inhibited cell differentiation and enhanced cell mineralization. In turn, MSCs proliferation and differentiation decreased significantly with greater or lower concentrations of the Pi supplement. Greater Pi concentrations also led to significant cell apoptosis [171].

In that way, bone tissue undergoes throughout life a process of remodeling via a tight coupling between bone formation from OBLs (derived from MSCs) and bone resorption by OCLs (which are hematopoietic in origin) [37]. It provides Ca^{2+} for CaR of stem cells near endosteal bone surface as proposed by Scadden [14] and Pi with own bioactivity. Further, bone topography changes permanently.

As a fact, not only ionic calcium but also phosphate as the products of metabolism of mineral bone matrix could affect chemically the stem cells. Ions with positive or negative charge influence the value of cell zeta-potential that is connected with the cell (trans)membrane one. In turn, membrane hyperpolarization promotes osteogenic (ALP gene expression, intracellular calcium level) differentiation of human MSCs unlike its depolarized state [172, 173].

On the other hand, there is a fatal disruption of pre-existing osteoblastic niches in the remodeling bone sites. Each site of trabecular or cortical bone is exposed to physiological remodeling each 3–10 years, on the average [75].

As a result, well-known clonal origin of hematopoiesis [174] could be stochastic process, as well as it can be stipulated by a reorganization of aged osteoblastic niche and HSCs activation by HIM stimuli. Herein, digital kinetics of HSCs egress from quiescent state caused by permanent change of bone topography may be calculated.

Thus, niches cannot be stable structure and niche territories could appear *de novo*. Bone is a native substrate for marrow MSCs and the surface topography of mineralized bone surface essentially affects the cell's fate [175]. Possibly, dynamic theory of hematopoietic and stromal niches, similarly to dynamic theory of hematopoiesis control [156, 176], waits in the wings.

It still remains unknown whether OBLs and MMSCs in different bone sites have distinct roles in HSCs regulation or not. Cortical and trabecular bones differ in their anatomical location, structure, and function. Cortical (compact) bone is located in the diaphyseal region of bone, is thick and smooth, and contacted with fat marrow. In contrast, trabecular (cancellous) bone in the metaphyseal region is rough and less dense, and promotes active hematopoiesis in red marrow. Mechanically, bone trabeculae distribute mechanical stresses and are usually absent from the diaphyseal bone where the cortical bone serves this function [177].

Recently Kiuru et al. [178] have determined sonic hedgehog (Shh)-mediated appearance of the bone trabeculae within the diaphysis of the femurs in postnatal mice. They suggest that overexpression of Shh morphogen is capable of shifting the function of the bone from a mechanical to a hematopoietic function with increasing surface area (the number of immature OBLs) and the hematopoietic niches, respectively.

Bone ECM synthesized by OBLs *in vitro* on titanium scaffolds can increase MMSCs osteogenic markers, such as ALP activity and calcium deposition [164].

From there, we hypothesized distinct physical effect of smooth and rough bone (predominantly, mineral bone matrix) surface on the quiescent or active status of the stem cell niche regulated by structural–functional changes in their HIM cells (MSCs, OBLs, OCLs, etc.) [136] and presented schematically in Figure 11.2. Blood mononuclear leukocytes (T cells, B cells, monocytes) modulate bone turnover in health, stress, and disease (for instance, osteogenesis imperfecta) [179, 180].

11.4 Topographical Stage of the Niche Concept

Historically, "niche" is generally used to describe the location of stem cells [8] in their specific sites of HIM. An anatomically defined, specifically constituted place represents the niche (highly specialized "microenvironmental" cues) for hematopoietic and other tissue-specific stem cells [181]. Nevertheless, anatomical structures in which HSCs interact with their specific microenvironment had not been still clear. An anatomical (morphofunctional) definition of the niche [111] raises immediately the problem of its suitable topographical position.

In 2003, two independent, simultaneous studies using genetic mutant mouse models led to the identification of osteoblastic cells as the key component of the HSCs niche [78, 124].

Of interest is the fact, topographical identification of HSCs osteoblastic niche is suggested from morphofunctional concept. First, Zhang et al., while examining the role of BMP signaling pathway in HSCs development, found histologically the attachment of long-term HSCs to a small subset of spindle-shaped SNO cells lining the inner cancellous/trabecular bone surface. SNO cells function was proposed as the key component of the trabecular (endosteal) niche for HSCs [8].

Second, Calvi et al. studied the signal transduction of the PTH receptor. PPR overexpression enhanced osteoblastic growth with parallel increase in the number of long-term HSCs in the marrow. The increase in long-term HSC populations was connected closely with enhanced Notch-1 signaling in HSCs, probably because of the enhanced expression of Jagged-1 receptors on OBLs. Both investigations point to the dependence of long-term HSCs on the endosteal OBLs.

A little latter, Arai et al. showed that Ang-1 expressed by OBLs activates Tie2 on the stem cells and promotes tight adhesion of stem cells to their niche. Presumably this adhesion results in HSCs quiescence and survival, resulting in stem cell maintenance and self-renewal [31, 133].

Some HPCs appear to contact the sinusoidal endothelium [182]. The clear interaction of putative HSCs with the sinusoidal endothelium suggests that endothelial cells create an alternative niche. The majority of HSCs resided in the perivascular region with only a minority (16%) at the periendosteal region [125].

To distinguish from the osteoblastic niche, the endothelial cell–containing vascular zone in the bone

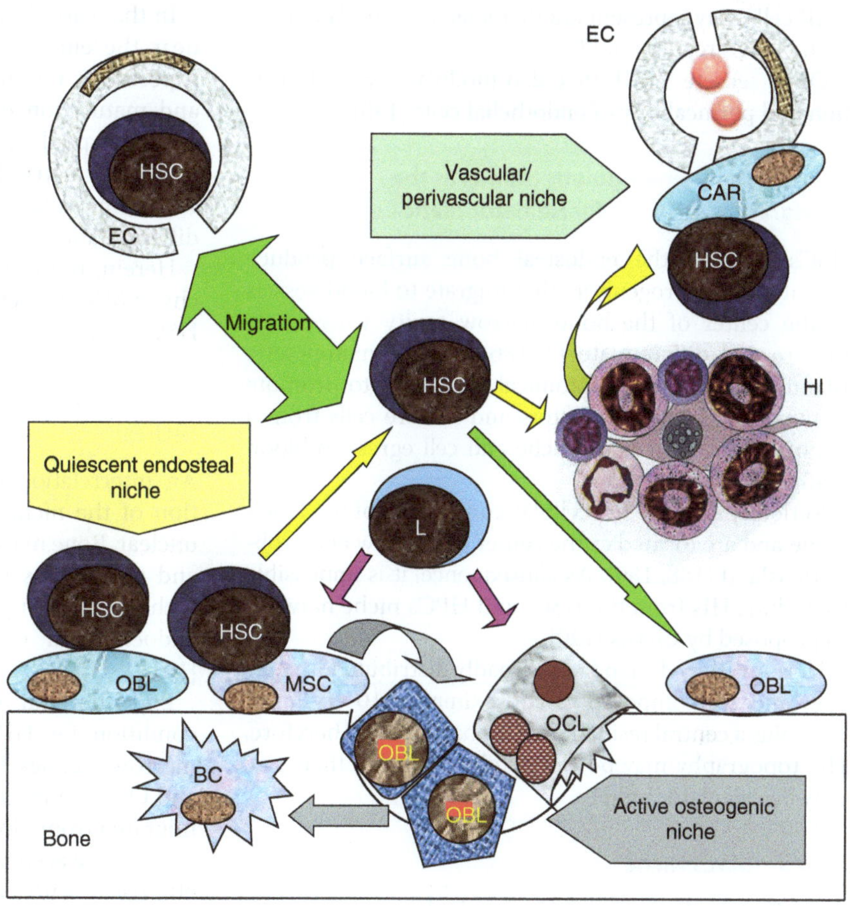

Figure 11.2 Schematic representation of niche dynamic reconstruction while bone remodeling in aging, fractures, and bone diseases passes. As shown, bone tissue undergoes permanent process of remodeling via bone resorption by osteoclasts coupled with bone formation by osteoblasts derived from MSCs. Blood leukocytes (T-lymphocytes, monocytes, etc.) are capable of modulating the bone remodeling under stress and pathological conditions, mainly. It leads to a disruption of preexisting quiescent niches in the reconstructed bone sites. As a result, active osteogenic niches can appear de novo. In turn, quit HSCs can target to other niches (HI, vascular niche) or emigrate from marrow. OBL niches can be seeded de novo by means of HSCs homing from blood. BC, bone cell (osteocyte); CAR cells, CXCL12-abundant reticular cells; EC, endothelial cells; HI, hematopoietic islets as a transit (?) niche for HPCs (hematopoietic progenitor cells); HSC, hematopoietic stem cell; L, leukocyte; MSC, mesenchymal stem cell; OBL, osteoblast; OCL, osteoclast.

marrow is termed the vascular niche [125, 132, 183]. However, this site would not meet the orthodox criteria for a niche (a site where HSCs self-renewal occurs) [37].

In summary, at least two topographically distinct niches supporting HSCs have been identified in the bone marrow: the osteoblastic (endosteal) niche and the endothelial (vascular) one. The osteoblastic niche may provide a quiescent microenvironment for HSCs maintenance. In contrast, the vascular niche facilitates HSCs transendothelial migration during mobilization or homing and may favor HSC proliferation and further differentiation [2].

However, the degree to which each niche contributes under normal or pathological conditions or during bioengineering is not clear.

11.4.1 Interconnection of Hematopoietic Niches

Both niches act together to maintain hemopoiesis or restore it after damage. The osteoblastic niche localized at the inner surface of the bone cavity and with abundant OBLs might serve as a reservoir for long-term HSCs storage in a quiescent state. Endothelial cells enhance proliferation of HSCs and play an important role in the hematopoietic pool maintaining. HSCs are associated with CAR cells in the sinusoidal region and are located between CAR and osteoblastic cells in the endosteal region, suggesting that those cells might be an important component of both the osteoblastic and the vascular niches in adult bone marrow [39, 184].

There is the current lack of knowledge of specific markers of vascular niche as compared with the accumulated evidence for the osteoblastic one [26]. Sacchetti et al. identified CD146$^+$ subendothelial cells residing in adult human bone marrow stroma on the sinusoidal wall that can generate both bone and HIM occurs via specific, dynamic interactions with developing sinusoids when transplanted under the skin of immunodeficient mice. They are the major producers of Ang-1 (a pivotal molecule of the both HSCs niche and of vascular remodeling). The functional relationships between transfer of the HIM *in vivo*, establishment of bone progenitors in the sinusoids, and angiogenesis were revealed. Hence,

CAR cells may represent another specific sites ("niches") of the HSCs regulation [38].

OBLs secrete VEGF that also modulates vascularization and permeability of endothelial cells [185].

11.4.2 The Hematopoietic Islands as the Topographical Niches for Hematopoietic Cells

HSCs residing the endosteal bone surface produce hematopoietic progenitors that migrate to blood vessels at the center of the bone marrow cavity where they mature and differentiate [2, 186, 187]. Hematopoietic islands (HIs) are the anatomical structures to promote a transit of HSCs, progenitors and mature cells from a hypothesized early stage niche and cell egress to blood [145].

Reticular cells are the cellular component of the HSCs niche and are located at the center of marrow erythroblastic island [188, 189]. As consequence, it is impossible to exclude HIs from the HSCs and HPCs niche network as proposed by Chasis [120].

Here, erythroid islands are broadly distributed in marrow, and are composed of approximately 10 erythroid cells plus a central resident macrophage [120]. Therefore, HIs topography may be closely observed and their size may be calculated simply.

11.4.3 MSCs Niche

The effective discussion and unreplied questions about the existence and functioning of MSCs niche has started recently in the scientific literature. What is the niche for the MSCs? Do HSCs and MSCs share the same niche end exchange signals to drive proliferation and differentiation? [74].

MSCs were found, with the use of the markers Stro-1 and CD146, lining blood vessels in human bone marrow and dental pulp [190]. These cells also expressed α-smooth muscle actin (α-SMA) and some even expressed 3G5, a pericyte-associated cell-surface marker as noted by Kolf et al. [24].

There are difficulties to localize the MSCs anatomical sites in the bone marrow cavity [60]. Doherty and Canfield have hypothesized that pericytes are in fact MSCs, because they can differentiate into OBLs, chondrocytes, and adipocytes [191]. Certain studies proposed a perivascular nature of the MSCs niche on the basis of the expression of α-SMA in MSCs isolated from all tissue types tested [59].

Proliferative capacity of human MMSCs was better maintained *in vitro* in hypoxic versus normoxic conditions (2% and 20% oxygen, respectively) [192]. Kolf et al. suggested hypoxia-induced enhancement of the proliferative capacity ("stemness") and the plasticity of MMSCs [24].

In that case, MMSCs niche thought to be else located near the endosteum with hypoxic milieu. Our recent experiment revealed *in vitro* osteogenic differentiation and maturation of human lung prenatal stromal cells (regional pool of MSCs) contacted short-termly with rough CP matrix [135]. The sockets in the bone matrix were conceived as active niches for MSCs osteoblastic differentiation and maturation.

Herein, the existence of structural-functional hierarchy of MMSC niches may be speculated by analogy with HSC ones.

11.4.4 Interrelation of Stromal and Hematopoietic Niches

An interrelation of an anatomical location and function of the niches for MMSCs and HSCs is currently unclear. Bone marrow MSCs may be both CD34-positive and negative as reviewed in [60]. Nevertheless, HSCs niche remodeling *in vivo* is conditioned at least by endochondral ossification [29] and bone formation [101].

Endochondral ossification is the most important condition for HIM development, including the bone marrow lacunes formation by recipient's macrophages and OCLs, and niches colonization by recipient's HSCs migrated from blood [29, 193].

The close accordance of ectopic growth of hematopoietic tissue with bone territories formed on the surface of artificial CP matrix was noted [103]. In this direction, $CD146^+$ CFU-Fs might play a pivotal role in the development of the MMSC and HSC niches by generating, or contributing to, structures (bone surfaces and sinusoidal abluminal surfaces) and functionally distinct cell types (OBLs and adventitial reticular cells) [38].

11.4.5 Dynamism of the Niches

In both the developing embryo and the adult, HSC niches vary in time, location, and composition [194]. Stem cell niches are the discrete and dynamic functional microenvironments that balance the stem cell activity to maintain tissue homeostasis and repair throughout the lifetime of an organism under diverse physiological (development and aging), reparative (acute trauma, lesion), and pathological (injury and disease) conditions [10].

The niche must be flexible domain and dynamic structure in order to coordinate stem cell behavior with homeostasis and repair [195]. Niche-derived signals are also critical for the engagement of specific programs in response to stress. Bone marrow stress can be induced by bleeding or by cell loss induced by toxic substances, including chemotherapeutic agents [3].

There are a few postulates in favor of niche dynamism [1]:

(1) stem cells can leave and return to their niches;
(2) a niche can remain vacant and exist independently of stem cells;
(3) a vacant niche can be occupied by excessive or transplanted stem cells and can provide for their functioning;
(4) a niche size allows a definite number of stem cells to be maintained;
(5) the niches control the number of stem cells in the body and protect it from excessive stem cell proliferation;
(6) stem cell niches are formed during ontogeny. The development can be described in terms of the formation of stem cells and their niches. In addition, permanent physiological remodeling of HIM can promote niche losing and change in HSCs and MSCs quiescent/active status (see Figure 11.2). A disruption of normal function and size of the stem cell niche may contribute to aging and disease onset and progression. Both spatial and temporal restrictions regulate the activity and number of niches.

Restoration and reversible expansion of the osteoblastic niche were observed after total body irradiation and were conditioned, in part, by proliferation of OBLs with subsequent hematopoietic regeneration [196]. Similarly, sinusoidal endothelial cells are capable of postradiation recovery and necessary for the recruitment and maintenance of HSCs pool [197].

When transplanted, leukemia cells initially localized on the surface of the OBLs in the inner vascular and diaphyseal region. The molecular mechanisms for the maintaining quiescence of normal HSCs may also facilitate a survival of leukemia stem cells. Under administration of a high dose of cytarabine leukemia cells clustered and adhered to the blood vessels, and they seemed receive also antiapoptotic signals from vascular niche [184].

Knowledge about the size of the stem cell niches will facilitate incorporation of the niche into stem cell-based therapies and regenerative medicine.

11.5 Quantitative Stage of the Niche Concept

There is complex hierarchical organization of the hematopoietic tissue. Thus, mouse marrow space can be approximately divided on 2600 cellular domains to regulate a production from stem to mature hematopoietic cells independently of each other, practically. Volume of each functional domain is equivalent of $50 \times 50 \times 50$ cells (nearly 10^8 μm^3) [198]. Naturally, domain includes HIs and niches. Delicate extracellular structure of the niche microterritory (MT) and its quantitative parameters are practically unknown.

Stem cells need to be tightly controlled through regulation of their proliferation, self-renewal and differentiation. Disruption of this regulation including the dynamic changes in the niche size can lead to severe consequences, such as age-related pathologies and cancer. Thus, the physiological niche size for germline stem cell in the adult flies is modulated by diet and age change [195].

Classically, the hematopoietic niche is the anatomical location or rather structural–functional site in which HSC resides and self-renew. The HSCs outside the niche do not self-renew and commence the process of differentiation to ultimately produce mature blood cells [37]. In this basis, HSCs niche requires the final size in order to cell could escape from it. The niche size is strongly controlled *in vivo* in order to maintain a constant number of HSCs and normal hematopoiesis [9, 199]. Otherwise, hematological disorders including leukemia occur.

At the modern state of the art, the most of investigations and reviews are mainly devoted to the changing in the niche regulation and signaling with the mathematical modeling of possible events, for example:

(1) The niche can contract and reexpand in response to altered Notch signaling in the *Drosophila* ovary [195].
(2) The niche size may control the differences in normal versus malignant cells living in and homing into the niche. Two questions arise; one is whether the leukemic stem cell occupies the same niche as the normal stem cell, and the other is whether the niche modifying agent can affect leukemic stem cells in the same way it does the normal cells [14].
(3) There are two regulators of a size of HSCs osteoblastic niche: PPR and BMP receptor 1A [78, 124].
(4) When the bone marrow MSCs were treated with platelet-derived growth factor (PDGF) and then transplanted into immunocompromised mice, the ratio of the niche size was 3.5-fold increase compared with nontreated transplants [200].
(5) The niche controlling mutated cells is larger since it is assumed mutated cells have more freedom in where they reside. It is likely that increasing the niche will have a major impact on tumor growth [6] causing critical imbalance between differentiation and stem cell self-renewal [201].
(6) ESCs niche size and composition regulate the balance between differentiation-inducing and differentiation-inhibiting factors. Two determinants of the hESC niche – colony size and cellular composition (number of undifferentiated and differentiated cells) – dramatically impact hESC fate and signaling [115].

In summary, the concept of the stem cell niche as specific anatomical locations assumes that the amount of space in microenvironments or niches is limited, the number of stem cells is also limited by the number that can fit in that space [7] plus feedback regulation by mature cells [6, 202].

Strangely little is known about the real niche size itself to count off its change in normal and pathological conditions. Future speculations are strongly needed for the experimental modeling of niche arising from its size, geometry, and topography.

Zhang et al. had determined per one histological cross-section of mouse femur nearly 50 niche-forming SNO cells contacted with a few hematological cells [78]. On the basis of this publication, Miura et al. [200] defined the osteoblastic niches as the bone marrow areas surrounded by the mononuclear spindle-shaped OBLs lining on the bone surfaces. The number of hematopoietic cells was determined by the nucleated cells counting in the bone marrow niche area.

No direct quantification of the niche size was specified by the authors. In our opinion, they studied the hematopoietic domains consisted of the number of the niches. At the same time, the area of one to two SNO cells as graphically modeling by Zhang et al. [78] has to include two dimensional (2D) size of the individual osteoblastic niche for HSCs.

Quantitative fluorescence microscopy was used by Peerani et al. [115] to assess the role of the microenvironment (ESC-derived extraembryonic endoderm) produced by human ESCs on the fate themselves. The localized cell density for each cell was computed by counting the number of cells that surrounded it within a radial threshold of 300 μm. This threshold was determined by empirically plotting Oct-4 (the octamer-binding transcription factor 4 gene plays a critical role in maintaining pluripotency during early mammalian embryonic development and self-renewal of ESCs) expression as a function of the localized cell density for radial thresholds ranging from 100 to 1000 μm and choosing the largest threshold that maintained a correlation. This analysis was consistent with the supposition of Francis and Palsson [203] that autocrine and paracrine effects are likely restricted to a few cell diameters around any given cell. The relative impact of ESCs endogenous regulators was local cell density (critical niche-size) dependent. Larger ESCs colonies with high local cell density microenvironments promote the maintenance of the undifferentiated phenotype (pluripotency) in human embryonic line [115].

A quantitative study would yield considerable insight into the properties of the individual ESCs niche. Likewise, we tried to determine optimal microterritory selected by embryonic cell [101, 204]. The line of prenatal stromal cells with $CD34^{-}CD44^{+}OCN^{-}$ phenotype prepared from the human lung (HLPSCs) was used due to the following reasons: (i) as embryonic cells, they supplied information about the early stages of niche self-organizing for their own self-renewal and differentiation [115, 175] and (ii) as stromal fibroblast-like cells, HLPSCs have an affinity to ECM.

During bone tissue remodeling *in vivo*, the stromal precursors colonize dish-shaped sockets with a depth up to 40 μm in the trabecular bone, formed by OCLs, and differentiate into OBLs actively synthesizing the bone matrix [75]. The most common strategy to differentiate MSCs is to use a combination of growth factors or biochemical cues [60]. Nevertheless, various studies have shown that ECM topography alone can induce or enhance the MSCs differentiation [205].

Currently, rough CP materials consisting of spherulites, valleys with small sockets and pores are the advanced ECM model of regenerating bone-mineralized matrix [101].

According to light microscopy, the area of socket in the microarc CP coating preferentially occupied *in vitro* by each ALP-positive HLPSC was about 302 μm^2, 86% of ALP-stained cells were seen in the sockets with areas of 100–625 μm^2. Scanning electron microscopy (SEM) showed that the cell occupied on average 217 μm^2 (118–316 μm^2 with consideration for standard deviation) or 42% its individual socket. These sockets were considered as microterritories (osteogenic niches) where HLPSCs differentiate and maturate into OBLs expressed ALP and osteocalcin (OC), and secreted OC into cultural medium [135, 204].

The niche for induction of osteogenic differentiation of MSCs was proposed as a structural and functional microregion and was named as "niche-relief." It can be characterized by an index calculated (in %) as the ratio of the total area of ALP-positive cell staining to the area of artificial socket occupied by one stained cell (microterritory [MT]): S_{ALP}/S_{MT} [135]. Maximal heterotopic remodeling of mouse bone/marrow system is noted *in vivo* on CP surface with optimal S_{ALP}/S_{MT} about 43% [206].

It is known that in the case of application of permanent electric field in the range of 0.1–1 V/mm, OBLs migrate quickly to negative electrode, and OCLs move to positive one [207]. A positive surface charge stimulates the differentiation of OCL-like cells [208]. In turn, the negative charge in the sockets (osteogenic niche) of CP surface was revealed in nano- and microscales [206, 209].

Optimal osteogenic magnitude of the electrostatic potential in rough CP surface was approximately 70–80 mV that can impact HSCs and MSCs transmembrane potential. It could be the physical mechanism mediating the influence of the surface topography on HLPSCs osteogenic maturation and differentiation [209]. Membrane hyperpolarization has been known to promote osteogenic differentiation of human MSCs unlike its depolarized state [172, 173].

The electric fields play a crucial role in the fate of stem cells because of its effects on zeta-potentials and cellular transmembrane (ion channels) [210]. Here, hyperpolarization of the negative membrane potential promotes osteogenic (ALP gene expression, intracellular calcium level) differentiation of human MSCs unlike its depolarized state [172] through intracellular signaling pathways.

Osteogenic differentiation of MSCs is a complex process that is tightly controlled by numerous signaling pathways and transcription factors [211]. Our data suggested optimal size of the bone matrix features as epigenetic regulator of MSCs behavior associated with osteogenic commitment that could be mediated by: (i) reduced promoter DNA methylation [212] and (ii) acetylation of H3 and H4 hystones associated with OC expression and osteogenic differentiation [213].

Finally, niche biology and function may impact on the ability to generate a larger number of stem cells or increase the efficiency of stem cells to engraft in the transplant setting [14]. Additional studies of factors that regulate the formation, activity, and the size of the stem cell niches are necessary in order to incorporate the niche concept into stem cell-based bioengineering and regenerative medicine. We presented primary physical, chemical, and biological steps to understand quantitative features of stromal and hemopoietic niches and to design them according to biomimetic principles. Of course, essential digital parameters of the niche can be received on the base of experimental modeling and bioengineering of stem microterritories.

11.6 Bioengineering Stage of the Niche Concept

The motivation that drives niche engineering is the question of how the extrinsic variables of the HIM can be realized in a controlled manner.

11.6.1 Biological Concept

First strategy of stem cell niche engineering is establishing the functional equivalents (physiological mechanisms, signaling) imitating the stem cell niche. Integral to niche engineering is dynamic control over soluble and surface-bound cytokines, ECM, cell–ECM and cell–cell interactions, mechanical forces, and physicochemical cues. There are a variety of approaches and devices to engineer, as well as to control individual niche components: soft lithography, microcontact printing, microfluidic techniques, ECM microarrays, etc. These approaches can be multiplexed to produce hybrid devices that simultaneously provide macroscopic (e.g. O_2-controlled bioreactors) and microscopic (e.g. micropatterned cocultures) control over the synthetic niche and the stem cell fate [194, 214].

Nevertheless, HSCs specific examples cannot be proper provided to illustrate a particular engineering strategy [194]. A reason is that a quantitative demarcation between individual microterritories (domain, niche) of stem cell and systemic HIM is still poorly understanding.

In this regard, round HIs seem to be suitable model and tool bar to compartmentalize *ex vivo* functional features of HSCs and HPCs niche, because their linear size may be estimated nearly 50–100 μm. Bigger micropattern and its other geometry will transform individual stem cell-niche interrelations. Large size of the niche increases a stem cell variability that is important for embryonic cells and tumor transformation of adult cells (see above).

There are essential differences between 2D and 3D cell cultures, in addition to differences in their behavior *in vivo* [215]. Deconstructing a complex 3D niche into 2D biomaterial model systems is a powerful and promising strategy for discovering new regulatory mechanisms governing stem cell biology. The structural, biophysical, and biochemical parameters of these model systems can be varied in myriad ways to identify and elucidate the effects of the components of putative stem cell niches on the stem cell function. Whereas 2D approaches allow well-controlled analysis of the impact on stem cells of individual components of the niche, 3D approaches, vice versa, should allow reconstruction, and realization of the complexity, of the natural tissue. For a more comprehensive review of such strategies, we refer our readers to review [216], where biochemical and biophysical properties of the artificial stem cell niches are *in vitro* describing the stem cell–ECM interactions, cell–cell interactions in two and three dimensions, as well biomaterials controlled delivery of niche signals and molecules.

In this regard, mimicking of MSCs and HSCs microenvironment is booming in 2D and 3D systems. The authors revealed 3D distribution of $CD34^+$ HSCs in the 2D HSCs/MSCs *in vitro* coculture system. First phase-dim (PD) compartment of hematopoietic cells migrated under the MSCs monolayer and showed "quiescent" cell-cycle activity and immature phenotype ($CD34^+CD38^-$). In contrast, phase-bright HSCs on the MSCs surface revealed significantly more proliferation and differentiation activities. The third compartment of nonadherent differentiated HSCs released from the MSCs surface into the supernatant [80]. The PD compartment beneath the MSCs layer seems to mimic the stem cell niche for immature hematopoietic cells.

11.6.2 ECM Mimicking by the Approaches in Materials Science

Biomaterials are rapidly being developed to display and deliver stem-cell-regulatory signals in a precise and near-physiological manner, and serve as powerful artificial microenvironments in which to study and instruct stem-cell fate both in culture and *in vivo*. Further synergism of cell biological and biomaterials technologies promises to have a profound impact on stem cell biology and provide insights that will advance stem cell based clinical approaches to tissue regeneration [216].

With the current growth rate in lab automation, rapid advancement in development of materials technology, and accelerated materials discovery for a fast-growing range of applications are expected [217]. Hereafter, the integration of biomaterials with existing induced pluripotent stem cells (iPSC) culture platforms could offer additional opportunities to better probe the biology and control the behavior of iPSCs or their progeny *in vitro* and *in vivo* [218].

The ability to better engineer artificial ECM that can control cell behavior, through physical as well as molecular interactions, may further extend our capabilities in engineering tissue substitutes from adult or ESCs [89, 219].

The biophysical properties of the HIM are important to understand the role of niche elements, including blood flow, matrix mechanical properties, geometry, topography, and the transmission of mechanical or other biophysical factors to the cell [155, 220]. The ECM of different tissues (bone, marrow, brain, muscle, etc.) is physically chemically diverse. To control the stem cells, biomaterial science mimics the properties of ECM.

Direct effects of matrix physical attributes have to be examined entirely. The majority of studies investigating the influence of physical factors on stem cells have focused on adult stem cell populations, such as MSCs or other connective tissue stem cells [220].

Herein, Wolff's law of bone growth and remodeling articulated in 1892 that changes in force applied to bone result in changes in its structure, mass, and strength. Apparently, it can be applied to an interconnection between ECM structure and cell structure, function, and commitment. Today, a set of key physicochemical parameters of artificial ECM that affect cells have already been identified, namely, architecture and mechanical properties [221], mechanical integrity, the rate of scaffold degradation, fluid transport [222], cell-recognizable surface chemical properties, the ability to induce signal transduction [223], surface free energy and wettability [224], surface electrical charge [225, 226], chemical composition [227], surface geometry, topography, and stiffness [228].

A wide variation in matrix stiffness for cells is known to influence focal-adhesion structure and the cytoskeleton [229, 230]. Mechanotransduction is modern direction to study stromal mechanocytes (fibroblasts, reticular cells) [231], as well lineage progenitors [232].

The MSCs surface as the major site of HSCs behavior affected various soluble and non-soluble signals [80]. Therefore, MSCs niche bioengineering can promote the designing of HSC microterritories.

Solid and soft tissues exhibit a range of stiffness, as measured by the elastic modulus (E). Stem cells may well possess more than the typical ensemble of force-coupled signaling pathways as a means to sensitize themselves to 3D microenvironments that range – physically – from flowing fluids and strained tissues to solid tissues of varied elasticity. Neurogenic markers of MSCs have been determined to be clearly highest on polyacrylamide gels with $E = 0.1–1\,\text{kPa}$. When MSCs are grown on firm gels that mimic the elasticity of muscle ($E = 8–17\,\text{kPa}$) and that are coated with collagen-I, myogenic markers are upregulated. When naive MSCs are grown on rigid gels ($E = 34\,\text{kPa}$) that mimic precalcified bone, the cells demonstrate osteogenic origin [232]. The authors showed that soluble induction factors tend to be less selective than matrix stiffness in driving specification, and cannot reprogram MSCs that are precommitted for weeks on a given matrix.

Lutolf et al. presented fine modeling *in vitro* of artificial niches for self-renewal divisions of single long-term HSCs with time-lapse microscopic analyses [233]. Soft (elastic modulus less than 1 kPa, [234]) cross-linked PEG (poly(ethylene glycol))-based inert hydrogel was used to simulate the soft and hydrated microenvironment of HSCs in the bone marrow. Nonadhesive for cells PEG hydrogel was attached to the bottom of tissue culture wells to mimic physicochemical properties of the niche. Since each well was supplemented with an individual proteins (Wnt3a or N-Cadherin), the several hundreds of single HSCs trapped within microwells (100–130 μm diameter) of a given well were all exposed to the same protein. Authors suggested that 3D effects of extrinsic N-Cadherin on HSCs self-renewal dissect the regulatory role of specific signals within a complex stem cell niche, and were likely to reflect its biological role in HSCs function in the niche.

In turn, a number of questions arise: what is topographical type of such niches (endosteal or vascular)? What is amount of HSCs to correspond to the microterritory of hematopoietic niche or hematopoietic domain? In our mind, this hydrogel microwell platform validates an interaction of migratory HSCs and ECM in the bone marrow milieu outside known hematopoietic niches. Thus, carefully made biomimetic materials with well-defined quantitative parameters can prime the control of specific progenitors mediated by epigenetic signals of the niche.

Size control is important to minimize gradients in oxygen and other physical or chemical factors that regulate stem cell fate [235]. It is designed *in vitro*, embryoid bodies with growing human ESCs can be sculpted to well-controlled diameters with polymer microwells [236].

Controlling *in vitro* the area of human MSCs contact with the help of micropatterned substrates, McBeath et al. [237] printed two-dimensional (2D) fibronectin "islands" and cultured for one week single MSCs per island. Authors found in proliferation-arrested MSCs induced adipogenesis on small fibronectin islands (1024 μm^2 that minimize matrix contact) and their osteogenesis on large islands (10 000 μm^2 that maximize contractile anchorage). Human MSCs allowed to adhere, flatten, and spread underwent osteogenesis, while unspread, round cells became adipocytes. Cell shape alone was concluded to drive the commitment of human MSCs to adipocyte or OBL fate by means of cytoskeletal tension.

According to our data, irregular distribution of $CD34^-CD44^+$ adherent HLPSCs was observed in 3D culture on rough CP scaffold-like coating. Fibroblast-like or flat cells with OCL-like (ACP – positive) phenotype were located on spherolites (top) of CP coatings. Round-shaped stromal cells with OBL-like (ALP) and OC staining manifested in the sockets (bottom) of CP surface [135].

Most probably, McBeath et al. established *in vitro* the minimal size of ECM domain to initiate MSCs osteogenic differentiation [237]. Indeed, adhesive circular micro domains (100–400 μm diameters) on glass cover slips may be manufactured by a maskless photolithography system. For all this, 200 μm circular domains were found to be the optimal diameter for the cardiac differentiation of murine ESCs in uniform sized aggregates [238].

Bone tissue growth in 3D porous CP ceramics has been known to be observed *in vivo* at pore's diameter of 100–800 μm [239–241], that corresponds to their approximate section areas of 8000–500 000 μm^2. In our mind, large pores played a role of synthetic micro domains for MSCs and HSCs, because the bone and marrow ectopic in-growth occurred [241].

Peerani et al. developed methods to culture human ESCs in defined microenvironments by micropatterning colonies on ECM substrate (Matrigel™) printed in distinct features. Poly(dimethylsiloxane) stamps with the diameter (*D*) of circular features from 200 to 800 μm and the distance between circular features from 500 to 1000 μm were fabricated using standard soft lithography techniques. ESCs were seeded as single cells onto the patterned substrates and cultured without any exogenous growth factors. Decreased pluripotency (enhanced differentiation) of human endocannabinoid systems (ECSs) was observed in $D = 200\,\mu m$. Colony size has been speculated to change the ratio of perimeter to internal cells as well as the levels and distribution of mechanical stress within a colony to influence gene expression and paracrine signaling feedback (growth differentiation factor 3 [GDF3]; BMP2) [115]. The authors concluded that the results presented in this work demonstrated a role of the niche size for human ESCs self-renewal control and provided a quantitative framework to test other niche-related factors in a systematic manner.

de Barros et al. developed *in vitro* a complex multicellular 3D spheroid model with human bone MSCs, undifferentiated (non-induced) or induced for one week into OBLs. After four days, MSCs formed spheroid structures of approximately 400 μm diameters (420 ± 23.7 μm; size correlated with 6–50 thousands of plated cells) with a complex 3D network similar to reticular cells in the marrow cavity. Mixed spheroids had osteoinduced MSCs at the center and non-induced MSCs around the spheroids simulated microterritory near subendosteal niches in the bone marrow. The aim was to create specialized regions, and by surrounding osteoinduced spheroids with MSCs authors sought to mimic the trabecular bone that is also surrounded by reticular cells. $CD34^+$ cells moving in and out of mixed spheroids occurred. Hematopoietic progenitors with restrained proliferation and migration were located in close proximity to osteoinduced MSCs [81].

To study a fate of HSCs pool, de Barros et al. simulated, apparently, large (domain) regions corresponded to pores in the bone materials described in [239].

Since 1964, Curtis and Varde [242] provided important effect of surface topography on the cell fate [243]. In principle, a lot of publications presented in part in [205] concerned the nano- and microtopographic modeling of systemic ECM to influence a cell fate. A wide range of cells (fibroblasts, OBLs, OCLs, nerve cells, MSCs, ESCs, etc.) respond to the surface micro- [243–245] and nanotopography [246, 247]; the main influencing factor *in vitro* is the latter topography and not the former [227, 248].

However, the biomechanical forces led to another results in *in vivo* conditions of subcutaneous test in mice. Only macroscale grooves of 1 mm width and depth on submicro-rough (average roughness index $R_a < 500\,nm$) CP surface promoted donor bone marrow survival and bone/marrow system remodeling. No smooth nanorough CP scaffolds affected ectopic MSCs and HSCs growth [136]. So, 3D structure (texture) of ECM has own potential to direct the stem cell fate [80].

Topographic cues of ECM altered the organization of various cytoskeletal components, including F-actin, vimentin, γ-tubulin, and α-tubulin, and the observed changes in proliferation and morphology were abolished by the effect of actin disrupting agents. Alternatively, the influence of nanotopographic features may be mediated through secondary effects, such as alterations in the effective stiffness perceived by the cell or differences in protein adsorption due to the structural features of the substrate [220].

Material architecture can be used to template ECM structure and to design the synthetic niche. Key elements of niche are known but the "cocktail" of biophysical mechanisms in the niche scale is not understood. The size of the niche and its composition regulate the balance between differentiation-inducing and differentiation-inhibiting factors of both ESCs and adult stem cells [115]. The achieved results are not unequivocal, and different conditions for fabricating scaffoldings were recognized as possible factors for the varying outcomes [249]. Thus, scientists are only just beginning to understand the niche–cell interactions [246].

Designing artificial matrices that can mimic the quantitative parameters of tissue microenvironment and regulate the appropriate differentiation of stem cells is a promising approach to therapeutic applications [24]. One of the limitations in stem cell research is the inability to scientifically reconstruct native niches, which makes it difficult to maintain stem cells *in vitro* [6] because signals from the niche affect stem-cell survival, self-renewal, and differentiation [2].

We have mimicked *in vitro* more individual endosteal microenvironment (niche) for MSCs with the help of rough CP materials. Costa et al. have recently demonstrated the capability of biomimetic HA coatings topography to influence the attachment and differentiation of OBLs and the resorptive activity of OCLs. OBL attachment and differentiation were stronger on more complex, microrough HA surfaces (roughness index $R_a \sim 2\,\mu m$) than on smoother topographies ($R_a \sim 1\,\mu m$). In contrast, OCL activity was greater on smoother than on microrough surfaces [250]. It is according with CP surface roughness to stimulate HLPSCs osteogenic differentiation *in vitro* [206].

Moreover, the microarc technology to simulate the architecture of porous bone by rough CP surface with $R_a = 2–3\,\mu m$ led *in vivo* to maximal ectopic remodeling of the bone/bone marrow system in mice [103, 251].

Thick microarc CP coating with $R_a = 1.5–6\,\mu m$ delivered a three-dimensional (3D) scaffold bone-like topography having a multilevel structure consisting of spherulites, valleys, sockets and pores that contains synthetic (artificial) microterritories for MSCs osteogenic differentiation and maturation as described above. Our manipulations with HLPSCs on such surface allowed defining the "niche-relief" and "niche-voltage" key concepts to design novel class of biomimetic materials for bone and marrow tissues bioengineering [206, 209].

At present, the osteogenic "niche-relief" may be primary site to regulate MSCs differentiation, because its size is at least 10-folds lower (see "Quantitative stage of niche concept") than stem cell domains designed by other authors. "Niche-potential" technology can be used as a tool for niche designing in smooth CaP surfaces to strengthen their integration with the bone tissue.

The key concept is that a biomaterial surface and volume can contain specific chemical and structural information that controls tissue formation, in a manner analogous to cell–cell communication and patterning during embryological development [89]. The application of stem cells in the bioengineering of new tissues and recovery of damaged ones is dependent on the use of an appropriate scaffold to maintain native 3D cell distribution and on the use of specific molecules to drive tissue-specific matrix [252]. Thus, 3D combination of systemic HIM components and integrated stem cell microterritories with clear quantitative and qualitative features seems to be more prospective approach to engineer the biomaterial (synthetic ECM) scaffolds as advanced stem cell niche carriers.

11.7 Concluding Remarks

The capability to sustain stem cells and tissues outside the body needs substantial improvement to achieve clinical applications. Isolated from tissues stem cells rapidly lose their status, function, and viability. The failure of stem cell function happens because the support network of microenvironment (other cell contacts, contacts to matrices and the captured insoluble adhesion proteins and support cells) does no longer exist. It is better to support cells inside privileged microenvironments, where they do not lose their special characteristics but, where their specialization can be programmed, maintained, and regulated *in vitro* and *in vivo* for a long time. Artificial life support systems dedicated to stem cells are being modeled on the structural design and composition of the ECM [253].

Niche hierarchy queries orthodox definition of HSCs niche as a place allowing the stem cell to proliferate and to retain its stemness and self-renewal capacity. At present, morphofunctional features of systemic HIM are still spreading to specialized microenvironment (niche) of HSCs. Required factors of ECM have been supposed to summarize stochastically in restricted region to influence stem cell behavior. For all this, a number of questions arise: what are necessary and sufficient sizes of such microterritory in systemic HIM to consider it as the niche? Do essential differences between the niche and ECM space exist?

Bioengineering provides vast prospective directions of the niche design as an approach to regenerative medicine. They connected with two principal strategies of niche technology.

Current extensive strategy is to employ biomaterials with surfaces and volumes designed to mimic and to combine numerous biological components of systemic HIM as potential niche factors. Such materials provide the scientific foundation for stochastic design of synthetic ECM to study stochastic stem cell reactions and to screen randomly the prospective scaffolds for regenerative medicine.

An increasingly prolific strategy has been to use the ECM directly, removed of its cells. Alternatively biomaterial copies are made of the ECM structure and function [253]. To have more regulation and control over cell responses it is necessary to be able to build tailor-made ECMs using a combination of natural molecules, purely synthetic molecules, and mixtures of the two. The most promising substrates that increasingly match native ECMs are protein polymers and synthetic polymers with oligopeptide additions; adhesion receptors; soluble and insoluble ligands that increase cell interactions and stimulate natural tissue remodeling [254, 255].

Promising intensive strategy is to define native sizes and initial matrix (anchor) of stem structural-functional microterritories, to modify step by step physicochemical and epigenetic features that influence the stem cells developmental program.

If cell niche is specific anatomical microterritory, its spatial restrictions must exist. Otherwise, its mechanisms are not distinguished from ones in systemic HIM. The dimension of microterritory seems to determine its intrinsic features as a niche space for stem cell, as a micro domain for cell population, and structural-functional units (liver acinus, renal corpuscle, etc.) of tissue. According to our opinion, the stem cell niche is distinct, structural-functional, energetically (thermodynamically) favorable microterritory in HIM contiguous space where quantitative parameters of a microenvironment promote qualitative control of the stem cell fate.

Individualized microenvironments using novel niche technology and extending the concept of hemopoietic and stromal niches may help to overcome the problems of stem cell transplantation and tissue bioengineering.

List of Abbreviations

5-FU	5-fluorouracil
α-SMA	α-smooth muscle actin
ACP	acid phosphatase
ALP	alkaline phosphatase
Ang-1	angiopoietin-1
BMPs	bone morphogenic proteins
BMSCs	bone marrow stromal cells
CaR	Ca^{2+}-sensing receptor
CAR	CXCL12-abundant reticular cells
CFU-E	colony-forming units of erythropoiesis
CFU-Fs	colony-forming units of fibroblast-like cells
CFU-GM	colony-forming units of granulomonocytopoiesis
c-Kit	v-kit Hardy-Zuckerman 4 feline sarcoma viral oncogene homolog
c-Myc	v-myc avian myelocytomatosis viral oncogene homolog
CP	calcium phosphate
C-X-C motif	CXCL12 ligand 12
E	elastic modulus
ECs	endothelial cells
ECM	extracellular matrix
ELP	early lymphoid progenitor cells
ESCs	embryonic stem cells
FGF-4	fibroblast growth factor-4
GAGs	glycosaminoglycans
G-CSF	granulocyte colony-stimulating factor
GDF3	growth differentiation factor 3
GM-CSF	granulocyte-macrophage colony-stimulating factor
HyA	hyaluronic acid
HA	hydroxyapatite
HIs	hematopietic islets
HIM	hemopoietic inductive microenvironment
HLPSCs	prenatal stromal cells prepared from the human lung
HPCs	hematopoietic progenitor cells
HSCs	hematopoietic stem cells
ICAM	intracellular cell adhesion molecule
IL	interleukin
iPSC	induced pluripotent stem cells
ISCT	International Society for Cellular Therapy
$Lepr^{+}$ cells	leptin receptor (Lepr)-expressing perivascular cells
LSK	lineage–$Sca\text{-}1^{+}c\text{-}Kit^{+}$
MAPK	mitogen-activated protein kinase
M-CSF	macrophage colony-stimulating factor
MMSCs	multipotent mesenchymal stromal cells
Mpl	protooncogene, thrombopoietin receptor
MSCs	mesenchymal stromal cells

mTOR	mammalian target of rapamycin
NE	norepinephrine
Notch1	a member of the type 1 transmembrane protein family, a human homolog of the *Drosophila* jagged receptor notch
NSCs	neural stem cells
OC	osteocalcin
OCLs	osteoclasts
Oct-4	the octamer-binding transcription factor 4 gene
OPG	osteoprotegerin
OPN	osteopontin
PD	phase-dim
PDGF	platelet-derived growth factor
PEG	poly(ethylene glycol)
PGE_2	prostaglandin E_2
PPR	parathyroid hormone-related peptide receptor
PTH	parathyroid hormone
RANK	receptor for RANKL
RANKL	receptor activator of nuclear factor kappa B ligand
RGD	arginine-glycine-aspartic acid
ROS	reactive oxygen species
SCF	stem cell factor
SDF-1	stromal cell derived factor-1
SEM	scanning electron microscopy
Shh	sonic hedgehog
SLAM	signaling lymphocytic activation molecule
SNO	N-cadherin positive/CD45 negative osteoblastic cells
SNS	sympathetic nervous system
TERT	telomerase reverse transcriptase
TGF	transforming growth factor
THPO	thrombopoietin
Tie2	a tyrosine kinase receptor
TNF	tumor necrosis factor
VCAM	vascular cell adhesion molecule
VEGF	vascular endothelial growth factor
VLA	very late antigen
Wnt	mammalian homolog of *Drosophila* wingless

References

1 Terskikh, V.V., Vasiliev, A.V., and Vorotelyak, E.A. (2007). Stem cell niches. *Biol. Bull.* **34** (3): 211–220.

2 Yin, T. and Li, L. (2006). The stem cell niches in bone. *J. Clin. Invest.* **116** (5): 1195–1101.

3 Lander, A.D., Kimble, J., Clevers, H. et al. (2012). What does the concept of the stem cell niche really mean today? *BMC Biol.* **10**: 19. https://doi.org/10.1186/1741-7007-10-19.

4 Cleavers, H. (2005). Stem cells, asymmetric division and cancer. *Nat. Genet.* **37**: 1027–1028.

5 Han, W., Yu, Y., and Liu, X.Y. (2006). Local signals in stem cell-based bone marrow regeneration. *Cell Res.* **16**: 189–195.

6 Gentry, S.N. and Jackson, T.L. (2013). A mathematical model of cancer stem cell driven tumor initiation: implications of niche size and loss of homeostatic regulatory mechanisms. *PLoS ONE* **8** (8): 71128. https://doi.org/10.1371/journal.pone.0071128.

7 Morrison, S.J., Shah, N.M., and Anderson, D.J. (1997). Regulatory mechanisms in stem cell biology. *Cell* **88**: 287–298.

8 Li, L. and Xie, T. (2005). Stem cell niche: structure and function. *Annu. Rev. Cell Dev. Biol.* **21**: 605–631.

9 Schofield, R. (1978). The relationship between the spleen colony-forming cell and the hematopopietic stem cell. A hypothesis. *Blood Cells* **4** (1–2): 7–25.

10 Voog, J. and Jones, D.L. (2010). Stem cells and the niche: a dynamic duo. *Cell Stem Cell* **6** (2): 103–115.

11 Wilson, A. and Trumpp, A. (2006). Bone-marrow haematopoietic-stem-cell niches. *Nat. Rev. Immunol.* **6**: 93–106.

12 Arai, F. and Suda, T. (2008). Quiescent stem cells in the niche. In: *The Stem Cell Research Community* (StemBook, ed). StemBook. https://doi.org/10.3824/stembook.1.6.1, http://www.stembook.org.

13 Simons, B. and Cleavers, H. (2011). Strategies for homeostatic stem cell self-renewal in adult tissues. *Cell* **1454**: 851–862.

14 Scadden, D.T. (2007). The stem cell niche in health and leukemic disease. *Best Pract. Res. Clin. Haematol.* **20** (1): 19–27.

15 Scadden, D.T. (2006). The stem-cell niche as an entity of action. *Nature* **441**: 1075–1079.

16 Wilkins, B.S. (1992). Histology of normal haemopoiesis: bone marrow histology I. *J. Clin. Pathol.* **45**: 645–649.

17 Trentin, J.J. (1971). Determination of bone marrow stem cell differentiation by stromal hemopoietic inductive microenvironments (HIM). *Am. J. Pathol.* **65**: 621–628.

18 Gancz, D. and Gilboa, L. (2013). Hormonal control of stem cell systems. *Annu. Rev. Cell Dev. Biol.* **29**: 137–162.

19 Tavassoli, M. (1975). Studies on hemopoietic microenvironments. *Exp. Hematol.* **3**: 213–226.

20 Boggs, S.S. (1999). The hematopoietic microenvironment: phylogeny and ontogeny of the hematopoietic microenvironment. *Hematology* **4** (1): 31–44.

21 de Saint-Georges, L. and Miller, S.C. (1992). The microcirculation of bone and marrow in the diaphysis of the rat hemopoietic long bones. *Anat. Rec.* **233**: 169–177.

22 Lichtman, M.A. (1981). The ultrastructure of the hemopoietic environment of the marrow: a review. *Exp. Hematol.* **9** (4): 391–410.

23 Lord, B.I. (1990). The architecture of bone marrow cell populations. *Int. J. Cell Cloning* **8**: 317–331.

24 Kolf, C.M., Cho, E., and Tuan, R.S. (2007). Mesenchymal stromal cells. Biology of adult mesenchymal stem cells: regulation of niche, self-renewal and differentiation. *Arthritis Res. Ther.* **9** (1): 204–219.

25 Suda, T., Arai, F., and Hirao, A. (2005). Hematopoietic stem cells and their niche. *Trends Immunol.* **26**: 426–433.

26 Jang, Y.Y. and Sharkis, S.J. (2007). A low level of reactive oxygen species selects for primitive hematopoietic stem cells that may reside in the low-oxygenic niche. *Blood* **110**: 3056–3063.

27 Holzwarth, C., Vaegler, M., Gieseke, F. et al. (2010). Low physiologic oxygen tensions reduce proliferation and differentiation of human multipotent mesenchymal stromal cells. *BMC Cell Biol.* **11**: 11. http://www.biomedcentral.com/1471-2121/11/11.

28 Brandi, M.L. and Collin-Osdoby, P. (2006). Vascular biology and the skeleton. *J. Bone Miner. Res.* **21**: 183–192.

29 Chan, C.K.F., Chen, C.C., Luppen, C.A. et al. (2009). Endochondral ossification is required for hematopoietic stem cell niche formation. *Nature* **457** (7228): 490–494.

30 Nakayama, N., Lee, J., and Chiu, L. (2000). Vascular endothelial growth factor synergistically enhances bone morphogenetic protein-4–dependent lymphohematopoietic cell generation from embryonic stem cells in vitro. *Blood* **95**: 2275–2283.

31 Taichman, R.S. (2005). Blood and bone: two tissues whose fates are intertwined to create the hematopoietic stem-cell niche. *Blood* **105** (7): 2631–2639.

32 Smith, J.N.P. and Calvi, L.M. (2013). Current concepts in bone marrow microenvironmental regulation of hematopoietic stem and progenitor cells. *Stem Cells* **31**: 1044–1050.

33 Calvo, W. (1967). The nerve supply of bone marrow of chicken and pigeon. *J. Morphol.* **123** (3): 445–490.

34 Calvo, W. and Forteza-Vila, J. (1970). Schwann cells of the bone marrow. *Blood* **36**: 180–188.

35 Yamazaki, K. and Allen, T.D. (1990). Ultrastructural morphometric study of efferent nerve terminals on murine bone marrow stromal cells, and the recognition of a novel anatomical unit: the "neuro-reticular complex". *Am. J. Anat.* **187**: 261–276.

36 Miller, M.R. and Kasahara, M. (1963). Observation on the innervation of human long bones. *Anat. Rec.* **145** (1): 13–23.

37 Purton, L.E. and Scadden, D.T. (2008). The hematopoietic stem cell niche. In: *The Stem Cell Research Community* (StemBook, ed). StemBook. https://doi.org/10.3824/stembook.1.28.1, http://www.stembook.org.

38 Sacchetti, B., Funari, A., Michienzi, S. et al. (2007). Self-renewing osteoprogenitors in bone marrow sinusoids can organize a hematopoietic microenvironment. *Cell* **131**: 324–336.

39 Sugiyama, T., Kohara, H., Noda, M., and Nagasawa, T. (2006). Maintenance of the hematopoietic stem cell pool by CXCL12-CXCR4 chemokine signaling in bone marrow stromal cell niches. *Immunity* **25**: 977–988.

40 Mendez-Ferrer, S., Michurina, T.V., Ferraro, F. et al. (2010). Mesenchymal and haematopoietic stem cells form a unique bone marrow niche. *Nature* **466**: 829–834.

41 Afan, A.M., Broome, C.S., Nicholls, S.E. et al. (1997). Bone marrow innervation regulates cellular retention in the murine haemopoietic system. *Br. J. Haematol.* **98**: 569–577.

42 Mendez-Ferrer, S., Lucas, D., Battista, M., and Frenette, P.S. (2008). Haematopoietic stem cell release is regulated by circadian oscillations. *Nature* **452**: 442–447.

43 Miller, M.L. and McCuskey, R.S. (1973). Innervation of bone marrow in the rabbit. *Scand. J. Haematol.* **10** (1): 17–23.

44 Spiegel, A., Shivtiel, S., Kalinkovich, A. et al. (2007). Catecholaminergic neurotransmitters regulate migration and repopulation of immature human $CD34^+$ cells through Wnt signaling. *Nat. Immunol.* **8**: 1123–1131.

45 Katayama, Y., Battista, M., Kao, W.M. et al. (2006). Signals from the sympathetic nervous system regulate hematopoietic stem cell egress from bone marrow. *Cell* **124**: 407–421.

46 Gol'dberg, E.D., Khlusov, I.A., Dygai, A.M., and Agafonov, V.I. (1993). The adrenergic mechanisms controlling the proliferation and differentiation of hematopoietic precursor cells under immobilization stress. *Bull. Exp. Biol. Med.* **116** (11): 457–460.

47 Dygai, A.M., Khlusov, I.A., Udut, V.V. et al. (1997). Regulating effect of sympathetic-adrenal system

on hemopoiesis suppressed by cytostatic drugs. *Pathophysiology* **4**: 175–181.

48 Khlusov, I.A., Dygai, A.M., and Gol'dberg, E.D. (1997). Adrenergic dependence of the proliferation of hemopoietic precursors under the influence of cytostatics. *Bull. Exp. Biol. Med.* **123** (6): 555–558.

49 Dexter, T.M., Allen, T.D., and Lajtha, L.G. (1977). Conditions controlling the proliferation of haemopoietic stem cells in vitro. *J. Cell. Physiol.* **91**: 335–344.

50 Weiss, L. (1976). The hematopoietic microenvironment of the bone marrow: an ultrastructural study of the stroma in rats. *Anat. Rec.* **186** (2): 161–184.

51 Zipori, D. (1989). Stromal cells from the bone marrow: evidence for a restrictive role in regulation of hemopoiesis. *Eur. J. Hematol.* **42** (3): 225–322.

52 Friedenstein, A.J. (1990). Bone marrow osteogenic stem cells. In: *Calcium Regulation and Bone Metabolism* (ed. D.V. Cohn, F.H. Glorieux, T.J. Martin, et al.), 353–361. Cambridge: Elsevier.

53 Dennis, J.E. and Caplan, A.I. (2004). Bone marrow mesenchymal stem cells. In: *Stem Cells Handbook* (ed. S. Sell), 107–117. Totowa, NJ: Humana Press Inc.

54 Dennis, J.E., Merriam, A., Awadallah, A. et al. (1999). A quadripotential mesenchymal progenitor cell isolated from the marrow of an adult mouse. *J. Bone Miner. Res.* **14**: 700–709.

55 Lo Celso, C., Fleming, H.E., Wu, J.W. et al. (2009). Live-animal tracking of individual haematopoietic stem/progenitor cells in their niche. *Nature* **457**: 92–96.

56 Xie, Y., Yin, T., Wiegraebe, W. et al. (2009). Detection of functional haematopoietic stem cell niche using real-time imaging. *Nature* **457** (7225): 97–01.

57 Owen, M. and Friedenstein, A.J. (1988). Stromal stem cells: marrow-derived osteogenic precursors. *Ciba Found. Symp.* **136**: 42–60.

58 Caplan, A.I. (1991). Mesenchymal stem cells. *J. Orthop. Res.* **9**: 641–650.

59 Da Silva Meirelles, L., Chagastelles, P.C., and Nardi, N.B. (2006). Mesenchymal stem cells reside in virtually all post-natal organs and tissues. *J. Cell Sci.* **119**: 2204–2213.

60 Aerts, F. and Wagemaker, G. (2006). Mesenchymal stem cell engineering and transplantation. In: *Genetic Engineering of Mesenchymal Stem Cells* (ed. J.A. Nolta), 1–44. The Netherlands: Springer.

61 Bianco, P. and Robey, P.G. (2004). Skeletal stem cells. In: *Handbook of Stem Cells*, vol. **2** (ed. R. Lanza), 415–424. New York: Academic Press.

62 Kfoury, Y., David, T., and Scadden, D.T. (2015). Mesenchymal cell contributions to the stem cell niche. *Cell Stem Cell* **16**: 239–253.

63 Kuznetsov, S.A., Krebsbach, P.H., Satomura, K. et al. (1997). Single-colony derived strains of human marrow stromal fibroblasts form bone after transplantation in vivo. *J. Bone Miner. Res.* **12**: 1335–1347.

64 Ho, A.D., Wagner, W., and Franke, W. (2008). Heterogeneity of mesenchymal stromal cell preparations. *Cytotherapy* **10**: 320–330.

65 Docheva, D., Popov, C., Mutschler, W., and Schieker, M. (2007). Human mesenchymal stem cells in contact with their environment: surface characteristics and the integrin system. *J. Cell. Mol. Med.* **11** (1): 21–38.

66 Armstrong, L., Lako, M., Buckley, N. et al. (2012). Editorial: our top 10 developments in stem cell biology over the last 30 years. *Stem Cells* **30**: 2–9.

67 Patki, S., Kadam, S., Chandra, V., and Bhonde, R. (2010). Human breast milk is a rich source of multipotent mesenchymal stem cells. *Hum. Cell* **23** (2): 35–40.

68 Via, A.G., Frizziero, A., and Oliva, F. (2012). Biological properties of mesenchymal stem cells from different sources. *Muscles Ligaments Tendons J.* **2** (3): 154–162.

69 Galmishe, M., Koteliansky, V., Briere, J. et al. (1993). Stromal cells from human long-term marrow cultures are mesenchymal cells that differentiate following a vascular smooth muscle differentiation pathway. *Blood* **82**: 66–76.

70 Pittenger, M.F., Mackay, A.M., Beck, S.C. et al. (1999). Multilineage potential of adult human mesenchymal stem cells. *Science* **284**: 143–147.

71 D'Ippolito, G., Schiller, P.C., Ricordi, C. et al. (1999). Age-related osteogenic potential of mesenchymal stromal cells from human bone marrow. *J. Bone Miner. Res.* **14**: 15–23.

72 Tuljapurkar, S.R., Jackson, J.D., Brusnahan, S.K. et al. (2012). Characterization of a mesenchymal stem cell line that differentiates to bone and provides niches supporting mouse and human hematopoietic stem cells. *Stem Cell Discovery* **2** (1): 5–14.

73 Zhou, X., Zhang, Z., Feng, J.Q. et al. (2010). Multiple functions of Osterix are required for bone growth and homeostasis in postnatal mice. *Proc. Natl. Acad. Sci. U.S.A.* **107**: 2919–2924.

74 Nardi, N.B. and da Silva Meirelles, L. (2006). Mesenchymal stem cells: isolation, in vitro expansion and characterization. *Handb. Exp. Pharmacol.* **174**: 249–282.

75 Riggs, B.L. and Melton, L.J. III, (1995). *Osteoporosis: Etiology, Diagnosis, and Management*, 2e. Philadelphia, PA and New York: Lippincott-Raven Publishers.

76 Mackie, E.J. (2003). Osteoblasts: novel roles in orchestration of skeletal architecture. *Int. J. Biochem. Cell Biol.* **35**: 1301–1305.
77 Frisch, B.J., Porter, R.L., and Calvi, L.M. (2008). Hematopoietic niche and bone meet. *Curr. Opin. Support. Palliat. Care* **2** (3): 211–217.
78 Zhang, J., Niu, C., Ye, L. et al. (2003). Identification of the haematopoietic stem cell niche and control of the niche size. *Nature* **425**: 836–841.
79 Stier, S., Ko, Y., Forkert, R. et al. (2005). Osteopontin is a hematopoietic stem cell niche component that negatively regulates stem cell pool size. *J. Exp. Med.* **201** (11): 1781–1791.
80 Jing, D., Fonseca, A.-V., Alakel, N. et al. (2010). Hematopoietic stem cells in co-culture with mesenchymal stromal cells – modeling the niche compartments in vitro. *Haematologica* **95**: 542–550.
81 de Barros, A.P.D.N., Takiya, C.M., Garzoni, L.R. et al. (2010). Osteoblasts and bone marrow mesenchemal stromal cells control hematopoietic stem cell migration and proliferation in 3D in vitro model. *PLoS ONE* **5** (2): e9093–e9111.
82 Martin, T.J. and Sims, N.A. (2005). Osteoclast-derived activity in the coupling of bone formation to resorption. *Trends Mol. Med.* **11**: 76–81.
83 Patt, H.M. and Maloney, M.A. (1972). Bone formation and resorption as a requirement for marrow development. *Proc. Soc. Exp. Biol. Med.* **140**: 205–207.
84 Teitelbaum, S.L. (2000). Bone resorption by osteoclasts. *Science* **289**: 1504–1508.
85 Ross, F.P. (2003). Cytokine regulation of osteoclast formation and function. *J. Musculoskel Neuron. Interact.* **3** (4): 282–286.
86 Lacey, D.L., Timms, E., Tan, H.L. et al. (1998). Osteoprotegerin ligand is a cytokine that regulates osteoclast differentiation and activation. *Cell* **93**: 165–176.
87 Surmenev, R., Surmeneva, M., Khlusov, I., and Pichugin, V. (2012). Hydroxyapatite nanostructured coatings prepared by radio-frequency magnetron sputtering deposition for medical implants: Properties and biomedical application. In: *Calcium Phosphate: Structure, Synthesis, Properties, and Applications* (ed. R.B. Heimann), 269–290. New York: Nova Science Publishers.
88 Blin-Wakkach, C., Rouleau, M., and Wakkach, A. (2014). Roles of osteoclasts in the control of medullary hematopoietic niches. *Arch. Biochem. Biophys.* **561**: 29–37.
89 Ratner, B.D., Hoffman, A.S., Schoen, F.J., and Lemons, J.E. (eds.) (2004). *Biomaterials Science: An Introduction to Materials in Medicine*, 2e. San Diego, CA, London: Elsevier Inc.
90 Rafii, S., Shapiro, F., Pettengell, R. et al. (1995). Human bone marrow microvascular endothelial cells support long-term proliferation and differentiation of myeloid and megakaryocytic progenitors. *Blood* **86**: 3353–3363.
91 Li, W., Johnson, S.A., Shelley, W.C., and Yoder, M.C. (2004). Hematopoietic stem cell repopulating ability can be maintained in vitro by some primary endothelial cells. *Exp. Hematol.* **32**: 1226–1237.
92 Cumano, A. and Godin, I. (2007). Ontogeny of the hematopoietic system. *Annu. Rev. Immunol.* **25**: 745–785.
93 Orkin, S.H. and Zon, L.I. (2008). Hematopoiesis: an evolving paradigm for stem cell biology. *Cell* **132**: 631–644.
94 Guerrouahen, B.S., Al-Hijji, I., and Tabrizi, A.R. (2011). Osteoblastic and vascular endothelial niches, their control on normal hematopoietic stem cells, and their consequences on the development of leukemia. *Stem Cells Int.* **2011**: 375857. https://doi.org/10.4061/2011/375857.
95 Sipkins, D.A., Wei, X., Wu, J.W. et al. (2005). In vivo imaging of specialized bone marrow endothelial microdomains for tumour engraftment. *Nature* **435**: 969–973.
96 Avecilla, S.T., Hattori, K., Heissig, B. et al. (2004). Chemokinemediated interaction of hematopoietic progenitors with the bone marrow vascular niche is required for thrombopoiesis. *Nat. Med.* **10** (1): 64–71.
97 Doan, P.L. and Chute, J.P. (2012). The vascular niche: home for normal and malignant hematopoietic stem cells. *Leukemia* **26**: 54–62.
98 Zhou, B.O., Yue, R., Murphy, M.M. et al. (2014). Leptin-receptor-expressing mesenchymal stromal cells represent the main source of bone formed by adult bone marrow. *Cell Stem Cell* **15**: 154–168.
99 Putnam, A.J. (2014). The Instructive role of the vasculature in stem cell niches. *Biomater. Sci.* **2** (11): 1562–1573.
100 Jacenko, O., Roberts, D.W., Campbell, M.R. et al. (2002). Linking hematopoiesis to endochondral skeletogenesis through analysis of mice transgenic for collagen X. *Am. J. Pathol.* **160**: 2019–2034.
101 Khlusov, I.A., Karlov, A.V., Sharkeev, Y.P. et al. (2005). Osteogenic potential of mesenchymal stem cells from bone marrow *in situ*: Role of physicochemical properties of artificial surfaces. *Bull. Exp. Biol. Med.* **140** (1): 144–152.
102 Khlusov, I.A., Karlov, A.V., Pozhen'ko, N.S. et al. (2006). Relationship between osteogenic characteristics of bone marrow cells and calcium phosphate

surface relief and solubility. *Bull. Exp. Biol. Med.* **141** (1): 99–103.

103 Gnedenkov, S.V., Sharkeev, Y.P., Sinebryukhov, S.L. et al. (2011). Formation and properties of bioactive surface layers on titanium. *Inorg. Mater. Appl. Res.* **2** (5): 474–481.

104 Frontini, A., Giordano, A., and Cinti, S. (2012). Endothelial cells of adipose tissues: a niche of adipogenesis. *Cell Cycle* **11** (15): 2765–2766.

105 Lee, Y.-H., Thacker, R., Hall, B. et al. (2014). Exploring the activated adipogenic niche: interactions of macrophages and adipocyte progenitors. *Cell Cycle* **13** (2): 184–190.

106 Rada, T., Reis, R.L., and Gomes, M.E. (2009). Adipose tissue-derived stem cells and their application in bone and cartilage tissue engineering. *Tissue Eng. Part B: Rev.* **15** (2): 113–125.

107 Morrison, S.J., Uchida, N., and Weissman, I.L. (1994). The Biology of hematopoietic stem cells. *Annu. Rev. Cell Dev. Biol.* **11**: 35–71.

108 Iwasaki, H. and Suda, T. (2010). Hematopoietic stem cells and their niche. In: *Hematopoietic Stem Cell Biology, Stem Cell Biology and Regenerative Medicine* (ed. M. Kondo), 37–55. New York: Humana Press.

109 Morrison, S.J. and Spradling, A.C. (2008). Stem cells and niches: mechanisms that promote stem cell maintenance throughout life. *Cell* **132** (4): 598–511.

110 Garrett, R.W. and Emerson, S.G. (2009). Bone and blood vessels: the hard and the soft of hematopoietic stem cell niches. *Cell Stem Cell* **4**: 503–506.

111 Boulais, P.E. and Frenette, P.S. (2015). Making sense of hematopoietic stem cell niches. *Blood* **125** (17): 2621–2629.

112 Crocker, P.R. and Gordon, S. (1985). Isolation and characterization of resident stromal macrophages and hematopoietic cell clusters from mouse bone marrow. *J. Exp. Med.* **162** (3): 993–1014.

113 Khlusov, I.A., Feduschak, T.A., and Khlusova, M.Y. (2013). Chemically inert nanoparticles affect hemopoietic and stromal cells microenvironments in vitro. *IFMBE Proc.* **38**: 209–212.

114 Bessis, M., Mize, C., and Prenant, M. (1978). Erythropoiesis: comparison of in vitro amplification. *Blood Cells* **4** (1–2): 155–174.

115 Peerani, R., Rao, B.M., Bauwens, C. et al. (2007). Niche-mediated control of human embryonic stem cell self-renewal and differentiation. *EMBO J.* **26** (22): 4744–4755.

116 Spradling, A., Drummond-Barbosa, D., and Kai, T. (2001). Stem cells find their niche. *Nature* **414**: 98–104.

117 Kincade, P.W., Igarashi, H., Medina, K.L. et al. (2002). Lymphoid lineage cells in adult murine bone marrow diverge from those of other blood cells at an early, hormone-sensitive stage. *Semin. Immunol.* **14** (6): 385–394.

118 Peschon, J.J., Morrissey, P.J., Grabstein, K.H. et al. (1994). Early lymphocyte expansion is severely impaired in interleukin 7 receptor-deficient mice. *J. Exp. Med.* **180** (5): 1955–1960.

119 Bessis, M. (1958). L'ilot erythroblastique, unite fonctionelle de la moelle osseuse. *Rev. Hematol.* **13**: 8–12.

120 Chasis, J.A. (2006). Erythroblastic islands: specialized microenvironmental niches for erythropoiesis. *Curr. Opin. Hematol.* **13**: 137–141.

121 Liesveld, J. (2012). Targeting myelogenous leukemia stem cells: role of the circulation. *Front. Oncol.* **2**: 86. https://doi.org/10.3389/fonc.2012.00086.

122 Colmone, A., Amorim, M., Pontier, A.L. et al. (2008). Leukemic cells create bone marrow niches that disrupt the behavior of normal hematopoietic progenitor cells. *Science* **322** (5909): 1861–1865.

123 Hölsken, A., Stache, C., Schlaffer, S.M. et al. (2014). Adamantinomatous craniopharyngiomas express tumor stem cell markers in cells with activated Wnt signaling: further evidence for the existence of a tumor stem cell niche? *Pituitary* **17** (6): 546–556.

124 Calvi, L.M., Adams, G.B., Weibrecht, K.W. et al. (2003). Osteoblastic cells regulate the haematopoietic stem cell niche. *Nature* **425**: 841–846.

125 Kiel, M.J., Yilmaz, O.H., Iwashita, T. et al. (2005). SLAM family receptors distinguish hematopoietic stem and progenitor cells and reveal endothelial niches for stem cells. *Cell* **121**: 1109–1121.

126 Kiel, M.J., Radice, G.L., and Morrison, S.J. (2007). Lack of evidence that hematopoietic stem cells depend on N-cadherin-mediated adhesion to osteoblasts for their maintenance. *Cell Stem Cell* **1**: 204–217.

127 Haug, J.S., He, X.C., Grindley, J.C. et al. (2008). N-cadherin expression level distinguishes reserved versus primed states of hematopoietic stem cells. *Cell Stem Cell* **2**: 367–379.

128 Wilson, A., Oser, G.M., Jaworski, M. et al. (2007). Dormant and self-renewing hematopoietic stem cells and their niches. *Ann. N.Y. Acad. Sci.* **1106**: 64–75.

129 Ogawa, M., Tajima, F., Ito, T. et al. (2001). CD34 expression by murine hematopoietic stem cells. Developmental changes and kinetic alterations. *Ann. N.Y. Acad. Sci.* **938**: 139–145.

130 Yang, L., Bryder, D., Adolfsson, J. et al. (2005). Identification of $Lin^{-}Sca1^{+}kit^{+}CD34^{+}Flt3^{-}$ short-term hematopoietic stem cells capable of rapidly reconstituting and rescuing myeloablated transplant recipients. *Blood* **105** (7): 2717–2723.

131 Cheshier, S.H., Morrison, S.J., Liao, X., and Weissman, I.L. (1999). In vivo proliferation and cell

cycle kinetics of long-term self-renewing hematopoietic stem cells. *Proc. Natl. Acad. Sci. U.S.A.* **96** (6): 3120–3125.

132 Kopp, H.G., Avecilla, S.T., Hooper, A.T., and Rafii, S. (2005). The bone marrow vascular niche: home of HSC differentiation and mobilization. *Physiology (Bethesda)* **20** (5): 349–356.

133 Arai, F., Hirao, A., Ohmura, M. et al. (2004). Tie2/angiopoietin-1 signaling regulates hematopoietic stem cell quiescence in the bone marrow niche. *Cell* **118**: 149–161.

134 Visnjic, D., Kalajzic, Z., Rowe, D.W. et al. (2004). Hematopoiesis is severely altered in mice with an induced osteoblast deficiency. *Blood* **103**: 3258–3264.

135 Khlusov, I.A., Khlusova, M.Y., Zaitsev, K.V. et al. (2011). Pilot in vitro study of the parameters of artificial niche for osteogenic differentiation of human stromal stem cell pool. *Bull. Exp. Biol. Med.* **150** (4): 535–542.

136 Khlusov, I.A., Shevtsova, N.M., MYu, K. et al. (2011). Niche-relief conception for stem cells as a basis of biomimetic approach to bone and hemopoietic tissues engineering. *Cell. Transplant. Tissue Eng.* **6** (2): 55–64.

137 Conboy, I.M., Conboy, M.J., Wagers, A.J. et al. (2005). Rejuvenation of aged progenitor cells by exposure to a young systemic environment. *Nature* **433**: 760–764.

138 Piccin, D., Tufford, A., and Morshead, C.M. (2014). Neural stem and progenitor cells in the aged subependyma are activated by the young niche. *Neurobiol. Aging* **35** (7): 1669–1679.

139 Sharpless, N.E. and DePinho, R.A. (2007). How stem cells age and why this makes us grow old. *Nat. Rev. Mol. Cell Biol.* **8**: 703–713.

140 Tlsty, T.D. and Coussens, L.M. (2006). Tumor stroma and regulation of cancer development. *Annu. Rev. Pathol.* **1**: 119–150.

141 Drummond-Barbosa, D. (2008). Stem cells, their niches and the systemic environment: an aging network (review). *Genetics* **180**: 1787–1797.

142 Zipori, D. (1992). The renewal and differentiation of hemopoietic stem cells. *FASEB J.* **6** (9): 2691–2697.

143 Forsberg, EC. and Smith-Berdan, S. (2009). Parsing the niche code: the molecular mechanisms governing hematopoietic stem cell adhesion and differentiation. *Haematologica* **94** (11): 1477–1481.

144 Zhang, C.C. and Lodish, H.F. (2008). Cytokines regulating hematopoietic stem cell function. *Curr. Opin. Hematol.* **15** (4): 307–311.

145 Sathyanarayana, P., Menon, M.P., Bogacheva, O. et al. (2007). Erythropoietin modulation of podocalyxin and a proposed erythroblast niche. *Blood* **110** (2): 509–518.

146 Adams, G.B., Martin, R.P., Alley, I.R. et al. (2007). Therapeutic targeting of a stem cell niche. *Nat. Biotechnol.* **25**: 238–243.

147 Fukuhara, S., Sako, K., Minami, T. et al. (2008). Differential function of Tie2 at cell–cell contacts and cell-substratum contacts regulated by angiopoietin-1. *Nat. Cell Biol.* **10**: 513–526.

148 Saharinen, P., Eklund, L., Miettinen, J. et al. (2008). Angiopoietins assemble distinct Tie2 signalling complexes in endothelial cell–cell and cell–matrix contacts. *Nat. Cell Biol.* **10**: 527–537.

149 Yoshihara, H., Arai, F., Hosokawa, K. et al. (2007). The niche regulation of quiescent hematopoietic stem cells through thrombopoietin/Mpl signaling. *Cell Stem Cell* **1**: 685–697.

150 Reya, T., Duncan, A.W., Ailles, L. et al. (2003). A role for Wnt signalling in self-renewal of haematopoietic stem cells. *Nature* **423**: 409–414.

151 Kirstetter, P., Anderson, K., Porse, B.T. et al. (2006). Activation of the canonical Wnt pathway leads to loss of hematopoietic stem cell repopulation and multilineage differentiation block. *Nat. Immunol.* **7**: 1048–1056.

152 Scheller, M., Huelsken, J., Rosenbauer, F. et al. (2006). Hematopoietic stem cell and multilineage defects generated by constitutive beta-catenin activation. *Nat. Immunol.* **7**: 1037–1047.

153 Nilsson, S.K., Johnston, H.M., Whitty, G.A. et al. (2005). Osteopontin, a key component of the hematopoietic stem cell niche and regulator of primitive hematopoietic progenitor cells. *Blood* **106**: 1232–1239.

154 Wilson, A., Murphy, M.J., Oskarsson, T. et al. (2004). c-Myc controls the balance between hematopoietic stem cell self-renewal and differentiation. *Genes Dev.* **18**: 2747–2763.

155 Discher, D.E., Mooney, D.J., and Zandstra, P.W. (2009). Growth factors, matrices, and forces combine and control stem cells. *Science* **324** (5935): 1673–1677.

156 Dygai, A.M. and Zhdanov, V.V. (2014). Theory of hematopoiesis control. In: *SpringerBriefs in Cell Biology*, vol. **5**, 1–93. Springer International Publishing.

157 Ingber, D.E. (2002). Mechanical signaling and the cellular response to extracellular matrix in angiogenesis and cardiovascular physiology. *Circ. Res.* **91**: 877–887.

158 Stabenfeldt, S.E., Brown, A.C., and Barker, T.H. (2010). Engineering ECM complexity into biomaterials for directing cell fate. In: *Studies in*

Mechanobiology, Tissue Engineering and Biomaterials, Biomaterials as Stem Cell Niche, vol. **2** (ed. G. Amit and K. Roy), 1–18. Berlin, Heidelberg: Springer-Verlag.

159 Gerecht, S., Burdick, J.A., Ferreira, L.S. et al. (2007). Hyaluronic acid hydrogel for controlled self-renewal and differentiation of human embryonic stem cells. *Proc. Natl. Acad. Sci. U.S.A.* **104** (27): 11298–11203.

160 Chung, C. and Burdick, J.A. (2008). Influence of three-dimensional hyaluronic acid microenvironments on mesenchymal stem cell chondrogenesis. *Tissue Eng. Part A* **15** (2): 243–254.

161 Huang, M.L., Smith, R.A.A., Trieger, G.W., and Godula, K. (2014). Glycocalyx remodeling with proteoglycan mimetics promotes neural specification in embryonic stem cells. *J. Am. Chem. Soc.* **136** (30): 10565–10568.

162 Salchert, K., Oswald, J., Streller, U. et al. (2005). Fibrillar collagen assembled in the presence of glycosaminoglycans to constitute bioartificial stem cell niches in vitro. *J. Mater. Sci. - Mater. Med.* **16** (6): 581–585.

163 Djouad, F., Delorme, B., Maurice, M. et al. (2007). Microenvironmental changes during differentiation of mesenchymal stem cells towards chondrocytes. *Arthritis Res. Ther.* **9** (2): R33.

164 Datta, N., Holtorf, H.L., Sikavitsas, V.I. et al. (2005). Effect of bone extracellular matrix synthesized in vitro on the osteoblastic differentiation of marrow stromal cells. *Biomaterials* **26** (9): 971–977.

165 Hynes, R.O. (2009). The extracellular matrix: not just pretty fibrils. *Science* **326**: 1216–1219.

166 Malanchi, I., Santamaria-Martinez, A., Susanto, E. et al. (2012). Interactions between cancer stem cells and their niche govern metastatic colonization. *Nature* **481**: 85–89.

167 Phadke, A., Chang, C.-W., and Varghese, S. (2010). Functional biomaterials for controlling stem cell differentiation. In: *Studies in Mechanobiology, Tissue Engineering and Biomaterials*, Biomaterials as Stem Cell Niche, vol. **2** (ed. G. Amit and K. Roy), 19–44. Berlin, Heidelberg: Springer-Verlag.

168 McNeil, S.E., Hobson, S.A., Nipper, V., and Rodland, K.D. (1998). Functional calcium-sensing receptors in rat fibroblasts are required for activation of SRC kinase and mitogen-activated protein kinase in response to extracellular calcium. *J. Biol. Chem.* **273**: 1114–1120.

169 Theman, T.A. and Collins, M.T. (2009). The role of the calcium-sensing receptor in bone biology and pathophysiology. *Curr. Pharm. Biotechnol.* **10** (3): 289–201.

170 Adams, G.B., Chabner, K.T., Alley, I.R. et al. (2006). Stem cell engraftment at the endosteal niche is specified by the calcium-sensing receptor. *Nature* **439**: 599–503.

171 Liu, Y.K., Lu, Q.Z., Pei, R. et al. (2009). The effect of extracellular calcium and inorganic phosphate on the growth and osteogenic differentiation of mesenchymal stem cells in vitro: implication for bone tissue engineering. *Biomed. Mater.* **4** (2): 025004. https://doi.org/10.1088/1748-6041/4/2/025004.

172 Sundelacruz, S., Levin, M., and Kaplan, D.L. (2008). Membrane potential controls adipogenic and osteogenic differentiation of mesenchymal stem cells. *PLoS ONE* **3** (11): e3737. https://doi.org/10.1371/journal.pone.0003737.

173 Sundelacruz, S., Levin, M., and Kaplan, D.L. (2009). Role of membrane potential in the regulation of cell proliferation and differentiation. *Stem Cell Rev* **5**: 231–246.

174 Kay, H.E.M. (1965). How many cell generations? *Lancet* **2**: 418–419.

175 Dellatore, S.M., Garsia, A.S., and Miller, W.M. (2008). Mimicking stem cell niches to increase stem cell expansion. *Curr. Opin. Biotechnol.* **19** (5): 534–540.

176 Gol'dberg, E.D., Dygai, A.M., Zhdanov, V.V., and Khlusov, I.A. (1999). Dynamic theory of hemopoiesis regulation. *Bull. Exp. Biol. Med.* **127** (5): 437–446.

177 Huiskes, R., Ruimerman, R., van Lenthe, G.H., and Janssen, J.D. (2000). Effects of mechanical forces on maintenance and adaptation of form in trabecular bone. *Nature* **405**: 704–706.

178 Kiuru, M., Hidaka, C., Hubner, R.-H. et al. (2009). Sonic hedgehog expands diaphyseal trabecular bone altering bone marrow niche and lymphocyte compartment. *Mol. Ther.* **17** (8): 1442–1452.

179 Pacifici, R. (2010). The immune system and bone. *Arch. Biochem. Biophys.* **503** (1): 41–53.

180 Saprina, T., Khlusov, I., and Borodulina, A. (2010). Change of properties of mononuclear leukocytes at patients with an osteogenesis imperfecta after operative treatment with using nanosized hydroxylapatite coatings. *Bone* **46** (Suppl. 1): S69–S70.

181 Adams, G.B. and Scadden, D.T. (2006). The hematopoietic stem cell in its place. *Nat. Immunol.* **7** (4): 333–337.

182 Cardier, J.E. and Barbera-Guillem, E. (1997). Extramedullary hematopoiesis in the adult mouse liver is associated with specific hepatic sinusoidal endothelial cells. *Hepatology* **26**: 165–175.

183 Wagers, A.J. (2005). Stem cell grand SLAM. *Cell* **121**: 967–970.

184 Ninomiya, M., Abe, A., Katsumi, A. et al. (2007). Homing, proliferation and survival sites of human

leukemia cells in vivo in immunodeficient mice. *Leukemia* **21** (1): 136–142.

185 Ferrara, N. and Davis-Smyth, T. (1997). The biology of vascular endothelial growth factor. *Endocr. Rev.* **18**: 4–25.

186 Gong, J.K. (1978). Endosteal marrow: a rich source of hematopoietic stem cells. *Science* **199**: 1443–1445.

187 Nilsson, S.K., Johnston, H.M., and Coverdale, J.A. (2001). Spatial localization of transplanted hemopoietic stem cells: inferences for the localization of stem cell niches. *Blood* **97**: 2293–2299.

188 Ben-Ishay, Z. (1974). Reticular cells in erythroid islands: their erythroblastophagocytic function. *J. Reticuloendothel. Soc.* **16** (6): 430–436.

189 Notsu, E., Sonoda, Y., and Sasaki, K. (2007). A histological study and three-dimensional reconstruction of F4/80-positive reticular cells and macrophages at the onset of murine bone marrow hematopoiesis. *Kaibogaku Zasshi* **82** (2): 53–60.

190 Shi, S. and Gronthos, S. (2003). Perivascular niche of postnatal mesenchymal stem cells in human bone marrow and dental pulp. *J. Bone Miner. Res.* **18**: 696–604.

191 Doherty, M.J. and Canfield, A.E. (1999). Gene expression during vascular pericyte differentiation. *Crit. Rev. Eukaryot. Gene Expr.* **9**: 1–17.

192 Grayson, W.L., Zhao, F., Izadpanah, R. et al. (2006). Effects of hypoxia on human mesenchymal stem cell expansion and plasticity in 3D constructs. *J. Cell. Physiol.* **207**: 331–339.

193 Friedenstein, A.J., Chailakhyan, R.K., Latsinik, N.V. et al. (1974). Stromal cells responsible for transferring the microenvironment of the hemopoietic tissues. Cloning in vitro and retransplantation in vivo. *Transplantation* **17**: 331–340.

194 Peerani, R. and Zandstra, P.W. (2010). Enabling stem cell therapies through synthetic stem cell–niche engineering. *J. Clin. Invest.* **120**: 60–70.

195 Bonfini, A., Wilkin, M.B., and Baron, M. (2015). Reversible regulation of stem cell niche size associated with dietary control of Notch signaling. *BMC Dev. Biol* **15**: 8. https://doi.org/10.1186/s12861-015-0059-8.

196 Dominici, M., Rasini, V., Bussolari, R. et al. (2009). Restoration and reversible expansion of the osteoblastic hematopoietic stem cell niche after marrow radioablation. *Blood* **114** (11): 2333–2343.

197 Hooper, A.T., Butler, J.M., Nolan, D.J. et al. (2009). Engraftment and reconstitution of hematopoiesis is dependent on VEGFR2-mediated regeneration of sinusoidal endothelial cells. *Cell Stem Cell* **4** (3): 263–274.

198 Patt, H.M. and Maloney, M.A. (1978). The bg^J/bg^J: W/W^v bone marrow chimera. A model for studying stem cell regulation. *Blood Cells* **4** (1–2): 27–35.

199 Weissman, I.L. (1994). Developmental switches in the immune system. *Cell* **76** (2): 207–218.

200 Miura, Y., Gao, Z., Miura, M. et al. (2006). Mesenchymal stem cell-organized bone marrow elements: an alternative hematopoietic progenitor resource. *Stem Cells* **24** (11): 2428–2436.

201 Rodriguez-Brenes, I., Komarova, N., and Wodarz, D. (2011). Evolutionary dynamics of feedback escape and the development of stem-cell driven cancers. *Proc. Natl. Acad. Sci. U.S.A.* **18** (47): 18983–18988.

202 Gentry, S., Ashkenazi, R., and Jackson, T. (2009). Maturity-structured mathematical model of mutation acquisition in the absence of homeostatic regulation. *Math. Modell. Nat. Phenom.* **4** (2): 156–182.

203 Francis, K. and Palsson, B.O. (1997). Effective intercellular communication distances are determined by the relative time constants for cyto/chemokine secretion and diffusion. *Proc. Natl. Acad. Sci. U.S.A.* **94**: 12258–12262.

204 Khlusov, I.A., Shevtsova, N.M., and Khlusova, M.Y. (2013). Detection in vitro and quantitative estimation of artificial microterritories which promote osteogenic differentiation and maturation of stromal stem cells. *Methods Mol. Biol.* **1035**: 103–119.

205 Teo, B.K.K., Ankam, S., and Yim, E.K.F. (2010). Stem cell interaction with topography. In: *Studies in Mechanobiology, Tissue Engineering and Biomaterials*, Biomaterials as Stem Cell Niche, vol. **2** (ed. G. Amit and K. Roy), 61–87. Berlin, Heidelberg: Springer-Verlag.

206 Khlusov, I.A., Yu, D., MYu, K. et al. (2013). Novel concepts of "niche-relief" and "niche-voltage" for stem cells as a base of bone and hematopoietic tissues biomimetic engineering. *IFMBE Proc.* **38**: 99–02.

207 Ferrier, J., Ross, S.M., Kanehisa, J., and Aubin, J.E. (1986). Osteoclasts and osteoblasts migrate in opposite directions in response to a constant electrical field. *J. Cell. Physiol.* **129** (3): 283–288.

208 Hamamoto, N., Hamamoto, Y., Nakajima, T., and Ozawa, H. (1995). Histological, histocytochemical and ultrastructural study on the effects of surface charge on bone formation in the rabbit mandible. *Arch. Oral Biol.* **40**: 97–06.

209 Khlusov, I.A., Khlusova, M.Y., Pichugin, V.F. et al. (2014). Artificial niches for stromal stem cells as a potential instrument for the design of the surface of biomimetic osteogenic materials. *Russ. Phys. J.* **56** (10): 1206–1211.

210 Li, G.R. and Deng, X.L. (2011). Functional ion channels in stem cells. *World J. Stem Cells* **3**: 19–24.
211 Teven, C.M., Liu, X., Hu, N. et al. (2011). Epigenetic regulation of mesenchymal stem cells: a focus on osteogenic and adipogenic differentiation. *Stem Cells Int* **2011**: 201371. https://doi.org/10.4061/2011/201371.
212 Villagra, A., Gutirrez, J., Paredes, R. et al. (2002). Reduced CpG methylation is associated with transcriptional activation of the bone-specific rat osteocalcin gene in osteoblasts. *J. Cell. Biochem.* **85** (1): 112–122.
213 Shen, J., Hovhannisyan, H., Lian, J.B. et al. (2003). Transcriptional induction of the osteocalcin gene during osteoblast differentiation involves acetylation of histones H3 and H4. *Mol Endocrinol* **17** (4): 743–756.
214 Ranga, A. and Lutolf, M.P. (2012). High-throughput approaches for the analysis of extrinsic regulators of stem cell fate. *Curr. Opin. Cell Biol.* **24** (2): 236–244.
215 Birgersdotter, A., Sandberg, R., and Ernberg, I. (2005). Gene expression perturbation in vitro–a growing case for three-dimensional (3D) culture systems. *Semin. Cancer Biol* **15**: 405–412.
216 Lutolf, M.P., Gilbert, P.M., and Blau, H.M. (2009). Designing materials to direct stem-cell fate. *Nature* **462**: 433–441.
217 Mei, Y. (2012). Microarrayed materials for stem cells. *Mater. Today (Kidlington)* **15** (10). https://doi.org/10.1016/S1369-7021(12)70196-7.
218 Tong, Z., Solanki, A., Hamilos, A. et al. (2015). Application of biomaterials to advance induced pluripotent stem cell research and therapy. *EMBO J* **34** (8): 987–908.
219 Metallo, C.M., Mohr, J.C., Detzel, C.J. et al. (2007). Engineering the stem cell microenvironment. *Biotechnol. Progr.* **23**: 18–23.
220 Guilak, F., Cohen, D.M., Estes, B.T. et al. (2009). Control of stem cell fate by physical interactions with the extracellular matrix. *Cell Stem Cell* **5** (1): 17–26.
221 Saha, K., Pollock, J.F., Schaffer, D.V., and Healy, K.E. (2007). Designing synthetic materials to control stem cell phenotype. *Curr. Opin. Chem. Biol.* **11**: 381–387.
222 Kobel, S. and Lutolf, M.P. (2011). Biomaterials meet microfluidics: building the next generation of artificial niches. *Curr. Opin. Biotechnol.* **22** (5): 690–697.
223 Dawson, E., Mapili, G., Erickson, K. et al. (2008). Biomaterials for stem cell differentiation. *Adv. Drug Delivery Rev.* **60**: 215–228.
224 Ponsonnet, L., Reybier, K., Jaffrezic, N. et al. (2003). Relationship between surface properties (roughness, wettability) of titanium and titanium alloys and cell behavior. *Mater. Sci. Eng., C* **23**: 51–60.
225 Ueshima, M., Tanaka, S., Nakamura, S., and Yamashita, K. (2002). Manipulation of bacterial adhesion and proliferation by surface charges of electrically polarized hydroxyapatite. *J. Biomed. Mater. Res.* **60**: 578–584.
226 Yu, D., Dvornichenko, M.V., Karlov, A.V. et al. (2009). Electrically functionalized hydroxyapatite and calcium phosphate surfaces to enhance immobilization and proliferation of osteoblasts in vitro and modulate osteogenesis in vivo. *IFMBE Proc* **25**: 245–248.
227 Martinez, E., Engel, E., Planell, J.A., and Samitier, J. (2009). Effects of artificial micro- and nano-structured surfaces on cell behaviour. *Ann. Anat.* **191**: 126–135.
228 Yu, L.M.Y., Leipzig, N.D., and Shoichet, M.S. (2008). Promoting neuron adhesion and growth. *Mater. Today* **11**: 36–43.
229 Bershadsky, A.D., Balaban, N.Q., and Geiger, B. (2003). Adhesion-dependent cell mechanosensitivity. *Annu. Rev. Cell Dev. Biol.* **19**: 677–695.
230 Discher, D.E., Janmey, P.A., and Wang, Y.L. (2005). Tissue cells feel and respond to the stiffness of their substrate. *Science* **310**: 1139–1143.
231 Tomasek, J.J., Gabbiani, G., Hinz, B. et al. (2002). Myofibroblasts and mechano-regulation of connective tissue remodelling. *Nat. Rev. Mol. Cell Biol* **3**: 349–363.
232 Engler, A.J., Sen, S., Sweeney, H.L., and Discher, D.E. (2006). Matrix elasticity directs stem cell lineage specification. *Cell* **126** (4): 677–689.
233 Lutolf, M.P., Doyonnas, R., Havenstrite, K. et al. (2009). Perturbation of single hematopoietic stem cell fates in artificial niches. *Integr. Biol. (Camb)* **1**: 59–69.
234 Lutolf, M.P. and Hubbell, J.A. (2005). Synthetic biomaterials as instructive extracellular microenvironments for morphogenesis in tissue engineering. *Nat. Biotechnol.* **23** (1): 47–55.
235 Parmar, K., Mauch, P., Vergilio, J.A. et al. (2007). Distribution of hematopoietic stem cells in the bone marrow according to regional hypoxia. *Proc. Natl. Acad. Sci. U.S.A.* **104** (13): 5431–5436.
236 Ungrin, M.D., Joshi, C., Nica, A. et al. (2008). Reproducible, ultra high-throughput formation of multicellular organization from single cell suspension-derived human embryonic stem cell aggregates. *PLoS ONE* **3** (2): e1565. https://doi.org/10.1371/journal.pone.0001565.
237 McBeath, R., Pirone, D.M., Nelson, C.M. et al. (2004). Cell shape, cytoskeletal tension, and RhoA

regulate stem cell lineage commitment. *Dev. Cell* **6** (4): 483–495.

238 Sasaki, D., Shimizu, T., Masuda, S. et al. (2009). Mass preparation of size-controlled mouse embryonic stem cell aggregates and induction of cardiac differentiation by cell patterning method. *Biomaterials* **30** (26): 4384–4389.

239 Gauthier, O., Bouler, J.-M., Aguado, E. et al. (1998). Macroporous biphasic calcium phosphate ceramics: influence macropore diameter and macroporosity percentage on bone ingrowth. *Biomaterials* **19** (1–3): 133–139.

240 Sous, M., Bareille, R., Rouais, F. et al. (1998). Cellular biocompatibility and resistance to compression of macroporous beta-tricalcium phosphate ceramics. *Biomaterials* **19**: 2147–2153.

241 Karlov, A.V. and Khlusov, I.A. (2000). Mikrostrukturische charakteristiken der poren, die osteoinduktiven eigenschaften der kalziumphosphatkeramik bilden. *Biomed. Tech.* **45** (1): 123–124.

242 Curtis, A.S. and Varde, M. (1964). Control of cell behavior: topological factors. *J. Natl. Cancer Inst* **33**: 15–26.

243 Curtis, A.S.G. and Wilkinson, C. (1998). Topographical control of cells. *Biomaterials* **18**: 1573–1583.

244 Boyan, B.D., Lossdorfer, S., Wang, L. et al. (2003). Surface microtopography regulates osteoblasts. *Eur. Cells Mater.* **6**: 22–27.

245 Meyer, U., Buchter, A., Wiesmann, H.P. et al. (2005). Basic reactions of osteoblasts on structured material surface. *Eur. Cells Mater.* **9**: 39–49.

246 Sniadecki, N.J., Desai, R.A., Ruiz, S.A., and Chen, C.S. (2006). Nanotechnology for cell-substrate interactions. *Ann. Biomed. Eng.* **34**: 59–74.

247 Ravichandran, R., Liao, S., Ng, C.C.H. et al. (2009). Effects of nanotopography on stem cell phenotypes. *World J. Stem Cells* **1**: 55–66.

248 Yim, E.K., Pang, S.W., and Leong, K.W. (2007). Synthetic nanostructures inducing differentiation of human mesenchymal stem cells into neuronal lineage. *Exp. Cell. Res.* **313** (9): 1820–1829.

249 Klein, C., de Groot, K., Chen, W. et al. (1994). Osseous substance formation induced in porous calcium phosphate ceramics in soft tissues. *Biomaterials* **15**: 31–34.

250 Costa, D.O., Prowse, P.D.H., Chrones, T. et al. (2013). The differential regulation of osteoblast and osteoclast activity by surface topography of hydroxyapatite coatings. *Biomaterials* **34**: 7215–7226.

251 Terleeva, O.P., Sharkeev, Y.P., Slonova, A.I. et al. (2010). Effect of parameters of microplasma modes and electrolyte composition on characteristics of calcium phosphate coatings on pure titanium for medical use. *Surf. Coat. Technol.* **205**: 1723–1729.

252 Huang, J.I., Yoo, J.U., and Goldberg, V.M. (2004). Orthopaedic applications of stem cells. In: *Handbook of Stem Cells*, vol. **2** (ed. H. Blau, D. Melton, M. Moore, et al.), 773–784. New York: Elsevier.

253 Green, D.W., Li, G., Milthorpe, B., and Ben-Nissan, B. (2012). Adult stem cell coatings for regenerative medicine. *Mater. Today* **15** (1–2): 60–66.

254 Hartgerink, J.D., Beniash, E., and Stupp, S.I. (2001). Self-assembly and mineralization of peptide-amphiphile nanofibers. *Science* **294** (5547): 1684–1688.

255 Stupp, S.I. (2010). Self-assembly and biomaterials. *Nano Lett.* **10** (12): 4783–4786.

12

Experimental and Pilot Clinical Study of Different Tissue-Engineered Bone Grafts Based on Calcium Phosphate, Mesenchymal Stem Cells, and Adipose-Derived Stromal Vascular Fraction

Ilia Y. Bozo[1,2,3], Grigory A. Volozhin[2], Vadim L. Zorin[1,3], Roman V. Deev[1,3,4], Sergey I. Rozhkov[2], Petr S. Eremin[3], Evgeniy N. Toropov[3], Andrey A. Pulin[3], Vasily I. Grachev[5], Ilya I. Eremin[3], and Vladimir S. Komlev[6,7]

[1] *Human Stem Cells Institute, Moscow, Russia*
[2] *A.I. Evdokimov Moscow State University of Medicine and Dentistry, Moscow, Russia*
[3] *A.I. Burnazyan Federal Medical and Biophysical Center, Moscow, Russia*
[4] *Kazan (Volga region) Federal University, Kazan, Russia*
[5] *X-ray Diagnostics Laboratories "3D Lab", Moscow, Russia*
[6] *A.A. Baikov Institute of Metallurgy and Materials Science, Russian Academy of Sciences, Moscow, Russia*
[7] *Institute of Laser and Information Technologies, Russian Academy of Sciences,, Moscow, Russia*

12.1 Introduction

Tissue engineering approaches in creation of optimized bone grafts find more and more applications and precedents of successful clinical translation [1–3]. The main indications for bone grafts application in dentistry, oral and maxillofacial surgery are jaw atrophy, bone defects after removal of benign and malignant tumors and pseudotumors, treatment of osteomyelitis and osteonecrosis, traumas, post-traumatic deformities, congenital anomalies, and maxillofacial deformities. Only in the United States, according to the data of the National Medical Statistics Center (2010), about 60 000 in-hospital operations were performed on facial bones. Moreover, about five million dental implants are annually placed in the United States [4]. Given that at least 20% of clinical cases require bone grafting, the high demand in bone grafts becomes obvious.

A treatment of patients with large bone defects is always a challenge, because bone substitutes without an osteoinductive potential appear to be not effective. The problem is partially solved with the use of bone autografts [5, 6]. Therefore, tissue-engineered bone substitutes could become an alternative to "the gold standard," enabling surgeons to limit or even abandon the use of bone autografts.

Generally, a tissue engineering approach implies the creation of a product composed by a scaffold and cells. The former promotes osteoconduction, i.e. fills in a bone defect, supports and maintains a newly forming bone tissue. Chemical similarity of synthetic calcium phosphates to the mineral component of bone matrix allows it to be applied successfully as bone substitutes. Among a number of calcium phosphates biomaterials with different phase compositions, tricalcium phosphate (TCP) ceramics are reliable, osteoconductive, and biodegradable materials, and some of them are registered and approved for clinical use. The cells provide osteogenecity – they restore a lost cambial reserve, proliferate and differentiate into osteoblasts. Furthermore, the cells possess a paracrine action producing a complex of biologically active substances that stimulate reparative regeneration [7, 8].

Autologous cells both "fresh" (non-manipulated) and expanded *in vitro* are most optimal in respect of safety and potential efficacy. In most cases, mesenchymal stem cells (MSCs), osteogenic cells of the periosteum, and a stromal vascular fraction of adipose (adSVF) tissue cells are used to make tissue-engineered bone grafts. However, considering the diversity of applied scaffolds, laboratory protocols, experimental models, and diagnostic methods and indications in clinical trials, it is difficult to compare the results published and give a preference to any particular cell type.

A source of cells for a tissue-engineered bone graft is highly important for its clinical translation. For example, bone marrow is a suitable source of the MSCs in traumatology and orthopedics; however, intra-oral tissues are more optimal in dentistry, oral and maxillofacial surgery [9]. Therefore, a number of authors suggest using a periodontal ligament, a tooth pulp or follicle, to derive the MSCs or cell populations with a similar therapeutic potential [10]. But in any of the above cases, manipulations to collect tissue are traumatic or feasible only in tooth removal. Thereupon, we consider the oral mucosa to be the most optimal source of cells for a

Bioceramics and Biocomposites: From Research to Clinical Practice, First Edition. Edited by Iulian Antoniac.

tissue-engineered bone graft. Gingival mesenchymal stem cells (gMSCs), like the MSCs from other tissue sources, are characterized by a high proliferative and secretory activity as well as osteogenic differentiation capacity [11].

In addition, adSVF is of particular interest as it has a heterogenic composition and an evident therapeutic potential, and it does not require an expansion *in vitro* [12]. This approach to use cells as "a fresh population" especially in combination with instrumental methods of cell derivation significantly facilitates the implementation of tissue-engineered bone grafts into clinical practice.

Therefore, our study was aimed to evaluate the safety and biological action in an experiment and the efficacy in a pilot clinical trial of several various tissue-engineered bone grafts composed by different scaffolds (TCP and octacalcium phosphates [OCPs]) and two autologous cell populations such as gMSCs and adSVF. A combination of each cellular component and the scaffold into a tissue-engineered construction was made both with and without fibrin glue ("Tissucol kit," BAXTER AG, Austria). The results of an experiment *in vivo* with tissue-engineered constructions based on OCP scaffold have been published previously [9].

12.2 Materials and Methods

12.2.1 Creation of Tissue-Engineered Constructions

12.2.1.1 TCP Manufacturing

TCP powder was synthesized in an aqueous medium by slow addition of diammonium phosphate [$(NH_4)_2HPO_4$] solution into calcium nitrate [$Ca(NO_3)_2 4H_2O$] solution, containing NH_4OH, under constant stirring. The pH of the mixture was about 7 with Ca/P molar ration of 1.5/1. After total addition of the reactants, the suspension was filtered, dried at 80 °C and sintered at 700 °C for 2 hours. TCP ceramics granules were prepared by the method described elsewhere [13]. The granules with diameter 1000 ± 100 μm were selected using standard sieves and were used for experiments. The sieved TCP ceramic granules were sterilized by heating at 120 °C for 2 hours.

12.2.1.2 OCP Manufacturing

For synthesis of starting calcium carbonate powders 30 g of CaO, 62 g of $(NH_4)_2CO_3$, and 300 ml of distilled water was added to a vessel for grinding. Grinding was carried out for 30 minutes at room temperature. After filtration, powders were washed and dried at 80 °C for 24 hours. Calcium carbonate granules were prepared according to the method described elsewhere [13]. Then the calcium carbonate ceramic granules were transformed to OCP as described elsewhere [9]. An aqueous solution was prepared by dissolving of 115 g of $NH_4H_2PO_4$ in 500 ml of distilled water at room temperature, pH 4.1 ± 0.1. 10 ± 1 g of calcium carbonate granules were added to the solution. The granules were shaked in a sealed glass vessel for 168 hours at 40 °C. After that the granules were thoroughly washed in distilled water at least five times and dried overnight at 37 °C. The obtained granules in amounts of 10 ± 1 g were placed in a second solution. Briefly, the second solution was prepared by dissolving 95.2 g of CH_3COONa in 700 ml of distilled water at 40 °C and pH 8.2 ± 0.2. The granules were again shaked in a sealed glass vessel for 168 hours at 40 °C. Then they were thoroughly washed in distilled water at least five times and dried overnight at 37 °C. The granules with diameter 1000 ± 100 μm were selected using standard sieves and were used for experiments. The sieved OCP ceramic granules were sterilized by heating at 120 °C for 2 hours.

12.2.1.3 Characterization of TCP and OCP Ceramic Granules

Phase composition of the samples was analyzed by conventional X-ray diffraction (XRD) technique (Shimadzu XRD-6000, Japan; Ni-filtered CuKα1 target, $\lambda = 1.541\,83$ Å). The samples were scanned at 2θ from 3° to 60° with a 0.02° step a preset time of five seconds. Scanning electron microscopy (SEM) apparatus (Tescan Vega II, Czech Republic), operated in secondary and backscattered electron modes, was used for microstructure analysis.

12.2.1.4 Obtaining of Rabbit Tissue Bioptates

All manipulations with rabbits were carried out according to Animal Welfare Act. In experimental part of the study, MSCs were isolated from a gingival mucosa and the SVF – from a rabbit inguinal adipose tissue. After premedication, (Sol. Atropini Sulfatis 0.04 mg/kg, Sol. Cephazolini 25 mg/kg) surgical operations were performed under local anesthesia (Sol. Lidocaini – 1%, 0.3 ml) with general sedation (0.4–0.8 ml Zoletil 100).

To obtain the MSCs a fragment of the attached mucosa with a size of 3 mm × 3 mm within the first left incisor was excised. To harvest an adipose tissue sample, a skin in the left inguinal region was dissected with a length of 2 cm. A volume of the inguinal fat up to 1 cm^3 was excised. A post-operative wound was sutured layer by layer with interrupted MonoSyn 4/0 stitches.

The tissue samples obtained were immediately placed in sterile tubes with a transport medium (DMEM F12, 2% FBS, Bioind., USA; 2 mM L-glutamine, StemCell Technology, USA; 200 U/ml penicillin and 200 mg/ml streptomycin, StemCell Technology, USA; 200 U/ml amphotericin; 100 U/ml gentamycin).

12.2.1.5 Obtaining of Rabbit gMSCs

A gingival bioptate was finely disintegrated with disposal sterile scalpels and incubated in 1 ml of 0.25% Try-EDTA at 37 °C for one hour. The enzyme was inactivated with a washing medium (low-glucose DMEM, StemCell Technology, USA; and 5% FBS, Biological Industries, Israel). The homogenate was precipitated at 300 g for seven minutes. The resulting suspension was incubated in 1 ml of 0.15% type II collagenase (Sigma, USA) at 37 °C for two hours. The enzyme was inactivated with 10 ml of the washing medium; the homogenate was precipitated at 300 g for seven minutes. The resulting precipitate was re-suspended in 10 ml of the "working medium" MesenCult (StemCell Technology, USA). An automated cell counter "Countess" (Invitrogen, USA) was used to define cell number and their viability evaluation. After that the cells were diluted in the working medium and placed in a flask in the amount of 3×10^5 cells/cm^2. The cells were expanded according to the standard technique of MSC culture. The cells were cultured up to three passages with changing the medium every third day.

12.2.1.6 Obtaining of Rabbit adSVF

A lipoaspirate was washed out twice with phosphate-buffered saline (PBS), and then cultured in 0.15% type II collagenase at 37 °C for 30 minutes. The enzyme was inactivated with a washing medium (low-glucose DMEM, StemCell Technology, USA) and 5% FBS. The cell suspension and the remaining tissue were filtered via a nylon filter (70 μm), precipitated at 300 g for seven minutes. The resulting precipitate was re-suspended in 10 ml of NaCl. An automated cell counter "Countess" was used for cells counting and their viability evaluation.

12.2.1.7 Tissue-Engineered Constructions

For experimental studies three variants of tissue-engineered bone grafts were made as follows: TCP + gMSC, TCP + fibrin glue + gMSC, and TCP + fibrin glue + adSVF. The latter variant was implemented as the second phase of the experimental study with the follow-up time points of 60 and 90 days which was carried out after analyzing the results of the first two series.

12.2.2 Experimental Studies *in Vivo*

12.2.2.1 Implantation of the Materials

Tissue-engineered bone grafts comprising TCP were tested in orthotopic conditions in male Chinchilla rabbits ($n = 24$, age 10–12 months) with a body weight of 2.0–2.5 kg in compliance with the international guidelines for the care and use of laboratory animals. Each rabbit underwent two similar symmetric full thickness defects of both parietal bones with a diameter of 10 mm. One of the three tissue-engineered constructions was engrafted into the right parietal bone defects, with the respective cell-free scaffolds implanted into the left one (the control groups).

After premedication (Sol. Atropini Sulfatis 0.04 mg/kg, Sol. Cephazolini 25 mg/kg) a linear dissection of soft tissues to the periosteum along the sagittal suture from the occipital bone tubercle anteriorly with length of 2–2.5 cm was made under infiltration anesthesia (Sol. Ultracaini 1.7 ml) with general sedation (0.4–0.8 ml Zoletil 100). Musculocutaneous-periosteal flaps were laterally retracted with exposure of a parietal bone surface. Using a trepan (an outer diameter of 10 mm) parietal bone defects were made without damaging the dura mater at continuous cooling irrigation with 0.9% NaCl. The bone defects were filled in with the study materials. An operation wound was sutured layer-by-layer with interrupted stitches (Vicryl 4/0). A closure of the dissected periosteum with interrupted sutures strongly fixed the implanted materials within the bone defects.

The animals were sacrificed with overdose of Zoletil 100 in 30, 60, and 90/120 days. The calvarium with the defect zones was removed and fixed in a 4% neutral buffered formalin solution.

12.2.2.2 X-ray Imaging

Microradiography and dental computed tomography (CT) (J. Morita 3D Accuitomo 170, J. Morita Corporation, Japan) were performed within the first week after obtaining the tissue materials without removing them from plastic jars with the fixative solution. The examination of all materials was performed by the same radiologist at the same exposure modes and parameters (voxel size 0.08 mm, 80 kV, 2 mA for CT). The microradiography findings were used for a qualitative evaluation of the results while the CT data – for a qualitative and quantitative assessment. A manual segmentation of the bone defect area (a cylinder with diameter of 10 mm and height of 1.2–1.5 mm depending on the parietal bone thickness) with the newly formed bone tissue was made in the software 3DSlicer (Brigham, USA), a tissue volume of the highlighted zone and an average density in Hounsfield units (HUs) were calculated in the "Label statistics" module.

12.2.2.3 Histological Analysis

The calvaria were decalcified in a Biodec-R solution (Bio-optica, Italy). Histological specimens were made under a standard technique. Slices were made on the frontal plane via the bone defect center. Microspecimens were stained with hematoxylin and eosin, as well as impregnated with silver nitrate ($Ag(NO_3)_2$) by Gordon. Histomorphometry was performed with the estimation of a newly formed bone tissue proportion in the bone defect central and peripheral zones. For this purpose a defect was divided into four 2.5 mm segments in the "Pannoramic Viewer" software (3DHISTECH, USA). Two marginal segments in sum composed the peripheral zone, two central ones forming the central area. A newly formed bone tissue proportion was determined separately in each of the two zones with the use of the "ImageJ" software (National Institutes of Health, USA).

12.2.3 A Pilot Clinical Study

12.2.3.1 Clinical Study Design

The clinical study was carried out as pilot, nonrandomized, noncomparative. The protocol was approved by the local Ethics Committee of the A.I. Burnazyan Federal Medical Biophysical Center.

The inclusion criteria were:

- age from 20 to 65 years inclusive;
- acquired (posttraumatic, postoperative) bone defect of the maxilla or mandible, or atrophy of the alveolar ridge;
- singed Informed Consent form.

The exclusion criteria were:

- co-existing decompensated somatic disorders;
- malignant tumors (including those in the history);
- an unexplained significant weight loss (>10% of the body weight for the previous year);
- alcohol addiction, use of narcotic or psychotropic agents;
- diabetes mellitus, thyroid, and parathyroid disorders (including those in the history);
- infectious diseases (HIV, hepatitis, syphilis, and others).

The safety criterion was the absence of adverse events and serious adverse events related to the use of tissue-engineered bone substitutes. A complete cure of jaw atrophy in the transplantation area or complete replacement of a bone defect by newly formed bone tissue with an average density of more than 450 ± 50 HU in four to six months after surgery was accepted as the primary efficacy criterion.

Thirteen patients participated in the study; they underwent bone grafting with the use of tissue-engineered bone substitutes (Table 12.1).

At the enrollment into the study (Visit 0) all the patients underwent a clinical examination, CT, and laboratory tests (hematology and blood biochemistry and urinalysis). After the enrollment (Visit 1) tissue sample harvesting (oral mucosa or adipose tissue) was carried out. The patients had surgery for bone defect replacement or alveolar bone augmentation using the tissue-engineered construction with gMSCs in 14 days and with adSVF on the same day. The patients were followed up for 12 months with clinical examination and CT. Some patients had dental implantation according to the treatment plan; in these cases newly formed bone tissue samples were taken for a histological examination.

12.2.3.2 Creation of Tissue-Engineered Bone Grafts

Tissue Sampling A biopsy of the oral mucosa was performed to obtain the MSCs. A fragment of the retromolar mucosa sized as 2 mm × 2 mm × 1 mm was excised with a scalpel under application anesthesia with Sol. Lidocaini 2% – 0.5 ml. The bioptate was placed in a transport medium (DMEM F12, 2% FBS, 2 mM L-glutamine, 200 U/ml penicillin and 200 mg/ml streptomycin, 200 U/ml amphotericin, 100 U/ml gentamycin) and delivered to the laboratory.

To obtain the adSVF, fat was aspirated from the hypogastrium. The skin in the umbilical region was linearly dissected with a length of 5–7 mm in parallel to the natural fold under endotracheal and local anesthesia with 20 ml of 0.5% Lidocaine solution. A cannula tightly connected to a syringe (20 ml) was inserted into the subcutaneous fat of the anterior abdominal wall via the dissection. The derived adipose tissue was placed in a transport medium (DMEM F12, 2% FBS, 2 mM L-glutamine, StemCell Technology, USA); 200 U/ml penicillin and 200 mg/ml streptomycin, 200 U/ml amphotericin, 100 U/ml gentamycin) and delivered to the laboratory within 30 minutes.

Cell Isolation All manipulations with a tissue and cell material were performed in accordance with the requirements of the GTP (Good Tissue Practice) and GLP (Good Laboratory Practice), as well as standard operating procedures established in the A.I. Burnazyan Federal Medical Biophysical Center.

The gingiva samples were kept at 4 °C for two to three hours in incubation medium: DMEM/F12 supplemented with 10% FBS and digested overnight at 37 °C by adding 0.2 mg/ml collagenase type II. To establish the primary explants of the gMSC culture, the digested material was washed twice with the same medium and placed in 25 cm^2 culture flasks in DMEM/F12 medium supplemented with 15% FBS. When confluent, the primary cells were trypsinized with 0.05% trypsin/EDTA solution. The cell culture medium was replaced every 72 hours. The sampling techniques to obtain adSVF comply with those described in the experimental part.

12.2.3.3 Bone Grafting

All the patients enrolled into the study underwent standard surgical interventions in accordance with the diagnosis and the treatment plan, i.e. sinus floor elevation,

Table 12.1 Patients and tissue-engineered bone grafts characteristics.

No.	Gender	Age	Disease	Scaffold	Fibrin glue (ml)	Cells	
						Type	Number
1	M	37	Benign tumor of the mandible	TCP	2	gMSCs	2×10^7
2	M	33	Alveolar ridge atrophy of the upper jaw	OCP	2	gMSCs	3.5×10^7
3	F	38	Alveolar ridge atrophy of the upper jaw	TCP	—	gMSCs	2.7×10^7
4	F	36	Nonunion of the mandible	TCP	2	adSVF	6×10^7
5	M	61	Benign tumor of the mandible	TCP	—	gMSCs	1×10^7
6	F	36	Defect of the alveolar ridge of the upper jaw	TCP	4	adSVF	8×10^7
7	M	62	Benign tumor of the mandible	—	2	adSVF	10×10^7
8	M	27	Postoperative deformity of the mandible	—	4	adSVF	8×10^7
9	F	38	Alveolar ridge atrophy of the upper jaw	TCP	—	gMSCs	2.7×10^7
10	M	43	Alveolar ridge atrophy of the upper jaw	TCP	—	gMSCs	2.6×10^7
11	M	57	Alveolar ridge atrophy of the mandible	TCP	—	gMSCs	1×10^7
12	M	22	Benign tumor of the mandible	TCP	4	gMSCs	7.8×10^7
13	M	33	Benign tumor of the mandible	TCP	4	adSVF	12×10^7

M – male and F – female.

dental implantation; excochleation of a fibrous dysplasia site; segmental resection of the maxilla or mandible for a histopathologically proven benign tumor; cystectomy; excision of a nonunion. The developed tissue-engineered constructions were implanted into bone defects and the sites of alveolar ridge atrophy during the above surgeries.

12.2.3.4 Clinical Examination

The process of postoperative wound healing and inflammation signs were evaluated in 2, 24, 48, 72 hours and 7 and 14 days after surgery. A pain level in the postoperative region was rated with the use of the Visual Analog Scale, edema was scored with the Numeric Rating Scale. The sutures were removed in 10–14 days after surgery.

12.2.3.5 X-ray Imaging

A dental panoramic radiograph and/or CT were carried out in the period of patients' enrollment into the study. In three to six months after surgery as well as after dental implantation CT was performed on the same tomograph and by the same radiologist as in the enrollment. The morphometry of newly formed bone tissue and measurements of its average density on serial sections (an interval – 0.5 mm) were performed on computer tomograms in the standard software with the use of the ROI (region of interest) tool.

12.2.3.6 Histological Analysis

The bioptates obtained with the trepan were decalcified in a Biodec-R solution (Bio-optica, Italy). Histological specimens were made under a standard technique and stained with hematoxylin and eosin.

12.2.4 Statistical Analysis

At the first stage for statistical analysis of the data obtained (newly formed bone tissue density in the defect region, a proportion of newly formed bone tissue in defect zones, a diameter of bone substitute granules) descriptive methods were applied such as the mean value, standard error of the mean, median, the interquartile range. Taking into consideration the nonparametric distribution of measurable characteristics, the nonparametric Kruskal–Wallis test was applied for the simultaneous comparison of more than two independent groups; the Mann–Whitney U-test with the Bonferroni correction was used to detect differences between two independent groups. The Wilcoxon test was applied to compare quantitative parameters within the same group at different time points of observation. A statistical significance value in all cases was accepted as $p < 0.05$.

12.3 Results

12.3.1 TCP and OCP Ceramic Granules

XRD observations of TCP and OCP ceramic granules confirmed that the major TCP and OCP phases are presented (data not shown). The scanning electron micrographs of TCP and OCP granule microstructures are presented on Figure 12.1. Both types of ceramics are quasi-spherical with large pores with the size around 500 μm. The size of the micropores is, on average, 0.1–50 μm for TCP and 0.1–20 μm for OCP granules.

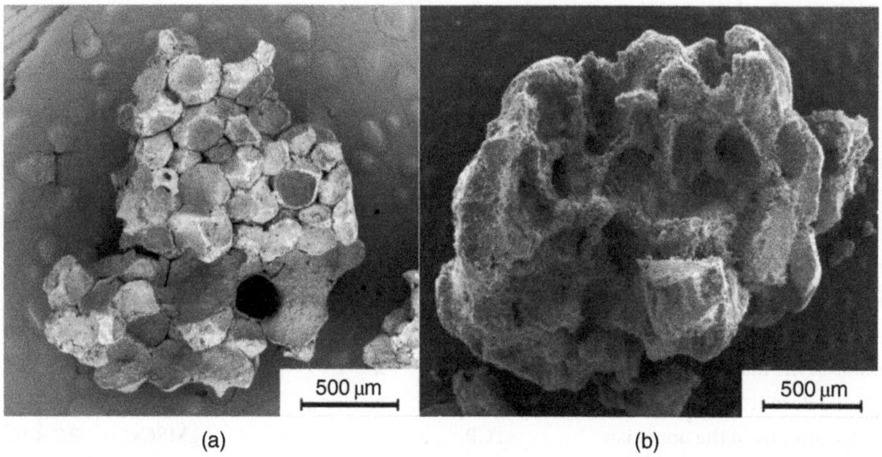

Figure 12.1 SEM images of TCP (a) and OCP (b) ceramic granules.

OCP (lamellar crystals), in comparison to TCP (globular crystals), exhibit a lamellar morphology.

12.3.2 Tissue-Engineered Bone Grafts

An average number of rabbit gMSCs obtained from each bioptate was $7.88 \pm 0.4 \times 10^6$, with human MSCs being $29.5 \pm 5.4 \times 10^6$. The number of cells isolated from adipose tissue was $45 \pm 6 \times 10^6$ in human and $5 \pm 1.1 \times 10^6$ in rabbits.

For experimental studies described in this article three variants of tissue-engineered bone grafts were made such as TCP + gMSC; TCP + fibrin glue + gMSC; TCP + fibrin glue + adSVF. The forth bone graft composed by OCP and gMSCs was tested in another experimental model [8]. For a clinical trial five different constructions were made, they are TCP + gMSC; TCP + fibrin glue + gMSC; TCP + fibrin glue + adSVF; OCT + fibrin glue + gMSC; and fibrin glue + adSVF.

In the clinical trial all materials in the amount required for bone grafting were delivered in an operation room directly prior to use.

12.3.3 Biological Activity Under Orthotopic Conditions

Two of 24 experimental animals died within the first three days after surgery due to early postoperative complication – a subdural hematoma, which is specific for this experimental model. The remaining animals were sacrificed as scheduled. Neither acute inflammation nor excessive swelling was observed in the postoperative region in any case.

12.3.3.1 Tissue-Engineered Bone Graft "TCP + gMSCs"

In 30 days after surgery, the defect margins were less distinctive in the experimental group than in the controls according to CT. Granules of the materials implanted were visualized as discrete regions with an increased radiodensity in both groups. An average density of newly formed bone tissue at this time point of observation was not statistically different, when being 1012.3 ± 152.6 HU in the experimental group and 1034.0 ± 144.8 HU in the control one (Figure 12.2). In 60 days in the experimental group the bone defects became irregular due to occurrence of regions with an increased density from the defect lateral side, fusing with the parietal bone edge. In the controls there were no such changes or they were minimally evident although the defects margins became less distinct in comparison with the previous time point. In 120 days after surgery in both groups there was an abrupt decrease of the newly formed bone tissue density mostly due to resorption of the granules of the bone substitutes implanted, i.e. 839.2 ± 119.5 and 787.5 ± 191.3 HU in the experimental and control groups, respectively. At the same time, regions with an increased density and homogeneous structure, merging from the parietal bone edges occupied most of the bone defects in both groups (Figure 12.2).

The histological examination revealed that most of the bone defect in both groups consisted of fibrous tissue in 30 days after surgery (Figure 12.3). Woven bone tissue formed mainly from the parietal bone edges, though there were signs of osteogenesis in the central area achieving 0.74% in one case in the experimental group and 0.24% in the control. In 60 days after transplantation of the tissue-engineered bone grafts, the average proportion of newly formed bone tissue achieved 41.5% in the peripheral zone, while in the control one it did not exceed 32.1% that is less in 1.3 times (Figure 12.4).

However, there were more regions of newly formed bone tissue around the substitute granules in the central zone in the control group than in the experimental one. No consolidation of a bone defect was achieved in either group by the latest time point of observation – there was a segment of connective tissue in the central part.

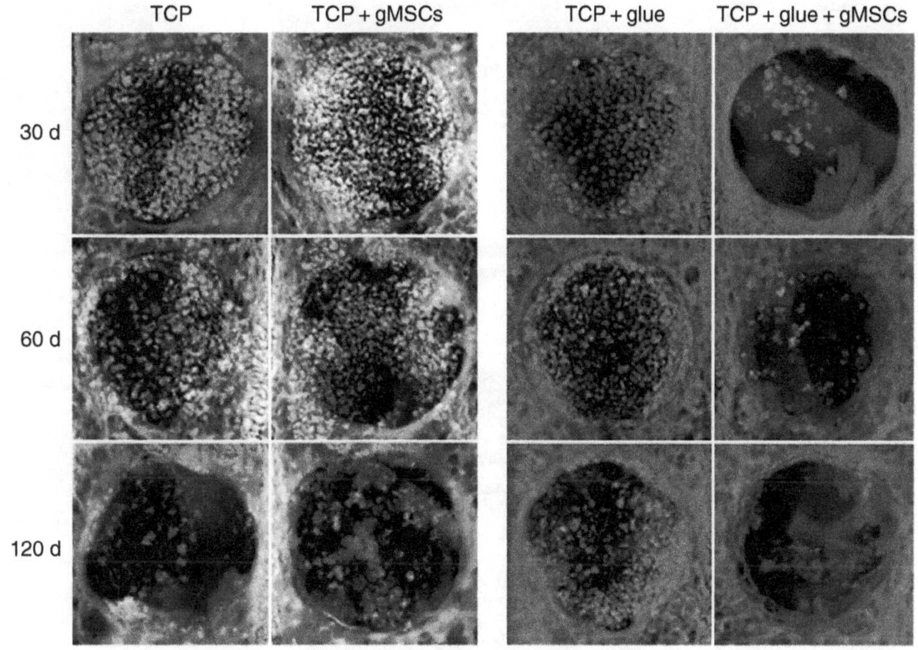

Figure 12.2 Rabbit parietal bone defects in different time points after implantation of the study material; microradiography.

However, regions of newly formed bone tissue both discrete and associated with substitute granules were detected along the defect entire length and characterized by complex morphology: the peripheral part was composed by lamellar bone tissue surrounding blood vessels, while the central zone bordering with connective tissue being woven bone. The formation of bone marrow between trabecules of the newly formed lamellar bone tissue and the substitute granules remained by this time was another specific histological finding in both groups (Figure 12.3).

12.3.3.2 Tissue-Engineered Bone Graft "TCP + fibrin glue + gMSCs"

In all time points of observation the X-ray examination detected much fewer substitute granules in the bone defects of the experimental group in comparison with the control one. Despite it, the bone defect margins were distinct and regular in 30 days after surgery, they became less distinguishable at the latest time points. In the control group substitute granules were clearly visualized in all time points by filling in a total defect volume (Figure 12.2). The newly formed bone tissue density gradually decreased from 1087.5 ± 137.3 to 921.6 ± 124.1 HU in the control, with there being an increase from 238.4 ± 83.8 HU at the time point of 30 days to 536.5 ± 146.1 HU in 120 days in the experimental group.

A histological examination confirmed the significantly fewer number of granules detectable in the defects of the experimental group. Despite that, a proportion of newly formed bone tissue in the peripheral zone was slightly higher after transplantation of the tissue-engineered bone graft than in the control group in all time points of observation. In the central zone reparative osteogenesis was more active in 30 and 60 days after surgery in the control group, though it was converse in 120 days after surgery. There was no complete restoration of the parietal bone continuity in any group. However, while almost each of the separate granules within the defect central part was surrounded by newly formed bone tissue, in the controls where there were significantly more fragments of the scaffold, only single granules were associated with the regions of reparative osteogenesis (Figure 12.3).

12.3.3.3 Tissue-Engineered Bone Graft "TCP + fibrin glue + adSVF"

There were no significant differences in the average tissue density within the bone defects in the experimental and control groups in both time-points of observation. The newly formed bone tissue density was slightly higher in the control – 959.3 ± 74.9 and 1020.0 ± 169.8 HU in 60 and 90 days, respectively, whereas it was 857.8 ± 139.4 and 990.4 ± 71.1 HU in the experimental group. It is specific that the defect margins were not clearly evident as early as in 60 days after surgery in both groups, with the tissue in the implantation zone in all cases being heteromorphic with discrete regions of increased density – more than 1500 HU (Figure 12.5).

The histological examination at the time point of 60 days detected evident peripheral newly formed bone tissue originating from parietal bone in both groups. The proportion of newly formed bone tissue was on average 44.7% and 49.1% of the total area of the regenerated

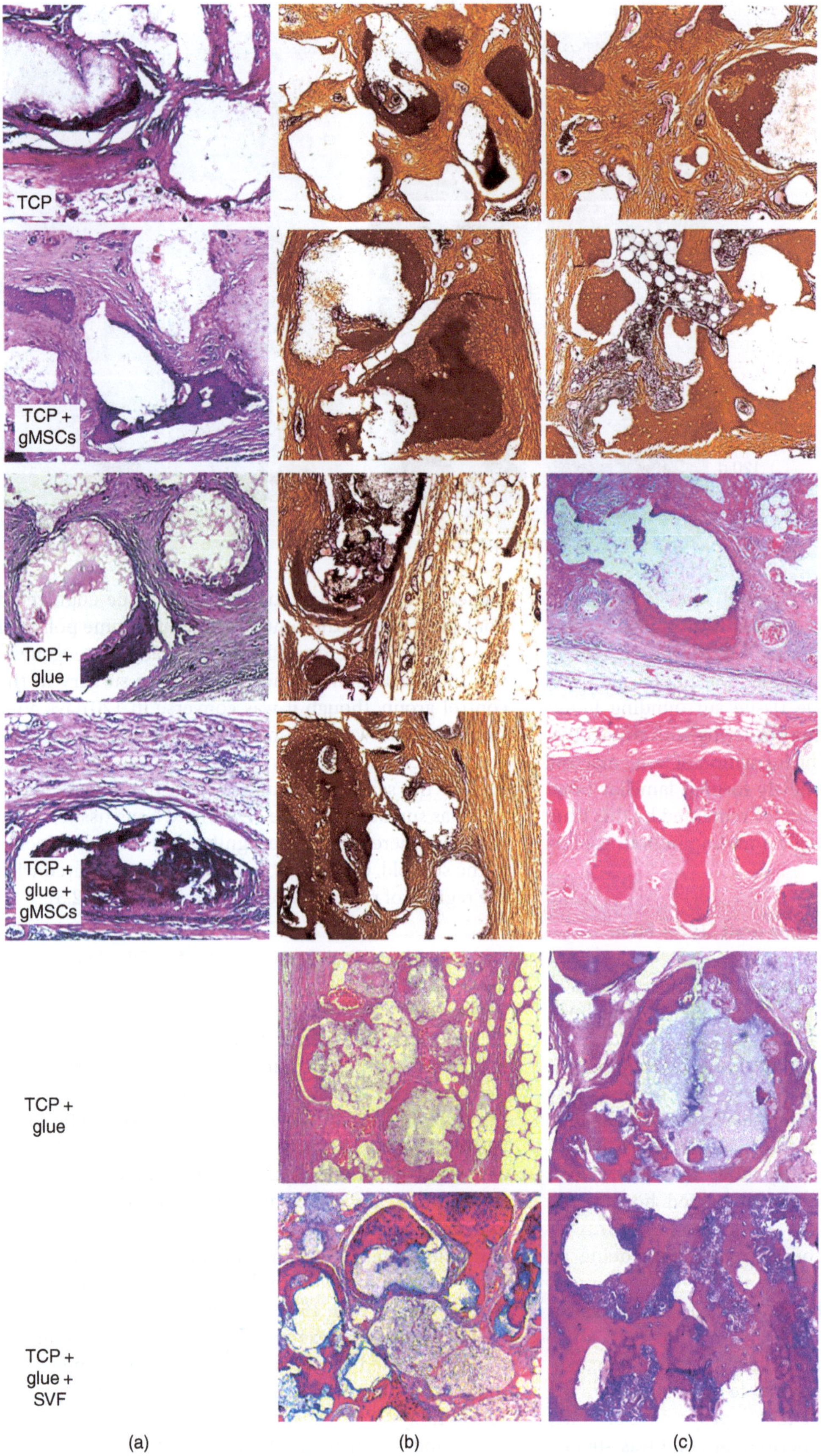

Figure 12.3 Rabbit parietal bone defects in different time points after implantation of the study materials: (a) 30 days, (b) 60 days, (c) 120 days and 90 days in case of the MSCs and adSVF, respectively. Material fragments, newly formed bone tissue, fibrous tissue. Staining: violet and pink – hematoxylin and eosin, brown – Gordon's silver staining.

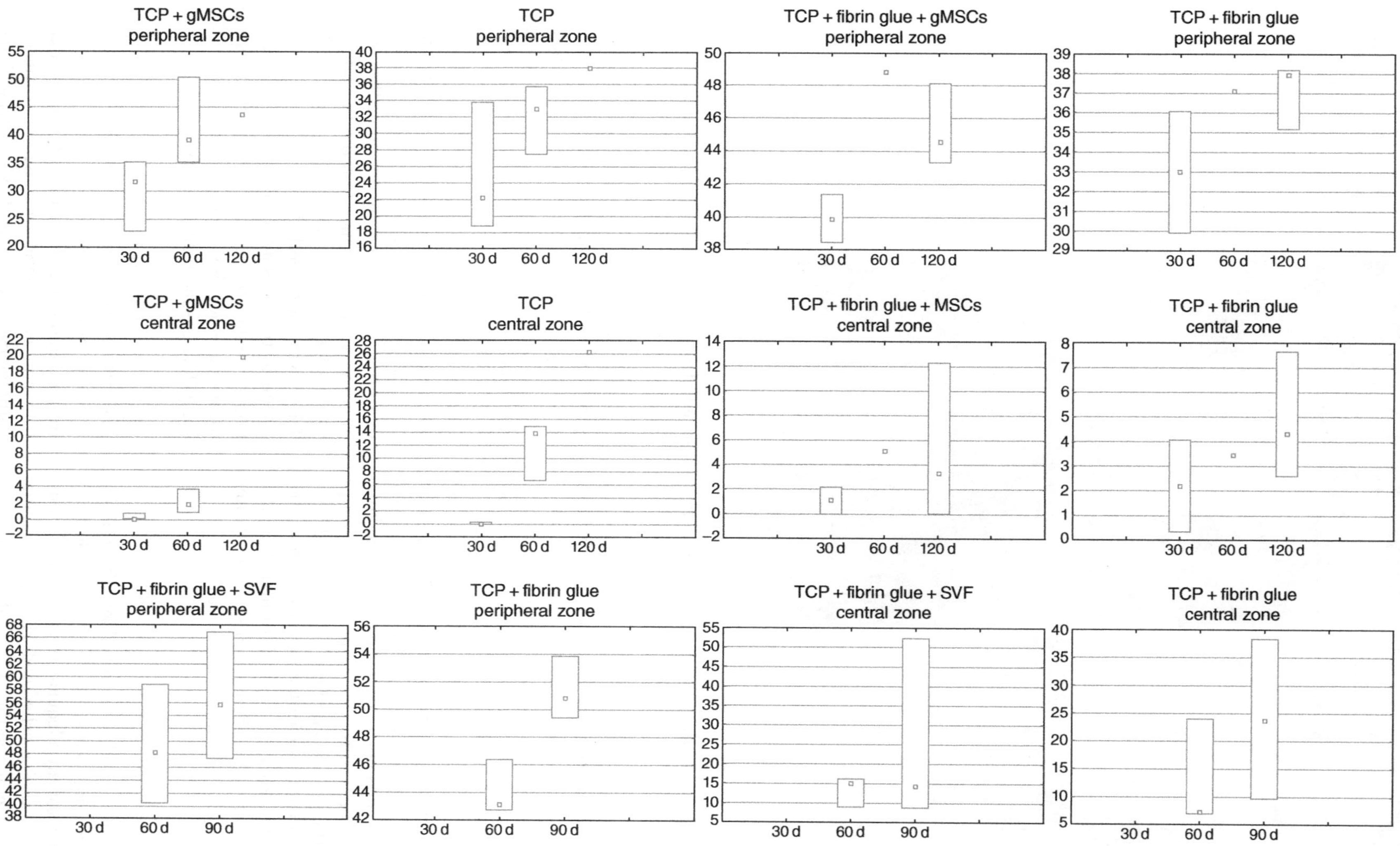

Figure 12.4 Proportions of newly formed bone tissue in the peripheral (a) and central (b) zone of bone defects. Middle point: median, box value: Min–Max.

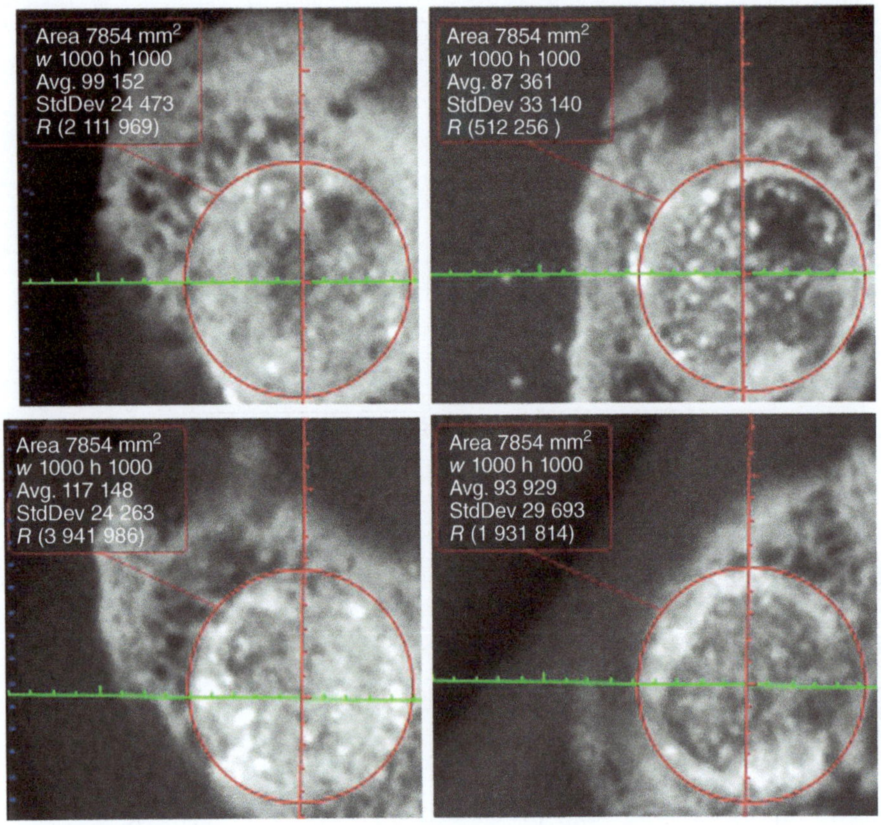

Figure 12.5 Rabbit parietal bone defects in different time points after implantation of the study material. Computed tomography, axial view.

peripheral zone defect in the controls and in the experimental group. Newly formed bone tissue was woven, partly remodeled in lamellar. The defect central part was filled by fibrous tissue. However, with implanting the tissue-engineered bone graft there was slightly more newly formed bone tissue around the substitute granules localized in the defect central zone (Figures 12.3 and 12.4). An average proportion of newly formed bone tissue in the central zone was 12.8% in the controls and 13.5% in the experimental group. These differences between the groups were also observed in 90 days after surgery, but they were statistically insignificant. In one animal there was a complete consolidation of the bone defect both in the control and experimental groups (Figure 12.3). The proportion of the newly formed bone tissue in the peripheral zone after transplantation of the tissue-engineered bone graft was by 6.4% more than that in the controls, with the difference in the central zone achieving 14.1% (Figure 12.4).

12.3.4 Safety and Efficacy in the Pilot Clinical Trial

An average age of the patients enrolled into the trial was 42.3 ± 14.2 years (nine males, four females) (Table 12.1). All the patients got an adequate treatment and completed the clinical trial as scheduled. Having undergone surgery under general anesthesia the patients received a standard complex therapy including a similar set of drugs (antibacterial, anti-inflammatory, desensitizing agents, analgesics) in a postoperative period.

Neither adverse events nor serious adverse events were observed in any patient. The postoperative period was typical for such interventions and occurred without complications. Pain and edema levels in the postoperative region complied with the severity of the operation without differences from an average for surgical interventions of this type. Maximum pain that control required analgesics was observed in the first day after surgery (6.1 ± 1.2), and significantly reduced to the third day (3.8 ± 0.7), that allowed discontinuing these drugs. Most intensive swelling occurred on the third day scoring up to 7.2 ± 1.4, however, it decreased significantly – up to 4.4 ± 2.3 by the seventh day.

Due to the diversity of pathology and the composition of tissue-engineered bone grafts it is reasonable to present operation protocols and results of the pilot clinical trial as individual clinical cases.

12.3.4.1 Clinical Case No. 1

The patient was enrolled with the diagnosis of cytologically proven fibrous dysplasia of the mandible frontal region (Figure 12.6). After an oral cavity sanation and endodontic treatment excochleation of the pathological tissues and immediate bone grafting

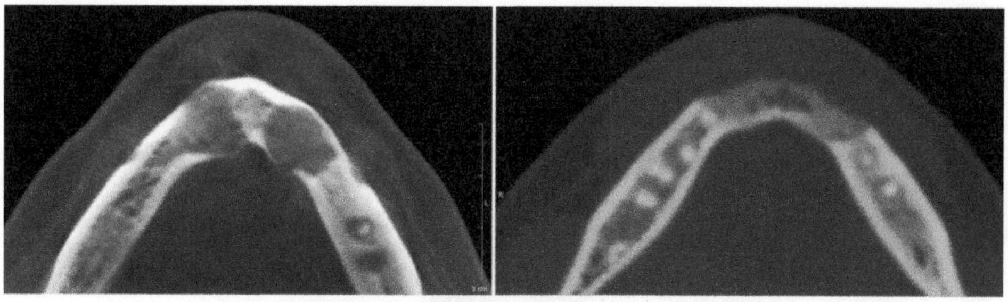

Figure 12.6 The mandible of Patient No. 1: (a) before treatment, (b) 4.5 months after treatment with the use of the tissue-engineered construction "TCP + fibrin glue + gMSCs." CT, axial view.

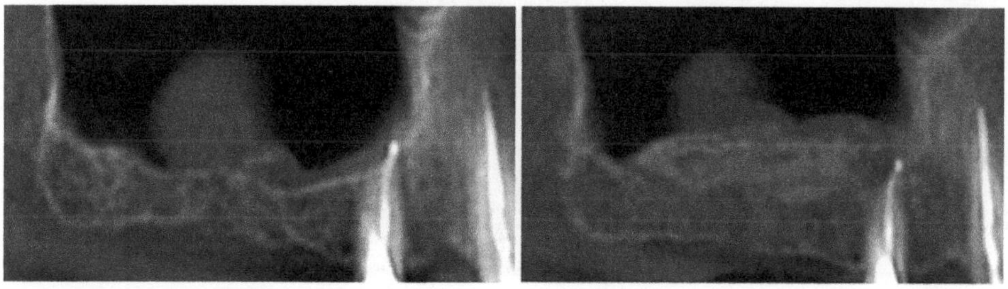

Figure 12.7 Patient No. 2: (a) access to the anterior lateral surface of the maxillary sinus; (b) filling of the space between the floor and the elevated sinus mucosa with a tissue-engineered construction.

with a tissue-engineered construction ($3\,cm^3$) composed by TCP, fibrin glue, and gMSCs were performed (Table 12.1).

An incision was made along the mucobuccal fold at the level of teeth 3.3–4.3 under endotracheal and local anesthesia, a mucoperiosteal flap was lifted, and a defect of the vestibular cortical lamina of the mandible visualized at the level of teeth 3.1–4.1. The defect was widened by grinding, abnormal tissues excised in full to the intact bone tissue with the resection of apexes of sealed frontal teeth roots. A formed defect of the mandible was filled in with the tissue-engineered construction. A postoperative wound was sutured with a continuous stitch (Novosyn 4/0).

Based on the control CT findings performed in 4.5 months after surgery the bone defect in the mandibular frontal region was replaced with irregular newly formed bone tissue, which average density was 682.7 ± 121.7 HU that corresponded to intact spongy bone (Figure 12.6). Regions with an increased density (from 930 to 1080 HU) were visualized in the defect central part. The integrity of the vestibular cortical plate has not been restored by this time point.

12.3.4.2 Clinical Case No. 2

The patient had atrophy of the maxillary alveolar process, partial secondary edentia of the maxilla and mandible. According to the CT a thickness of the maxillary alveolar process on the right side in projection of the lost molars was 4.3–5.7 mm (Figure 12.7).

A staged plan of combined treatment was formulated and included bone grafting, dental implants placement and a subsequent prosthetic treatment. During the treatment first stage within the clinical trial right sinus lifting was performed with the use of a tissue-engineered construction based on OCP, fibrin glue, and the MSCs (Table 12.1).

An incision via the alveolar crest and then vertically on the level of mesially located tooth were made under local anesthesia and the mucoperiosteal flap was lifted. A surface of the anterior lateral wall of the maxillary sinus was exposed and a window with a diameter of 5 mm formed. Schneider membrane was carefully elevated and a collagen membrane placed underneath. A tissue-engineered construction was transplanted into the space provided (Figure 12.8). A bone window was closed by a collagen membrane, and then soft tissues were sutured with Vicryl 5/0.

Based on the CT findings in 4.5 months after sinus-lifting with the use of the tissue-engineered bone graft the thickness of the maxillary alveolar process achieved 11.4–17.7 mm due to newly formed bone tissue within the zone of the material implanted. The newly formed bone tissue completely integrated with

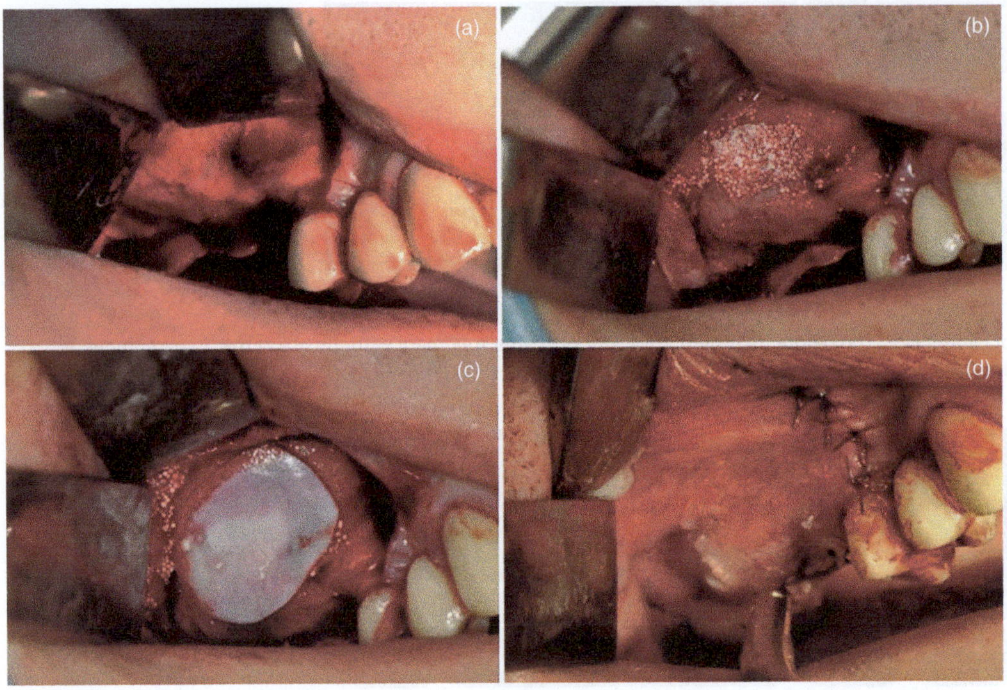

Figure 12.8 Patient No. 3: (a) CT 4.5 months after bone grafting, (b) CT after placement of dental implants; (c) a newly formed bone tissue within the area of implanting tissue-engineered construction "TCP + gMSC", (d) final aspect after suture.

the underlying bone and was relatively homogeneous, had an average density of 829.3 ± 89.8 HU, which slightly exceeded an intact spongy bone (Figure 12.7).

A successful bone grafting enabled to perform dental implantation in six months after surgery. At present, a prosthetic treatment with implants has been successfully performed.

12.3.4.3 Clinical Case No. 3

The patient had atrophy of the alveolar process, partial secondary edentia of the left maxilla. Atrophy was so pronounced that the alveolar process height was 1 mm in some parts. The patient underwent sinus floor elevation on the left side under the standard protocol, described above with implantation of a tissue-engineered bone graft composed by TCP and gMSCs without fibrin glue.

The postoperative period was typical for such interventions. In 5.5 months after surgery a growth of the left maxillary sinus floor achieved 9.7–12.1 mm. The newly formed bone tissue was heteromorphic due to detectable discrete radio-opaque granules with a high density of 1254 ± 117.4 HU. No hyperplastic reaction of the sinus floor mucosa was observed (Figure 12.9a). In 8.5 months after operation three dental implants were placed, two of them within the bone grafting zone (Figure 12.9b). The newly formed bone tissue density in that time point was 1358.6 ± 138.5 HU, significantly exceeding spongy bone. Successful osteointegration of implants enabled to perform an adequate prosthetic treatment.

During dental implants placement a fragment of newly formed bone tissue was taken with a trepan for a histological examination. Trabecules of newly formed lamellar bone tissue including those connected with singular granules of the tissue-engineered bone graft were detected (Figure 12.10).

12.3.4.4 Clinical Case No. 4

The patient had a postoperative deformity of the facial lower region, nonunions within the fixation areas of a rib bone autograft and the mandible. A resection of the mandible from the frontal region to the right ramus due to fibrous dysplasia was made in 2010. In a regional hospital two unsuccessful attempts of mandibular microsurgical reconstruction with the use of vascularized fibular bone autografts were undertaken. Both interventions resulted in vascular anastomosis failure. In 2011, a reconstruction of the mandible was performed with a free rib bone autograft fixed with four titanium miniplates by two in proximal and distal regions. In 1.5 years after surgery no significant resorption of the bone autograft was observed, but, nonunions were formed within the zones of distal and proximal fixation with 5–7 mm diastases between bone fragments (Figure 12.11a).

The patient underwent reconstructive surgery on the mandible with a removal of metal constructions, excision of nonunions scar tissues, and bone grafting

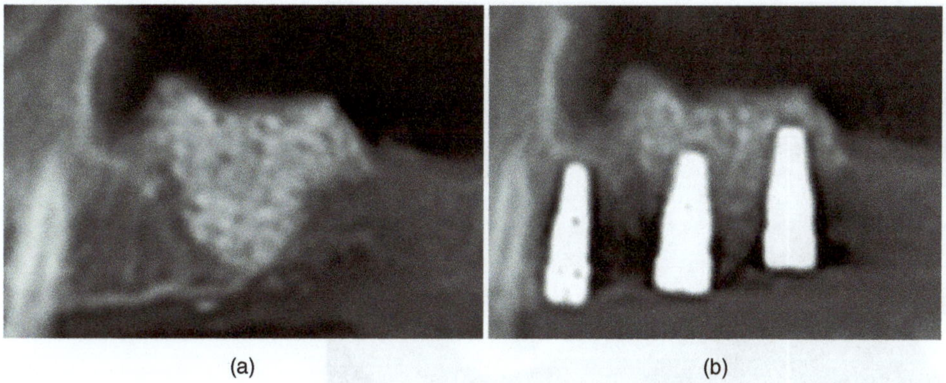

Figure 12.9 The maxillary left sinus floor of Patient No. 3: (a) 4.5 months after bone grafting, (b) after placement of dental implants. CT, sagittal view.

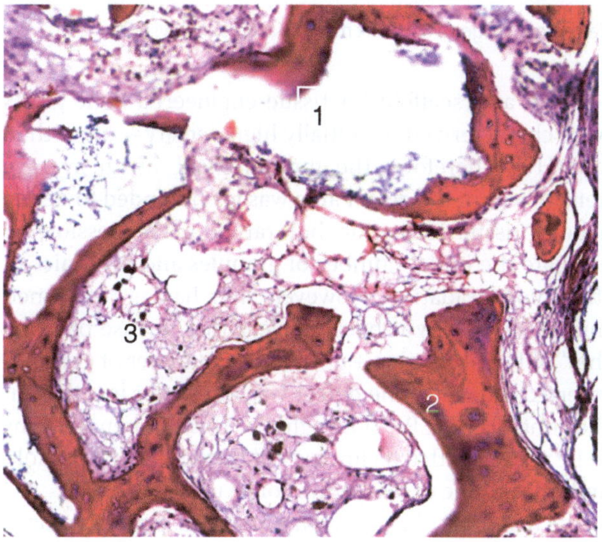

Figure 12.10 Newly formed bone tissue within the area of implanting tissue-engineered construction composed by TCP and gMSCs, clinical case No. 3: (1) the substitute fragment; (2) newly formed bone tissue; (3) fibrous tissue. Staining: hematoxylin and eosin.

with a tissue-engineered substitute "TCP + fibrin glue + adSVF" (Table 12.1).

Lipoaspiration was performed according to the above procedure to obtain adSVF under combined endotracheal anesthesia. The postoperative scar in the right submandibular region was excised. Soft tissues were processed to the periosteum. The bone was exposed only in the autograft fixation sites to minimize the effect on its blood supply. The miniplates were removed. Fibrous tissue was excised, bone surfaces processed. The bone autograft was positioned correctly and fixed with four straight miniplates and miniscrews (with a length of 5 and 7 mm, and a diameter of 2 mm). Diastases (from 2 to 3 mm) between mandibular fragments and the bone autograft were filled in with the tissue-engineered construction. Postoperative wound were sutured by layers with Vycril 4/0, Surgipro 4/0.

The postoperative period was typical for such interventions, without signs of inflammation. In six months after surgery the control CT detected no consolidation within the proximal and distal bone autograft fixation (Figure 12.11b). Diastases did not exceed 2 mm. A slight mobility was detected within the nonunion in the mandibular frontal region. The patient was re-operated with the use of another bone substitute and better fixation with miniplates.

12.4 Discussion

12.4.1 Experimental Part

Despite significant technological advances in the development of tissue-engineered bone grafts, there are still lots of issues to be solved that are related to the selection of a scaffold, a cell type, number, sources, processing to the stage of combining with a scaffold material, the combination protocols, as well as the objective evaluation of a biological activity *in vivo*.

Therefore, our aim was to conduct a large-scale pilot study to evaluate a number of various tissue-engineered bone grafts differing by composition and manufacturing technologies. The study was focused to assess the biological action of each variant in a standard experimental model and to determine the effect reproducibility in different clinical conditions rather than to compare different materials with each other.

Given the specificity of maxillofacial surgery we have selected gMSCs and adSVF as optimal cell populations, i.e. those cell types that can be easily obtained by a maxillofacial surgeon. At the same time, the chosen cell components of tissue-engineered bone grafts are absolutely different that is of additional interest for a pilot study. The former are a relatively pure cell population standardized

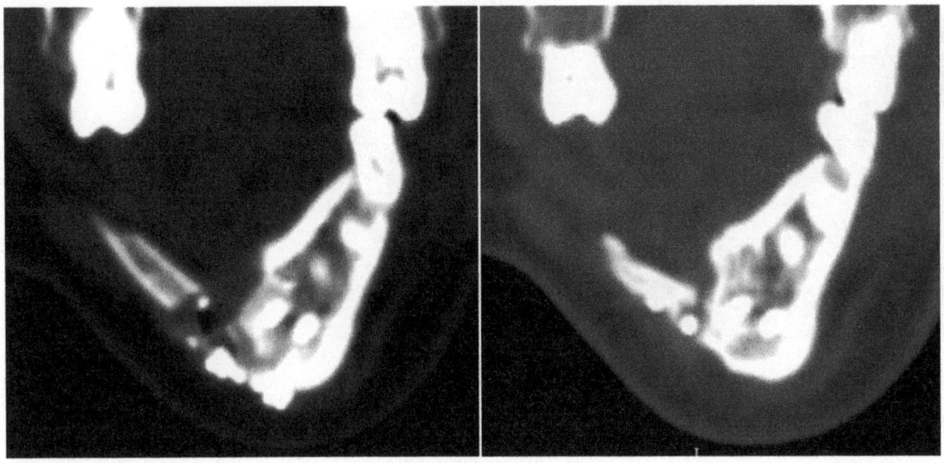

(a) (b)

Figure 12.11 Non-union in the mandible frontal region of Patient No. 4: (a) before surgery; (b) in six months after surgery; CT.

in qualitative and quantitative criteria and expanded *in vitro* [14]. The latter are a primary cell population of various cytogenesis, which are related with the adipose tissue microvasculature. A therapeutic application of these cells is possible immediately after isolation including the setting with the use of instrumental processing [15].

There is a number of experimental models *in vivo*, including those with standardized protocol and study methods that enable to determine a biological action of bone grafts [16]. However, in our opinion, rabbit parietal bone defects are the most relevant model for maxillofacial surgery. Firstly, parietal bones, as most of the maxillofacial bones, are characterized by endesmal osteogenesis [17]. Secondly, the calvarium is not exposed to loading that makes it possible to avoid the use of additional fixing structures (for example, miniplates), capable to affect the reparative regeneration. Thirdly, the presence of natural "membranes" such as the dura mater and the periosteum allows avoiding the use of membranes required in other experimental models to hold granules within a bone defect zone. And, finally, cranial defects with a size of more than 10 mm are "critical" even when periosteum is maintained because the parietal bones cannot be restored completely without additional optimizing impact. However, this experimental model is technically complex due to the proximity to the vital anatomical structures. Therefore, death of 10–12% of animals could be expected because of subdural hematoma formation. In our study 8% of animals died for this reason.

The experimental part was performed in two stages. During the first one, the tissue-engineered bone grafts containing the MSCs were studied in three time points of observation such as 30, 90, and 120 days. X-ray imaging methods had limited value as the TCP granules selected as a scaffold for tissue-engineered bone grafts were characterized by initially high density – more than 1600 HU. Therefore, the measurement of an average density within the defect area was less intended to define a bone tissue formation but rather made possible to evaluate the initial number of granules and dynamics of their biodegradation. However, after having performed microradiography it became clear that in case of using the "TCP + fibrin glue + gMSCs" the number of granules inserted into the bone defect was one order less than in the controls ("TCP + fibrin glue"). This difference seems to be related with a technology of combining the scaffold and cells, a glue excess in the construction.

The histological analysis was essential. Separate quantitative measurements of osteogenesis (bone formation) in the peripheral and central areas of bone defects, especially in the time points of 30 and 60 days were of importance in evaluating the biological effect of materials. Thus, the activation of bone formation from periphery confirms the material osteoconductive properties while the detection of bone tissue formation regions in the central part may give evidence of not only osteoconduction but also an osteoinductive potential of the substitute. It was found that both in experimental and control groups the most evident signs of osteogenesis were detected in the peripheral zone. No connective tissue layer formed between the substitute granules located herein and the newly formed bone tissue. This, in combination with the lack of inflammation signs and lymphocytic infiltration, confirm the biocompatibility of the study materials. Most of newly formed bone tissue in the peripheral zone was observed "TCP + gMSCs" group (Figure 12.4). At the same time most of newly formed bone tissue was detected in the central zone on the latest time points of observation when TCP was used. It seems to be due to the higher baseline number of substitute granules implanted into the bone defects in this group caused by the lack of additional components (fibrin glue), capable to reduce a proportion of the scaffold in a total volume of the bone defect. A lot of granules provided more pronounced osteoconductive properties enabling the newly formed bone tissue from the peripheral zone to achieve the central as early as in 60 days. Despite that no complete consolidation of the bone defect occurred in either group of the first experiment stage *in vivo*, a slightly larger volume of newly formed bone tissue was detected with the use of the tissue-engineered bone grafts ("TCP + gMSCs," "TCP + fibrin glue + gMSCs") in comparison with the respective controls although there were fewer substitute granules in experimental groups, especially in the group with "TCP + fibrin glue + gMSCs."

Considering the results of the first stage and disadvantages associated with a small amount of a solid scaffold we have modified the technology in the group implanted with the adSVF by reducing the amount of fibrin glue. Based on the CT results of the second stage of experimental study, the number of granules and an average density in HU in the experimental group were only slightly inferior to the control one (Figure 12.5). This study involved only two time points of observation – 60 and 90 days – as the most important in the evaluation of a biological action of the bone grafts in this experimental model. Even in 60 days, a proportion of newly formed bone tissue both in the peripheral and central zones was found out to be higher than in the controls. Moreover, the restoration of the parietal bones was observed by the time point of 90 days. At the same time, when using the "TCP + fibrin glue + SVF" construction the consolidation was complete, while small areas of connective tissue remained in the controls that divided the newly formed bone tissue into segments.

Thus, a two-staged experimental study revealed that the tissue-engineered bone grafts had no negative effects. A biological action of the constructions developed was to activate reparative osteogenesis mainly near to bone edges. The intensity of stimulating effects was superior to those in the controls, although the differences were not statistically significant. The induction of bone tissue formation was more intense in case of using the adSVF, it was observed even in the defect central part. This effect may be related to an optimization of the technology to make bone substitute materials containing a glue component as increasing the proportion of a solid scaffold rather than the differences in a biological action of the MSCs and adSVF that requires additional studies.

It should be noted that most of the published results of using tissue-engineered bone grafts based on the MSCs *in vivo* are successful, while the efficacy of constructions for bone grafting based on the SVF are ambiguous. For example, in the study performed by Kim et al. a tissue-engineered bone graft from polylactic glycolic acid (PLGA) and an autologous SVF did not exert an optimizing biological action on reparative regeneration of bone tissue in a rabbit radial bone defect [18]. However, in our study the material containing fibrin glue and the SVF has demonstrated a marked osteoinductive potential.

12.4.2 Clinical Part

The successful results of the experimental study facilitated the initiation of a pilot clinical trial. When planning this clinical study we have not intentionally restricted the inclusion criteria to any singular pathology. Being convinced in the safety of the technology and constructions developed, we wanted to identify the indications when tissue-engineered bone grafts would be most effective. Moreover, having identified the peculiarities of the biological action of various tissue-engineered bone grafts in the previous experiment *in vivo* we decided not to choose the best one for the pilot clinical trial. Such selection is impossible only on the basis of the experimental data as neither evident positive biological effect in an experiment ensures the clinical efficacy, nor the moderate level of the required biological action *in vitro* or *in vivo* excludes the possibility to achieve the successful treatment results. Therefore, we used five different tissue-engineered bone grafts in our clinical trial.

Patients with jaw pathology of different genesis such as atrophy, benign tumors, and pseudotumors as well as post-traumatic deformities (Table 12.1) were enrolled into the trial. In some clinical cases (such is the case 4) the situation was especially complex, and the achievement of a successful result was determined not only and not so much by a bone graft as co-existing factors, the history and a surgical technique. This diversity of indications to use and tissue-engineered graft variants is specific for pilot clinical trials in maxillofacial surgery [2].

Neither adverse events nor serious adverse events were observed in any patient that confirmed the safety of the tissue-engineered bone grafts developed to the full extent. However, in evaluating the efficacy ambiguous results were obtained, which depend upon the indications chosen as it was expected.

In particular, different bone grafts were most effective in the treatment of jaw atrophy ($n = 5$) and in sinus floor elevation. Taking into account a high density of the newly formed bone tissue in four to six months after surgery, it can be stated that not all the scaffold fragments resorbed by that time. Indeed, the histological examination of the bioptate obtained when placing dental implants detected substitute granules in the newly formed bone tissue. However, as in the experimental study there was no connective tissue layer between them and the newly formed bone tissue. In the other words, the material was completely integrated that enabled to carry out dental implantation and a prosthetic treatment, i.e. to achieve the successful treatment results. The results obtained for these indications correspond with the other data published, which demonstrated the efficacy of various tissue-engineered bone grafts [2, 19].

In case of benign tumors, defects, nonunions and post-traumatic deformities ($n = 8$), the results are determined not only by the bone graft efficacy but also by bone defect extend, radical removal of the involved tissues, patients' bad habits, co-existing pathology, and other factors that have a negative impact on bone tissue formation. In our trial, the abnormalities specified had the sizes that allowed radical surgical interventions such as cytoectomy, excochleation of a fibrous dysplasia site, or segmental resection with maintaining the jaw continuity. The clinical trial protocol did not specify a resection of the mandible without maintaining its continuity, when bone grafting would require the application of additional fixative items such as a titanium mesh or reconstructive plates [20]. As for the previous indications there was a heteromorphic newly formed bone tissue within the transplantation zone; its density exceeded spongy bone due to the presence of radio-opaque granules in its composition.

The treatment failed only in 1 of 13 clinical cases (case 4) and a re-operation was required in half a year. When analyzing this case, we derived the following: two nonunions within the fixation area of a rib bone autograft to the mandibular ramus and body, two previous unsuccessful reconstructive microsurgeries with the fibula flaps, and more than 15 years of smoking, and we have concluded that the patient was not the best candidate for bone grafting with a tissue-engineered construction.

Thus, it was found in the pilot clinical trial that the developed tissue-engineered constructions demonstrating a favorable biological action in experiments *in vivo* are effective for the treatment of patients with jaw atrophy and bone defects after removal of benign tumors and pseudotumors. Post-traumatic deformity, nonunions, and jaw reconstruction with the use of additional items for fixation require additional studies.

Based on the results of this study and the conclusions we have initiated the initiative clinical trial of one of the tissue-engineered bone grafts developed and for the only indication to use, namely "TCP + gMSCs", in sinus lifting procedure [21].

Acknowledgments

The study was funded by grants of the Russian Science Foundation (project No. 15-13-00108, the development of the initial materials for this study and project No. 14-25-00166, the experimental and pilot clinical study).

References

1 Gómez-Barrena, E., Rosset, P., Lozano, D. et al. (2015). Bone fracture healing: cell therapy in delayed unions and nonunions. *Bone* **70C**: 93–101.

2 Sándor, G.K., Numminen, J., Wolff, J. et al. (2014). Adipose stem cells used to reconstruct 13 cases with cranio-maxillofacial hard-tissue defects. *Stem Cells Transl. Med.* **3**: 530–540.

3 Giannotti, S., Trombi, L., Bottai, V. et al. (2013). Use of autologous human mesenchymal stromal cell/fibrin clot constructs in upper limb non-unions: long-term assessment. *PLoS One* **8**: e73893.

4 report, A. (2013). *Turning a New Page*. Straumann http://www.straumann.com/content/dam/internet/straumann_com/Resources/investor-relations/annual-report/2013/STMN-2013-Annual-Report.pdf.

5 Tosco, P., Tanteri, G., Iaquinta, C. et al. (2009). Surgical treatment and reconstruction for central giant cell granuloma of the jaws: a review of 18 cases. *J. Craniomaxillofac. Surg.* **37**: 380–387.

6 Mitsimponas, K.T., Iliopoulos, C., Stockmann, P. et al. (2014). The free scapular/parascapular flap as a reliable method of reconstruction in the head and neck region: a retrospective analysis of 130 reconstructions performed over a period of 5 years in a single department. *J. Craniomaxillofac. Surg.* **42**: 536–543.

7 Sanz, A.R., Carrión, F.S., and Chaparro, A.P. (2015). Mesenchymal stem cells from the oral cavity and their potential value in tissue engineering. *Periodontology* **2000**, **67**: 251–267.

8 Knight, M.N. and Hankenson, K.D. (2013). Mesenchymal stem cells in bone regeneration. *Adv. Wound Care (New Rochelle)* **2**: 306–316.

9 Zorin, V.L., Komlev, V.S., Zorina, A.I. et al. (2014). Octacalcium phosphate ceramics combined with gingiva-derived stromal cells for engineered functional bone grafts. *Biomed. Mater.* **9**: 055005.

10 Estrela, C., Alencar, A.H., Kitten, G.T. et al. (2011). Mesenchymal stem cells in the dental tissues: perspectives for tissue regeneration. *Braz. Dent. J.* **22**: 91–98.
11 Zorin, V.L., Zorina, A.I., Eremin, I.I. et al. (2014). Comparative analysis of osteogenic potential of multipotent mesenchymal stromal cells derived from oral mucosa and bone marrow. *Genes Cells* **9** (1): 50–57.
12 Farré-Guasch, E., Prins, H.J., Overman, J.R. et al. (2013). Human maxillary sinus floor elevation as a model for bone regeneration enabling the application of one-step surgical procedures. *Tissue Eng. Part B Rev.* **19**: 69–82.
13 Komlev, V.S., Barinov, S.M., and Koplik, E.V. (2002). A method to fabricate porous spherical hydroxyapatite granules intended for time-controlled drug release. *Biomaterials* **23**: 3449–3454.
14 Dominici, M., Le Blanc, K., Mueller, I. et al. (2006). Minimal criteria for defining multipotent mesenchymal stromal cells. The international society for cellular therapy position statement. *Cytotherapy* **8**: 315–317.
15 Dong, Z., Fu, R., Liu, L., and Liu, F. (2013). Stromal vascular fraction (SVF) cells enhance long-term survival of autologous fat grafting through the facilitation of M2 macrophages. *Cell Biol. Int.* **37**: 855–859.
16 ASTM F2721-09 (2009). Standard guide for pre-clinical in vivo evaluation in critical size segmental bone defects. West Conshohocken, PA: Astm International. http://www.astm.org/Standards/F2721.htm (accessed 21 August 2017).
17 Maruyama, T. (2011). Development of the skeletal system in utero. *Clin. Calcium.* **21**: 1299–1305.
18 Kim, A., Kim, D.H., Song, H.R. et al. (2012). Repair of rabbit ulna segmental bone defect using freshly isolated adipose-derived stromal vascular fraction. *Cytotherapy* **14**: 296–305.
19 Drobyshev, A.Y., Rubina, K.A., Sisoeva, V.Y. et al. (2011). Clinical study of tissue-engineered construction based on autologous stromal cells of adipose tissue in patients with bone deficiency in the regions of maxilla alveolar processus and mandible alveolar part. *Vest. Exp. Clin. Surg.* **IV**: 764–772.
20 Sándor, G.K., Tuovinen, V.J., Wolff, J. et al. (2013). Adipose stem cell tissue-engineered construct used to treat large anterior mandibular defect: a case report and review of the clinical application of good manufacturing practice-level adipose stem cells for bone regeneration. *J. Oral Maxillofac. Surg.* **71**: 938–950.
21 Grigory A. Volozhin, Ilya I. Eremin (2014). Effectiveness and safety of method of maxilla alveolar process reconstruction using synthetic tricalcium phosphate and autologous MMSCs. http://www.clinicaltrial.gov/ct2/show/NCT02209311?term=FMBA+Burnasyan&rank=5.

13

Bone Substitutes in Orthopedic and Trauma Surgery

Lupescu Olivera[1] and Iulian Antoniac[2]

[1] Department of Orthopaedics, Faculty of Medicine, "Carol Davila" University of Medicine and Pharmacy of Bucharest, 37 Dionisie Lupu Street, District 2, 020021 Bucharest, Romania
[2] Department of Metallic Materials Science, Physical Metallurgy, Faculty of Material Science and Engineering, Politehnica University of Bucharest, 313 Splaiul Independentei, District 6, JA 104-106 Building, 060042 Bucharest, Romania

13.1 Introduction

Bone substitutes (BS) represent synthetic, inorganic, or biologically organic combinations which can be inserted for treating bone defects (BDs) instead of autogenous or allogenous bone graft (BG).

Although concern for bone healing existed even in ancient medicine [1], history of bone grafting starts with the Dutch surgeon Job van Meekeren who, in 1668, healed a soldier with a war wound (skull) with a piece of bone from a dog [2]. Although the soldier was permanently excommunicated for being part dog, the success of the procedure opened the way for those interested in this field, so, in 1821, the first autograft was recorded in Germany. More than 100 years later, in 1965, Ulrist reported the osteointegration properties of bone morphogenetic proteins (BMPs) [3]; since then research has focused on finding solutions for the problem of bone loss.

Nowadays, bone grafting is the second most common transplantation tissue (blood being the most common) [4] and, in 2006, more than 500 000 bone-grafting procedures where performed in the USA, with the estimation of a double number on a global basis [5] (http://www.aaos.org/research/committee/biologic/bi_se_2006-1.pdf).

Since literature about BS is quite abundant, this chapter will not perform a comprehensive literature review, but a selection of the main practical aspects from the point of view of the orthopedic surgeon, underlining the elements with clinical significance, important for daily practice. Clinical cases will be presented as examples suggestive for benefits and indications of BS, since the finality of using these devices is early and total recovery of the patients with skeletal pathology involving bone gaps.

13.2 Principles of Bone Grafting

The concept of bone grafting, although not new, has still to be clarified; it is a common misconception that it means "filling a bone gap," since the purpose of grafting is much more complex: to re-create the bone where it was lost, to re-establish the continuity of the bone, which must act properly; that is why, in our opinion, it has to be clearly understood by all those involved in it that bone grafting means much more than filling the empty space, it means restoring the bone so as to able to perform its physiological functions, and the materials used for it must have certain properties able to build functional bone.

Unlike many human tissues which heal with a connective tissue scar, bone has, even in adult life, the ability to heal by producing bone, as it does after fractures. So since the final purpose of grafting is bone restoration, the principles to be followed are those of bone healing; according to the nowadays accepted "diamond concept" [6] the prerequisites for any bone to heal are the following:

- *Cells*: A large variety of cells are involved in fracture healing; the most important are the multipotent mesenchymal cells, which are recruited at the fracture site and transformed into osteoblasts [7]; inflammatory cells, as well as osteoclasts, have their own roles in bone grafting integration, as they have in postfracture bone healing.
- *Scaffolds*: In normal bone, the extracellular matrix provides the natural scaffold for all the cellular activities.
- *Growth factors*: The hematoma that appears after the fracture usually contains large quantities of factors called "signaling molecules," with different roles in bone healing; the most important are interleukins (IL-1, IL-6), fibroblast growth factor (FGF),

Bioceramics and Biocomposites: From Research to Clinical Practice, First Edition. Edited by Iulian Antoniac.

platelet-derived growth factor (PDGF), vascular endothelial growth factor (VEGF), transforming growth factor β (TGF β) superfamily members, tumor necrosis factor-α (TNF-α), and insulin-like growth factor (IGF) that are able to induce a cascade by which certain cells are activated to promote healing [8]. These substances are produced by endothelial cells, platelets, monocytes, macrophages, as well as by the mesenchymal stem cells, and the mesenchymal derived cells: the osteoblasts, the chondrocytes, the osteocytes, and the osteoblasts themselves. The most significant clinical relevance is that of some of the bone morphogenetic proteins (BMP-2 and BMP-7), members of the TGF β superfamily, already introduced in practice [9, 10].
- *Vascularity*: Since oxygen is the unique element vital for any survival cell or organism, its presence is crucial for the bone, as for any other tissue of the human body. An avascular environment will impair all the processes taking place during graft integration, as hypoxia and secondary acidosis maintain inflammation, disturbs collagen synthesis and deviates the cellular activity from osteogenesis to chondrocyte production so that bone is not produced any more [6].

These explain why all circumstances affecting one or another vascular segment of the affected area (arteries, arterioles, microcirculation, postcapillary venules, or veins) increase the risk of healing disturbances by different mechanism – by direct ischemic hypoxia, when the arterial segment is affected and by stasis when the venous return suffers; due to its severity and limited treatment possibilities, a special attention must be paid to angiopathies, such as the one associated to diabetes, or to chronic smoking; these situations, and many others like them, irreversibly damage the smallest arteries, thus impairing cellular oxygen supply with no possibility of compensation, because they are in the most distal position. If one such circumstance is identified in a patient with bone loss, careful assessment must be performed because the failure and risk of bone grafting procedures are considerable.

Mechanical stability is as important as any of the previous factors, since the maturation of the callus from woven to lamellar bone depends on this stability. Lack of stability results in persistent bleeding and impaired healing, but care must be taken so as to avoid extensive surgical approaches and invasive procedures and implants, as in these cases, the balance between biology and mechanical stability is mandatory for successful bone grafting [11].

These five conditions were described by Giannoudis as "biological chamber," meaning that for the graft to be integrated and transformed into functional bone, a proper environment must be created by surgery, and all the other therapeutic methods [12]. This environment must provide all the five elements previously described, otherwise, the result can be uncertain. The "diamond concept" must guide all therapeutic interventions for bone grafting, so preoperative planning must identify all potential factors that can negatively affect one of these elements or another and to neutralize its action before surgery is performed, otherwise a high risk of failure must be taken into consideration.

13.3 Causes of Bone Defects in Orthopedic Surgery

Numerous circumstances, such as trauma, infections, and tumors, can produce bone gaps; a comprehensive etiological classification is complicate and beyond the purpose of this book; since indications for a certain method of grafting are not established following the cause of the BD, but the characteristics of the remaining tissue, the most frequent indications for bone grafting will be described not from the point of view of surgical principles, but regarding the type of the properties of the environment.

1. Bone tumors require complete excision following oncological rules followed by grafting procedures and implant stabilization/prosthetic devices; in this situation, autografts are limited to small size defects, usually resulting from benign tumors excision, while large bone defects can require allografts; the indications for BS in these circumstances have to be established regarding the risk of recurrence (in malignant tumors), associated oncological treatments, as well as the ability to fit to the implants [13].
2. Bone loss following revised arthroplasties became an issue of modern orthopedic surgery due to increased number of arthroplastic procedures; poor bone stock, due to osteoporosis (most of these procedures are associated with increased age), and osteolysis induced by mechanical stress and biological factors (chronic inflammation) require grafting materials able to sustain the functional loading while interacting with massive implants which not only that can affect integration but also considerably increase the risk of infection [14, 15].

   The causes of implant loosening have been thoroughly studied, thus identifying the chronic inflammation as the central point of the process; this is started by the wear debris of polymethyl-methacrylate (PMMA), metal, ceramics, which initiate a biological and immunological response, activating of PMMA, metal, ceramics, which initiate a biological and immunological response, activating macrophages and IL-1, IL-6,

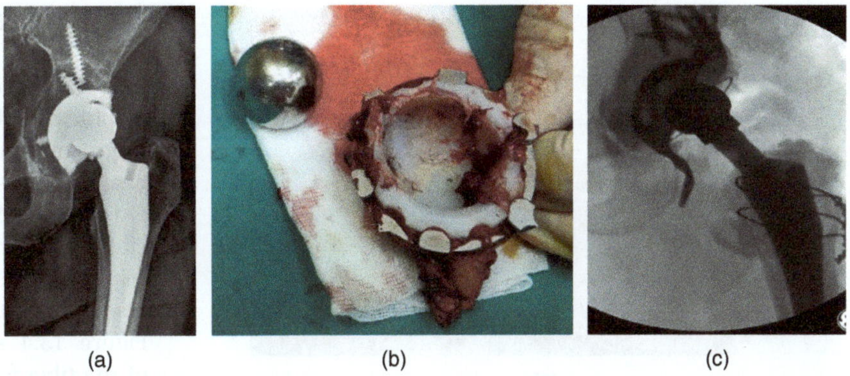

Figure 13.1 Aseptic loosening of total hip prosthesis with bone defect (a) generated by PMMA wear debris (b); postoperative result after grafting and revision arthroplasty (c).

Il-10, and TNF-α; the inflammatory cells then secrete metallo-proteinase which inhibit the bone-formatting cells, stimulate orthoclastic resorption as well as fibroblastic activity; bone gaps and excessive fibrous tissue occur and the stability of the implant is severely damaged; once the implant starts to move, a vicious circle is built, since progressive bone lysis is induced by micromovements; allowing further implant loosening, and so on [16]. Figure 13.1 shows a case, female, 68 years old, with aseptic loosening; the initial X-ray shows osteolysis around both the acetabular and the femoral component; intra-operative, PMMA cup deterioration with large amount of wear debris were found; auto-graft augmented cemented revision arthroplasty was performed.

3. Bone infections need thorough debridement and complete excision of the infected tissues, after proper identification (usually requiring imagistic complex evaluation), since incomplete sterilization of the infection site will be certainly followed by septic recurrence; due to their characteristics, indications of BS in osteitis must be carefully assessed, especially that all healing processes are impaired by infection and even osteogenetic compounds have limited or no activity in a septic environment; therefore, grafting using BS in these situations must be performed only when the infection has been totally cured and using materials with maximum biological integration, since local viability is affected by chronic inflammation [17–19].
4. Surgical treatment of deformities or malunions – whenever the axis of the length of a certain bone generates a functionally significant disturbance of the skeleton and surgery is indicated, restoring osteotomies (with or without lengthening procedures associated) are followed by a bone defect. In these situations, BS can be used when there are no sequential procedures to be performed (such as distraction); since the main problem in these situations is maintaining the correction, optimal loading resistance has to be considered when choosing the substitute.
5. Trauma generates several conditions resulting in BD especially that the severity of injuries increased due to increased energy of traumatic agents (as consequence of increased speed vehicles, challenging working conditions, etc.). As estimated in 2010, in the United States, 280 000 hip fractures, 700 000 vertebral, and 250 000 wrist fractures occur each year, with a cost of $10 bill [16].

The most important circumstances to be discussed are the following:

(a) *High-severity injuries* (especially open fractures) affect the bone and increase the risk of healing disturbances, and the incidence of nonunion is 20% for high-energy fractures, compared with 5% for all the fractures [19].
High-energy trauma generates multifragmentary (comminuted) fractures, and soft tissues injuries as well, thus interrupting in a significant manner the blood flow of the bone. In the ultimate situations when fragments of bone are totally isolated, almost floating, with no muscular or periosteal connection, these are practically ischemic tissues which have to be primarily removed, otherwise, they will become infected and transformed into sequesters. Bone defect is to be expected in these cases, and bone grafting procedures are to be planned, so the fixation devices and the soft tissue coverage procedures must be adapted to these requirements. Figure 13.2 shows a IIIB (Gustillo–Andersen) open fracture-dislocation of the ankle, where some fragments from the peroneum where extruded through the wound, thus resulting in a bone defect (a). Initial stabilization was performed using an ExFix, tension band on the internal malleola and Kirschner wire for the peroneum (b). The peroneal defect is to be grafted after soft tissue healing, once the infection risk has decreased.
(b) Fractures in cancellous bone often result in *bone impaction*. Since these fractures are mainly situated in the periarticular, this has a significant impact

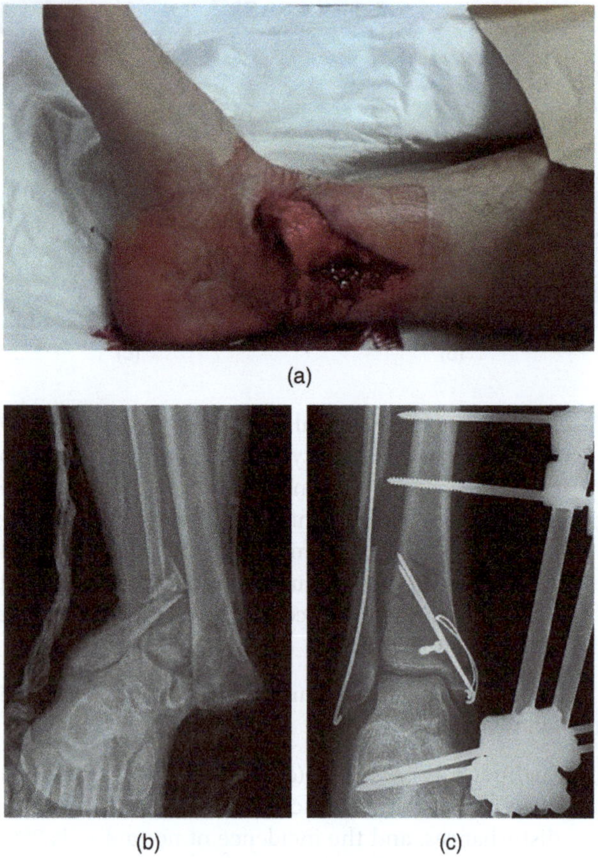

Figure 13.2 Clinical (a) and X-ray aspect (b) IIIB open fracture-dislocation of the ankle; primary stabilization with peroneal defect (c).

because it alters the functional anatomy of the joint. In these situations, optimal reduction of the fractures involves restoring physiological axes and angles of the joint, so that the impacted areas have to be brought back to their normal position, thus resulting in a subjacent bone defect. Some of the most frequent impacted fractures are the proximal tibial (plateau) fractures, where, due to an abnormal position of the knee in the moment of impact (valgus or a varus), the internal or external part of the plateau can be depressed [20–23].

Figure 13.3 presents a case of comminuted proximal tibial fracture with depression, needing elevation and grafting of the gap that resulted from reduction (elevation of the depressed surface in order to restore the articular surface).

(c) Treatment of *pseudarthrosis* (absence of fracture healing) requires bone grafting maneuvers; when bone defect is associated with impaired local vitality (such as in atrophic pseudarthrosis), osteogenic support is mandatory, usually provided by using an autograft. When local vitality is satisfactory, either an osteoinductive or an osteoconductive agent (or an association of both) can be used, augmented or not with autograft, so as to promote healing. Bone gaps have to be considered even when treating hypertrophic pseudarthrosis, because the nonunited bone fragments are sclerotic, and they do not promote healing unless they are excised until the healthy bone is reached. More than that, the medullary canal is closed, limiting the endosteal vascular supply to the injury site, thus requiring opening of the canal and resection of the obstructive sclerotic part of bone. Figure 13.4 shows a hypertrophic pseudarthrosis of the tibia following multiple surgeries for a shank fracture; treatment was surgical, requiring excision, grafting, and stable fixation.

(d) Treatment of posttraumatic malunions often need bone grafting. Posttraumatic complications producing severe functional alterations require surgery because any bone deformity impairs the normal activity of the adjacent joints thus generating different degrees of incapacity. In order to restore the normal joint function, correctional osteotomies are performed, with consecutive bone gaps which need grafting [24]. Figure 13.5 shows a case with a malunion after a distal radial fracture. Due to functional impairment generated by dorsal angulation and shortening of the radius, surgical correction was indicated. Distal radius osteotomy with lengthening and volar tilting resulted in a bone defect that was filled with a bone substitute based on calcium phosphate, followed by stabilization with a volar plate.

The most severe cases of bone loss are those which combine two or more of the causes anteriorly mentioned. One example is that of septic prosthetic loosening, when the bacterial action initiates the ostelysis, thus enhancing the mechanical and biological triggers of the implant-induced chronic inflammation. In these situations, the bone defect affects not only the integrity of the joint, but even the function of the limb and the daily activities of the patient.

Figure 13.6 presents a case with severe bone loss due to a complicated total hip arthroplasty. It is to be noted that the osteoporosis of the patient (78 years) that might have contributed to the poor outcome. One year after a total hip replacement, the patient was again operated for pelvic protrusion of the acetabular cup with septic loosening, since the microbiological evaluation demonstrated a Meticilino-Resistant *Staphylococcus aureus* (MRSA), the most frequent bacteria associated with implant infections. The prosthesis was removed and a spacer was used for temporary stabilization. Revision surgery failed due to septic loosening, and after multiple surgery, the aspect shows massive bone loss both on the

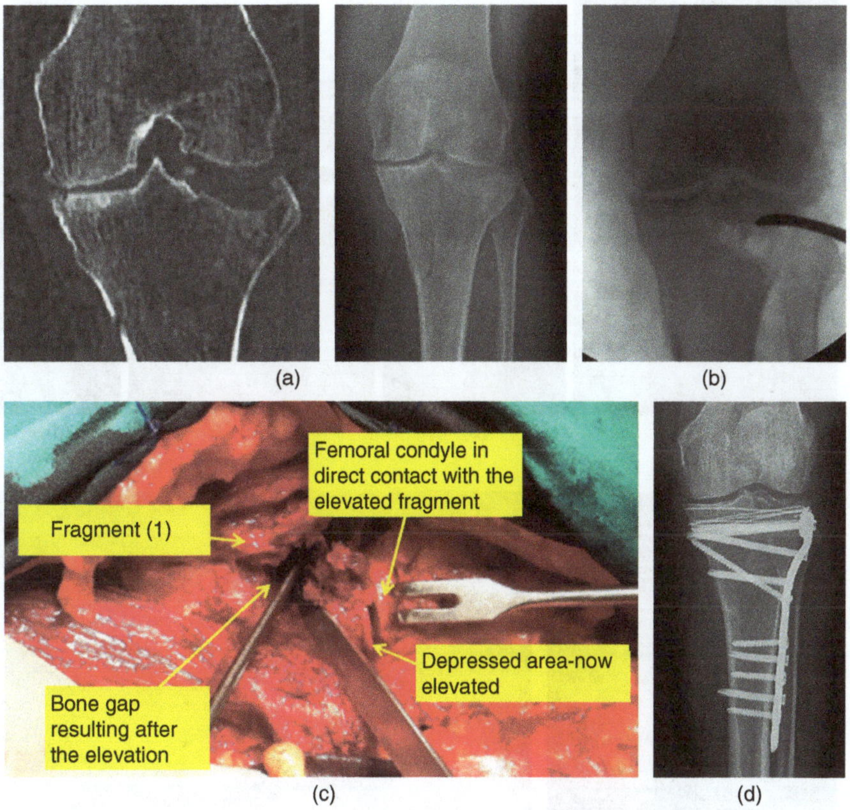

Figure 13.3 Tibial plateau fracture with depression – X-ray and CT (a), intra-operative elevation (b), generating a bone defect (c), autograft and stabilization with titanium locked plate (d).

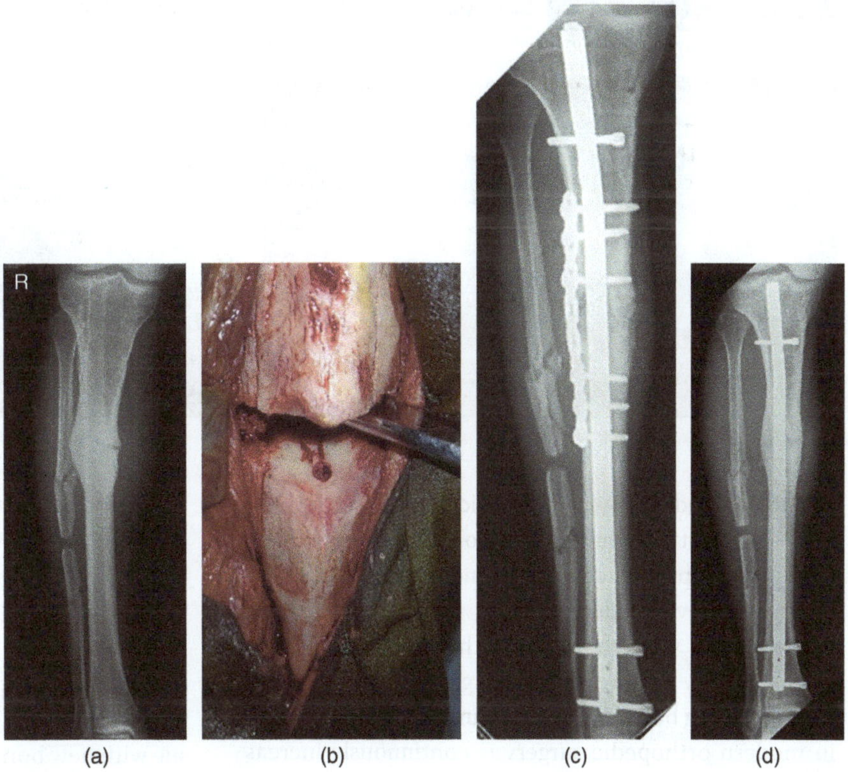

Figure 13.4 Posttraumatic pseudarthrosis multiply operated: X-ray (a) shows enlarged sclerotic bone on the fracture site, while the intraoperative aspect (b) suggests low possibilities of osteogenic activity of the bone; the bone defect was grafted and the fracture fixed in a stable manner (c) with healing (d).

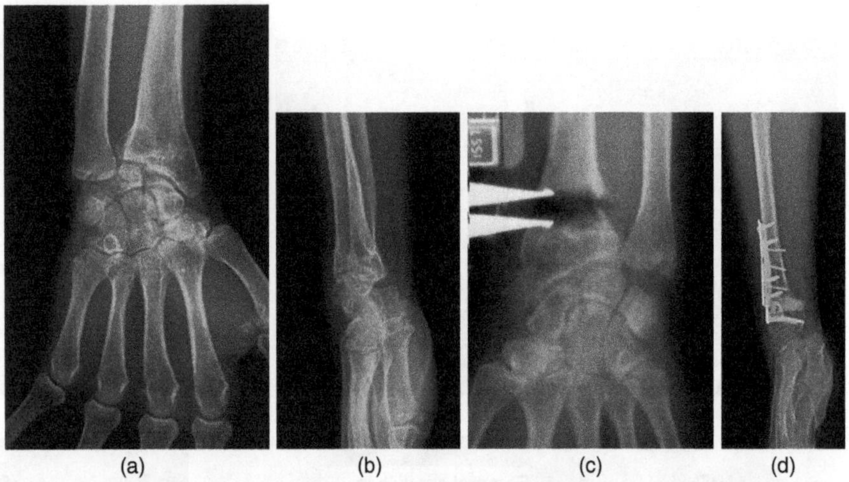

Figure 13.5 Posttraumatic deformity (a) needing osteotomy with bone defect (b); grafting with bone substitute (c); and stabilization with plate (d).

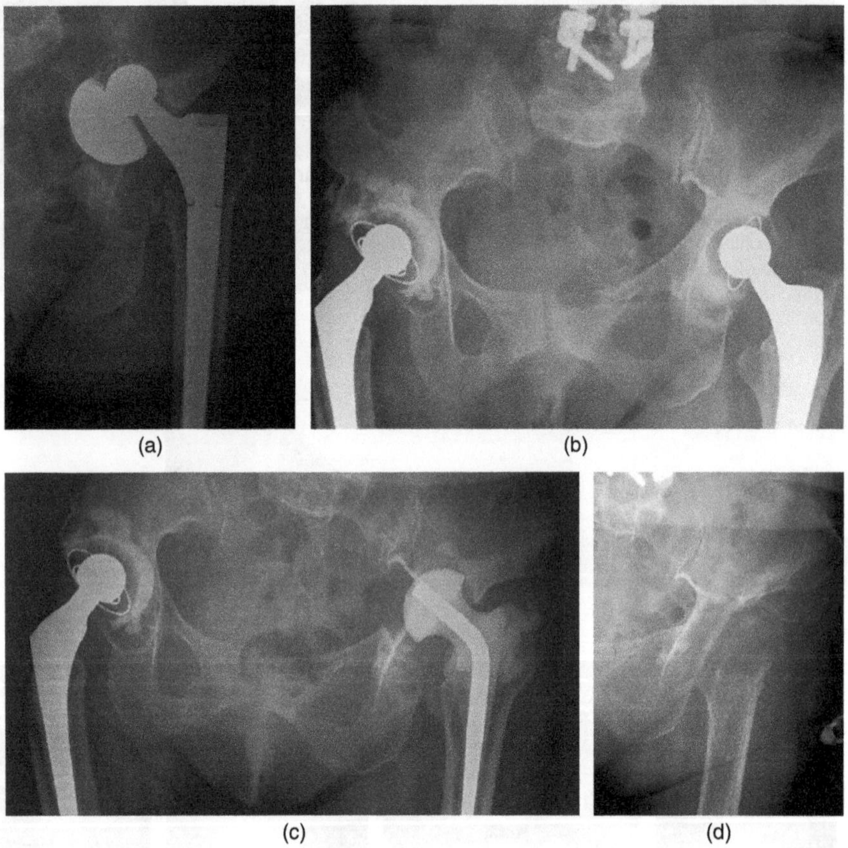

Figure 13.6 Pelvic protrusion (a) with septic complication (b) followed by temporary procedures (back), resulting in massive bone loss (c); X rays (d) revealed the osteolysis in the acetabular and femoral part of the joint.

acetabular and on the femoral side of the joints. Due to the quantity of the graft, autografting alone is not enough and preoperative planning should include BS and special revision devices.

These cases were chosen since they are representative of the variety of circumstances generating bone loss, thus requiring bone grafting. The interest for this subject in modern orthopedic surgery is continuously increasing as a response to the primary objective of skeletal surgery – early functional recovery of the patients and improving the quality of our patients' life.

13.4 Properties of Bone Substitutes

Graft incorporation has been defined as the process of "envelopment and interdigitation of the donor bone tissue with new bone deposited by the recipient" depending both on the status of the host and of the graft.

In order to describe the BS, some properties have been standardized as landmarks for BS activity, and from the point of view of the orthopedic surgeon, the main aspects used in clinical practice to choose, describe, and use a BS are the following.

1. Biocompatibility is essential for the clinical outcome since it refers to all the interactions between the BS and the host. The chemical structure of the BS determines whether it is integrated or rejected, pending on the immune reactions. An optimal biocompatibility has been described for calcium phosphate, collagen, and hydroxyapatite (HA), as well as for some inorganic materials, such as bioglasses, magnesium (phosphate), and calcium (sulfate, carbonate, and silicate) salts. A good cellular recognition has also been demonstrated for chitosan, alginate, cellulose, gelatin, collagen, and keratin, all of them being high molecular weight polymers, rapidly degradable, thus stimulating healing [25].
2. Osteointegration and thus the ability to restore functional bone depends on the main activity of the bone substitute, which can be
   - Osteogenesis is the formation of new bone by the cells contained within the graft. It is an **active** process involving the cells of the **graft,** able to survive and produce bone, finalized with synthesis of new bone.
   - Osteoinduction is a chemical process in which molecules contained within the graft (BMPs) convert the patient's cells into cells capable of forming bone. It is also an **active process,** but it involves **the host cells,** which are recruited and differentiated, thus stimulating bone healing.
   - Osteoconduction is a physical effect where the graft becomes a scaffold on which the cells of the host cells form new bone. It is a **passive phenomenon** which refers to scaffolds that supports migration of the **host** cells and capillaries and bone formation due to its 3D structure. The osteoconductive ability is mainly related to the porous structure of the graft, and less to its chemical and physical properties [26–28].
3. Resorption rate is important since for most of the BS, their integration starts with resorption and sometimes the products resulting from degradation enhance healing; still, some of the BS have a very low resorption rate, and can be considered permanent, such as calcium phosphate.

The resorption rate varies widely, it depends on composition so some products may be combined to optimize resorption rate; it is also dependent on porosity and geometry and ideally, resorption should be contemporary or immediately followed by mature bone generation, so as during the process of graft integration the bone should maintain its resistance. The term "resorption" (and the related ones-absorption, biodegradation) refers to the disappearance of the BS form the grafted site, regardless the mechanism of this process. It must be underlined that, unlike BS, when integration takes place after resorption, autografts are characterized by concomitant resorption and vascular ingrowth process called "creeping substitution."

Due to the impact of resorption upon the activity of BS, controlling the dynamics of this process is of great importance, and two methods have been described for that

- Optimizing the geometry of the BS – refers to the dimension and the position of the pores/channels which are interconnected, and which must enable the vascular and cellular ingrowth (more than 0.005 mm diameter), a good example being pore incorporation into injectable calcium phosphate cement.
- Optimizing the chemistry of the BS includes introduction of more degradable sequences or variation of polymer crystallinity, either by combining different sequences or by incorporating cleavage sequences for targeted enzymes. Depending on the basic structure of the BS, corrosion stabilizers can be used for metal allies, and thermodynamic controllers are used for ceramics. For example, research has provided modalities to start from HA, which is practically inert, to reactive compounds: β-TCP (tricalcium phosphate) combined with HA, getting to "biphasic calcium phosphate" (BCP), α-TCP, octocalcium phosphate (OCP), dicalcium phosphate dehydrate (DCPD, "brushite"), and anhydrous dicalcium phosphate (DCP) [29, 30].

Resorption rate is also dependent on the form in which the BS is handled: granules (0.5–1 mm diameter), porous blocks or sponges, hardening paste, and nonhardening paste (putty), the last two consisting of a highly viscous gellum including granules. The form also influences the indications since the form must cover the bone defect in an appropriate manner. The main form-dependent characteristics are the following:

- The granules need direct access so that they can be applied in an open bone gap with the possibility of migration into the surrounding tissue. Despite their lack of mechanical stability, they have the advantage that the resorption/formation processes take place throughout the defect.
- The macroporous blocks are also resorbed throughout the defect, adaptable to closed or open defects, and they have a better mechanical strength, but their shape limits the adaptability to the defect.
- The cement paste is to be used only in closed bone gaps; with a good mechanical resistance, the

resorption and formation is peripheral, but the handling has to be carefully performed, as it can harden too fast or might be poorly injectable.
- The putty is designed both for closed and open spaces, and depending on the composition, resorption starts at the periphery or throughout the material and the handling depends on the mixing process [31–33].

Different types of resorption have been described, such as

- Dissolution – for calcium sulfate hemihydrate (CSH)
- Dissolution and/or converted into apatite for DCPD, while for the ceramics, limited resorption is based on limited dissolution
- Cell-mediated processes for calcium phosphates (DCP, OCP, β-TCP, BCP, β-CPP) – by the osteoclasts, which release small amounts of hydrochloric acid, change the pH and hence induce dissolution. The components of these products – calcium and phosphate – interfere with bone metabolism: phosphate ions influence osteoblastic activity, apoptosis, osteopontin generation, and mineralization rate, while calcium ions regulate both osteoblast proliferation and osteoclastic activity. Due to these activities, the resorption of TCP can be considered a self-regulating mechanism since the calcium and phosphate ions generated by osteoclastic activity influence the osteoclastic activity in return.
- Corrosion for magnesium and iron alloys.
- Hydrolysis for synthetic polymers (PLA, PLGA, etc.) in an aqueous environment.
- Transporting to lymph nodes for cellulose.
- Enzymatic lysis for hyaluronan (hyaluronidae), fibrin (plasmin), collagen (collagenase), and chitosan (lysozyme).
- Combined mechanisms dissolution *in vivo* and re-crystallizing into apatite – for DCPD.
- Resorption does not appear when the BS is represented by sintered HA, tantalum, and titanium [26, 34, 35].

The resorption abilities are correlated with the drug-delivery capacities of each product, generating the interest of loading resorbable structures with different drugs/ions to be delivered, such as silicon, strontium, or zinc, but these ions also change the chemical properties, thus the profile of the final product [36].

4. Mechanical properties vary widely; this refers to resistance to compression and torsion and can be influenced by the structure of the material, as well as by the processing methods. Dependent on composition:

(i) Calcium phosphate cement has highest compressive strength
(ii) Cancellous bone compressive strength is relatively low
(iii) Many substitutes have compressive strengths similar to cancellous bone
(iv) All designed to be used with internal fixation

Mechanical stability is required as BS is designed to overtake the function of bones, which are supposed to have high mechanical loading. For the BS to be successful, it must be able not only to sustain forces comparable to those sustained by the bone it replaces but also to provide a balanced behavior of rigidity/elasticity as close to that of the normal skeleton. Still, the biogradable polymers, especially polylactic-co-glycolic acid (PLGA), are largely used as BS although they have no mechanical strength, but used as scaffolds.

Porosity should be high enough to allow space for integration processes, such as cellular growth and extracellular matrix regeneration. At the same time, the space distribution of the pores should be similar to that of the original bony structure, so there is the scaffold to guide the cells to recreate the initial spatial design. Micropores (less than 10 μm) allow capillary ingrowth, while macropores (150–900 μm) allow nutrient suppliable to reproduce the desired structure [27, 37, 38].

Depending on their properties, BS can act as

- Expanders for autogenous bone graft, such as in large defects or in multiple level spinal fusion
- Enhancers to improve success of autogenous bone graft, and
- Substitutes to replace autogenous bone graft [39, 40].

This concept is important since it underlines the complexity of the process of bone grafting, which does not at all mean that some material will cover a missing part of the bone; the proper perception is a bilateral interaction.

The graft generates a certain reaction from the host, hence an inflammatory process at the beginning, then a cascade of processes starting with osteolysis [41], continuing with bone healing mechanisms, including, for osteoinductive grafts, cell differentiation. It must be underlined that each step of this process has its own importance – the inflammation is responsible for the chemotactic phenomena; otherwise, the healing process cannot start without cells; on the other hand, an excessive osteolysis will reduce the chances of success for the graft, since integration is highly improbable under these circumstances.

13.5 Types of Bone Substitutes

Since bone grafts have various properties, several classifications have been achieved in order to reflect their clinical significance, potential indications, and contraindications [42].

Osteoconductive agents act as scaffolds; from the point of view of the orthopedic surgeon, the main classes with this type of action are the following:

1. *Polymers*: Can be natural or synthetic; the natural polymers, such as type I collagen, fibrin, hyaluronic acid, and chitosan have limited indications due to their low mechanical strength, although they have very good biocompatibility and osteoconductivity.
   The synthetic biodegradable ones have different properties and are used mainly as scaffolds; some of them, like poly-lactide-co-glycolide (PDLGA) and polycaprolactone (PCL) can be less used for drug delivering mechanisms, as they undergo bulk degradation; on the opposite side, due to their more predictable delivery curve, the surface-eroding polymers (polyanhydrides) are preferred as carriers for factors and other substances (antibiotics, chemotherapic drugs, etc.) [43].
2. *Ceramics*: This term describes an inorganic, nonmetallic material with a crystalline structure. Usually they have a high compressive strength and low ductility, thus opposing deformation but being highly sensitive to failure due to their brittle characteristics because their compressive modules often exceed that of the trabelcular bone, some ceramics, such as calcium phosphates, calcium sulfates, and bioactive glass, have been used as scaffolds. Their biomimetic activities are the result of their capacity of precipitation and deposition (of CP) or of their protein-binding affinities (calcium sulfate) [44].
3. *Metallics*: Porous titanium and tantalum have a 3-D interconnected porous structure comparable to that of the trabecular bone. They are highly biocompatible, resistant to corrosion, not biodegradable; their elastic modules is somehow similar to that of the trabecular bone although the relatively stiffness of titanium can produce stress-shielding problems and subsequent implant loosening. Due to all these elements, these two materials are preferred for coating the prosthetic implants, where bone ingrowth is crucial for secondary prosthetic stability [45].
4. *Demineralized bone matrix (DBM)*: Keeps the trabecular structure of the original bone, theoretically able to replicate the 3D architecture of the bone [46].
5. *Osteoinductive agents*: The ability to contain growth factors is offered by far less agents than the previous group. These are represented by growth factors-derived BMPs, Bone Marrow Aspirate (BMA), and gene therapy-generated products [47–49]. Since for the moment, only BMPs are used in clinical practice, these are going to be briefly discussed in this chapter.
6. *Composites*: Represent combinations of materials with different properties, thus having the ability to offer individual advantages enhancing the properties of the associated structures. To give some examples, the mechanical properties of polymers (as scaffolds) are enhanced by combining them with CP, while combining polymers with ceramics optimize the brittleness of the ceramic and the ability to deliver different substances. In the same manner, the osteointegration would be better if titanium (otherwise, a rather bioinert material) is combined with HA and osteoinductive properties are added by combining BMA with DBM or HA [50]. Table 13.1 presents the main characteristics of BS, underlining the characteristics with clinical significance; it is less important to choose a BS from a certain **group**, but a BS with certain **characteristics** [51, 52].

13.6 Choosing the Bone Graft

Although it seems an easy task, choosing the ideal BS in clinical practice is a multifactorial task, since a lot of factors influence it. Even if it refers to the BS, it is not related only with the substitute, but to the host also. Several factors have been identified as a "check-list" for establishing which material fits best for a certain bone gap.

Host-related factors

(a) *The intended clinical application*: For example, if the bone gap is closed and the desired technique is to keep it closed, an injectable form must be used. If the grafting site has enough cells, like in the metaphyseal areas, an osteoconductive BS should be enough in order to obtain graft integration.
(b) *Defect size and total bone mass required*: Can be approximated using the computed tomography (CT) scan.

Graft-related

(c) *Biomechanics*: If mechanical strength of the graft is required, a high-resistance product will be chosen, and not a collagen-based graft, for example.
(d) *Chemical composition*: It is a crucial factor, since it determines most of the grafting material properties.
(e) Desired bioactivity.
   - *Osteoconductive*: When only a scaffold is considered to be necessary, an osteoconductive material should be used; for that, there must be no doubt upon the vitality of the grafting site.
   - *Osteoinductive*: When the cell stock and the scaffold are both enough, active, and only growth factors are necessary, an osteoinductive material can be used (such as in delayed healing, when there is no bone loss, but a slow healing).

Table 13.1 Bone substitutes commercial names and main characteristics.

Name	Material	Delivery	OC; OI	Properties	Indications	Level of evidence
Apapore	HA	Granules	OC	25% interconnected microporosity	Low load: small voids, autograft extender	$n = 1$ (III)
Allogran – N	HA	Granules	OC	Nonresorbable	High load: impaction grafting as autograft extender, revision hip arthroplasty	$n = 1$ (III)
Allogran-R	HA	Granules	OC	Resorbable	Void filler, spines, delayed union, can be used in presence of infection	
Calcibon	HA	Granules and cement	OC	Resorbtion at 24 wk; porosity 30–40%	Use with BMA, autograft or platelet rich plasma (PRP) in metaphyseal chancellors defects	$n = 3$ (II, III)
Endobon	HA	block, cylinder, granules	OC	Resorbable; porosity 60–80%	Tibial plateau, distal tibial, calcaneal, distal radial fractures, bone tumor surgery	
ENGIpore	HA	granules, blocks	OC	Porosity 90%, resorbed over 6–18 mo	Trauma, revision arthroplasty surgery, spinal surgery, bone void filler	
Nanostim	HA	Granules	OC+OI		Spinal surgery and fusion	
Hydroset	HA	Cement	OC		Injectable; not load-bearing	
Collapat II	Collagen HA	Fleece	OC	Resorbable; hemostatic properties	Aseptic enclosed metaphyseal defects; best mixed with blood, bone marrow or PRP	
Healos	Collagen HA	Sponge, matrix	OC	Resorbable mineralized porous collagen matrix	Mix with bone marrow; spinal surgery	$n = 5$ (III, IV)
RegenOss	Collagen HA	Patch strips	OC	Resorbable over 6–12 mo	Long bone Fx, revision hip arthoplasty to fill acetabular defects, spinal fusion	
SINT life	Mg-HA	Granules, paste/putty	OC		Bone void filler; trauma and spinal surgery. High tibial osteotomy for patients with osteoarthritis of the knee	$n = 1$ (III)
OpteMx	HA and TCP	Granules, sticks	OC	Resorbable; 70% porosity	Bone voids, tumors, spine	
OsSatura BCP	80% HA and 20% Beta TCP	Granules	OC	Rapidly resorbable; 50% interconnected porosity	Mix with blood products; contained defects; load sharing	
Repros	60% HA and 40% Beta TCP	Granules, blocks	OC	Non-load-bearing; 80% porosity	Bone void filler with autograft extender. Mix with blood products	
Mastergraft	15% HA and 85% Beta TCP	Granules	OC	Resorbable	Bone void filler in trauma and spinal surgery	
BCP granules	35% HA and 65% Beta TCP	Granules	OC		Bone void filler in trauma and spinal surgery	
Bonesave	20% HA and 80% Beta TCP	Granules	OC	50% surface porosity	Bone void filler; revision hip surgery; spinal fusion surgery	$n = 2$ (III, IV)
Tri-Calcit	70% HA and 30% TCP. Synthetic	Granules, blocks	OC	70% macroporosity	Bone void filler in trauma surgery	
Conduit TCP	Beta TCP	Granules	OC	Resorbable	Enclosed metaphyseal defects; mix with blood, bone marrow or PRP	

(Continued)

Table 13.1 (Continued)

Name	Material	Delivery	OC; OI	Properties	Indications	Level of evidence
OsSaturaTCP	Beta TCP	Granules	OC	Resorbable; 70% interconnected porosity	Mix with blood products. Contained defects. Load sharing	
Integra Mozaik	Beta TCP and BMA	Putty/strip	OC	80% Beta TCP and 20% purified collagen		
ChronOS	Beta TCP	Granules, blocks	OC	Resorbable at 6–18 mo; porosity 70%	Nonload bearing; void filler in areas where cancellous bone is required rather than cortical bone; trauma, spinal and reconstruction surgery	$n = 3$ (II, IV)
Cellplex TCP	TCP	TCP granules and BMA	OC	Resorbable; allows early load-bearing	Trauma surgery; bone void filler	
CycLOS	Beta TCP and fermented sodium hyaluronate	Putty, granules	OC	Resorbable	Bone void filler; nonload bearing applications	
Vitoss	Beta TCP, 20% Type 1 Collagen	Foam	OC + OI	Resorbable; 90% porosity	Spinal and trauma surgery	$n = 7$ (I, II, III, IV)

Name	Material	Delivery	OC; OI	Properties	Indications	Level of evidence
Alpha-BSM	Calcium phosphate	Paste	OC	Resorbable; porosity 50–60%	Trauma; early weight-bearing	$n = 2$ (I)
CarriGen	Calcium phosphate	Paste	OC	Resorbable; porosity 65%	bone void filler in pelvis, extremities and spine	
Beta-BSM	Calcium phosphate	Paste	OC	Resorbable	Trauma and bone void filler	
Gamma-BSM	Calcium phosphate	Paste	OC	Resorbable	Trauma and bone void filler	
BoneSource	Calcium phosphate	Cement	OC	Not load bearing; porosity 46%	Void filler in tibial plateau Fx and proximal femoral voids in revision hip surgery with distal stem fixation	$n = 4$ (II)
Norian SRS	Calcium phosphate	Cement	OC	Resorbable; remodeling by 76 wk; early weight bearing; porosity 60%	Distal radius, proximal and distal tibia, acetabulum Fx, proximal humerus	$n = 22$ (I, II, III, IV)
Stimulan	Calcium sulfate	Pellets, paste	OC	Resorbable	Low load, can be used in presence of infection as fully resorbed	
Osteoset	Calcium sulfate	Pellets, beads	OC	Resorbable	Spinal surgery, trauma, benign cysts, and adult reconstruction	$n = 8$ (II, III, IV)
BonePlast Quick Set	Calcium sulfate	Paste	OC	Resorbable	Bone void filler	
Calceon 6	Calcium sulfate	Pellets	OC	Bioresorbable		
MIIG X3	Calcium sulfate	Paste	OC	Resorbable	Trauma surgery, tibial plateau Fx, metaphyseal defects	$n = 2$ (IV)
GeneX	Calcium phosphate + calcium sulfate	Paste, putty	OC	Resorbable	Scaphoid nonunions, trauma, bone void filler	$n = 1$ (IV)
Actifuse	Calcium phosphate + silicon	Granules	OC + OI	Porosity 80%	Low load (spinal surgery, small voids)	$n = 3$ (IV)
Actifuse ABX	Calcium phosphate + silicon	Putty	OC + OI	Contains 96% scaffold	Low load (spinal surgery, small voids)	

(Continued)

Table 13.1 (Continued)

Name	Material	Delivery	OC; OI	Properties	Indications	Level of evidence
Osteoset II DBM	Calcium sulfate and DBM	Pellets	OC	Resorbable; rapid remodeling	Spinal surgery, trauma, benign cysts and adult reconstruction; AVN of femoral head when combined with autograft	$n = 2$ (III, IV)
Ignite	DBM, Calcium sulfate, BMA	Paste	OC + OI	Resorbable	Nonunion where no callus is seen at 6–8 wk; delayed union with well-fixed hardware; contraindicated in infected cases or when bone gap > 3 mm	
ProDense	75% Calcium phosphate (TCP) and 25% calcium sulfate	Paste	OC	Resorbable	Bone void filler -calcaneal, tibial plateau, distal radius, proximal humerus; benign bone cysts; osteotomy and decompression surgery	$n = 1$ (IV)
ProStim	ProDense + DBM	Paste	OC + OI	Resorbable	Bone void filler -calcaneal, tibial plateau, distal radius, proximal humerus; benign bone cysts; osteotomy and decompression surgery	
Name	**Material**	**Delivery**	**OC;OI**	**Properties**	**Indications**	**Level of evidence**
Bonus II **DBM**	DBM	Paste	OC+OI	Non load-bearing	Injectable; use with BMA; in nonunions, revisions, ankle fusion	—
Equiva Bone	DBM+CP	Paste	OC+OI	Resorbable	Void filler in trauma and spine surgery	
Optecure	DBM	Putty	OI+OC	Nonload bearing	Mix with blood or autograft	
Opteform	DBM	Paste	OI+OC	Nonload bearing	Bone void filler	
Optefil	DBM	Paste	OI+OC	Nonwater soluble Bioresorbable; osteogenesis when mixed with autogenous bone graft	Bone void filler	
Optium DBM	DBM	Gel/Putty	OI+OC	Nonload bearing; calcium <8%	Spinal fusions, tumors, fractures	
Accell Connexus	DBM	Putty in syringe	OI+OC	Nonload bearing	Spinal fusion, revision surgery	$n = 1$ (III)
Dynagraft II	DBM	Putty/gel	OI+OC	Nonload bearing	Graft extender	
Orthoblast	DBM	Putty/paste	OI+OC	Nonload bearing; macro/microporosity=1/1	Fusions	$n = 3$(III)
Osteofil DBM	DBM	Paste; moldable strips	OI+OC	Bioresorbable	Bone void filler	
Progenix	DBM	Putty	OI+OC	Bioresorbable	Bone void filler; bone graft substitute/extender	
DBX	DBM	Putty	OI+OC	Nonload bearing	Void filler	
Grafton	DBM	Matrix, putty, gel, paste	OI+OC	Nonload bearing	Fusions, arthrodesis	$n = 15$ (II, III, IV)
BioSet	DBM	Paste, putty strips	OI+OC	Bioresorbable	Bone void filler	
Viagraf	DBM	Putty, paste, gel	OI+OC	Bioresorbable	Bone void filler	

(Continued)

Table 13.1 (Continued)

Name	Material	Delivery	OC; OI	Properties	Indications	Level of evidence
Puros DBM	DBM	Putty, putty with chips	OI+OC	Bioresorbable		
InterGro	DBM	paste, putty, mix with HA composite granules	OI+OC	Bioresorbable	Bone void filler; bone graft extender	
AlloFuse	Heat sensitive copolymer with DBM	injectable gel and putty	OI+OC	Bioresorbable	Bone void filler; bone graft extender	
IC Graft Chamber	DBM particles and cancellous chips	Lyophilized	OI+OC	Bioresorbable; use with blood, PRP or bone marrow		
Plexure	DBM + Polyactide-*co*-glycolide	Wedge, granules, block	OI+OC	Resorbable	Void filler, oncology bone surgery, tibial plateau Fx, arthroplasty surgery	
Allomatrix	DBM + calcium sulfate carrier (Osteoset)	Paste, chips	OI+OC	Nonload bearing	Void filler in tumors, trauma, lumbar spine surgery	$n = 5$ (III, IV)
Name	**Material**	**Delivery**	**OC; OI**	**Properties**	**Indications**	**Level of evidence**
Cortoss	Bioactive glass cement	Paste	OC	Non-resorbable	Kyphoplasty vertebroplasty; trauma surgery; bone void filler	$n = 4$ (I, II, III, IV)
Colloss	Collagen lyophilisate	Fleece	OC	Resorbable after a few weeks	No primary stability	
Targobone E	Colloss and teicoplanin	Fleece with antibiotic	OC	Resorbable after a few weeks	No primary stability, marketed for use in infection	
Plexure	DBM and polylactide-co-glycolide	Granules, wedge, blocksheat	OC + OI	Resorbable	Void filler	
Infuse	rhBMP-2 protein on absorbable collagen sponge	Multiple kit sizes	OI	Bioresorbable carrier; chemotaxis of stem cells; indirect osteogenesis	Fusion with spinal cage, open tibia Fx with IM nail	
OP-1	rhBMP-7 with Type 1 bone collagen	Lyophilized powder	OI	Bioresorbable scaffold	Long bone nonunions	
Trinity evolution	Viable cellular bone matrix		OC + OI	Osteogenesis	Regulated as a human tissue	
NovaBone	Bioactive silicate	Particulate, putty and morsels	OC + OI	Bioresorbable	Bone void filler	
Allopure	Sterile femoral/tibial allograft	Wedges	OC		Regulated as a human tissue	
Cancello-pure	Bovine bone	Wedges	OC		Bone void filler	
CopiOs Bone void filler	Dibasic calcium phosphate and Type 1 collagen	Sponge, paste	OC	Bioresorbable; accelerated healing; osteogenesis when mixed with BMA	Bone void filler; must be used with BMA	
CopiOs cancellous bone graft	Bovine bone	Chips, cubes and wedges	OC		Bone void filler	

BSM, bone substitute materials (α-BSM® is a biomimetic endothermically setting apatitic calcium phosphate bone substitute material); SRS, skeletal repair system

- *Osteogenic*: The osteogenic grafts are able to provide cells that are by themselves able to generate bone. From all the grafts, only the autografts have this property.

(f) *Desired resorption rate*: Depends on the structure of the material and influences the interaction between the bone and the graft – the longer the resorption is, the reduced the interaction between the graft and the host is, some of the grafts, such as calcium phosphate based, being considered permanent.

(g) *Handling characteristics*: The more complicated is handling a bone substitute, a more complicated procedure it needs, thus diminishing the clinical interest for it.

(h) *Associated side effects*: Refers especially to the local tolerability, since systemic reactions are rarely described after bone grafting.

(i) Availability and cost must be taken into consideration due to the relative high price of BS.

(j) Ethical issues have to be considered especially toward the grafting process itself, since religious or other type of considerations, as well as personal beliefs could influence the adherence of the patient to the treatment [53, 54].

In conclusion, the ideal bone substitute should have the following characteristics:

- should be able to re-create bone
- biocompatible, bioresorbable, and generating minimal fibrous reaction
- should be osteoconductive, osteoinductive, or better osteogenetic
- structurally similar to bone, with an optimal resorption rate, rapidly integrated, easily molded into the defect into a short time
- with optimal mechanical resistance
- safe – no risk of transmitting infectious diseases
- manageable, easily traceable *in vivo* radiolucent and easily available
- thermally nonconductible
- cost-effective [55]

It must be underlined that, since the success of grafting depends not only on the graft, but on the host, as well, certain actions can be taken so as to improve the result, such as

- quit smoking [56, 57],
- improve nutrition
- treat comorbidities, such as diabetes [58]
- treat infection, which can be associated with certain presumed methods, such as
  - Hyperbaric oxygen
  - Electrical stimulation
  - Low-intensity ultrasound
  - Low-power laser [59, 60]
  - Limited weight bearing, which has been until now demonstrated to have a positive effect, but without randomized prospective studies which should clearly stipulate their advantages

The main types of BS with clinical implications are going to be briefly described, insisting on the clinical relevant facts and properties.

13.7 Demineralized Bone Matrix (DBM)

DBM is produced from cortical bone, by decalcification, and then, processed so as to reduce the immune host response and the risk of infection, as well. Included by some authors in the category of allografts, DBM was first described in 1975 [61], now being widely available, representing 50% of all allografts performed in the United States [62].

Through demineralization, the bone retains less than 5% calcium, but because it keeps the trabecular collagenous structure from the original bone, theoretically able to replicate the 3D architecture of the bone, it can act as an osteoconductive scaffold, guiding the host cells to populate it, to grow, and to differentiate.

It is quickly revascularized, therefore, can be used as a suitable carrier for autologous bone marrow [62].

Since proteins and growth factors are contained in the extracellular matrix, they are not entirely lost due to demineralization; different amounts of BMP, IGF, TGF, and FGF can stimulate osteogenic stem cells to migrate and become active and can induce revascularization, thus conferring DBM-limited osteoinductive properties.

Although the osteoinductive capacity is higher than that of allografts, especially that, once the mineral matrix is removed, the growth factors (including BMPs) become more available, but it has to be underlined that the biological properties of DBM largely depends on the donor and can be affected by processing and storage methods (including sterilization), such as techniques using alcohol or some acids (acetic, lactic, and nitric) [63].

DBM has been produced as injectable bone paste, gel, putty, flexible strips, and moldable paste with bone chips (increasing the osetoconductivity).

Due to mineral loss, it has very low structural strength and that is why it is mainly used as an expander, or as a filler, rather than a graft substitute, in a mechanically stable environment (either as a small bone cavity with enough cortical resistance, or as implant stabilization) [64, 65].

Successful procedures using DBM were reported when it was used combined with: autologous bone marrow, calcium sulfate, collagen, hyaluronic acid, or autologous bone graft, but little available data support the use of DBM alone as a bone substitute [65, 66].

Other disadvantages of DBM are related to the variations of characteristics (due to different donors and different processing methods), especially those of the levels of BMP2 and BMP7 [67] as well to the still existing risk of antigenic response and infection transmission (including HIV).

13.8 Bone Morphogenetic Proteins (BMPs)

Although they were originally described in the 1960s by Urist [3] (while generating DBM) as substances able to induce ectopic bone formation, BMPs became a useful tool for bone grafting. They represent a heterogeneous group of proteins belonging to the TGFβ family (with the exception of BMP1, which is a metalloproteinase), with multiple implications in embryogenesis and postnatal skeletal events [1, 2].

Their main characteristic is that of osteoinduction, and it was *in vitro* demonstrated that they act on the multipotent mesenchymal cells, by binding to their cell receptors and induce their proliferation and differentiation to the chondrogenic and osteogenic lines, and stimulate angiogenesis. The osteoinductive capacities were confirmed by preclinical and clinical studies which demonstrated fusion rates between 80% and 99%, comparable to that of autogenous grafting, especially when combined with collagen [4, 8].

Wang and Sampath [68, 69] demonstrated that rhBMP 2 and 7 induce bone formation thorough a process similar to endochondral ossification (even in ectopic sites), while fracture healing acceleration by subcutaneous injection of rhBMP2 was demonstrated by Einhorn [8, 9]. Later studies of Bostrom and his team showed a biphasic straining activity of rhBMP2 upon callus formation – the first stage when stimulating the mesenchymal cells differentiation, and the second stage while the fibrocartilage was invaded by osteoblasts in order to form the definitive callus [68].

Until now, from approximately 20 BMPs discovered, only recombinant human BMP2 and BMP7 have been approved for clinical use: products containing BMP2 are indicated in open tibia fracture and lumbar fusion [69–71], while BMP7 is recommended for tibia nonunions [71, 72]. They provide doses considerable higher (10–100-fold) than those of native BMPs, and there are still many unclear aspects regarding BMPs, especially those related to the variation of their effect depending on the donor and the method of processing [73]. Although the concern for neoplastic changes proved to be unfounded, some adverse effects were still described:

- Ectopic bone formation in adjacent soft tissues (muscles, nerves, and vessels)
- Immune reactions with antibody formation due to which they are contraindicated in certain sites, such as cervical spine [74].

An interesting thing must be underlined regarding BMPs in osteoporotic fractures: although the involvement of BMPs into the bone metabolism made Urist describe osteoporosis as "a bone-morphogenetic auto-immune disorder" [75], and genetic polymorphisms in BMP-2 were demonstrated to be responsible for familiar osteoporosis [76], BMP-2 has been related only to the achievement of peak bone mass, and not with the osteolytic activity and bone loss, thus explaining the lack of data related to BMPs in the treatment of osteoporotic fractures [77].

Due to their price (higher than other BS), BMPs cannot be routinely used, but they should be taken into consideration in young patients with high risk of developing a nonunion. In such a situation, the cost of BMPs would be significantly lower than that of treating a nonunion, thus justifying the prophylactic use of these substances.

Since they act directly upon the defect site, BMPs have to be delivered, thus being associated with carriers, which should have certain properties:

- a slow releasing mechanism, thus allowing the BMP to act gradually and constantly, the initial extract of BMP is hydrophobic, and the process of purification makes it more hydrophilic, increasing its dispersion and allowing the osteoinductivity to become active shortly after implantation. A slow releasing carrier limits the ectopic activity and focuses the bone generation activity to the desired site.
- biologically and immunologically inert.
- quickly absorbed from the defect site, but provide enough mechanical strength to withstand loading until bone is restored.
- scaffold-like activity (supporting angiogenetic and cell proliferation mechanisms).
- easily handled, stored, and sterilized [25].

Different types of carriers can be divided into

(a) Natural polymers: DBM and collagen
Yasko demonstrated a 100% union rate in experiments in rats using DBM-carried rhBMP-2. Starting from their promising results obtained using autologous bone graft supplemented with BMP, Johnson and coworkers demonstrated the same optimal results in patients with resistant nonunions [77–79]. As for collagen, although the results are affected by the mechanical disadvantages (low compression

strength), the delivery pattern of collagen has proven to be superior to that of HA, TCP, glass beads, and PMMA, but the potential antigenicity and infectious and viral contamination impairs the use of DBM and collagen as well [80].

(b) Synthetic polymers have been explored despite their inflammatory-inducing effects and extensive absorption time. After the results delivered by Ferguson, showing new bone formation 16 weeks after grafting in an animal with a bovine bioabsorbable polymeric material-polylactic-co-glycolic acid (BPM-PLGA) carrier, research focused on finding more quickly degrading polymers, so as not to interfere with bone formation [80]. Animal experiments performed by Kirker-Head and his team using rhBMP2 combined with PDLGA particles (150–500 μm) and autologous blood demonstrated fracture healing with woven and then lamellar bone production [69]. Depending on the polymerization process, the molecular weight differs, so does the aspect of PLA/BMP or (poly-L-lactic acid) PLLA/BMP products, but it was demonstrated that only polylactic acid (PLA) with a molecular weight of 650 was able to ensure the optimal BMP delivery for bone formation, with an optimal degradation speed of the polymer. Furthermore, when adding a 200-Da polyethylene glycol (PEG), bone and bone marrow were generated three weeks after implantation, with an increased amount of bone resulting. Supplementing the composite with HA transformed the initial viscous composite into a paste, able to act as a matrix [77]. Studies demonstrated that the properties of BMP-synthetic polymers are influenced not only by the molecular weight of the polymer, but by the shape of the resulting product, so careful customization of the product to the characteristics of the defect is mandatory.

(c) Ceramics – Koempel et al. and then Tsuruga et al. demonstrated that BMP augmented porous and HA (200–500 μm pore size) augmented bone formation, with the highest bone formation when the pores had 300–400 μm diameter., inducing high rates of union despite the disadvantages of porous HA – slow degradation, brittleness, lack of osteoinduction, and low mechanical strength [72, 81].

Augmenting the composition of BMP – collagen with HA-generated osteoconductive and osteoinductive properties, especially when the pores of HA were 200–400 μm diameter, when increased speed of callus formation as well as increased mechanical strength were demonstrated [72, 82].

In conclusion, growth-factor derived BMPs offer osteoinductive support useful in healing disturbances especially when associated with other osteocoindutive structures, so as to achieve a complex with maximal activity able to provide success in bone grafting [82].

13.9 Calcium Phosphate and HA

Hydroxyapatite (HA) $Ca_5\ (PO_4)_3OH$ or $Ca_{10}\ (PO_4)_6OH_2$ is a natural compound. It represents up to 70% of the dry weight of bone [1]. It is the crystalline form of the TCP.

Compared to the natural product, synthetic HA has a similar structure to that of the natural product and has osteoconductive properties, but the speed of resorption is much lower [13, 20].

It is produced from marine coral exoskeletons that are hydrothermically converted to HA, the natural mineral composition of bone, which has a porosity closely resembling the porosity of human cancellous bone, manufactured in many forms, such as granules and porous blocks, usually combined with TCP [29, 79].

The hydroxyl and phosphate groups of HA can be replaced with carbonate, silicate, and magnesium so that sustained attempts to increase the bioactivity and osteoconductive properties of synthetic products and so as to get closer to the properties of the natural products.

This effort resulted in biomimetic ceramic substitutes, such as alginate, strontium, silicon, carbonate, magnesium, and substituted synthetic HA.

Tricalcium phosphate $Ca_3(PO_4)_2$ (TCP) – is a bioceramic which is less stronger than synthetic HA, but it more hydrosoluble and it resorbs faster; from the two forms (α and β), the β form has been used in fusing procedures, as well as a component of bioabsorbable screws [83, 84].

BCPs, resulted from blending different ceramics, try to adapt biomechanical properties and resorption rate to create a favorable balance [81, 85].

Calcium Phosphate Cement is a white powder containing TCP, calcium carbonate, and monocalcium phosphate; mixed with water, it becomes a paste which can be used for filling bone defects. It hardens quickly (20 minutes) if pH is normal, and the reaction is isothermal, producing no damage to the surrounding tissues. Hardening results in an apatite-like material with a compressive strength at least equal to that of cancellous bone, but after 48 hours. The mechanical properties of the cement depend on the amount of different calcium products; usually, the compressive strength is high, 10–100 MPa, while the tensile strength is only 1–10 MPa. Due to their very low resorption rate, these materials can be considered permanent [86–88].

13.10 Bioactive Glasses

Represent a class of bioactive glass (BS) including synthetic and biocompatible materials with osteoconductive activity and high antibacterial and angiogenetic properties [89]. Studies have demonstrated not only an optimal bone integration but also their efficiency in treating bone infections, by the following mechanism:

- The dissolution of the ceramics in the wet environment releases alkali and alkaline earth ions, thus rapidly increasing the osmotic pressure and especially the pH up to 11.65, explaining the bactericidal effect on (as shown *in vitro*) all the pathogens tested (including the most pathogenic bacteria, multiresistant to antibiotics). The correlation between the pH changes and the antibacterial effect is demonstrated by the fact that neutralizing the pH, this effect disappears [90, 91]. A sequence of reactions within the glass and at its surface are responsible for bone bonding.
  - Na^+ in the glass is rapidly exchanged with H^+ and H_3O^+ form the surrounding tissue, thus the hydroxyl structure silanol (SiOH) is generated at the surface of the BS and, after repolimerization, a layer of SiO_2 appears.
  - Due to migration of ionic calcium and phosphoric groups to the surface and their crystallization, a HA layer is generated on top of the silicon layer.
  - The interactions between the HA layer and the surrounding tissue initiate bone formation; the GF and the osteoprogenitor cells will generate the extracellular matrix and new bone.

The bioglasses stimulate the release of angiogenetic factors and promote angiogenesis. Studies have shown that a fibroblast-reach environment induces the secretion of tubules, essential for cell proliferation, cell migration, vessel branching, and interconnecting activity; due to their angiogenetic potential, and the bioglasses represent an alternative to GF with the same action [92].

Due to the fact that it has strong antibacterial properties, silicon-based bioglass is used with good results in treating bone infections, an aspect which will be discussed later.

13.11 Polymers-Based Bone Graft Substitutes

The mechanical, physical, and chemical properties of polymers are totally different from other BS, yet they have been studied and used because of many advantages as it will be discussed [93]. They have osteoconductive properties and can be classified into natural and synthetic polymers, and these, in turn, into resorbable and nonresorbable substitutes.

(a) Natural polymers include polysaccharides (chitin and chitosan) and polypeptides (collagen). They have a remarkable biocompatibility, but poor mechanical strength in wet environment and relatively high resorption speed [39].
Collagen – is the most important natural polymer in bone.
Different combinations of collagen and osteoconductive carriers have proven to be as effective as autograft when mixed with autologous bone marrow. Chapman demonstrated that tricalcium-phosphate-collagen graft can be successfully used in treating long bone fractures properly stabilized, as mesenchymal cells from the autologous bone marrow provided enough osteoprogenitor cells [94–97].
Due to its lack of mechanical strength, collagen is rarely used as a bone substitute alone, but in combinations in which its biological scaffold properties allow the other substances to become osteoinductive or even osteogenetic, if autograft is used in combination with collagen-based substitutes. More than that, due to its properties, collagen-based materials can be used as carriers for different substances, especially antibiotics, a matter of great importance in treating bone infections, which became more frequent and severe, with high morbidity and social cost, therefore, requiring new therapeutic approaches. For this reason, some aspects regarding BS in osteitis are going to be separately discussed later on [98, 99].

(b) Synthetic polymers have the advantage of a relative uniformity of composition and properties, thus creating a predictable effect. Due to their processing method, the concern for immunogenicity is less than for the natural products (such as bacterially produced polyhydroxybutyrate [PHB] and polyhydroxybutyrate-co-hydroxy-valerate [PHBV]), but they can still contain low quantities of impurities which can affect their bioacceptability [100].
The degradable (resorbable) polymers raise the problem of an adequate resorption speed, so as to match with that of bone production, but they give the injured site the possibility to heal itself with no foreign body retained. The most studied bioresorbable polymers are the polyesters:

- *PLA*: It is a semicrystalline product, slowly biodegradable (more than 24 months).
- *Polyglycolic acid* (*PGA*): It is highly crystalline, with a relatively short *in vivo* stability, degradable in 6–12 months.
- *PLGA*: It has a tunable degradation rate (1–12 months), faster than other substances from the same class.
- *PCL*: It is semicrystalline, with a good tissular compatibility, with a slow degradation rate (over 24 months) [101, 102].
- With less clinical use can also been described:
- High-density polyethylene (HDPE), which is biostable, nondegradable, and bioinert inorganic filler
- *PHB*: It is bioerodible, with high strength, but brittle; it has a slow degradation time

- *PHBV*: It is bioerodible, has a better ductility than PHB, a slow degradation time; it is less crystalline; and the content of hydroxyl-valerate can affect its properties.

The resorption process may take place via a bulk or a surface erosion, which is important especially for the mechanical properties of the substitute: surface-eroding polymers can be used as scaffolds, while bulk-eroding components can abruptly lose their mechanical strength.

Since most of the polymers have an incomplete profile – either less mechanical strength, or lower bioactivity, they are usually associated with other components able to enhance their mechanical and biological characteristics up to the desired ones. The density, phase purity, crystallinity, and size of primary particles have a crucial importance for the properties of the final product.

PLA and PLGA have been studied and used alone or in different combinations, with the goal of obtaining a bioacceptable, nonimmunogenic, nontoxic, and serializable product, with a reasonable price and able to be processed so as to get accurately sized and shaped devices. A special mention is the necessity for the polymer to have thermal properties allowing for processing and mechanical properties allowing functional loading [103–105].

13.12 Bone Substitutes in Treating Bone Infections

Chronic bone infections have certain characteristics which severely limit the therapeutic options:

- The infected bone is practically avascular, thus impenetrable for all the blood-delivered substances; it is isolated from the rest of the bone and impairs healing since it continuously "delivers" bacteria which maintain chronic inflammation and inhibit the reparatory processes.
- The surrounding fibrous tissue has low blood flow and inflammatory characteristics, thus being unable to protect the bone, or to induce healing.
- So, in chronic osteitis, total excision of the infected structures is mandatory for a successful treatment and alternative antibiotic delivery systems have to be used in order to deliver active concentrations to the tissues.
- Excision refers bone to soft tissue and the affected bone, thus bone gaps usually result from this excision step of treatment. Grafting this type of bone gaps is difficult since the risk of recurrence is considerable. That is why most of BS are contraindicated in osteitis. Systemic antibiotherapy has limited value, so different methods of local delivery have been searched for, especially because the carrier itself must be biocompatible and resorbable, so as not to enhance the inflammatory reaction.

The most studied of the biocompatible carriers so far has been collagen, especially materials made from bovine collagen. As for the antibiotics, gentamicin has been added to the collagen matrix, resulting in the so-called gentamicine containing collagen implants (GCCI) [106], which were introduced in 1985 [107] for the prevention of surgical site infections (SSI) [108].

The main advantages of GCCI are the following:

- Rapid and complete biodegradation (by collagenases), with no foreign-body reaction and no need for surgical removal, as for the antibiotic-coated spacers [109].
- Active doses of Gentamicine, considerably higher than those inhibiting Gentamicine-resistant bacteria [110, 111].
- Anti-edematous capacity, due to its ability to absorb exudates [112], but at the same time maintaining the humidity of the environment [112].
- The possibility of molding so completely filling the gap and adherence to its walls [113].
- Sealing the bone thus protecting it from secondary infection.
- Osteoconductive activity due to the network aspect of the structure, which allows cell penetration and new tissue formation. In addition, due to the combination with autograft, the osteoinductive and osteogenetic properties become active [114–116].

Based on type-1 collagen matrix obtained from bovine Achilles tendon, an example of GCCI is Collatamp G, consisting of a fully resorbable, lyophilized collagen sponge (280 mg collagen) saturated with 200 mg gentamicin (1.3 mg gentamicin base per square centimeter of collagen). It combines the wound-healing and haemostatic properties of collagen with the antimicrobial activity of Gentamicine.

The sponge may be cut or rolled, and, once introduced, studies have identified three stages of releasing the antibiotic, creating a "minivan aspect curve": an initial high and rapid release of Gentamicine, raising the local concentration of antibiotic up to 2000 μg/ml within 24 hours [5]; then, a secondary release phase from partial closed porosity (peak around day 3), and, finally, prolonged, later release from partially immobilized drug (peak between days 4 and 5), thus generating a constant antimicrobial environment[117–120].

Considering that reports showed that it might reduce the rate of SSIs more than 50% [121, 122]. and that no adverse effect has been reported for collagen or Gentamicine, this type of BS can be considered useful tools in treating bone infections.

The following clinical case demonstrates the advantages of using this type of GCCI: the patient, 19 years

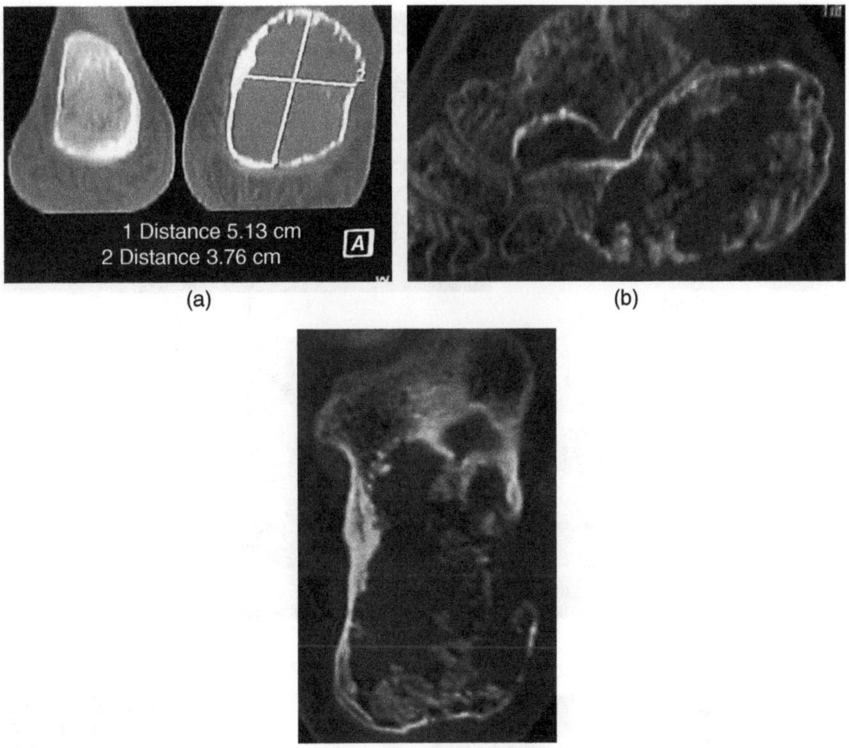

Figure 13.7 CT aspect of the calcaneal osteolysis – frontal (a), sagital (b), and horizontal (c) view.

old, was admitted after multiple failed surgeries for calcaneal osteolysis, with intermittent fistula appearance. Although inconstant results of the microbiological tests impaired previous treatments, complete bone excision was performed, followed by grafting using Collagen-based Collatamp augmented with autograft. (Figure 13.7). The outcome was favorable, both clinical (no pain, full weight bearing, no septic recurrences), and radiological (bone healing). (Figure 13.8)

The following aspects are to be discussed:

- Due to multiple failed surgery, it was clear that remaining and resistant infection was responsible for the septic recurrence, thus complete excision was mandatory, since osteolysis was primarily generated by sepsis.
- Because of [123, 124] prolonged vascular and metabolic changes (infection-induced hypoxemia), antibiotic blood delivery was insufficient and inconstant, with concentrations potentially generating even resistance of the bacteria through adaptive changes.
- The bone gap needed grafting after the infection was stopped, since autonomous healing was impossible.

In this type of cases, the collagen sponge stimulate healing by creating a matrix on which bone formation is induced. It has also hemostatic effect and the antibiotic is directly delivered to the infection site, following a pre-established and controllable curve, thus optimal antimicrobial concentrations are achieved. So the osteoconductive properties are completed with osteogenetic and osteoinductive capacities of the cancellous autograft, in the same, protecting the tissues from further septic episodes. Since the matrix is fully resorbable, it does not interfere with further bone formation and allows the new bone to completely restore the bone gap.

Another type of material used in treating bone infections belongs to the bioactive bioglass category. BonAlive is a bone substitute −100% synthetic and biodegradable, with the following composition SiO_2 53%, Na_2O 23%, CaO 20%, P_2O5 4% (by weight). In contact with an aqueous solution BonAlive® develops a silica-gel layer that acts as a template for calcium phosphate precipitation, thus enabling bonding of BonAlive to the surrounding bone. Besides, its actions are bacterial growth inhibiting, bioactive, and osteostimulative properties.

It has bioactive properties, as the surface of the granules bond chemically to bone, and it is highly osteoconductive, as it is able to stimulate the recruitment and differentiation of osteoblasts, which are activated to produce new bone [125]. It also has osteoconductive properties, working as a scaffold that allows bone growth into its 3D structure, thus having the role of support for the osteoblast cells so that bone grows onto and between the biomaterial granules.

More than that, the antibacterial activity of BonAlive is efficient upon a wide range of clinically relevant aerobic

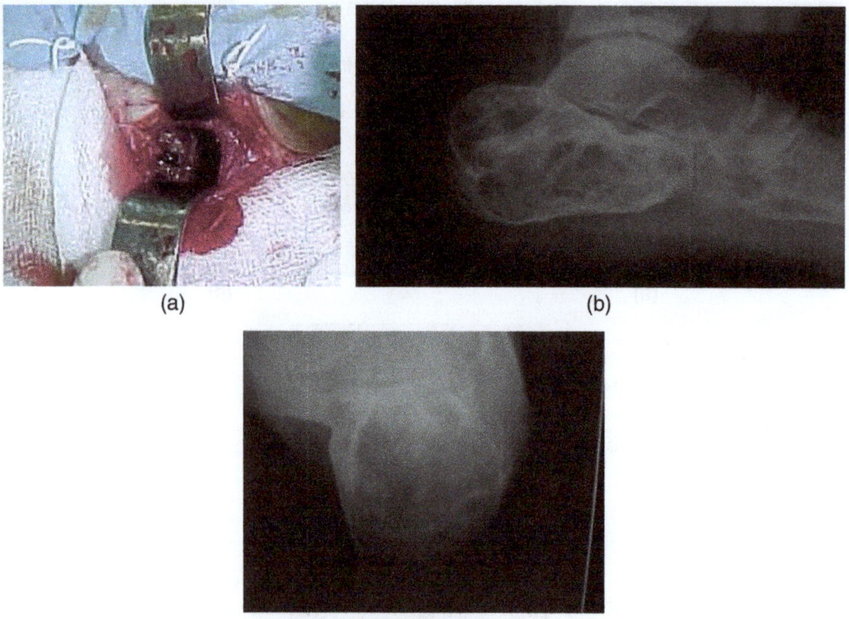

(a) (b) (c)

Figure 13.8 Intraoperative aspect (a) and favorable outcome – radiological – sagital (b) and frontal (c) views.

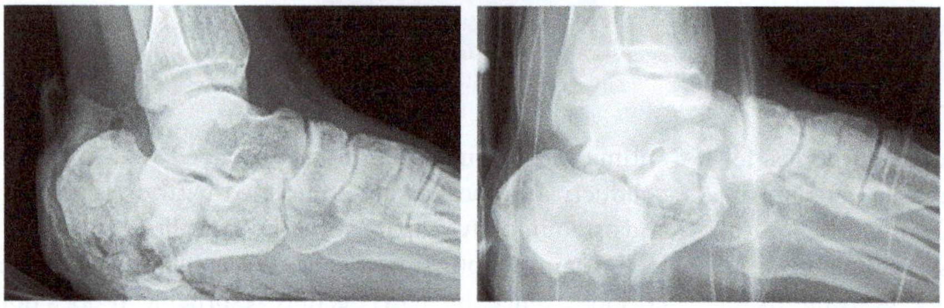

Figure 13.9 Bilateral infected open calcaneal fracture-preoperative X-ray.

and anaerobic bacteria species through *in vitro* studies, due to increased pH (produced by sodium release) and increased osmotic pressure (ions like Na, Ca, P, and Si) [126, 127].

The following case illustrates the therapeutic benefit of this bioactive glass in infected fractures. The patient was admitted with bilateral open calcaneal fracture contaminated with *St. aureus*. Figure 13.9 shows initial bilateral X-ray, with marked comminution.

Surgical treatment was performed; within surgery, extensive soft tissue injury, with periosteal stripping from the external cortex, debris and foreign debris were found. Necrotic tissue was excised. Lavage was performed, and then the fractures were reduced and stabilized. Figure 13.10 shows the bone gap resulting from the postoperative reduction of the fractures. The gravity of the case consisted especially of the infection, let alone that the fracture was bilaterally.

Under these circumstances, choosing the BS was a difficult task, as the presence of infection represented a contraindication for most of these products [128–130]. One of the very few which have bactericidal activity is the silicon-based bioactive glass, which was used bilaterally to graft the calcaneal bones.

The outcome was favorable (Figure 13.11) showing bone healing, and at the same time, infection was cured. It must be underlined that grafting was performed after thorough and repeated debridement of the wound, after granulation tissue appeared.

The problem of the bone infections was tackled separately first of all due to the increasing number of bone defect resulting from osteitis, as well as due to severe therapeutic problems which orthopedic surgeons must face in these cases.

13.13 Conclusion

Bone grafting is a complex process aiming at the restoration of a bone able to fulfill its functional tasks, meaning much more than filling. The success of bone grafting depends on the host and on the graft as well – preparing the patient from a local and a general point of view by minimizing the factors which impair graft integration,

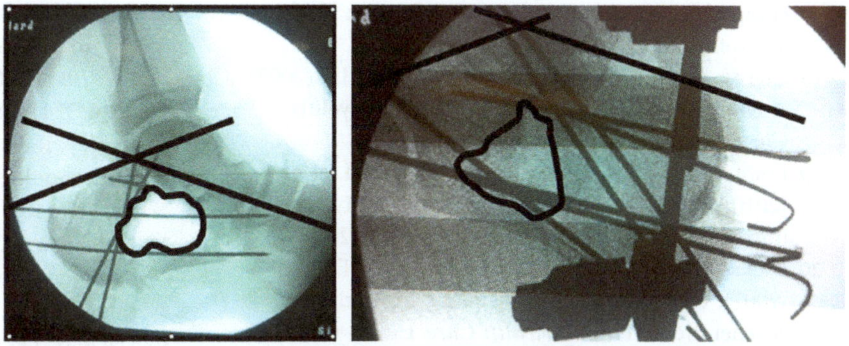

Figure 13.10 Postoperative bilateral result, with bone gap, contaminated with *St. aureus*.

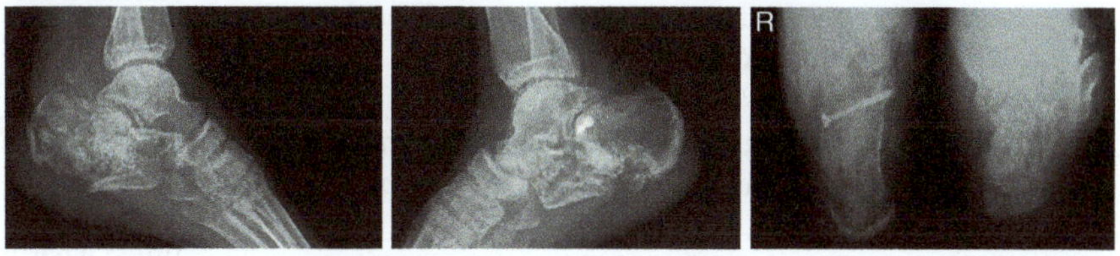

Figure 13.11 Bioactive glass was used for grafting – optimal result with healing without infection.

and also properly choosing the graft are prerequisites for a favorable outcome. The BS is to be chosen considering all the aspects related to their composition, but mainly to their characteristics, which must correspond to the characteristics of the host. The most actual tendency is that of obtaining and using BG with properties as close to those of autograft (still considered the golden standard).

References

1 Donati, D., Zolezzi, C., Tomba, P., and Vigano, A. (2007). Bone grafting: historical and conceptual review, starting with an old manuscript by Vittorio Putti. *Acta Orthop.* **78**: 19–25.
2 de Boer, H.H. (1988). The history of bone grafts. *Clin. Orthop. Relat. Res.* **226**: 292–298.
3 Urist, M.R. (1965). Bone: formation by autoinduction. *Science* **150**: 893–899.
4 Giannoudis, P.V., Dinopoulos, H., and Tsiridis, E. Bone substitutes: an update. *Injury* **36** (3): S20–S27.
5 Schlickewie, W. and Schlickewie, C. (2007). The use of bone substitutes in the treatment of bone defects—the clinical view and history. *Macromol. Symp.* **253** (1): 10–23.
6 Giannoudis, P.V., Einhorn, T.A., and Marsh, D. (2007). Fracture healing the diamond concept. *Injury* **38** (Suppl. 4): S3–S6.
7 Brighton, C.T. and Hunt, R.M. (1991). Early histological and ultrastructural changes in medullary fracture callus. *J. Bone Joint Surg. Am.* **73**: 832–847.
8 Einhorn, T.A. (1998). The cell and molecular biology of fracture healing. *Clin. Orthop. Relat. Res.* S7–S21.
9 Einhorn, T.A. (2003). Clinical applications of recombinant human BMPs: early experience and future development. *J. Bone Joint Surg. Am.* **85-A** (Suppl. 3): 82–88.
10 Tsiridis, E., Upadhyay, N., and Giannoudis, P. (2007). Molecular aspects of fracture healing: which are the important molecules? *Injury* **38** (Suppl. 1): S11–S25.
11 Perren, S.M. (1979). Physical and biological aspects of fracture healing with special reference to internal fixation. *Clin. Orthop. Relat. Res.* **138**: 175–196.
12 Calori, G.M. and Giannoudis, P.V. Enhancement of fracture healing with the diamond concept: the role of the biological chamber. *Injury* **42** (11): 1191–1193.
13 Nishida, J. and Shimamura, T. (2008). Methods of reconstruction for bone defect after tumor excision: a review of alternatives. *Med. Sci. Monit.* **14** (8): RA107–RA113.
14 Holt, G., Murnaghan, C., Reilly, J., and Meek, R.M.D. (2007). The biology of aseptic osteolysis. *Clin. Orthop. Relat. Res.* **460**: 240–252.
15 Jones, L.C. and Hungerford, D.S. (1987). Cement disease. *Clin. Orthop. Relat. Res.* **225**: 192–206.
16 Brydone, A.S., Meek, D., and Maclaine, S. (2010). Bone grafting, orthopaedic biomaterials, and the clinical need for bone engineering. *Proc. IMechE Part H* **224** (12): 1329–1343.
17 Romanò, C.L., Romanò, D., Logoluso, N., and Drago, L. (2011). Bone and joint infections in adults: a

comprehensive classification proposal. *Eur. Orthop. Traumatol.* **1**: 207–217.

18 Cierny, G. III,, Mader, J.T., and Penninck, J.J. (2003). A clinical staging system for adult osteomyelitis. *Clin. Orthop. Relat. Res.* **414**: 7–24.

19 Lindfors, N.C., Hyvönen, P., Nyyssönen, M. et al. (2010). Bioactive glass S53P4 as bone graft substitute in treatment of osteomyelitis. *Bone* **47**: 212–218.

20 Dickson, G.B.F., Marsh, D., Harkin-Jones, E. et al. (2007). Orthopaedic tissue engineering and bone regeneration. *Technol. Health Care* **15**: 57–67.

21 Tscherne, H. and Lobenhoffer, P. (1993). Tibial plateau fractures. Management and expected results. *Clin. Orthop. Relat. Res.* **292**: 87–100.

22 Goff, T., Kanakaris, N.K., and Giannoudis, P.V. (2013). Use of bone graft substitutes in the management of tibial plateau fractures. *Injury* **44** (Suppl. 1): S86–S94.

23 Veitch, S.W., Stroud, R.M., and Toms, A.D. (2010). Compaction bone grafting in tibial plateau fracture fixation. *J. Trauma* **68**: 980–983.

24 Macarini, L., Murrone, M., Marini, S. et al. (2004). Tibial plateau fractures: evaluation with multidetector-CT. *Radiol. Med.* **108**: 503–514.

25 Larsson, S. and Hannink, G. (2011). Injectable bone-graft substitutes: current products, their characteristics and indications, and new developments. *Injury* **42** (Suppl. 2): S30–S34.

26 Greenwald, A.S., Boden, S.D., Goldberg, V.M. et al. (2001). Bone-graft substitutes: facts, fictions, and applications. *J. Bone Joint Surg. A* **83** (2): 98–103.

27 Sung, H., Meredith, C., Johnson, C., and Galis, Z.S. (2004). The effect of scaffold degradation rate on three-dimensional cell growth and angiogenesis. *Biomaterials* **25** (26): 5735–5742.

28 Moore, S.T., Katz, J.M., Zhukauskas, R.M. et al. (2011). Osteoconductivity and osteoinductivity of Puros(R) DBM putty. *J. Biomater. Appl.* **26** (2): 151–171.

29 Klein, C.P., Driessen, A.A., de Groot, K., and van den Hooff, A. (1983). Biodegradation behavior of various calcium phosphate materials in bone tissue. *J. Biomed. Mater. Res.* **17** (5): 769–784.

30 Schwartz, Z. and Boyan, B.D. (1994). Underlying mechanisms at the bone-biomaterial interface. *J. Cell. Biochem.* **56** (3): 340–347.

31 Carvalho, A.L., Faria, P.E.P., Grisi, M.F.M. et al. (2007). Effects of granule size on the osteoconductivity of bovine and synthetic hydroxyapatite: a histologic and histometric study in dogs. *J. Oral Implantol.* **33** (5): 267–276.

32 Blokhuis, T.J. and Arts, J.J.C. (2011). Bioactive and osteoinductive bone graft substitutes: definitions, facts and myths. *Injury* **42** (Suppl. 2): S26–S29.

33 Rau, J.V., Antoniac, I., Cama, G. et al. (2016). Bioactive materials for bone tissue engineering. *BioMed Res. Int.* **2016**: 3741428, 3 p. https://doi.org/10.1155/2016/3741428.

34 Kenley, R.A., Yim, K., Abrams, J. et al. (1993). Biotechnology and bone graft substitutes. *Pharm. Res.* **10** (10): 1393–1401.

35 Finkemeier, C.G. (2002). Bone-grafting and bone-graft substitutes. *J. Bone Joint Surg. A* **84** (3): 454–464.

36 Davidas, J.P. (2014). Looking for a new international standard for characterization, classification and identification of surfaces in implantable materials: the long march for the evaluation of dental implant surfaces has just began. *POSEIDO* **2** (1): 1–5.

37 Hannink, G. and Arts, J.J.C. (2011). Bioresorbability, porosity and mechanical strength of bone substitutes: what is optimal for bone regeneration? *Injury* **42** (2): S22–S25.

38 Figueiredo, M., Henriques, J., Martins, G. et al. (2010). Physicochemical characterization of biomaterials commonly used in dentistry as bone substitutes—comparison with human bone. *J. Biomed. Mater. Res. Part B* **92** (2): 409–419.

39 Campana, V., Milano, G., Pagano, E. et al. (2014). Bone substitutes in orthopaedic surgery: from basic science to clinical practice. *J. Mater. Sci. - Mater. Med.* **25** (10): 2445–2461.

40 Lindfors, N.C. and Aho, A.J. (2003). Granule size and composition of bioactive glasses affect osteoconduction in rabbit. *J. Mater. Sci. - Mater. Med.* **14** (4): 365–372.

41 Knight, M.N. and Hankenson, K.D. (2013). Mesenchymal stem cells in bone regeneration. *Adv. Wound Care* **2** (6): 306–316.

42 Reichert, J.C., Saifzadeh, S., Wullschleger, M.E. et al. (2009). The challenge of establishing preclinical models for segmental bone defect research. *Biomaterials* **30** (12): 2149–2163.

43 Nair, L.S. and Laurencin, C.T. (2007). Biodegradable polymers as biomaterials. *Prog. Polym. Sci.* **32** (8–9): 762–798.

44 Zakaria, M., Zein, S.H.S., Othman, M.R. et al. (2013). Nanophase hydroxyapatite as a biomaterial in advanced hard tissue engineering: a review. *Tissue Eng. Part B: Rev.* **19** (5): 431–441.

45 Witte, F., Kaese, V., Haferkamp, H. et al. (2005). In vivo corrosion of four magnesium alloys and the associated bone response. *Biomaterials* **26** (17): 3557–3563.

46 Irinakis, T. (2011). Efficacy of injectable demineralized bone matrix as graft material during sinus

elevation surgery with simultaneous implant placement in the posterior maxilla: clinical evaluation of 49 sinuses. *J. Oral Maxillofac. Surg.* **69** (1): 134–141.
47 Wang, Z., Guo, Z., Bai, H. et al. (2013). Clinical evaluation of β-TCP in the treatment of lacunar bone defects: a prospective, randomized controlled study. *Mater. Sci. Eng., C* **33** (4): 1894–1899.
48 Chu, T.-M.G., Warden, S.J., Turner, C.H., and Stewart, R.L. (2007). Segmental bone regeneration using a load-bearing biodegradable carrier of bone morphogenetic protein-2. *Biomaterials* **28** (3): 459–467.
49 Place, E.S., Evans, N.D., and Stevens, M.M. (2009). Complexity in biomaterials for tissue engineering. *Nat. Mater.* **8** (6): 457–470.
50 Kang, Y., Scully, A., Young, D.A. et al. (2011). Enhanced mechanical performance and biological evaluation of a PLGA coated β-TCP composite scaffold for load-bearing applications. *Eur. Polym. J.* **47** (8): 1569–1577.
51 Kurien, T. and Pearson, R.G. (2013). Bone graft substitutes currently available in orthopaedic practice; the evidence for their use. *Bone Joint J.* **95-B**: 583–597.
52 AATB (2010). Summary of typical bone-graft substitutes that are commercially available. http://www.aatb.org/aatb/files/ccLibraryFiles/Filename/000000000323/BoneGraftSubstituteTable2010.pdf (accessed 13 November 2018).
53 Laurencin, C., Khan, Y., and El-Amin, S.F. (2006). Bone graft substitutes. *Expert Rev. Med. Devices* **3** (1): 49–57.
54 Roberts, T. and Rosenbaum, J. (2012). Bone grafts, bone substitutes and orthobiologics. *Organogenesis* **8** (4): 114–124.
55 Giannoudis, P.V., Chris Arts, J.J., Schmidmaier, G., and Larsson, S. (2011). What should be the characteristics of the ideal bone graft substitute? *Injury* **42** (Suppl. 2): S1–S2.
56 Miller, S. (2014). How smoking can hinder fracture healing. *Emergency Nurse* **22** (4): 28–30.
57 Sloan, A., Hussain, I., Maqsood, M. et al. (2010). The effects of smoking on fracture healing. *Surgeon* **8** (2): 111–116.
58 Kayal, R.A., Tsatsas, D., Bauer, M.A. et al. (2007). Diminished bone formation during diabetic fracture healing is related to the premature resorption of cartilage associated with increased osteoclast activity. *J. Bone Miner. Res.* **22** (4): 560–568.
59 Fávaro-Pípi, E., Ribeiro, D.A., Ribeiro, J.U. et al. (2011). Low-level laser therapy induces differential expression of osteogenic genes during bone repair in rats. *Photomed. Laser Surg.* **29** (5): 311–317.
60 Leonida, A., Paiusco, A., Rossi, G. et al. (2013). Effects of low-level laser irradiation on proliferation and osteoblastic differentiation of human mesenchymal stem cells seeded on a three-dimensional biomatrix: in vitro pilot study. *Lasers Med. Sci.* **28** (1): 125–132.
61 Urist, M., Mikulski, A., and Boyd, S. (1975). A chemosterilized antigenextracted autodigested alloimplant for bone banks. *Arch Surg.* **110** (4): 416–428.
62 Kinney, R.C., Ziran, B.H., Hirshorn, K. et al. (2010). Demineralized bone matrix for fracture healing: fact or fiction? *J. Orthop. Trauma* **24** (Suppl. 1): S52–S55.
63 Khan, S.N., Cammisa, F.P. Jr.,, Sandhu, H.S. et al. (2005). The biology of bone grafting. *J. Am. Acad. Orthop. Surg.* **13**: 77–86, PMID: 15712985.
64 Lindsey, R.W., Wood, G.W., Sadasivian, K.K. et al. (2006). Grafting long bone fractures with demineralized bone matrix putty enriched with bone marrow: pilot findings. *Orthopedics* **29** (10): 939–941.
65 Grabowski, G. and Cornett, C.A. (2013). Bone graft and bone graft substitutes in spine surgery: current concepts and controversies. *J. Am. Acad. Orthop. Surg.* **21** (1): 51–60.
66 Song, S.-H., Kim, S.-G., Kim, S.-E., and Song, H.-R. (2015). Is DBM beneficial for the enhancement of bony consolidation in distraction osteogenesis? A randomized controlled trial. *BioMed Res. Int.* **2015**: 281738, 8 p. https://doi.org/10.1155/2015/281738.
67 Roberts, T. and Rosenbaum, A. (2012). Bone grafts, bone substitutes and orthobiologics: the bridge between basic science and clinical advancements in fracture healing. *Organogenesis* **8** (4): 114–124.
68 Wang, E.A., Rosen, V., D'Alessandro, J.S. et al. (1990). Recombinant human bone morphogenetic protein induces bone formation. *Proc. Natl. Acad. Sci. U.S.A.* **87**: 2220–2224.
69 Sampath, T.K., Maliakal, J.C., Hauschka, P.V. et al. (1992). Recombinant human osteogenic protein-1 (hOP-1) induces new bone formation in vivo with a specific activity comparable with natural bovine osteogenic protein and stimulates osteoblast proliferation and differentiation in vitro. *J. Biol. Chem.* **267**: 20352–20362.
70 Khan, S.N., Bostrom, M.P., and Lane, J.M. (2000). Bone growth factors. *Ortho. Clin. North Am.* **31** (3): 375–387.
71 Kirker-Head, C.A., Gerhart, T.N., Armstrong, R. et al. (1998). Healing bone using recombinant human bone morphogenetic protein 2 and copolymer. *Clin. Orthop. Relat. Res.* **349**: 205–217.

72 Koempel, J.A., Patt, B.S., O'Grady, K. et al. (1998). The e!ect of recombinant human bone morphogenetic protein-2 on the integration of porous hydroxyapatite implants with bone. *J. Biomed. Mater. Res.* **41**: 359–363.

73 Garrison, K.R., Donell, S., Ryder, J. et al. (2007). Clinical effectiveness and cost-effectiveness of bone morphogenetic proteins in the non-healing of fractures and spinal fusion: a systematic review. *Health Technol. Assess.* **11** (30): 1–150.

74 Shields, L.B., Raque, G.H., Glassman, S.D. et al. (2006). Adverse effects associated with highdose recombinant human bone morphogenetic protein-2 use in anterior cervical spine fusion. *Spine* **31** (5): 542–547.

75 Mussano, F., Ciccone, G., Ceccarelli, M. et al. (2007). Bone morphogenetic proteins and bone defects: a systematic review. *Spine* **32** (7): 824–830.

76 Gao, T.J., Lindholm, T.S., Kommonen, B. et al. (1996). Enhanced healing of segmental tibial defects in sheep by a composite bone substitute composed of tricalcium phosphate cylinder, bone morphogenetic protein, and type IV collagen. *J. Biomed. Mater. Res.* **32**: 505–512.

77 Wu, X., Shi, W., and Cao, X. (2007). Multiplicity of BMP signaling in skeletal development. *Ann. N.Y. Acad. Sci.* **1116**: 29–49.

78 Yasko, A.W., Lane, J.M., Fellinger, E.J. et al. The healing of segmental bone defects, induced by recombinant human bone morphogenetic protein (rhBMP-2). A radiographic, histological, and biomechanical study in rats. *J. Bone Joint Surg. Am.* **74**: 659–670, Published Erratum appears in: *J. Bone Joint Surg. Am.* 1992; 74 (7): 1111.

79 Johnson, E.E., Urist, M.R., and Finerman, G.A. (1988). Repair of segmental defects of the tibia with cancellous bone grafts augmented with human bone morphogenetic protein. A preliminary report. *Clin. Orthop. Relat. Res.* 249–257.

80 Urist, M.R., Hudak, R.T., Huo, Y.K., and Rasmussen, J.K. (1985). Osteoporosis: a bone morphogenetic protein auto-immune disorder. *Prog. Clin. Biol. Res.* **187**: 77–96.

81 Tsuruga, E., Takita, H., Itoh, H. et al. (1997). Pore size of porous hydroxyapatite as the cell-substratum controls BMPinduced osteogenesis. *J. Biochem.* **121**: 317–324.

82 Miyazono, K., Maeda, S., and Imamura, T. (2005). BMP receptor signaling: transcriptional targets, regulation of signals, and signaling crosstalk. *Cytokine Growth Factor Rev.* **16** (3): 251–263.

83 Johnson, E.E., Urist, M.R., and Finerman, G.A. (1992). Resistant nonunions and partial or complete segmental defects of long bones. Treatment with implants of a composite of human bone morphogenetic protein (BMP) and autolyzed, antigen-extracted, allogeneic (AAA) bone. *Clin. Orthop. Relat. Res.* 229–237.

84 Reddi, A.H. (1998). Role of morphogenetic proteins in skeletal tissue engineering and regeneration. *Nat. Biotechnol.* **16**: 247–252.

85 Ferguson, D., Davis, W.L., Urist, M.R. et al. (1987). Bovine bone morphogenetic protein (BMP) fraction-induced repair of craniotomy defects in the rhesus monkey (*Macaca speciosa*). *Clin. Orthop. Relat. Res.* **219**: 251–258.

86 Giannoudis, P.V. and Einhorn, T.A. (2009). Bone morphogenetic proteins in musculoskeletal medicine. *Injury* **40** (Suppl. 3): S1–S3.

87 Nauth, A., Giannoudis, P.V., Einhorn, T.A. et al. (2010). Growth factors: beyond bone morphogenetic proteins. *J. Orthop. Trauma* **24** (9): 543–546. https://doi.org/10.1097/BOT.0b013e3181ec4833.

88 Janicki, P. and Schmidmaier, G. (2011). What should be the characteristics of the ideal bone graft substitute? Combining scaffolds with growth factors and/or stem cells. *Injury* **42** (Suppl. 2): S77–S81.

89 Larsson, S. and Hannink, G. (2011). Injectable bone-graft substitutes: current products, their characteristics and indications, and new developments Injury. *Int. J. Care Injured* **42**: S30–S34.

90 Coelho, P.G., Coimbra, M.E., Ribeiro, C. et al. (2009). Physico/chemical characterization and preliminary human histology assessment of a β-TCP particulate material for bone augmentation. *Mater. Sci. Eng., C* **29** (7): 2085–2091.

91 Dai, L.Y. and Jiang, L.S. (2008). Single-level instrumented posterolateral fusion of lumbar spine with beta-tricalcium phosphate versus autograft: a prospective, randomized study with 3-year follow-up. *Spine* **33** (2): 1299–1304.

92 Komlev, V.S., Barinov, S.M., Bozo, I.I. et al. (2014). Bioceramics composed of octacalcium phosphate demonstrate enhanced biological behavior. *ACS Appl. Mater. Interfaces* **6** (19): 16610–16620.

93 Ebrahimi, M., Pripatnanont, P., Monmaturapoj, N., and Suttapreyasri, S. (2012). Fabrication and characterization of novel nano hydroxyapatite/beta-tricalcium phosphate scaffolds in three different composition ratios. *J. Biomed. Mater. Res. Part A* **100** (9): 2260–2268.

94 Blokhuis, T.J. and Chris Arts, J.J. (2011). Bioactive and osteoinductive bone graft substitutes: definitions, facts and myths. *Injury* Bone Substitutes: A Comprehensive Overview **42** (Suppl. 2): S1–S90.

95 Wang, S., Wang, X., Draenert, F.G. et al. (2014). Bioactive and biodegradable silica biomaterial for bone regeneration. *Bone* **67**: 292–304.

96 Bernstein, A., Niemeyer, P., Salzmann, G. et al. (2013). Microporous calcium phosphate ceramics as tissue engineering scaffolds for the repair of osteochondral defects: histological results. *Acta Biomater.* **9** (7): 7490–7505.

97 Andersson, O.H. and Kangasniemi, I. (1991). Calcium phosphate formation at the surface of bioactive glass in vitro. *J. Biomed. Mater. Res.* **25**: 1019–1030.

98 Andersson, O.H., Karlsson, K.H., and Kangasniemi, K. (1990). Calcium-phosphate formation at the surface of bioactive glass in vivo. *J. Non-Cryst. Solids* **119**: 290–296.

99 Hench, L.L. and Paschall, H.A. (1973). Direct chemical bond of bioactive glass-ceramic materials to bone and muscle. *J. Biomed. Mater. Res.* **7**: 25–42.

100 Nandi, S.K., Roy, S., Mukherjee, P. et al. (2010). Orthopaedic applications of bone graft & graft substitutes: a review. *Indian J. Med. Res.* **132**: 15–30.

101 Wagner-Ecker, M. and Voltz, P. (2013). The collagen component of biological bone graft substitutes promotes ectopic bone formation by human mesenchymal stem cells. *Acta Biomater.* **9** (7): 7298–7307.

102 Ricciardi, B.F. and Bostrom, M. (2013). Bone graft substitutes: claims and credibility. *Semin. Arthroplasty* **24** (2): 119–123.

103 Maté-Sánchez de Val, E., Mazõn, P., Guirado, J.L.C. et al. (2014). Comparison of three hydroxyapatite/β-tricalcium phosphate/collagen ceramic scaffolds: an in vivo study. *J. Biomed. Mater. Res. Part A* **102** (4): 1037–1046.

104 Haugh, M.G., Jaasma, M.J., and O'Brien, F.J. (2009). The effect of dehydrothermal treatment on the mechanical and structural properties of collagen-GAG scaffolds. *J. Biomed. Mater. Res. Part A* **89** (2): 363–369.

105 Barradas, A.M.C., Yuan, H., van Blitterswijk, C.A., and Habibovic, P. (2011). Osteoinductive biomaterials: current knowledge of properties, experimental models and biological mechanisms. *Eur. Cells Mater.* **21**: 407–429.

106 Noah, E.M., Chen, J., Jiao, X. et al. (2002). Impact of sterilization on the porous design and cell behavior in collagen sponges prepared for tissue engineering. *Biomaterials* **23** (14): 2855–2861.

107 Fuchs, J.R., Nasseri, B.A., and Vacanti, J.P. (2001). Tissue engineering: a 21st century solution to surgical reconstruction. *Ann. Thorac. Surg.* **72** (2): 577–591.

108 Xu, C., Su, P., Chen, X. et al. (2011). Biocompatibility and osteogenesis of biomimetic bioglass-collagen-phosphatidylserine composite scaffolds for bone tissue engineering. *Biomaterials* **32** (4): 1051–1058.

109 Uemura, T., Dong, J., Wang, Y. et al. (2003). Transplantation of cultured bone cells using combinations of scaffolds and culture techniques. *Biomaterials* **24** (13): 2277–2286.

110 Wahl, D.A., Sachlos, E., Liu, C., and Czernuszka, J.T. (2007). Controlling the processing of collagen-hydroxyapatite scaffolds for bone tissue engineering. *J. Mater. Sci. - Mater. Med.* **18** (2): 201–209.

111 Kozłowska, J. and Sionkowska, A. (2015). Effects of different crosslinking methods on the properties of collagen-calcium phosphate composite materials. *Int. J. Biol. Macromol.* **74**: 397–403.

112 Salvatore, L., Madaghiele, M., Parisi, C. et al. (2014). Crosslinking of micropatterned collagen-based nerve guides to modulate the expected half-life. *J. Biomed. Mater. Res. Part A* **102** (12): 4406–4414.

113 Sugiura, H., Yunoki, S., Kondo, E. et al. (2009). In vivo biological responses and bioresorption of tilapia scale collagen as a potential biomaterial. *J. Biomater. Sci., Polym. Ed.* **20** (10): 1353–1368.

114 Park, S.-N., Lee, H.J., Lee, K.H., and Suh, H. (2003). Biological characterization of EDC-crosslinked collagen-hyaluronic acid matrix in dermal tissue restoration. *Biomaterials* **24** (9): 1631–1641.

115 Geiger, M. and Friess, W. (2000). Crosslinking of porous collagen carrier systems by dehydrothermal treatment. *Proceedings of the 3rd World Meeting APV/APGE*, Berlin, Germany.

116 Wang, C., Meng, G., Zhang, L. et al. (2012). Physical properties and biocompatibility of a core-sheath structure composite scaffold for bone tissue engineering in vitro. *J. Biomed. Biotechnol.* **2012**: 579141, 9 p.

117 Gunatillake, P., Mayadunne, R., and Adhikari, R. (2006). Recent developments in biodegradable synthetic polymers. *Biotechnol. Annu. Rev.* **12**: 301–347.

118 Cascone, M.G., Barbani, N., Cristallini, C. et al. (2001). Bioartificial polymeric materials based on polysaccharides. *J. Biomater. Sci.* **12** (3): 267–281.

119 Ciardelli, G., Chiono, V., Vozzi, G. et al. (2005). Blends of poly-(ε-caprolactone) and polysaccharides in tissue engineering applications. *Biomacromolecules* **6** (4): 1961–1976.

120 Roether, J.A., Boccaccini, A.R., Hench, L.L. et al. (2002). Development and in vitro characterisation of novel bioresorbable and bioactive composite materials based on polylactide foams and Bioglass® for tissue engineering applications. *Biomaterials* **23** (18): 3871–3878.

121 Koushki, N., Katbab, A.A., Tavassoli, H. et al. (2015). A new injectable biphasic hydrogel based on partially hydrolyzed polyacrylamide and nanohydroxyapatite as scaffold for osteochondral regeneration. *RSC Adv.* **5** (12): 9089–9096.

122 Lewandrowski, K.-U., Gresser, J.D., Wise, D.L., and Trantolo, D.J. (2000). Bioresorbable bone graft substitutes of different osteoconductivities: a histologic evaluation of osteointegration of poly(propylene glycol-co-fumaric acid)-based cement implants in rats. *Biomaterials* **21** (8): 757–764.

123 Lanao, R.P.F., Jonker, A.M., Wolke, J.G.C. et al. (2013). Physicochemical properties and applications of poly(lactic-co-glycolic acid) for use in bone regeneration. *Tissue Eng. Part B: Rev.* **19** (4): 380–390.

124 Mishra, P.K., Ashoub, A., Salhiyyah, K. et al. (2014). Role of topical application of gentamicin containing collagen implants in cardiac surgery. *J. Cradiothorac. Surg.* **9**: 122–126.

125 Stermberger, A., Grimm, H., Bader, F. et al. (1997). Local treatment of bone and soft tissue infections with the collagen-gentamicin sponge. *Eur. J. Surg. Suppl.* **578**: 17–26.

126 Friberg, Ö., Svedjeholm, R., Söderquist, B. et al. (2005). Local gentamicin reduces sternal wound infections after cardiac surgery: a randomized controlled trial. *Ann. Thorac. Surg.* **79**: 153–162.

127 Chvapil, M. (1977). Collagen sponge: theory and practice of medical applications. *J. Biomed. Mater. Res.* **11**: 721–741.

128 Drosos, G.I., Touzopoulos, P., Ververidis, A. et al. (2015). Use of demineralized bone matrix in the extremities. *World J. Orthop.* **6** (2): 269–277.

129 Pieske, O., Wittmann, A., Zaspel, J. et al. (2009). Autologous bone graft versus demineralized bone matrix in internal fixation of ununited long bones. *J. Trauma Manag. Outcomes* **3**: 11.

130 Styrkarsdottir, U., Cazier, J.B., Kong, A. et al. (2003). Linkage of osteoporosis to chromosome 20p12 and association to BMP2. *PLoS Biol.* **1**: e69.

Index

Bioceramics and Biocomposites: From Research to Clinical Practice, First Edition. Edited by Iulian Antoniac.

d

e

f

g